1996
YEAR BOOK OF
SURGERY®

Statement of Purpose

The YEAR BOOK Service

The YEAR BOOK series was devised in 1901 by practicing health professionals who observed that the literature of medicine and related disciplines had become so voluminous that no one individual could read and place in perspective every potential advance in a major specialty. In the final decade of the 20th century, this recognition is more acutely true than it was in 1901.

More than merely a series of books, YEAR BOOK volumes are the tangible results of a unique service designed to accomplish the following:

- to *survey* a wide range of journals of proven value
- to *select* from those journals papers representing significant advances and statements of important clinical principles
- to provide *abstracts* of those articles that are readable, convenient summaries of their key points
- to provide *commentary* about those articles to place them in perspective

These publications grow out of a unique process that calls on the talents of outstanding authorities in clinical and fundamental disciplines, trained literature specialists, and professional writers, all supported by the resources of Mosby, the world's preeminent publisher for the health professions.

The Literature Base

Mosby and its Editors survey more than 1,000 journals published worldwide, covering the full range of the health professions. On an annual basis, the publisher examines usage patterns and polls its expert authorities to add new journals to the literature base and to delete journals that are no longer useful as potential YEAR BOOK sources.

The Literature Survey

The publisher's team of literature specialists, all of whom are trained and experienced health professionals, examines every original, peer-reviewed article in each journal issue. More than 250,000 articles per year are scanned systematically, including title, text, illustrations, tables, and references. Each scan is compared, article by article, to the search strategies that the publisher has developed in consultation with the 270 outside experts who form the pool of YEAR BOOK editors. A given article may be reviewed by any number of editors, from one to a dozen or more, regardless of the discipline for which the paper was originally published. In turn, each editor who receives the article reviews it to determine whether or not the article should be included in the YEAR BOOK. This decision is based on the article's inherent quality, its probable usefulness to readers of that YEAR BOOK, and the editor's goal to represent a balanced picture of a given field in each volume of the YEAR BOOK. In addition, the editor indicates when to include figures and tables from the article to help the YEAR BOOK reader better understand the information.

Of the quarter million articles scanned each year, only 5% are selected for detailed analysis within the YEAR BOOK series, thereby assuring readers of the high value of every selection.

The Abstract

The publisher's abstracting staff is headed by a seasoned medical professional and includes individuals with training in the life sciences, medicine, and other areas, plus extensive experience in writing for the health professions and related industries. Each selected article is assigned to a specific writer on this abstracting staff. The abstracter, guided in many cases by notations supplied by the expert editor, writes a structured, condensed summary designed so that the reader can rapidly acquire the essential information contained in the article.

The Commentary

The YEAR BOOK editorial boards, sometimes assisted by guest commentators, write comments that place each article in perspective for the reader. This provides the reader with the equivalent of a personal consultation with a leading international authority—an opportunity to better understand the value of the article and to benefit from the authority's thought processes in assessing the article.

Additional Editorial Features

The editorial boards of each YEAR BOOK organize the abstracts and comments to provide a logical and satisfying sequence of information. To enhance the organization, editors also provide introductions to sections or individual chapters, comments linking a number of abstracts, citations to additional literature, and other features.

The published YEAR BOOK contains enhanced bibliographic citations for each selected article, including extended listings of multiple authors and identification of author affiliations. Each YEAR BOOK contains a Table of Contents specific to that year's volume. From year to year, the Table of Contents for a given YEAR BOOK will vary depending on developments within the field.

Every YEAR BOOK contains a list of the journals from which papers have been selected. This list represents a subset of the more than 1,000 journals surveyed by the publisher and occasionally reflects a particularly pertinent article from a journal that is not surveyed on a routine basis.

Finally, each volume contains a comprehensive subject index and an index to authors of each selected paper.

The 1996 Year Book Series

Year Book of Allergy, Asthma, and Clinical Immunology: Drs. Rosenwasser, Borish, Gelfand, Leung, Nelson, and Szefler

Year Book of Anesthesiology and Pain Management: Drs. Tinker, Abram, Chestnut, Roizen, Rothenberg, and Wood

Year Book of Cardiology®: Drs. Schlant, Collins, Engle, Gersh, Kaplan, and Waldo

Year Book of Chiropractic®: Dr. Lawrence

Year Book of Critical Care Medicine®: Drs. Parrillo, Balk, Calvin, Franklin, and Shapiro

Year Book of Dentistry®: Drs. Meskin, Berry, Kennedy, Leinfelder, Roser, Summitt, and Zakariasen

Year Book of Dermatologic Surgery®: Drs. Swanson, Glogau, and Salasche

Year Book of Dermatology®: Drs. Sober and Fitzpatrick

Year Book of Diagnostic Radiology®: Drs. Federle, Clark, Gross, Latchaw, Madewell, Maynard, and Young

Year Book of Digestive Diseases®: Drs. Greenberger and Moody

Year Book of Drug Therapy®: Drs. Lasagna and Weintraub

Year Book of Emergency Medicine®: Drs. Wagner, Dronen, Davidson, King, Niemann, and Roberts

Year Book of Endocrinology®: Drs. Bagdade, Braverman, Horton, Kannan, Landsberg, Molitch, Morley, Nathan, Odell, Poehlman, Rogol, and Ryan

Year Book of Family Practice®: Drs. Berg, Bowman, Davidson, Dexter, and Scherger

Year Book of Geriatrics and Gerontology®: Drs. Beck, Burton, Rabins, Reuben, Roth, Shapiro, and Whitehouse

Year Book of Hand Surgery®: Drs. Amadio and Hentz

Year Book of Hematology®: Drs. Spivak, Bell, Ness, Quesenberry, Wiernik, and Blume

Year Book of Infectious Diseases®: Drs. Keusch, Barza, Bennish, Klempner, Skolnik, and Snydman

Year Book of Infertility and Reproductive Endocrinology: Drs. Mishell, Lobo, and Sokol

Year Book of Medicine®: Drs. Bone, Cline, Epstein, Greenberger, Malawista, Mandell, O'Rourke, and Utiger

Year Book of Neonatal and Perinatal Medicine®: Drs. Fanaroff and Klaus

Year Book of Nephrology, Hypertension, and Mineral Metabolism: Drs. Coe, Curtis, Favus, Henderson, Kashgarian, Luke, and Myers

Year Book of Neurology and Neurosurgery®: Drs. Bradley and Wilkins

Year Book of Neuroradiology: Drs. Osborn, Eskridge, Grossman, Hudgins, and Ross

Year Book of Nuclear Medicine®: Drs. Gottschalk, Blaufox, McAfee, Wackers, and Zubal

Year Book of Obstetrics and Gynecology®: Drs. Mishell, Herbst, and Kirschbaum

Year Book of Occupational and Environmental Medicine®: Drs. Emmett, Frank, Gochfeld, and Hessl

Year Book of Oncology®: Drs. Simone, Bosl, Cohen, Glatstein, Ozols, and Tallman

Year Book of Ophthalmology®: Drs. Cohen, Augsburger, Eagle, Flanagan, Grossman, Laibson, Maguire, Nelson, Rapuano, Sergott, Tasman, Tipperman, and Wilson

Year Book of Orthopedics®: Drs. Sledge, Cofield, Dobyns, Griffin, Poss, Springfield, Swiontkowski, Wiesel, and Wilson

Year Book of Otolaryngology–Head and Neck Surgery®: Drs. Paparella and Holt

Year Book of Pain: Drs. Gebhart, Haddox, Jacox, Janjan, Marcus, Rudy, and Shapiro

Year Book of Pathology and Laboratory Medicine: Drs. Mills, Bruns, Gaffey, and Stoler

Year Book of Pediatrics®: Dr. Stockman

Year Book of Plastic, Reconstructive, and Aesthetic Surgery®: Drs. Miller, Cohen, McKinney, Robson, Ruberg, and Whitaker

Year Book of Podiatric Medicine and Surgery®: Dr. Kominsky

Year Book of Psychiatry and Applied Mental Health®: Drs. Talbott, Ballenger, Breier, Frances, Meltzer, Schowalter, and Tasman

Year Book of Pulmonary Disease®: Drs. Bone and Petty

Year Book of Rheumatology®: Drs. Sergent, LeRoy, Meenan, Panush, and Reichlin

Year Book of Sports Medicine®: Drs. Shephard, Drinkwater, Eichner, Torg, Col. Anderson, and Mr. George

Year Book of Surgery®: Drs. Copeland, Bland, Deitch, Eberlein, Howard, Luce, Seeger, Souba, and Sugarbaker

Year Book of Thoracic and Cardiovascular Surgery®: Drs. Ginsberg, Wechsler, and Williams

Year Book of Ultrasound®: Drs. Merritt, Carroll, and Fleischer

Year Book of Urology®: Drs. DeKernion and Howards

Year Book of Vascular Surgery®: Dr. Porter

1996

The Year Book of SURGERY®

Editor-in-Chief
Edward M. Copeland, III, M.D.
*The Edward R. Woodward Professor and Chairman, Department of Surgery,
University of Florida College of Medicine; Director, University of Florida
Shands Cancer Center, Gainesville, Florida*

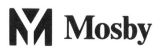 Mosby

St. Louis   Baltimore   Boston   Carlsbad   Chicago   Naples   New York   Philadelphia   Portland
London   Madrid   Mexico City   Singapore   Sydney   Tokyo   Toronto   Wiesbaden

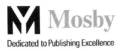

Mosby
Dedicated to Publishing Excellence

A Times Mirror
Company

Vice President and Publisher, Continuity Publishing: Kenneth H. Killion
Director, Editorial Development: Gretchen C. Murphy
Assistant Developmental Editor, Continuity: Vivienne Heard
Acquisitions Editor: Gina G. Wright
Illustrations and Permissions Coordinator: Steven J. Ramay
Manager, Continuity–EDP: Maria Nevinger
Project Manager, Editing: Jill C. Waite
Senior Project Manager, Production: Max F. Perez
Freelance Staff Supervisor: Barbara M. Kelly
Director, Editorial Services: Edith M. Podrazik, B.S.N., R.N.
Information Specialist: Kathleen Moss, R.N.
Circulation Manager: Lynn D. Stevenson

Printed in the United States of America
Composition by Reed Technology and Information Services, Inc.
Printing/binding by Maple-Vail

Mosby–Year Book, Inc.
11830 Westline Industrial Drive
St. Louis, MO 63146

Editorial Office:
Mosby–Year Book, Inc.
161 N. Clark Street
Chicago, IL 60601

International Standard Serial Number: 0090-3671
International Standard Book Number: 0-8151-7795-X

Editors

Victor E. Pricolo, M.D.

Associate Professor of Surgery, Brown University School of Medicine; Chief of Gastrointestinal Surgery, Rhode Island Hospital, Providence, Rhode Island

H. Hank Simms, M.D.

Associate Professor of Surgery, Brown University School of Medicine; Chief, Division of Surgical Critical Care, Department of Surgery, Rhode Island Hospital, Providence, Rhode Island

Table of Contents

Journals Represented

Mosby and its Editors survey more than 1,000 journals for its abstract and commentary publications. From these journals, the Editors select the articles to be abstracted. Journals represented in this YEAR BOOK are listed below.

American Journal of Infection Control
American Journal of Medical Quality
American Journal of Medicine
American Journal of Orthopedics
American Journal of Pathology
American Journal of Physiology
American Journal of Respiratory and Critical Care Medicine
American Journal of Roentgenology
American Journal of Surgery
American Surgeon
Anaesthesia and Intensive Care
Anesthesia and Plastic Surgery
Annals of Internal Medicine
Annals of Otology, Rhinology and Laryngology
Annals of Plastic Surgery
Annals of Surgery
Annals of Surgical Oncology
Annals of Thoracic Surgery
Annals of Vascular Surgery
Annals of Disease in Childhood
Archives of Otolaryngology-Head and Neck Surgery
Archives of Surgery
Australian and New Zealand Journal of Medicine
Blood
British Journal of Cancer
British Journal of Surgery
British Medical Journal
Burns
Canadian Association of Radiologists Journal
Canadian Journal of Surgery
Canadian Medical Association Journal
Cancer
Cancer Research
Chest
Clinical Infectious Diseases
Clinical Science
Critical Care Medicine
Digestive Diseases and Sciences
Diseases of the Colon and Rectum
European Journal of Cancer
European Journal of Pediatric Surgery
European Journal of Surgery
European Journal of Vascular and Endovascular Surgery
Gastroenterology
Gastrointestinal Endoscopy
Gynecologic Oncology
Head and Neck

Human Pathology
Injury
Intensive Care Medicine
International Journal of Artificial Organs
International Journal of Cancer
International Journal of Radiation, Oncology, Biology, and Physics
Israel Journal of Medical Sciences
Journal of Burn Care and Rehabilitation
Journal of Cardiovascular Surgery
Journal of Clinical Anesthesia
Journal of Clinical Endocrinology and Metabolism
Journal of Clinical Oncology
Journal of Clinical Ultrasound
Journal of Computer Assisted Tomography
Journal of Family Practice
Journal of Laryngology and Otology
Journal of Medical Genetics
Journal of Pediatric Surgery
Journal of Pediatrics
Journal of Surgical Research
Journal of Thoracic and Cardiovascular Surgery
Journal of Trauma
Journal of Trauma: Injury, Infection, and Critical Care
Journal of Vascular Medicine and Biology
Journal of Vascular Surgery
Journal of the American College of Cardiology
Journal of the American College of Surgeons
Journal of the American Medical Association
Journal of the National Cancer Institute
Journal of the Royal College of Surgeons of Edinburgh
Lancet
Laryngoscope
Metabolism: Clinical and Experimental
Microsurgery
Neurosurgery
New England Journal of Medicine
Otolaryngology–Head and Neck Surgery
Pediatric Pulmonology
Pediatrics
Plastic and Reconstructive Surgery
Radiology
Science
Southern Medical Journal
Stroke
Surgery
Transplantation
Transplantation Proceedings
World Journal of Surgery
Wound Repair and Regeneration

STANDARD ABBREVIATIONS

The following terms are abbreviated in this edition: acquired immunodeficiency syndrome (AIDS), cardiopulmonary resuscitation (CPR), central nervous system (CNS), cerebrospinal fluid (CSF), computed tomography (CT), deoxyribonucleic acid (DNA), electrocardiography (ECG), health maintenance organization (HMO), human immunodeficiency virus (HIV), intensive care unit (ICU) intramuscular (IM), intravenous (IV), magnetic resonance (MR) imaging (MRI), and ribonucleic acid (RNA).

NOTE

The YEAR BOOK OF SURGERY is a literature survey service providing abstracts of articles published in the professional literature. Every effort is made to assure the accuracy of the information presented in these pages. Neither the editors nor the publisher of the YEAR BOOK OF SURGERY can be responsible for errors in the original materials. The editors' comments are their own opinions. Mention of specific products within this publication does not constitute endorsement.

To facilitate the use of the YEAR BOOK OF SURGERY as a reference tool, all illustrations and tables included in this publication are now identified as they appear in the original article. This change is meant to help the reader recognize that any illustration or table appearing in the YEAR BOOK OF SURGERY may be only one of many in the original article. For this reason, figure and table numbers will often appear to be out of sequence within the YEAR BOOK OF SURGERY.

1 General Considerations

Introduction

The role of medical students in a managed care environment has been questioned but seldom studied. As it turns out, medical students may represent a cost-efficient workforce on a surgical service, and patients enjoy student participation. Patient care doesn't suffer from resident sleep deprivation as measured by an increase in complications as a correlate to lack of sleep. The current recommendations from the Surgical Residency Review Committee for the resident work week is 80 hours, yet residents may still get only 2 hours of sleep per on-call night. Reducing work hours during the week has not eliminated sleepless nights; in fact, it may have increased sleeplessness while on call. Women surgeons are happy with their career choices, but comparison with men is difficult since male surgeons have not had their lifestyles scrutinized as in depth as have women surgeons. Hepatitis B continues to be a much greater health hazard for surgeons than does HIV, and there is a vaccine for it—if only surgeons could be convinced to become vaccinated.

Much concern over a surplus of physicians in the future exists. In fact, if the current trend continues into the early 21st century, there may be a relative shortage of general surgeons. All surgical specialties have held the number of annually issued board certificates almost constant since 1982, whereas credentialed medical specialists have increased dramatically and may be more vulnerable to an acute reduction in specialty service needs. Medical schools have not yet decreased the number of medical students matriculating into the first year class; thus the physician pipeline remains wide open. Medical specialization has been de-emphasized in the curriculum, but the net effect on specialty overproduction will remain unknown for several more years. Likewise, competition between family physicians and nonphysician clinicians may dictate fewer physician generalists than currently anticipated. Downsizing medical schools will be a hotly debated issue, especially since foreign medical graduates continue to occupy 25% of the physicians in graduate medical education programs in the United States (not yet addressed is the question of whether or not there are too many graduate medical education programs). Some medical schools may be eliminated simply because funding, previously from practice income, will no longer be available and no alternative funding source exists. In the end, market forces that are unresponsive to the Association of American Medical Colleges may dictate the number of viable medical schools and, consequently, the number of medical students. In surviving medical schools, significant "re-engineering" will be required because of economic constraints. The nonproductive faculty member will face reassignment or elimination, volunteer clinical faculty within a managed care network will be more involved in medical education, and a small but well-defined medical school faculty will be responsible for "core" education.

Reimbursement for surgical procedures has decreased dramatically and is often not relative to the work effort involved in care of the patient. For example, hepatic trisegmentectomy is paid by Medicare at a disproportionately low rate based on the technical skill and time needed to do the procedure. Dr. James Maloney has devised a reimbursement system that meets established national criteria and reimburses based on skill level required and treatment intensity.

Canadians have had a cost containment medical delivery system for some time now, but easy access to medical care may be limited, especially in rural areas. General practitioners have been able to safely substitute for anesthesiologists when required to do so. Even in the Canadian system, however, patients were dissatisfied by the inconvenience of "early" hospital discharge (0.57 days vs. 1.63 days) after hernia repair. Canadians are accustomed to cost containment yet desired overnight admission for hernia repair. The reaction to cost containment strategies by the American public is only beginning. Will we be more or less tolerant of the inconvenience of managed care as compared with Canadians? Patient complications secondary to cost containment measures may negate the savings derived from a specific cost containment strategy. Regionalization of high-risk procedures such as pancreaticoduodenectomy may, however, reduce the mortality rate, costly complications, and days of hospitalization. If health care is rationed in this country, will the elderly be denied appropriate surgical treatment? Certainly, outcome data in the elderly indicates that the majority of them are returned home with a pain-free existence after most surgical procedures.

Laparoscopic cholecystectomy has lowered the threshold for elective cholecystectomy in the Medicare age group, the result of which has been a decreased incidence of complicated cholecystectomies in the elderly and an overall reduction in mortality rate from all cholecystectomies in this age group. Therefore, the increased frequency of this surgical procedure may have reduced the overall cost of managing cholecystitis. Factored into this equation, however, must be additional complications from the new procedure such as major vascular injuries from trocar insertion.

Several definitive articles are included that address the controversial topics of intrahospital transport of critically ill patients, transfusion requirements in surgical ICU patients, number of days required to withhold warfarin to ensure a normal international normalized ratio, and the safety of estrogen and progestin hormone replacement therapy relative to breast cancer risk. Each article describes practical guidelines that are clinically applicable. Last, I have included a marvelous article on surgical knots, something we use all the time and evaluate seldom.

Edward M. Copeland III, M.D.

Patients' Attitudes Toward the Involvement of Medical Students in Their Care
York NL, DaRosa DA, Markwell SJ, Niehaus AH, Folse R (Southern Illinois Univ, Springfield)
Am J Surg 169:421–423, 1995   1–1

Introduction.—Studies involving various patient groups suggest overall satisfaction with the care given by medical students and residents. Randomly selected patients in a surgical unit were interviewed to determine variables that influence patient attitudes toward students.

Patients and Methods.—The 88 patients were assessed and followed by surgery students rotating through a 10-week clerkship. Faculty members from the department of surgery interviewed 4 to 6 patients for each of 16 surgery students during the study period. The 12 interview questions dealt with the patients' perceptions of the attitudes and abilities of the medical students. In-depth comments were sought on the benefits of having a student participate in patient care, particularly in the area of increased information.

Results.—Six students received honors in the surgical rotation, 9 passed, and 1 remediated the clerkship. The patients had a mean age of 63 years and an average hospital stay of 7.4 days. Half of the patients who had previous hospital admissions reported prior contact with medical students. Patient responses to the survey showed an overwhelmingly favorable attitude toward the students. The patients found the students to be informative, attentive, and concerned with their well-being, and more than 92% "agreed" or "strongly agreed" when asked whether they had benefited from student involvement. Mean patient ratings did not differ for male and female medical students or for those who received honors vs. those who passed. Patients hospitalized for more than 1 week were more likely to rate the medical student as confident and relaxed.

Conclusion.—As with previous studies, patients appreciated the medical students' involvement in their care. Students are able to show genuine concern about patient outcome and spend more time answering questions than other members of the health care team. Such positive interactions can increase patient or "consumer" satisfaction with the health care system.

▶ Medical students add to the efficiency of a surgical service rather than detract from it. They are certainly adequate help in the operating room and can first assist on simple cases. In an outpatient setting, the medical student can evaluate a new patient while you see multiple postoperative patients whose maladies are of minimal teaching value. Hospitalized patients enjoy the attention and concern from the students who, in the current hospital environment, are seldom called upon to "hurt" the patients by nasogastric tube insertion, venipuncture, or other invasive maneuvers (although training of students has suffered from this lack of contact). Within the training environment, students represent a cost-effective workforce who benefit educationally (if not taken advantage of).

In contrast, students are often thought to be an efficiency liability on medical services. An interesting study would be to compare the teaching techniques of surgeons and internists for knowledge imparted and career choices stimulated.

E.M. Copeland III, M.D.

Are Postoperative Complications Related to Resident Sleep Deprivation?

Haynes DF, Schwedler M, Dyslin DC, Rice JC, Kerstein MD (Tulane Univ, New Orleans, La)
South Med J 88:283–289, 1995   1–2

Introduction.—A number of recent articles have examined the potential adverse effects of sleep loss on residents and on the quality of care they deliver. The findings of these studies have been contradictory, however, partly because of the different ways in which the effects of sleep deprivation were measured. Perioperative complications of surgical procedures were retrospectively correlated with the resident surgeon's call status.

Methods.—Included in the analysis were all emergency and elective procedures done by residents on 4 surgical services during a 40-month period. A complication was defined as any intraoperative or postoperative effect or outcome reported to the weekly death and complications conference. If more than 1 complication was reported for an operation, the more severe or life-threatening event was considered. Residents were considered subject to sleep deprivation when they were required to remain in house for the duration of the 24-hour call day. Residents' sleep habits during on-call and off-duty nights were also surveyed.

Results.—During the study period there were 6,371 procedures done by resident surgeons; 351 cases (5.51%) involved a surgical complication. The lowest incidence of complications occurred during non–sleep-deprived periods, whereas the highest incidence of complications was recorded during periods defined as sleep-deprived. Yet the overall incidence of complications in relation to call status was low, ranging from 4.62% to 6.71%. When the complications were divided into emergency and nonemergency categories, however, the incidence of complications for emergency operations was approximately 3 times that of nonemergency operations. The highest rate of complications for emergency procedures (11.7%) was found in the non–sleep-deprived state. Complication rates were higher for upper-level residents than for junior residents and interns. The resident sleep survey showed a mean of last-call sleep of 1.8 hours.

Conclusion.—Surgical residents work an average of 87 hours per week; sleep deprivation might increase the incidence of postsurgical complications. Yet it appears that residents are able to overcome the effects of fatigue, perhaps by a heightened awareness and an increase in stress hormone levels.

▶ Although no significant differences in postoperative complications could be determined for operations done by sleep-deprived vs. non–sleep-deprived residents, only 1.8 hours of sleep in a 24-hour period must affect cognitive judgment (a much more difficult measure to obtain). The interesting correlate in this study is the 80-hour work week with the 1.8 hours of sleep when on call. A resident who is on call 1 night out of 4 must usually cross-cover patients who are unknown, thus necessitating an evaluation of every patient problem regardless of its chronicity. If a call schedule could be constructed whereby residents covered only patients for whom they were primarily responsible during the day, predictably more than 1.8 hours of sleep would be possible. Residents might spend more than 80 hours a week in the hospital, but a great deal more of that time would be spent asleep. The result would be a rested resident on the post–call day, resulting in a better educational experience for the resident and potentially better patient care. If a hospital emergency room is busy enough to disrupt an in-house call schedule, the institution should consider a separate emergency call schedule.

E.M. Copeland III, M.D.

Women Surgeons: Career and Lifestyle Comparisons Among Surgical Subspecialties
Mackinnon SE, Mizgala CL, McNeil IY, Walters BC, Ferris LE (Washington Univ, St Louis, Mo; Univ of Toronto)
Plast Reconstr Surg 95:321–329, 1995   1–3

Introduction.—Although the number of women entering medical school continues to increase, surgical specialties remain dominated by men. A survey of career and lifestyle patterns among Canadian women surgeons was prompted by the need to recruit more women into surgical training programs.

Methods.—The survey population included all women listed as members and practicing in Canada with The Royal College of Surgeons of Canada and La Corporation Professionelle des Médecins du Québec as of March 1990. Of the 459 surgeons who could be located, 419 responded to the questionnaire. The 93-item survey included personal history, medical training, professional productivity, and quality-of-life issues.

Results.—For analysis, 4 categories of surgical subspecialties were identified: obstetrics-gynecology (41%), ophthalmology (21%), general surgery (12%), and "others" (26%). Marital status did not differ significantly among the 4 major subspecialties, although general surgeons were most likely (58%) and ophthalmologists least likely (32%) to remain childless. Women in obstetrics-gynecology and general surgery had a significantly longer work week, and those in ophthalmology had the shortest hours. Women in all subspecialties had a tendency toward low academic rank; only 33 of 419 respondents were associate professors. Most of the surgeons had delayed childbearing until completion of training. Women surgeons retained the primary responsibility for running the household. Approximately 60% of the surgeons in the general, obstetrics-gynecology, and "other" categories reported that their career had compromised their family and personal life. Nevertheless, there was a high level of satisfaction (84.1 to 91%) with quality of life among all 4 surgical subspecialties.

Conclusion.—Overall, 88% of women surgeons were happy with their decision to pursue a career in surgery and felt that they had successfully combined a productive career with a rewarding family and personal life. Only 6.5% were separated or divorced. When asked whether discrimination occurred during the selection process for residency, only 15% perceived such attitudes.

▶ It would be interesting to obtain responses from men to the same questionnaire. I would predict that career has compromised the family and personal life of men as well and that no more than 88% of men are happy with the decision to pursue a surgical career. Women are pursuing a career in surgery with increasing frequency and, in my opinion, are as competitive as men. The excellent women as candidates for general surgery training may be more likely to be ranked higher on the intern matching list than equally qualified male applicants. The reverse may also be true.

E.M. Copeland III, M.D.

Serosurvey of Human Immunodeficiency Virus, Hepatitis B Virus, and Hepatitis C Virus Infection Among Hospital-Based Surgeons
Panlilio AL, Shapiro CN, Schable CA, Mendelson MH, Montecalvo MA, Kunches LM, Perry SW III, Edwards JR, Srivastava PU, Culver DH, Weisfuse IB, Jorde U, Davis JM, Solomon J, Wormser GP, Ryan J, Bell DM, Chamberland ME, and the Serosurvey Study Group (Centers for Disease Control and Prevention, Atlanta, Ga; Mount Sinai School of Medicine, New York; New York Medical College, Valhalla; et al)
J Am Coll Surg 180:16–24, 1995   1–4

Background.—Surgeons continue to experience frequent blood contact despite the adoption of universal precautions. Such exposure carries a risk for infection with HIV, hepatitis B virus (HBV), hepatitis C virus (HCV), and other blood-borne pathogens. To estimate the prevalence of infection with HIV, HBV, and HCV, an anonymous seroprevalence survey was conducted among hospital-based surgeons practicing in areas with moderate to high rates of HIV infection and AIDS.

Methods.—The serosurvey was conducted from October 1991 through July 1992. Eligible participants were all surgeons in training or in practice in general surgery, obstetrics and gynecology, and orthopedics at the 21 selected hospitals. Voluntary enrollment for serologic testing extended from January through July 1992. Data collected included the surgeons' practice characteristics and nonoccupational risk factors for HIV infection. Counseling was available before and after blood testing.

Results.—Of the 2,887 surgeons eligible for the serosurvey, 1,427 completed the background survey, and 770 participated in the testing for HIV antibody, HCV antibody, and markers of HBV infection. Most of the participants (86%) reported operating on patients with HIV infection or AIDS. One of the 770 serosurvey participants was found to be HIV-seropositive. This surgeon did not report nonoccupational risk factors but had performed surgery on at least 100 patients with HIV infection or AIDS and at least another 100 patients with risk factors for HIV infection or AIDS. None of the 20 surgeons who reported nonoccupational HIV risk factors were HIV-positive. Three of 129 participants with past or current HBV infection had chronic HBV infection; all were negative for hepatitis B e antigen. Risk factors identified for HBV infection were not receiving hepatitis B vaccine (odds ratio, 14.7) and practicing surgery for at least 10 years (odds ratio, 2.2). Half of the 199 surgeons who reported receiving no vaccine had serologic results indicating susceptibility to HBV infection. Surgeons who received 3 doses of vaccine were significantly less likely to have evidence of HBV infection than those who had received fewer than 3 doses. Seven surgeons had anti-HCV.

Conclusion.—Occupational blood contact was reported in 1.8 of 100 operative procedures by this group of surgeons practicing in metropolitan areas with a moderate to high AIDS incidence. Although the rate of undetected HIV infection was low (.14%), HBV infection remains a problem. The overall prevalence of HBV serologic markers among these surgeons was 17%; the prevalence among the United States general population is 5%.

▶ Once again, the chance of contracting hepatitis B virus as a blood-borne pathogen was far more of a risk than contracting HIV, even in hospitals with a moderate to high HIV incidence. Of the participants in this study, only 55% reported receiving at least 3 doses of hepatitis B vaccine, 88% of whom had seromarkers consistent with appropriate immunity. Common sense would dictate that surgeons avail themselves of an effective vaccine against a potentially lethal disease. I wonder why they don't do it?

E.M. Copeland III, M.D.

Calculating the Workforce in General Surgery

Jonasson O, Kwakwa F, Sheldon GF (American College of Surgeons, Chicago; Univ of North Carolina, Chapel Hill)

JAMA 274:731–734, 1995   1–5

Introduction.—Most surveys and analyses of the physician and specialist workforce report a large surplus of general surgeons and predict an even greater surplus in the future. A 1991 study conducted by Abt Associates, however, suggests that a shortfall of as much as 15% in the general surgical workforce may occur by the year 2010. Data from 4 different sources were analyzed in an attempt to provide a reasonable estimate of the patient care and resident physician workforce practicing general surgery in 1994.

Methods.—Sources of information were the American College of Surgeons' *Longitudinal Study of Surgical Residents: 1992–1993;* the American Medical Association's *Physician Characteristics and Distribution in the United States,* 1994 edition; the American Board of Medical Specialties' (ABMS) database on general surgeons; and the American Board of Surgery recertification data from the files of diplomates since 1968. Each source was analyzed separately. In the case of the 1994 *Physician Characteristics and Distribution* document, only surgeons listed as practicing abdominal, critical care, general, and traumatic surgery were included.

Results.—The mean number of residents graduating from general surgery programs has been 1,004 per year since 1981. After eliminating those who proceed to further specialization, approximately 600 general surgeons enter the workforce each year. The ABMS database identified 22,740 certified general surgeons aged 65 years or younger with no additional subspecialty certification. Together with approximately 1,000 engaged in the certification process, the total number of general surgeons is estimated to range between a minimum of 19,520 and a maximum of 21,953 (Table). With adjustment for death, retirement, and moving abroad, 19,917 appears to be a reasonable estimate of the maximum number of practicing certified general surgeons and 18,775 is a reasonable estimate for the minimum number.

Conclusion.—Although the number of physicians completing general surgical residencies has remained stable since 1982, approximately 40% enter a subspecialty field. Thus little accrual of general surgeons occurs when death and retirement are taken into consideration. If the subspecialization trend continues, the general surgery workforce may be reduced below needed levels.

► The conclusions from this study are good news for general surgeons since the prevailing opinion in the managed care arena has been an overabundance of all specialists. The number of certificates issued by virtually all surgical specialty boards has been relatively constant for the past 10 years, whereas medical specialty certificates, especially in gastroenterology and

TABLE.—Calculations of the General Surgery Workforce

General Surgery Workforce	AMA Physician Masterfile*	ABMS Listing	ABS
Maximum Scenario Calculation			
Total listed	38 239	22 740	18 917
Add			
In process of certification	0	1000	1000
Subtract			
Federally employed surgeons	1578†	1341†‡	0
51% Nonclinical general surgeons	525§	446‡§	0
65% Residents and fellows	5771‖	0	0
Surgeons aged ≥65 y	3283¶	0	0
75% Surgical subspecialists	3428**	0	0
100% Specialty residents and fellows	152††	0	0
Maximum General Surgeons	**23 502**	**21 953**	**19 917**
Minimum Scenario Calculation			
Total listed	38 239	22 740	18 917
Add			
In process of certification	0	1000	1000
Subtract			
Federally employed surgeons	1578†	1341†‡	0
100% Nonclinical general surgeons	1030	876	0
100% Residents and fellows	8879	0	0
Surgeons aged ≥62 y	4740¶‡‡	2003	0
100% Surgical subspecialists (including residents and fellows)	4723	0	0
All nonrecertified	0	0	1142§§
Minimum General Surgeons	**17 289**	**19 520**	**18 775**

* From *Physician Characteristics and Distribution in the United States, 1994 Edition.* Chicago, American Medical Association, 1994.

† "Federal surgeons" is derived from Tables A-2 and B-5, *Physician Characteristics and Distribution in the United States, 1994 Edition.*

‡ Approximately 85% of general surgeons are certified by the American Board of Surgery (T.W. Biester, M.S., written communication, July 1994).

§ Nonclinical surgeons indicate that most of their time is spent in administration, research, teaching, or other nonclinical activities. They are assumed to spend 51% of their time in nonclinical activities and 49% in patient care (Table B-6, *Physician Characteristics and Distribution in the United States, 1994 Edition*).

‖ Each resident is assumed to be equivalent in service to 0.35 of a full-time practicing surgeon (Graduate Medical Education National Advisory Committee: *Summary Report to the Secretary, Department of Health and Human Services.* Hyattesville, Md, Health Resources Administration, Publication HRA 81-651, 1980).

¶ The number of general surgeons aged 65 years or older (3,955 [Table B-5]) has been reduced by 17%, the number of surgical subspecialists included in the "General Surgery" category (cardiovascular, head and neck, pediatric, and vascular surgeons) (*Physician Characteristics and Distribution in the United States, 1994 Edition*).

** Subspecialty surgeons included in the "General Surgery" category may spend a portion of their time providing general surgery services. This is estimated to be no more than 25% of the time spent.

†† Subspecialy residents spend 100% of their time in the subspecialty program and do not provide general surgery services.

‡‡ The mean and median age of retirement of general surgeon fellows of the American College of Surgeons and certified general surgeons is 62 years (F. Padberg, M.D., written communication, November, 1994). As many general surgeons retire before the age of 62 years as retire after the age of 62.

§§ Certified general surgeons who did not recertify and whose certificates have expired. All are assumed to have ceased practice.

Abbreviations: AMA, American Medical Association; ABMS, American Board of Medical Specialties; ABS, American Board of Surgery.

(Courtesy of *JAMA,* September 6, vol 274, pp 731–734, Copyright 1995, American Medical Association.)

cardiology, have escalated dramatically. There are a lot of procedures that multiple specialist claim, e.g., thyroidectomy, laminectomy, head and neck oncologic procedures, endoscopy, hand surgery, and maxillofacial trauma. Cost savings may emanate from directing patients needing these procedures to a limited number of surgeons concentrated in only a very few specialties.

E.M. Copeland III, M.D.

Managed Health Care: Implications for the Physician Workforce and Medical Education
Rivo ML, for the Council on Graduate Medical Education (Council on Graduate Med Education, Rockville, Md)
JAMA 274:712–715, 1995   1–6

Objective.—A 1992 report of the Council on Graduate Medical Education suggested that shortages of generalist and minority physicians, specialty physician surplus, and poor geographic distribution would lead to problems in the provision of high-quality, affordable health care to all Americans. The rise of managed care since that time prompted another report examining the impact of managed care on the physician workforce and on medical education.

Findings.—Most areas of the country have seen rapid growth in managed care in both the public and private sectors, and this trend is likely to continue or accelerate in the future. As service volume becomes less phy-

---

TABLE 1.—Definitions of 6 Representative Organizational Forms of Health Care Delivery Listed by Intensity of Management From Least Managed to Most Managed

Organizational Form	Definition
Indemnity plan with fee for service	Complete freedom of choice to patients. Insurer reimburses physicians on a fee-for-service basis.
Managed indemnity plan	Free choice and fee for service, but insurer exercises some degree of utilization control to manage costs.
Preferred provider organization	Insurer channels patients to "preferred" physicians who are usually paid discounted fee for service. The insurer, not the physician, usually accepts financial risk for performance.
Independent practice association	Insurer channels patients to physicians usually solo or in small groups who have agreed to some financial risk for performance. Payment may be either captitation or fee for service with financial incentives based on performance.
Network independent practice association	Similar to independent practice association but consists of a network of larger group practices. Payment is usually capitation to each group, which then pays the physicians.
Staff/group health maintenance organization	The classic, prepaid, large multispecialty group practice. Patients are covered only for care delivered by the health maintenance organization. The physicians are usually salaried and work either for the plan (staff-model health maintenance organization) or for a physician group practice (group-model health maintenance organization) that has an exclusive contract with the plan.

Not shown are hybrid arrangements such as open-ended and point-of-service arrangements whereby patients in a preferred provider organization, independent practice association, or staff/group HMO may have some insurance coverage for care outside the providers approved by the insurer.

(Adapted from Moore GT: *The Impact of Managed Care on the Medical Education Environment.* Rockville, Md, Council on Graduate Medical Education Environment, Nov 1993. Courtesy of JAMA, September 6, vol 274, pp 712–715, Copyright 1995, American Medical Association.)

sician directed and more service directed (Table 1), physicians' practice styles are becoming more collaborative and cost-effective. The rise of managed care is likely to increase the previously cited concerns about the physician workforce. The oversupply of specialists and subspecialists is further increasing in the face of a modest need for more generalists. By the 21st century—regardless of whether a managed care or a fee-for-service approach prevails—there is a real potential for physician unemployment or underemployment.

The same forces that have encouraged the growth of managed care are also affecting the medical education system and its teaching institutions. Financial support for undergraduate and graduate medical education is likely to erode, thus reducing its quality. Increased competition is likely to decrease the clinical income of many teaching hospitals, which has traditionally supported medical education. In response, teaching hospitals are finding many different ways of shifting toward managed care. Although managed care is likely to enhance to shortcomings of the current medical education system, it will also provide new opportunities to improve physician training, particularly for cost-effective practice in a managed care setting. Finally, many different factors are making it difficult for medical education entities and managed care organizations to address problems related to the physician workforce and medical education priorities. If cuts are to be made in Medicare graduate medical education funding, funds should be targeted to train physicians in the settings, specialties, and skills they need to meet the needs of Medicare beneficiaries and the public at large.

Summary.—The rapid growth of managed care will have an important impact on the physician workforce and on the future of medical education. Attention is needed to ensure that physicians are receiving the training they need to work in a managed care environment.

▶ Medical schools have not yet decreased enrollment to eliminate the predicted oversupply of physicians in the 21st century. Instead, the strategy seems to be to divert students into family practice rather than into a specialty. Likewise, applicants to medical schools have not decreased, nor has the quality of the student applicant diminished. In fact, never has the competition in some schools, including ours, been more keen. The driving force for most students to enter the field of medicine is the allure of helping our fellow man. There is no reason to think that managed care will diminish this desire, and in fact, it hasn't.

E.M. Copeland III, M.D.

Perspectives on the Physician Workforce to the Year 2020
Cooper RA (Med College of Wisconsin, Milwaukee)
JAMA 274:1534–1543, 1995   1–7

Objective.—There is increasing concern about a surplus of physicians in the United States, where fears of a shortage 2 decades ago prompted a

TABLE 2.—Physician Supply and Demand, 1993–2020

Variable	1993	2000	2010	2020
Supply				
Practicing physicians	474 (183)	568 (204)	704 (227)	755 (219)
Residents and fellows	102 (39)	97 (35)	94 (30)	94 (27)
Patient care physicians	576 (222)	665 (238)	798 (257)	849 (247)
Resident-adjusted patient care physicians	540 (208)	631 (226)	765 (247)	816 (237)
Demand				
Patient care physicians	532 (205)	600 (215)	703 (227)	829 (241)
Surplus [deficit]				
Patient care physicians	8 (3)	31 (11)	62 (20)	[13] ([4])
Patient care physicians, %	1.4	4.9	8.1	[1.6]

Note: Numbers of physicians are in thousands, with numbers per 100,000 population in parentheses.
(Courtesy of *JAMA*, November 15, vol 274, pp 1534–1543, Copyright 1995, American Medical Association.)

doubling of the capacity to train new physicians. This survey assesses the supply and demand for physicians up to the year 2020. Future surpluses will depend in the main on how physicians are distributed geographically and also on the degree to which patients expect services from physicians that will also be offered by an increasing number of nonphysician clinicians (NPCs).

Perspectives.—Demand for physician services was examined by analyzing HMO experiences. Second, the distribution of physicians was studied in each state to compare regional utilization patterns with national norms. Finally, the future supply of NPCs and their impact on physician services were addressed.

Supply and Demand.—The estimated need for physicians in 1993 was estimated at 205 per 100,000 population, and demand is expected to increase 18% by 2020 (Table 2). The supply of physicians is expected to increase more rapidly than demand at first and create a 5% surplus of patient care physicians in 2000 and an 8% excess (62,1000 physicians) in 2010. Later the gap will narrow. Presently the per capita distribution of physicians varies more than 2-fold between states (Fig 2). Some states already have surpluses, whereas shortages persist in others. The supply of NPCs is increasing, and by 2010 they are expected to reach a level equal to 60% of the number of patient care physicians.

Demographics.—The average number of patient visits per week has decreased about 15% in the past 15 years. Presently, 22% of practicing physicians are older than 55 years, and this figure will rise to 38% in 2020. At the same time, the proportion of women physicians will increase from 19% to 35%. Many physicians are assuming an employed status, and on average, those employed work fewer hours per week. It seems likely that both physician work efforts and the intensity of medical practice will continue to decline.

Summing Up.—There is no evidence of a substantial national surplus of physicians. Geographic distribution will be the chief determinant of whether a given region will have a surplus. In time, the major factor will

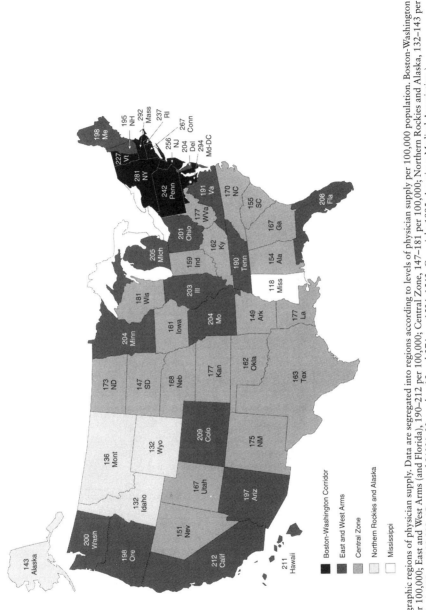

FIGURE 2.—Geographic regions of physician supply. Data are segregated into regions according to levels of physician supply per 100,000 population. Boston-Washington Corridor, 227–294 per 100,000; East and West Arms (and Florida), 190–212 per 100,000; Central Zone, 147–181 per 100,000; Northern Rockies and Alaska, 132–143 per 100,000; and Mississippi, 118 per 100,000. (Courtesy of *JAMA*, November 15, vol 274, pp 1534–1543, Copyright 1995, American Medical Association.)

be the extent to which patients continue to prefer to see physicians for services that will also be available from an increasing group of NPCs.

▶ This article approaches the physician "surplus" from a different perspective than most and suggests that in the year 2020, the determinant of physician surplus will continue to be geographic distribution. Other factors will affect the physician workforce, such as earlier retirement since there will be a larger proportion of older physicians (greater than 55 years), an increase in part-time physicians, and more reliance on NPCs. Students entering medical school today need to consider career paths in which they cannot be replaced by either emerging technology or NPCs. For example, will NPCs do the majority of family practice in the future?

E.M. Copeland III, M.D.

The Health Work Force, Generalism, and the Social Contract
Sheldon GF (Univ of North Carolina, Chapel Hill)
Ann Surg 222:215–228, 1995   1–8

Introduction.—In the near future, health system change is expected to occur through physician workforce reform. Our future population will contain more elderly people, who have a higher incidence of chronic disease and require more frequent visits to physicians than do younger people. The elimination of some diseases will result in longer life expectancy, but this may increase health care costs. Managed care with capitation will affect care of the elderly. Health professionals practicing in our future must deal with a knowledge-based economy, limitations on health care availability, and a managed health care system. The number and types of health care providers required by this system should be carefully analyzed.

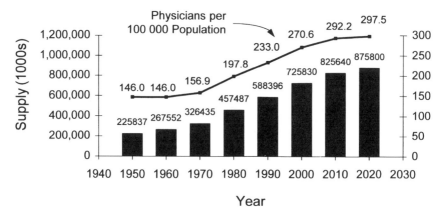

FIGURE 4.—The supply of active physicians has increased to 233 per 100,000 and is projected to continue increasing into the 21st century. Education of the workforce and its orientation toward an aging, knowledge-based, information-rich society will require planning. (Courtesy of Sheldon GF: The health work force, generalism, and the social contract. *Ann Surg* 222:215–228, 1995.)

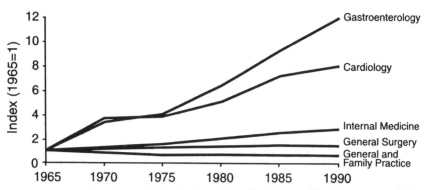

FIGURE 6.—Trends in the growth of selected specialties. Specialty growth has been uneven, with, for example, a 1,073% increase in gastroenterology and a 740% increase in cardiology since 1965. (Courtesy of Sheldon GF: The health work force, generalism, and the social contract. *Ann Surg* 222:215–228, 1995.)

Physician Number.—It is estimated that the ratio of physician to population will rise in the near future (Fig 4) and lead to a physician surplus. The advent of manged health care will lead to a reduction in demand for physicians. In addition to the graduates of American medical schools, international medical graduates also immigrate to fill postgraduate spots in medical schools. The United States is in danger of becoming a safety valve for the overproduction of physicians in other countries. The physicians most vulnerable to unemployment would be recent graduates and women. Downsizing graduating medical classes and reduction of selected specialities could help prevent this problem.

Conclusions.—The ratio of generalist physicians to the population is currently similar to that of other industrialized societies. Most industrialized societies have overproduced physicians, particularly some types of specialists such as those in internal medicine. General surgery is currently balanced but tending toward a deficit (Fig 6). The output of American medical schools and graduate medical programs must be reduced to prevent a future surplus, although each specialty must be considered individually. Universally funded health care with a single payer system should be a national priority.

▶ This abstract is from the Presidential Address delivered by George Sheldon, M.D., to the membership of the American Surgical Association in 1995. He emphasizes the significance of the problem of foreign medical school graduates overpopulating the U.S. medical system. For example, international graduates represent 22% of practicing physicians in the United States, 25% of the physicians in graduate medical education, and 40% of all slots in the 1994 National Residency Matching Program in internal medicine. Downsizing of U.S. medical schools may be a difficult "pill to swallow" when these figures are widely publicized.

E.M. Copeland III, M.D.

Potential Effects of Managed Care on Specialty Practice at a University Medical Center

Billi JE, Wise CG, Bills EA, Mitchell RL (Univ of Michigan, Ann Arbor)
N Engl J Med 333:979–983, 1995 1–9

Introduction.—Because the growth of managed care is likely to result in decreased demand for specialty services and decreased use of academic medical centers (with preference for community hospitals), academic medical centers will have to serve a larger population to maintain adequate referrals to specialists. The number of HMO enrollees needed to maintain the current level of revenue for specialists was estimated by using 3 models.

Methods.—The rates of utilization and payment and the faculty number at the University of Michigan Medical Center in its independent practice association HMO in 1992 were used as the reference points. The size of the HMO membership needed to preserve these reference points was estimated by using an all-services model (in which it was supposed that the academic medical center provided all specialty services to the enrollees), a network model (in which it was supposed that the academic medical center provided only referral services to the enrollees), and a combined model (in which the academic medical center provided all specialty services to 100,000 enrollees in the HMO and only referral services to the remaining enrollees). Medicare enrollees were excluded from the analysis.

Results.—To sustain the 1992 level of specialty revenue and faculty members, the required enrollments would be more than 250,000 with the all-services model (Table 3) and more than 1 million with the network model. If all specialty services were provided to 100,000 HMO members and referral services were provided to an additional 500,000 HMO members in the combined model, substantial faculty cuts would be necessary in all specialty departments (Table 4). The largest faculty reductions would be necessary in internal medicine, radiology, anesthesiology, and pathology and would exceed 50% in some departments.

Discussion.—Managed care presents a much greater financial risk for providers of specialty care than for providers of primary care. Large academic medical centers will be unable to create an HMO or network that is large enough to support the current levels of specialty care. These findings also imply that unrealistically large numbers of primary care physicians will have to be acquired by an HMO or network to preserve the current level of specialty services at academic medical centers. These findings may be considered conservative if Medicare beneficiaries are encouraged to enroll in managed care plans.

▶ Clinical income has been used in the past to support the research and education missions of U.S. medical schools. There are faculty members who have these missions as their major responsibility. By necessity in the immediate future, clinical income will not be readily available as a method of funding these 2 very important missions.

TABLE 3.—Managed Care Enrollees Needed to Maintain the 1992 Level of Professional Specialty Revenue at the University

Specialty	All-Services Model		Network Model		Combined Model	
	No. of Enrollees	No. per Faculty Member	No. of Enrollees	No. per Faculty Member	No. of Enrollees*	No. per Faculty Member
Anesthesiology	471,223	13,351	1,283,677	36,365	1,111,263	31,485
Dermatology	275,116	47,460	4,195,523	723,366	2,770,523	477,940
Internal medicine	409,163	6,940	5,273,652	89,460	4,084,763	69,284
Neurology	591,712	57,434	4,881,626	473,944	4,156,626	403,459
Obstetrics and gynecology	157,179	10,091	2,847,706	182,780	1,135,942	72,928
Ophthalmology	563,041	40,405	1,714,714	123,095	1,510,169	108,373
Otolaryngology	363,087	63,110	1,984,875	345,196	1,538,209	267,364
Pathology	542,099	30,213	11,926,176	664,781	9,826,176	547,646
Pediatrics	2,010,943	33,138	Not available	Not available	Not available	Not available
Physical medicine	387,785	32,576	1,163,356	97,761	963,356	80,927
Radiation oncology	530,013	106,128	6,095,155	1,221,474	5,045,155	1,010,225
Radiology	357,972	7,913	5,727,550	126,604	4,227,550	93,450
Emergency services	168,797	25,869	5,063,910	775,484	2,163,910	331,630
General surgery	595,583	54,702	3,527,684	323,938	3,035,376	278,788
Neurosurgery	1,463,046	268,252	2,560,330	469,785	2,485,330	455,690
Orthopedic surgery	526,099	62,986	2,008,743	240,568	1,726,925	206,752
Pediatric surgery	2,124,289	531,604	Not available	Not available	Not available	Not available
Plastic surgery	801,691	152,997	865,826	165,234	857,826	163,710
Thoracic surgery	1,600,464	289,561	4,201,219	759,714	4,038,719	730,698
Urology	533,151	98,084	1,821,600	334,853	1,579,933	290,661
Vascular surgery	837,294	466,844	1,196,134	668,231	1,153,277	643,024

* Assumes that all specialty services for 100,000 enrollees are provided by the academic medical center.
(Reprinted by permission of *The New England Journal of Medicine* from Billi JE, Wise CG, Bills EA, et al: Potential effects of managed care on specialty practice at a university medical center. *N Engl J Med* 333:979–983, Copyright 1995, Massachusetts Medical Society.)

TABLE 4.—Actual Number of Full-Time-Equivalent Clinical Faculty Members at the University in 1992 as Compared With the Estimated Number Needed to Provide Managed Care Services or Network Referrals

SPECIALTY	NO. OF ACTUAL CLINICAL FACULTY MEMBERS	NO. NEEDED TO SERVE 100,000 ENROLLEES	NO. NEEDED TO SERVE 100,000 ENROLLEES AND PROVIDE NETWORK REFERRALS FOR 500,000 OTHERS
Anesthesiology	35.3	7.5	21.2
Dermatology	5.8	2.1	2.8
Internal medicine	59.0	14.4	20.0
Neurology	10.3	1.7	2.8
Obstetrics and gynecology	15.6	9.9	12.6
Ophthalmology	13.9	2.5	6.5
Otolaryngology	5.8	1.6	3.0
Pathology	17.9	3.3	4.1
Pediatrics	60.7	3.0	Not available
Physical medicine	11.9	3.1	8.2
Radiation oncology	5.0	0.9	1.4
Radiology	45.2	12.6	16.6
Emergency services	6.5	3.9	4.5
General surgery	10.9	1.8	3.4
Neurosurgery	5.5	0.4	1.4
Orthopedic surgery	8.4	1.6	3.7
Pediatric surgery	4.0	0.2	Not available
Plastic surgery	5.2	0.7	3.7
Thoracic surgery	5.5	0.3	1.0
Urology	5.4	1.0	2.5
Vascular surgery	1.8	0.2	1.0

(Reprinted by permission of *The New England Journal of Medicine* from Billi JE, Wise CG, Bills EA, et al: Potential effects of managed care on specialty practice at a university medical center. *N Engl J Med* 333:979–983, Copyright 1995, Massachusetts Medical Society.)

Faculty members with primarily clinical responsibilities who are nonproductive require identification and either reassignment to productive activities or elimination from the system. A ratio of income from all sources to salary earned would be a fair guideline for compensating both clinical and basic science faculty members. Likewise, such a guideline would be market sensitive.

Academic institutions must be price competitive within their geographic location; once this goal is accomplished, then institutional reputation may be marketable within the health care industry. Downsizing is inevitable, and the specific responsibilities of faculty members must be identified. Surgical research and education must be fostered, particularly at a time when gene identification and therapy have broadened the research vista in multiple medical disciplines. Within every medical school faculty certain individuals are more adept at the educational mission, and their peers are willing to allow them to have the majority share of the educational resources. Therefore, the faculty members who are not as actively involved in the educational mission will be required to support it financially. This might mean a restructuring of salaries for everyone.

E.M. Copeland III, M.D.

A Rational Process for the Reform of the Physician Payment System
Maloney JV Jr (Univ of California, Los Angeles)
Ann Surg 222:134–145, 1995   1–10

Introduction.—Traditionally, the monetary value of work is negotiated and reimbursed in terms of dollars per unit of time after determining the economic value of outputs. Despite its intention to reimburse physicians on the basis of time and intensity of work, the resource-based relative value scale (RBRVS) for physician payment will have hourly reimbursement rates that are unrelated to the intensity of work and income that is unrelated to hours worked by 1996. A consensus method of payment was studied as an alternative to the RBRVS. It is proposed that the consensus method would reintroduce time as a basic measure of work, establish a rational differential for the value of an hour's time in each specialty, use the national Medicare charge data for all services by all physicians to maintain budget neutrality, and add the current geographic determinants of overhead and malpractice costs to physician payment to arrive at charges.

Study Design.—A pilot survey was conducted among 300 physicians who were selected such that the representation of each specialty was proportional to the total number certified by the clinical specialty boards of the American Board of Medical Specialties during the past 10 years. Unlike the RBRVS system, which involves mathematical transformation of raw data to establish specialty work values, the physicians assigned dimensionless numbers to the relative value of work in 15 specialties based on the definition of work intensity by Hsiao et al. as "time modified by mental effort, clinical judgment, technical skill, and physical effort under stress." Hourly reimbursement rates for each specialty were determined by the Physician Payment Review Commission by dividing annual income by weekly work hours for a work year of 47 weeks. Work hours, reimbursement rates, and annual income on the customary, prevailing, and reasonable system (CPR, pre-1992), the RBRVS system, and the proposed consensus system were compared.

Results.—Under the consensus method, primary care specialties are rated more highly as a group than in the RBVRS system (Table 1). General surgery and orthopedics have similar relative values in the consensus method, whereas general surgery shares with internal medicine the lowest relative value of all specialties with the RBRVS system. Furthermore, the consensus method demonstrates a direct linear correlation of income with both length of the physician's work week and intensity of effort. In contrast, neither the CPR nor the RBRVS system showed a correlation between income and hours of labor (Fig 1). With the CPR system, some specialties such as dermatology and ophthalmology achieve high income by a higher-than-consensus reimbursement rate that offsets a short work week, whereas others such as general surgery have a lower income despite high intensity and a long work week. Analysis of special-interest groups indicates that a global surgical fee for surgeons results in an hourly rate

TABLE 1.—Specialty Work Hours, Annual Income, and Reimbursement Rates

SECTIONS	I CPR				II Hsiao				III HCFA				IV Consensus				V Equal Pay	
COLUMNS A	B	C	D	E	F	G	H	I	J	K	L	M	N	O	P	Q	R	S
Specialties	Code	Work Hrs/Wk	Income $/Yr	Reimbursement Rate (36–94) $/Hr	Code	Impact	Income $/Yr	Reimbursement Rate (45–98) $/Hr	Code	Impact	Income $/Yr	Reimbursement Rate (44–84) $/Hr	Code	Work Value (1–20)	Reimbursement Rate (44–84) $/Hr	Income $/Yr	Code	Income $/Yr
Orthopedics	OR	49.8	219,100	94	OR	+5%	230,100	98	DRM	0%	156,000	84	NS	18.9	84	223,900	NS	162,600
Ophthalmology	OPH	38.9	167,900	92	DRM	-45%	132,600	71	OR	-11%	195,000	83	GS	14.4	72	184,800	GS	156,500
Neurosurgery	NS	56.7	236,400	89	OB	+5%	165,800	70	NS	-18%	193,800	73	OB	13.1	69	162,800	IM	152,800
Dermatology	DRM	39.6	156,000	84	FP	+65%	150,500	66	OPH	-21%	132,600	72	CRD	12.7	68	169,000	CRD	151,700
Cardiology	CRD	52.9	186,500	75	OTO	-5%	136,400	64	OTO	+3%	147,900	69	OR	12.6	68	159,200	GI	147,400
Gastroenterology	GI	51.4	179,800	74	GP	+65%	130,000	60	CRD	-17%	154,800	62	OTO	11.5	65	139,300	OB	143,900
Obstetrics/Gynecology	OB	50.2	157,900	67	IM	+35%	141,600	57	GI	-18%	147,400	61	OPH	10.2	61	110,900	OR	142,800
Otorhinolaryngology	OTO	45.6	143,600	67	PSY	+5%	105,000	51	NEU	-4%	119,800	52	IM	9.5	60	153,300	NEU	141,600
Neurology	NEU	49.4	124,800	54	OPH	-45%	92,300	50	FP	+28%	116,700	51	GI	9.3	59	142,500	FP	139,600
General Surgery	GS	54.6	135,000	53	GS	-15%	114,800	45	PSY	+3%	103,000	50	NEU	8.5	57	132,400	PD	133,000
Psychiatry	PSY	44.2	100,000	48	CRD	—	—	—	GP	+27%	100,100	46	PD	7.5	55	119,900	GP	131,900
Pediatrics	PD	46.4	98,900	$45	GI	—	—	—	GS	-13%	117,400	46	FP	6.1	51	116,700	OTO	130,700
Internal Medicine	IM	53.3	104,900	42	NS	—	—	—	IM	+5%	110,100	44	GP	6	51	110,300	PSY	126,700
Family Practice	FP	48.7	91,200	40	NEU	—	—	—	OB	—	—	—	PSY	4.1	46	95,500	DRM	113,500
General Practice	GP	46	78,800	36	PD	—	—	—	PD	—	—	—	DRM	3.3	44	81,900	OPH	111,500

Section I CPR contains the data of the Physician Payment Review Commission (PPRC) for the year 1988 under the previous customary prevailing and reasonable system (CPR). Sections II Hsiao and III HCFA (Health Care Financing Commission) show the intended change from CPR in 1996 resulting from these 2 versions of the resource-based relative value scale (RBRVS). Section IV Consensus is the result of the proposed method for valuing of work intensity by the criteria of Hsiao et al. Section V Equal Pay is the hypothetical income if all physicians were paid the average reimbursement rate of $61 per hour.

Column A, specialties rank-ordered by reimbursement rate (column E) under the CPR payment system; column C, average work hours per week by specialty PPRC data; columns E, I, and M, hourly reimbursement rates determined by multiplying the weekly work hours (column C) by a 47-week work year and dividing the product into annual income (columns D, H, and L) for payment systems I, II, and III; reimbursement rates in column E are actual, whereas those in column M reflect work values determined at the result of the intended impact of the RBRVS on specialty income in 1996, assuming that specialty-specific work hours do not change and that the RBRVS has its intended impact; columns F, J, and N, altered rank ordering of specialties based on computed reimbursement rates in columns I, M, and P, respectively; column G, percent intended impact of the Hsiao version of the RBRVS on specialty income; column H, annual income under the Hsiao version of the RBRVS, calculated by multiplying CPR income (column D) by the Hsiao impact (column G); column I, reimbursement rate (reflecting work value/intensity by Hsiao), calculated by dividing the annual income (column H) by the annual work hours, as above; column K, percent intended impact by the HCFA version of the RBRVS on specialty income; column L, annual income under the HCFA version of the RBRVS, calculated by multiplying CPR income (column D) by the HCFA impact (column K); column M, reimbursement rate under the HCFA RBRVS, calculated from HCFA income and annual work hours, as above; column O, average work value in each specialty expressed on a 20-point scale (raw data) in a pilot consensus program; column P, relative reimbursement rates (work values based on the 4 criteria of Hsiao obtained by scaling the raw data in column O to the same spread of reimbursement rates ($45–98) that characterize the 1996 HCFA fee schedule; column Q, annual income under the consensus payment method, calculated by multiplying the consensus determined reimbursement rate (column P) by the specialty-specific annual work hours, as above; column R, rank-ordered specialties based on annual income if physicians in all specialties were reimbursed at the same $61 per hour rate; column S, annual income under the "equal pay" system was calculated by multiplying $61 by the specialty-specific annual work hours, as above.

Differences in rank ordering under the consensus system are generally not statistically significant if based on a difference of less than $2 in reimbursement rate. The cost of programs to the government or society cannot be predicted from tabular data without reference to the BMD database because specialty services must be weighted according to the frequency with which they are used.

(Courtesy of Maloney JV Jr: A rational process for the reform of the physicians payment system. Ann Surg 222:134–145, 1995.)

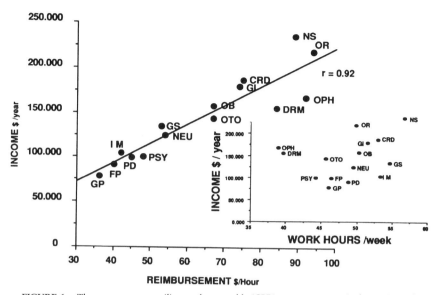

FIGURE 1.—The customary, prevailing, and reasonable (CPR) payment system is shown. Procedure-oriented specialties dominate the higher reimbursement rates and higher annual incomes. Specialties below the regression line (ophthalmology, dermatology, otolaryngology, psychiatry, and general practice) have an income less than anticipated by their reimbursement rate because of their short work week. The incremental income earned by those above the line is achieved by long work hours. Because annual income is the product of the hourly reimbursement rate and hours worked, income is expected to correlate with both. The *inset* shows no correlation between work hours and annual income, which suggests a defect in the CPR system. Specialty abbreviations are given in Table 1. The ordinate is scaled in 1988 dollars. (Courtesy of Maloney JV Jr: A rational process for the reform of the physicians payment system. *Ann Surg* 222:134–145, 1995.)

that is not different from that of nonsurgeons and that "equal pay" favors the procedural specialties because they work longer hours.

Conclusion.—The proposed consensus method makes a possible rational payment system for physicians. It meets the original intent of the RBRVS to reimburse physicians on the basis of the resource input of time as modified by the criteria of Hsiao et al.

▶ The methodology used by Jim Maloney to establish relevance makes entirely too much sense to ever be adopted.

E.M. Copeland III, M.D.

Role of the General Practitioner in the Delivery of Surgical and Anesthesia Services in Rural Western Canada
Chiasson PM, Roy PD (Dalhousie Univ, Halifax, NS, Canada)
Can Med Assoc J 153:1447–1452, 1995   1–11

Background.—The rural population of western Canada is dispersed in smaller communities in an extremely large area, and the often inclement weather adds to the likelihood that it may be very difficult or impossible to urgently transfer patients. This situation makes it important to know whether high-quality surgical care is available outside the urban setting. There is growing interest in "generalist" general surgeons as an alternative to tertiary care, which is not feasible in this setting. Communities have relied on these practitioners to perform gynecologic, orthopedic, obstetric, and reconstructive as well as general surgery.

Objective.—A questionnaire regarding surgical and anesthesia services was sent to the administrators of 148 rural hospitals in British Columbia, Alberta, Yukon Territory, and Northwest Territories. Responses were available for 101 hospitals having 50 or fewer beds that serve a population no larger than 15,000.

Findings.—Surgical services were available at 55% of the 101 hospitals analyzed. They were provided by general practitioners (GPs) at 45 of these hospitals and by GPs having limited additional training in surgery at 33 institutions. Fifteen hospitals relied totally on GPs having limited training in surgery. General practitioners provided anesthesia services at 45 of the 56 hospitals, and in all cases, they had some added training in anesthesia. At 36 hospitals only GPs provided anesthesia services. Only 7 hospitals had full-time anesthetists. Three fourths of all administrators claimed that their community's basic surgical needs were being adequately served. This was the case for several hospitals that did not provide surgical services but were located within 75 km of a referral center.

Implication.—General practitioners have a major role in providing surgical services in rural western Canada. It may be a good idea to establish surgical fellowships for designated GPs working in rural settings. They would be analogous to those already established in anesthesia and emergency medicine.

▶ Rural Canada, according to this article, is in a time warp, never having emerged from the time of general practitioners providing both anesthetic and surgical services. Interestingly, the hospital administrators in these areas report the surgical needs of the community to be met. The procedures done included appendectomies, hernia repair, cesarean section, closed fracture reduction, tonsillectomy, and excisional breast biopsy. The quantity of procedures and quality of care provided were not addressed. These data are of major importance, for if quality is satisfactory, the data would provide a benchmark in modern times of the success of the general practitioner surgeon.

E.M. Copeland III, M.D.

Caremap Management in Low-Severity Surgery: A Comparative Trial
Wilson DE, Noseworthy TW, Grace MG (Univ of Alberta, Edmonton, Canada)
J Am Coll Surg 181:49–55, 1995   1–12

Background.—Caremap management refers to a multidisciplinary health care approach used to identify the optimal clinical guidelines for managing defined patient groups and acheiving cost-effective patient outcomes. Caremap management was compared with traditional treatment in a large series of patients undergoing surgery for hernia.

Study Design.—A controlled, prospective study was performed to compare traditional treatment of 141 patients with caremap management of 110 patients undergoing inguinal herniorrhaphy. The 2 groups were matched for age, gender, and surgical procedure and compared for hospital length of stay (LOS), resource consumption, and outcome. Patient satisfaction was assessed by telephone interview.

Results.—The caremap patients had a significant reduction in average LOS and number or laboratory tests performed. There were no significant differences in readmission rate, reutilization of health care services, or complications between the 2 treatment groups. However, there was a strong preference in the caremap group for an additional day of hospitalization to regain mobility and confidence and to reduce the burden on family member caregivers. There was a significantly lower requirement for home assistance in the traditional care group.

Conclusions.—The use of caremap clinical guidelines reduced the length of hospital stay and number of laboratory tests in a group of patients undergoing inguinal herniorrhaphy without adverse effects. However, patients in the caremap group expressed a desire for longer hospital stays to stabilize their condition and reduce the need for home assistance.

▶ This study was conducted in Canada with patients who had standard open hernia repairs under general anesthesia. Clinical pathway managment (caremap) was compared with traditional management. Length of stay was reduced from 1.63 days to 0.57 days, but quality of care was negatively affected. Patients preferred to stabilize while in the hospital and were anxious at home. From a pure outcomes perspective, the 2 methods were the same and caremap was less expensive. One wonders, however, whether the American public is prepared to give up certain comforts of low-severity illness and whether families are willing to tolerate the concomitant frustrations that ensue from the managed care process. The Canadians were quite annoyed by the inconvenience. I don't think Americans know yet what they are buying into. Only recently has patient acceptance of managed care strategies become a topic of the national news media, and the reports have not been totally complimentary. We are entering some interesting times!

E.M. Copeland III, M.D.

Costs of Potential Complications of Care for Major Surgery Patients
Kalish RL, Daley J, Duncan CC, Davis RB, Coffman GA, Iezzoni LI (Harvard Med School, Boston; Veterans Affairs Med Ctr, West Roxbury, Mass; Yale Univ, New Haven, Conn; et al)
Am J Med Qual 10:48–54, 1995   1–13

Background.—Nearly all health services carry some risk. Some patients are known to be at greater risk for complications than others. Certain complications can be prevented by improving surgical technique, refining risk assessment, improving patient monitoring, and generally providing better care. Health care costs could be lowered by minimizing the risk for and possibly preventing complications.

Methods.—Computerized hospital discharge data were analyzed in 372,680 adults undergoing major surgery in 404 acute care centers in California in 1988. Eleven percent of the patients had at least 1 potential in-hospital complication.

Findings.—Patients with complications were older and more likely to die in the hospital than patients without complications. Length of hospitalization in the 2 groups was 13.5 and 5.4 days, respectively. Total hospital charges were $30,896 for those with complications and $9,239 for those without. After adjusting for demographic, clinical, and hospital variables, total hospital charges for those with complications were a mean $16,023 higher than for those without complications. Including all patients, complications were associated with more than $647 million in additional total charges.

Conclusions.—Even after many patient and hospital variables were taken into consideration, in-hospital complications were associated with much greater total hospital charges. This increase exceeded 96%. Preventing or minimizing complications will be challenging, particularly when the final goal is cost savings.

▶ This extremely valuable study quantifies what all of us know from clinical practice—complications are expensive. Continuous quality improvement teams that involve the hospital and physician personnel providing care for patients in a particular clinical pathway will need to carefully monitor changes in patient management aimed at lowering costs. Changes in instruments, materials, drugs, and monitoring frequency have the potential to create subtle or dramatic changes that might result in complications going unrecognized. Such complications secondary to cost containment measures are obviously counterproductive in a competitive market and subject patients to unnecessary additional risks.

E.M. Copeland III, M.D.

The Effects of Regionalization on Cost and Outcome for One General High-Risk Surgical Procedure
Gordon TA, Burleyson GP, Tielsch JM, Cameron JL (Johns Hopkins Med Insts, Baltimore, Md)
Ann Surg 221:43–49, 1995   1–14

Introduction.—The delivery of care at a selected number of provider sites is termed regionalization and has been considered as a means of cost-effective delivery of tertiary care. Today, community hospitals can provide services once reserved for tertiary care centers because of the abandonment of certificate-of-need requirements. The costs of a high-risk procedure was compared in a high-volume regional center and low-volume centers.

Methods.—One high-volume regional provider performed 54% of all the pancreaticoduodenectomies (Whipple procedure) in Maryland, with the remaining 46% being performed in 38 other hospitals in the state. This procedure has a statewide mortality rate of 7.7% as compared with an overall surgical mortality rate of 2.2%. Data were obtained from the discharge summaries reported to the Maryland Health Services Cost Review Commission (MHSCRC) from 1988 through mid 1993. Cost and outcomes were compared between the regional center and the other 38 hospitals.

Results.—According to the MHSCRC, complete data were available on 501 discharges from the 39 hospitals. Patients at the regional center were most likely to have been transferred from another facility, have commercial insurance, be white, and have diabetes or hypertension as secondary diagnoses. The hospital mortality rate was 6 times greater in the low-volume centers even after adjustment for age, gender, race, method of payment, admission source, and comorbidity (Table 2). Mortality rate and patient volume were inversely related. The mortality rate at the regional center was 2.2% vs. 19.1% at centers that performed 5 or fewer cases over the 5-year period. Overall length of stay, length of stay in the ICU, and total charges were reduced at the regional center. The regional center averaged $5,455 less for all discharges and $6,727 less for live discharges (see table 2). In addition, the charges at the regional center decreased and then remained stable. The low-volume centers raised costs over the 5-year period.

Conclusion.—The experienced team had a standardized approach to the procedure and made less use of imaging examinations, laboratory tests, and supplies, and their patients had a shorter length of stay. The study was

TABLE 2.—In-Hospital Mortality, Length of Stay, and Charges Among Persons Undergoing Whipple Procedures in Maryland Hospitals

	Regional Provider	38 Other Maryland Hospitals	Crude Difference	P Value	Adjusted Difference*	P Value
In-hospital mortality	2.2%	13.5%	11.3%	< 0.001	11.4%	< 0.001
Relative risk	1.0	6.1				
(95% CI)		(2.9, 12.7)				
Mean length of stay						
All discharges	23.0	27.1	4.1	0.04	4.2	0.05
Live discharges	22.5	27.9	5.4	< 0.001	5.7	< 0.001
Mean ICU length of stay						
All discharges	2.2	4.1	1.9	< 0.001	1.7	0.004
Live discharges	1.8	3.8	2.0	< 0.001	1.9	< 0.001
Mean total charges						
All discharges	$26,204	$31,659	$5,455	< 0.001	$5,011	< 0.001
Live discharges	$24,478	$31,205	$6,727	< 0.001	$6,758	< 0.001

* Adjusted for age, race, gender, source of payment, source of admission, and comorbidity.
(Courtesy of Gordon TA, Burleyson GP, Tielsch JM, et al: The effects of regionalization on cost and outcome for one general high-risk surgical procedure. *Ann Surg* 221:43–49, 1995.)

limited to in-hospital mortality, had no information on the severity of the patient's condition before admission, and had no information on the number of diagnostic procedures performed before admission. There can be a substantial impact on the cost and outcome of complex procedures if performed at regional centers. Further research should identify those procedures most appropriately performed at regional centers and develop the specific clinical indications for referral to such a center.

▶ The mortality rate of 2.2% for the regional center (Johns Hopkins) and 19.1% for other centers performing 5 or fewer pancreaticoduodenectomies during a 5-year period means that the occasional Whipple procedure should be discouraged. I suspect there are community hospitals that compare favorably with referral centers (i.e., university hospitals) simply because the community surgeons do enough Whipple procedures to remain competent (at least more than 1 per year). Also, other referral centers may not have a mortality rate as low as that of Johns Hopkins Hospital, even though the physicians have a special interest in pancreatic carcinoma. Conversely, the data could be used to argue for strict regionalization of technically challenging procedures that beget serious complications, which also require special expertise to diagnose and manage. The data, at least for the State of Maryland, are powerful in this regard.

E.M. Copeland III, M.D.

Surgery in Nonagerians: Morbidity, Mortality, and Functional Outcome
Ackermann RJ, Vogel RL, Johnson LA, Ashley DW, Solis MM (Mercer Univ, Macon, Ga)
J Fam Pract 40:129–135, 1995
1–15

Introduction.—The population older than 65 years of age has about twice the number of operations as the group aged 45–64 years. Longevity and improvements in surgical and anesthetic techniques suggest that even more operations will be performed on the elderly, the fastest growing segment of the American population. There are many factors to consider when operating on very old patients, such as the short life span, quality-of-life issues, and mortality and morbidity rates. Because little research has been devoted to surgery in the elderly, there is little training or written material in surgical texts about the advantages and disadvantages.

Methods.—The minimum age for this prospective series was 90 years. A total of 116 patients had 134 major procedures. Only the first operation was reported. Demographic data, residence, functional and ambulatory status, and discharge status were recorded. Mortality and survival curves were computed.

Results.—The patients ranged in age from 90 to 103 years. Ninety-two patients were women, 75 were white, 63 were admitted from a nursing home, and 77 had normal or minimal impairment of functional status. The

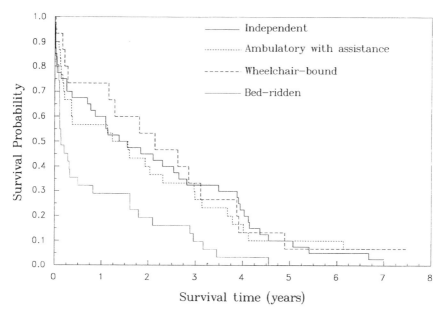

FIGURE 3.—Postsurgical survival outcomes for 116 nonagenarians at various levels of ambulatory status. (Courtesy of Ackermann RJ, Vogel RL, Johnson LA, et al: Surgery in nonagerians: Morbidity, mortality, and functional outcome. *J Fam Pract* 40:129–135, Copyright 1995. Reprinted by permission of Appleton & Lange, Inc.)

most common procedure was repair of a hip fracture, followed by gangrene of the lower extremity and small-bowel obstruction. There were 19 deaths from the 1st to the 62nd postoperative day, mostly from cardiac arrest (6 of 19). The overall perioperative mortality rate was 19.8%, it was highest (33.3%) for patients who had abdominal procedures. Survival was significantly longer in patients who were admitted from a family residence (1.6 years) then in those admitted from a nursing home (0.7 years). Patients with minimal or no functional impairment survived longer than those with more severe impairment. Bedridden patients had a poor survival rate (Fig 3). All patients who were admitted from a nursing home were returned to the nursing facility. Thirteen of the 45 patients who were admitted from a family residence were discharged to a nursing home whereas the remainder went back to their family residence. Eighty-four of the 97 survivors maintained their functional status, and the others declined in status.

Conclusion.—Once the patient survives the postoperative period, the mortality rate of the very old is similar to that of the general population. Chronologic age is a poor criterion for determining whether surgery is appropriate. The 1-year survival rate for independent patients was 63% vs. 34% for nursing home patients. Caution should be used in suggesting surgery for the very old. This was a select and robust group. With advancing dementia, providing comfort measures may be more compassionate than complex surgical procedures.

▶ The decision to operate on a person 90 years of age or older can be difficult. Although the outcome may be somewhat unpredictable, it is often very rewarding. A 63% 1-year survival rate for independent individuals, the majority of whom are returned to the home, sets a good standard and serves as a goal for patients who require operations such as hip fracture, bowel obstruction, and amputation.

In my experience, healthy elderly patients will do well postoperatively if no complications ensue. The elderly tolerate complications poorly, and one complication often begets another. Therefore, maximizing the patient*s tolerance for anesthesia and surgery preoperatively becomes of paramount importance, e.g., pulmonary function, ideal volume replacement, and nutritional repletion. A pain-free existence should be the first goal; for example, an impacted fracture of the femoral neck in a nonambulatory patient might best be left alone.

E.M. Copeland III, M.D.

Falling Cholecystectomy Thresholds Since the Introduction of Laparoscopic Cholecystectomy
Escarce JJ, Chen W, Schwartz JS (Univ of Pennsylvania, Philadelphia)
JAMA 273:1581–1585, 1995   1–16

Introduction.—Since the introduction of laparoscopic cholecystectomy in 1989, several reports have documented a sharp increase in the frequency of cholecystectomy. Medicare hospital claims data for Pennsylvania were reviewed to determine whether the increase in cholecystectomy rates was similar in young and elderly cohorts and whether changes in rates were accompanied by lower clinical thresholds for surgery.

Methods.—Data were obtained from all Medicare discharges in Pennsylvania from 1986 to 1993 for patients aged 65 or older who underwent cholecystectomy. The stage of gallstone disease at the time of surgery, type of admission, patient age, and patient comorbidities were noted for each patient. Postoperative mortality 30 days after cholecystectomy was calculated.

Results.—Cholecystectomy rates in elderly Medicare beneficiaries in Pennsylvania were stable in the years preceding introduction of the laparoscopic cholecystectomy procedure. Cholecystectomy rates for elderly patients increased by 22% from 1989 to 1993. The proportion of uncomplicated gallstone disease decreased by an average of 0.25% per quarter before introduction of the laparoscopic procedure. However, the proportion of patients with uncomplicated disease undergoing cholecystectomy increased significantly after the laparoscopic procedure was introduced. Neither the age distribution of patients undergoing cholecystectomy nor the proportion of patients without comorbidities changed significantly throughout. Of 16,334 patients who underwent cholecystectomy after introduction of the laparoscopic procedure, 57.5% and 42.5% had laparoscopic cholecystectomy and open cholecystectomy, respectively. Postoperative 30-day mortality rates decreased significantly after the introduction of laparoscopic cholecystectomy.

Conclusion.—Patients with laparoscopic cholecystectomy were more likely to be younger, were less likely to have complicated disease or be admitted urgently or emergently, had fewer comorbidities, and had a lower 30-day mortality rate. It was not possible to determine whether the introduction of laparoscopic cholecystectomy was responsible for lower clinical thresholds for cholecystectomy.

▶ An interesting trend in Medicare patients (after the introduction of laparoscopic cholecystectomy)—an increase in uncomplicated cholecystectomies, a decrease in complicated cholecystectomies, and a reduction in the mortality rate for cholecystectomy. Are these trends related? Probably so. The gallbladder is not around to get a disease-related complication, and laparoscopic cholecystectomy is a less morbid operation than open cholecystectomy. There has been some criticism of surgeons for lowering the threshold for cholecystectomy. In fact, liberal use of cholecystectomy may eliminate an expensive health hazard, i.e., complicated biliary tract disease.

E. M. Copeland III, M. D.

Major Vascular Injuries During Laparoscopic Procedures
Nordestgaard AG, Bodily KC, Osborne RW Jr, Buttorff JD (Cascade Vascular Assoc, Tacoma, Washington)
Am J Surg 169:543–545, 1995   1–17

Background.—Although laparoscopy has proved to be a safe, effective, and well-tolerated procedure, complications and failures can occur. Major vascular complications, although uncommon, carry a risk of serious morbidity or mortality when they do occur. Experience with 5 major vascular injures occurring during laparoscopic procedures is reported, as are the findings of previously described major vascular injuries.

Patients and Findings.—Five major vascular injuries occurred in 3 women aged 31 to 39 years and 1 man aged 76 years over a 3-year period. All injuries were sustained during pelvic laparoscopy, which was performed for diagnostic reasons in 2 patients and for tubal ligation and hernia repair in 1 patient each. Vascular injuries were detected during laparoscopy in 3 patients, with immediate vascular surgery consultation required in 1 patient. Injuries to the iliac artery were noted in 3 patients. The iliac vein and the inferior epigastric artery were also injured in 1 patient each. In 2 patients, the mechanism of injury was the trocar. In the remaining 2 patients, vascular injuries were caused by sharp dissection for lysis of adhesions. Polytetrafluoroethylene (PTFE) interposition, PTFE patch angioplasty, resection and primary anastomosis, and ligation were used to repair arterial injures in 1 patient each, and lateral venorrhaphy was used for venous repair. Three patients recovered without complications. The fourth patient had an ischemic cerebral accident necessitating an extended stay in the rehabilitation unit.

Twenty previous major vascular injuries have been reported in the literature, all of which occurred as a result of the pneumoperitoneum needle or trocar insertion. The terminal aorta, cava, and iliac arteries and veins were most commonly injured, and most injures were managed by direct suture repair. Prompt identification of injuries was associated with patient recovery, whereas 3 of 8 patients with delayed injury recognition died.

Conclusions.—Although rare, major laparoscopic-related vascular injuries are serious and can be fatal. When such injures occur, prompt conversion to an open procedure and utilization of proper vascular surgical methods are needed to re-establish arterial and venous continuity and reduce complications and fatal outcomes.

▶ Vascular injuries during laparoscopy are uncommon. However, procrastination in opening the abdomen to gain control can be lethal. I chose this abstract to remind the reader of the complication and to implore surgeons to have a low threshold for exploratory laparotomy if there is suspicion of a major vascular injury. Surgeons should be alert to prevent vascular injury during trocar insertion and during dissection around major vessels. The iliac vessels, predictably, are the most vulnerable.

E.M. Copeland III, M.D.

High-Risk Intrahospital Transport of Critically Ill Patients: Safety and Outcome of the Necessary "Road Trip"
Szem JW, Hydo LJ, Fischer E, Kapur S, Klemperer J, Barie PS (Cornell Univ, New York)
Crit Care Med 23:1660–1666, 1995   1–18

Rationale.—It is often necessary to transport critically ill patients within the hospital to ensure optimal care, but moving ICU patients has been accompanied by a high rate of potentially serious complications. A prospective cohort study was planned at a 780-bed urban teaching hospital to ascertain the actual effects of transport-related complications on morbidity and mortality.

Methods.—Of 759 surgical ICU patients, 175 were moved out of the unit for testing or surgery. Acute Physiology and Chronic Health Evaluation (APACHE) II and III scores were estimated 24 hours after admission to the ICU. High-risk patients were designated as those requiring positive end-expiratory pressure (PEEP) of more than 5 cm H_2O or a continuous infusion of either dobutamine or norepinephrine. The course and outcome were compared with those in APACHE-matched control patients.

Management During Transport.—A physician, usually a second-year surgery resident, was always present during intrahospital transport. A respiratory therapist or anesthesiologist was available to re-establish mechanical ventilation. The patient's ventilator was used for transport if PEEP of more than 15 cm H_2O was required. Portable monitors provided the same physiologic data as were available in the ICU. Patients were moved in their own beds.

Results.—Complications developed in 6.3% of the low-risk and 5.5% of the high risk patients. Nevertheless, mortality was significantly higher for transported patients than for controls (28.6% vs. 11.4%). No deaths resulted directly from transport. More than half (51.4%) of the high-risk transport patients died, significantly more than their APACHE-matched controls. Mortality, however, was not significantly greater than that predicted. Regardless of the risk level, transport patients remained in the surgical ICU 3 times longer than APACHE-matched control patients.

Discussion.—Increased mortality in this study was related not to transport itself but to a high degree of critical illness mandating intervention outside the ICU. Complications are frequent but may well be acceptable if outside intervention is considered necessary.

▶ Although transported patients had a higher mortality and a longer ICU stay than matched control patients who were not transported, these increases were not related to transportation and no mortality resulted from the transport. A very important component of this study was the resident and respiratory therapist or anesthesiologist who accompanied the patient during transport. My selection of this study for inclusion was specifically to make this point. The accompanying medical personnel are most likely responsible for safety of the transport and for ensuring that the appropriate tests are obtained upon arrival at the testing site. To attempt to transport patients as ill as those in this study without appropriate accompaniment could be disastrous.

E.M. Copeland III, M.D.

Transfusion Requirements in Critical Care: A Pilot Study

Hébert PC, for the Canadian Critical Care Trials Group (Univ of Ottawa, Ontario, Canada)
JAMA 273:1439–1444, 1995   1–19

Background.—Critically ill patients commonly have anemia, which results in the frequent use of red blood cell (RBC) transfusions. In such patients, however, no optimal, safe lower limit to the transfusion threshold has been established. In addition, transfusion practice can vary significantly among practitioners. The mortality and morbidity associated with restrictive and liberal RBC transfusion strategies in critically ill patients were compared.

Methods.—Sixty-nine normovolemic critically ill patients were enrolled in the multicenter, prospective, randomized trial. The patients had been admitted to 1 of 5 tertiary-level ICUs and had hemoglobin values of less than 90 g/L within 72 hours. Patients were randomly assigned to a liberal transfusion group, in which hemoglobin values were maintained between 100 and 120 g/L, or a restrictive transfusion group, in which hemoglobin values were maintained between 70 and 90 g/L.

Findings.—Mean daily hemoglobin values were 90 g/L in the restrictive transfusion group and 109 g/L in the liberal transfusion group. In the restrictive group, 2.5 units per patient was given as compared with 4.8 units in the liberal transfusion group for a relative reduction of 48% in RBC units transfused per patient. Thirty-day mortality rates were 24% and 25% in the restrictive and liberal transfusion groups, respectively. Intensive care unit mortality, 120-day mortality, and organ dysfunction scores were also similar. Survival analysis comparing time to death in the 2 groups also showed no significant differences.

Conclusions.—Transfusion strategy did not affect mortality or the development of organ dysfunction in this study. Thus a more restrictive approach to RBC transfusion in critically ill patients may be safe. However, because this study did not have the statistical power to detect small but clinically significant differences, further research is needed.

▶ A difference between a hemoglobin level of 1.9 g/dL may be insignificant when comparing complications secondary to different hemoglobin concentrations. The important observation in this study is the significant difference in number of transfusions per patient necessary to increase the hemoglobin value from 9 to 10.9 g/dL. The results of the study aid in developing clinical pathways that involve transfusion of normovolemic patients. The cost and complications of an additional 2-unit transfusion are substantial.

In a hypovolemic patient with acute hemorrhage, a hemoglobin level of 9 g/dL may not be acceptable. The value may be spuriously high if the dilutional effect from the intravascular incorporation of extracellular fluid has not occurred. Intravascular volume may be dangerously low with no reserve for continued bleeding.

E.M. Copeland III, M.D.

Temporary Discontinuation of Warfarin Therapy: Changes in the International Normalized Ratio
White RH, McKittrick T, Hutchinson R, Twitchell J (Univ of California, Davis)
Ann Intern Med 122:40–42, 1995   1–20

Background.—Long-term warfarin therapy must frequently be withheld before dental and surgical procedures. However, few data are available to establish the optimal interval between discontinuation of therapy and surgery. The rate of decrease of the international normalized ratio (INR) was measured after temporary withdrawal of warfarin therapy.

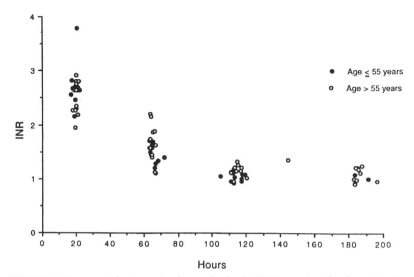

FIGURE 1.—Decrease in the international normalized ratio (*INR*) over time after discontinuation of warfarin therapy. The measured INR is depicted as a function of time after the last dose of warfarin. (Courtesy of White RH, McKittrick T, Hutchinson R, et al: Temporary discontinuation of warfarin therapy: Changes in the international normalized ratio. *Ann Intern Med* 122:40–42, 1995.)

Method.—Twenty-two patients receiving a fixed evening dose of warfarin who were considered suitable for temporary discontinuation of therapy were studied. Those with a history of widely fluctuating warfarin requirements or with a complex dosing regimen were excluded. Serial plasma samples were drawn for INR measurements at 20, 65, 115, and 185 hours after the last dose of warfarin. In 5 patients, the INR was measured twice daily for 5 days.

Results.—For patients with a mean steady-state INR of 2.6, the mean INR at 65 hours after stopping warfarin therapy was 1.6. Twenty of the 22 patients (91%) had an INR greater than 1.2. On day 3, a mean of 66.5 hours after the last dose of warfarin, 10 of the patients (55%) had an INR greater than 1.5, whereas only 2 (9%) had an INR less than 1.2. On day 5, 115 hours after discontinuation of therapy, all but 5 patients had an INR less than 1.2, and by day 8, all except 2 had INRs that were less than 1.2 (Fig 1). In the 5 patients who were studied in detail, the INR was seen to increase exponentially and had a half-life that ranged from 0.52 to 1.2 days; the onset of maximal decrease began 24 to 36 hours after warfarin therapy was discontinued. Age was found to be a significant independent predictor of smaller decreases in the INR between days 1 and 3.

Conclusion.—The INR decreases exponentially 24–36 hours after the last dose of warfarin, with wide interpatient variation in the rate of decrease. Age is correlated with a slower rate of decrease. To ensure that the INR at the time of surgery is less than 1.2, it is advisable to withhold warfarin therapy for 96–115 hours in patients with a steady-state INR between 2.0 and 3.0. In patients with a higher steady-state INR, it is necessary to wait longer.

▶ This study adds data to what has often been guesswork. Withholding warfarin for 5 days reduced all study patients with initial INRs of 2–3 to an acceptable INR of 1.5 or less. Older patients or patients with initial INRs greater than 3 may take even longer. If withholding warfarin for 5 days is medically acceptable, then there is no reason to re-evaluate the INR at an earlier date. If 5 days is unacceptable, than vitamin K or heparin should be considered.

E.M. Copeland III, M.D.

Combined Estrogen and Progestin Hormone Replacement Therapy in Relation to Risk of Breast Cancer in Middle-Aged Women
Stanford JL, Weiss NS, Voigt LF, Daling JR, Habel LA, Rossing MA (Fred Hutchinson Cancer Research Ctr, Seattle; Univ of Washington, Seattle)
JAMA 274:137–142, 1995   1–21

Background.—The use of combined progestin and estrogen for hormone replacement therapy (HRT) has increased among U.S. women. Although this combination may in theory alter the incidence of breast cancer, few epidemiologic data are available on the association of combined estrogen-progestin HRT and breast cancer.

Methods.—Five hundred thirty-seven 50- to 64-year-old women with breast cancer and 492 randomly selected women with no history of breast cancer were included in the case-control study. All were residents of 1 county in western Washington State.

Findings.—Sixty-one percent of the control group and 57.6% of the breast cancer patients had used some type of postmenopausal hormone. The 21.5% of patients and 21.3% of control subjects who had ever used combined estrogen-progestin HRT had no increased risk of breast cancer. When compared with hormone nonusers, women who had used estrogen-progestin for 8 years or more had a decreased breast cancer risk.

Conclusions.—The use of combination estrogen-progestin HRT is apparently unrelated to an increased risk of breast cancer in middle-aged women. Further research is needed to determine whether the incidence of breast cancer is altered many years after estrogen-progestin HRT is begun, especiially among long-term users.

▶ The association between breast cancer and the ingestion of estrogen or progesterone, either alone or in combination, is in constant evolution. This study shows no association with the combination in middle-aged women, including those with a prior benign breast biopsy or a positive family history of breast cancer. Large population studies need to continue, however, since the ultimate effect of long-term use of hormone replacement on the incidence of breast cancer remains unknown. For now, replacement therapy probably has more beneficial effects (prevention of osteoporosis and cardiovascular diseases) than the risk of increasing the incidence of breast cancer, possibly with the exception of patients who have multiple first-degree relatives with breast cancer and/or biopsy-proven severe atypical hyperplasia. Even in postmenopausal women who are disease free from breast cancer in the distant past, the risk/benefit of replacement therapy may be skewed toward prescribing it.

E.M. Copeland III, M.D.

Understanding Surgical Knot Security: A Proposal to Standardize the Literature

Dinsmore RC (Eisenhower Army Med Center, Fort Gordon, Augusta, Ga)
J Am Coll Surg 180:689–696, 1995   1–22

Background.—Little work has been done on the knot handling properties of various suture materials. Because the tensile strength of sutures is severalfold greater than their shear strength, shear forces are generally responsible for rupture, and knots are the most common shear point. Tensile force is converted to shear force at the point that the suture bends into the body of the knot.

Objective.—Current knowledge about the efficiency of surgical knots (Fig 2) was surveyed by reviewing the relevant literature.

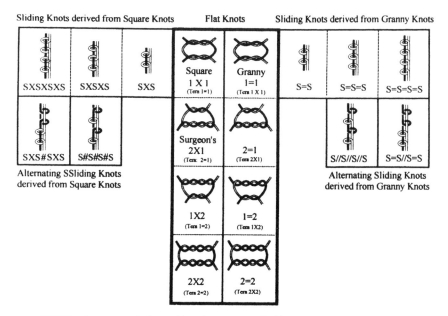

FIGURE 2.—Structure and relationships of common surgical knots.

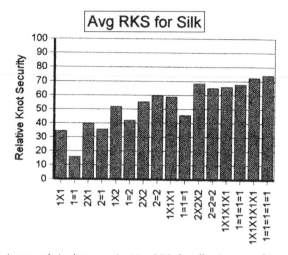

FIGURE 6.—Average relative knot security (*Avg RKS*) for silk. (Courtesy of Dinsmore RC: Understanding surgical knot security: A proposal to standardize the literature. *J Am Coll Surg* 180:689–696, 1995. By permission of the *Journal of the American College of Surgeons.*)

Nomenclature.—Only studies that reported data in terms of relative knot security (RKS) were considered. Relative knot security is the knot-holding capacity (KHC) expressed as a percentage of the tensile strength of the suture. In the illustrations, an "equals" sign indicates that the next throw turns in the same direction as the one preceding it, and an "X" means that it turns in the opposite direction.

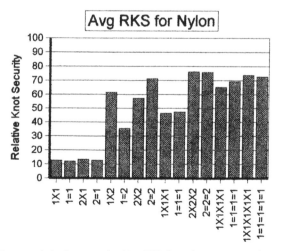

FIGURE 7.—Average relative knot security (*Avg RKS*) for nylon. (Courtesy of Dinsmore RC: Understanding surgical knot security: A proposal to standardize the literature. *J Am Coll Surg* 180:689–696, 1995. By permission of the *Journal of the American College of Surgeons.*)

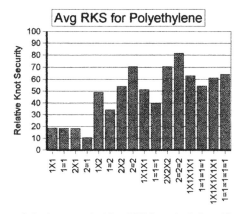

FIGURE 8.—Average relative knot security (*Avg RKS*) for polyethylene. (Courtesy of Dinsmore RC: Understanding surgical knot security: A proposal to standardize the literature. *J Am Coll Surg* 180:689–696, 1995. By permission of the *Journal of the American College of Surgeons*.)

Findings.—A plot of average RKS for various suture materials reveals 2 broad groups: material in which the type of knot strongly influences the RKS and others in which it has a minimal effect (Figs 6 through 16). For flat knots with a single turn per throw, square throws (1×1) outperformed granny throws (1=1). The same was the case for knots in which the first throw had 1 turn and the second, had 2. The opposite was the case for knots with 2 turns per throw (2×2). For material in which the type of knot strongly affected RKS, a generally linear increase in RKS was noted as the knots became more complex, up to 4–5 single throws. This pattern

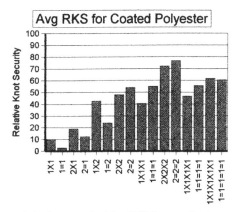

FIGURE 9.—Average relative knot security (*Avg RKS*) for coated polyester. (Courtesy of Dinsmore RC: Understanding surgical knot security: A proposal to standardize the literature. *J Am Coll Surg* 180:689–696, 1995. By permission of the *Journal of the American College of Surgeons*.)

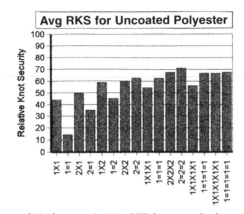

FIGURE 10.—Average relative knot security (*Avg RKS*) for uncoated polyester. (Courtesy of Dinsmore RC: Understanding surgical knot security: A proposal to standardize the literature. *J Am Coll Surg* 180:689–696, 1995. By permission of the *Journal of the American College of Surgeons*.)

did not hold for knots in which the second throw consisted of 2 turns, which are much more efficient than those consisting of a single turn per throw. The increase in efficiency with complexity was less evident when RKS was only minimally affected by the type of knot.

Implications.—Both the type of knot and the type of suture material are important elements determining the security of sutures. Knots in which the second throw consists of 2 turns are relatively very efficient. Nevertheless, these studies do not accurately simulate in vivo conditions. It is probably valid to extrapolate them, but this remains to be demonstrated.

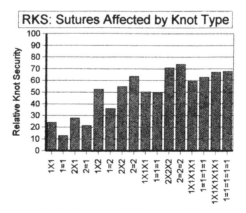

FIGURE 11.—Average relative knot security (*RKS*) sutures affected by knot type. (Courtesy of Dinsmore RC: Understanding surgical knot security: A proposal to standardize the literature. *J Am Coll Surg* 180:689–696, 1995. By permission of the *Journal of the American College of Surgeons*.)

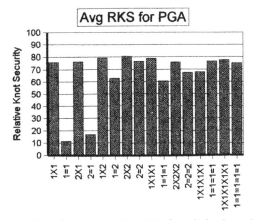

FIGURE 12.—Average relative knot security (*Avg RKS*) for polyglycolic acid (*PGA*). (Courtesy of Dinsmore RC: Understanding surgical knot security: A proposal to standardize the literature. *J Am Coll Surg* 180:689–696, 1995. By permission of the *Journal of the American College of Surgeons*.)

▶ It is quite worthwhile for the surgeon to spend some time reviewing the contents of the figures presented herein. Almost all types of suture material are represented, and knot security is clearly affected by the number and type of throws used in the knot. For example, do not use 2 throws followed by a single throw, and 2 throws repeated 3 times produces a strong knot with all suture material. You might be surprised by the data presented in this study when evaluating the knot strength of your favorite suture.

E.M. Copeland III, M.D.

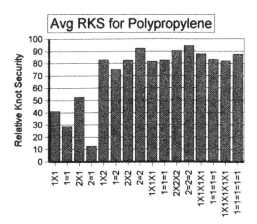

FIGURE 13.—Average relative knot security (*Avg RKS*) for polypropylene. (Courtesy of Dinsmore RC: Understanding surgical knot security: A proposal to standardize the literature. *J Am Coll Surg* 180:689–696, 1995. By permission of the *Journal of the American College of Surgeons*.)

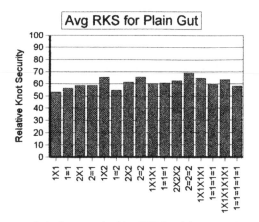

FIGURE 14.—Average relative knot security (*Avg RKS*) for plain catgut. (Courtesy of Dinsmore RC: Understanding surgical knot security: A proposal to standardize the literature. *J Am Coll Surg* 180:689–696, 1995. By permission of the *Journal of the American College of Surgeons.*)

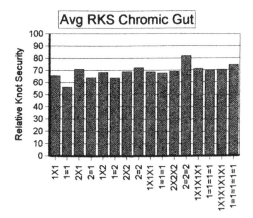

FIGURE 15.—Average relative knot security (*Avg RKS*) for chromic catgut. (Courtesy of Dinsmore RC: Understanding surgical knot security: A proposal to standardize the literature. *J Am Coll Surg* 180:689–696, 1995. By permission of the *Journal of the American College of Surgeons.*)

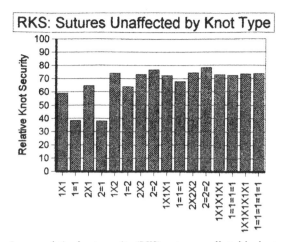

FIGURE 16.—Average relative knot security *(RKS)*: sutures unaffected by knot type. (Courtesy of Dinsmore RC: Understanding surgical knot security: A proposal to standardize the literature. *J Am Coll Surg* 180:689–696, 1995. By permission of the *Journal of the American College of Surgeons.*)

2 Critical Care

Introduction

One phenomenon that has always amazed me is how long it takes between the time a therapy is proved to be effective by published studies and the time this therapy becomes widely accepted by the medical community. For most drugs, the lag phase between proof of effectiveness and widespread use averages 5 to 8 years. The reason for this well-documented phenomenon is not fully clear, but the potential adverse effect of this delay on patient care is clear. One increasingly common method used to decrease the time between the accumulation of information and the utilization of this information by practicing physicians is the consensus conference. Consequently, I have included in this year's selection of articles the results of 2 consensus conferences dealing with adult ICU patients. The first presents practice parameters for IV analgesia and sedation in the ICU, while the second presents practice parameters for sustained neuromuscular blockade. Both are very important. Wide dissemination of practice parameters for the care of comatose head-injured patients would appear to be an important goal based on the results of a survey examining the current level of care these patients receive. In this study, Ghajar et al. found a wide disparity between the best-available level of care and the level of care actually administered at a significant number of the centers surveyed. This study highlights the disparity between what is proved to be the best therapy from well-controlled clinical trials and what is done. Another controversial and emotionally laden subject included in this year's selections for which opinion and survey data are available is the decision to limit or stop ICU therapy in futile circumstances.

Human errors in the ICU. How often and when do they occur? A prospective study designed to answer this question documented that they occur surprisingly frequently, and the most common cause appeared to be verbal miscommunication. This study highlights the importance of clear communication in preventing potentially adverse patient events. Miscommunication can also occur between man and machine. For example, not uncommonly, pulmonary capillary wedge pressure measurements are at odds with clinical judgment, especially in our sickest patients. Although extremely helpful, pulmonary arterial wedge pressure (PAWP) measurements do have their limitations in accurately predicting whether cardiac output can be improved by increasing preload (i.e., giving volume), especially in patients with altered myocardial compliance or pulmonary hypertension, as well as in patients receiving positive-pressure ventilation. As reported by Durham et al., one potential solution to this problem is the use of a modified Swan-Ganz catheter that allows measurement of right ventricular end-diastolic volume since ventricular volume is a better predictor of cardiac output than ventricular pressure (PAWP). That routine prophylactic administration of low-dose dopamine improves renal function appears to be another misconception based on a prospective randomized double-blinded clinical trial. That is, although dopamine increases urine output in septic and critically ill patients, it does not improve renal function, i.e., it acts as an expensive diuretic. Another controversy that continues concerns maximization of oxygen delivery. Thus not to be remiss, I have included an article evaluating the risks and benefits of maximizing oxygen delivery in ICU patients.

What is the current prognosis for patients with acute respiratory failure? The answer to that question is covered in a prospective evaluation of outcome in 1,426 patients treated in 25 critical care units. Unfortunately, the results of this study do not show much progress over the last 10 to 20 years as far as survival is concerned. Recognition of the limitations of current therapy have prompted searches for new or better ways to treat patients with severe but potentially reversible acute respiratory failure. Since one such new approach is liquid ventilation with perfluorocarbon solutions, 2 experimental studies dealing with this topic were chosen. An area in which there is some reason to be optimistic, although the evidence is anecdotal, is the use of corticosteroids for the treatment of refractory late adult respiratory distress syndrome. Because enteral feeding is important but at times difficult in mechanically ventilated patients, the observation that erythromycin is effective in increasing gastric motility in mechanically ventilated patients was chosen because of its potential clinical importance.

What is in a name? The answer is quite a lot when it comes to determining prognosis or setting enrollment criteria for clinical trials. Thus 2 studies were chosen, 1 on the natural history of systemic inflammatory response syndrome and 1 defining a multiple organ dysfunction score. The final articles chosen represent a variety of topics ranging from the heat shock response to the pretreatment of patients with monophosphoryl lipid A to induce endotoxin tolerance. All these articles have something important to say.

Edwin A. Deitch, M.D.

Practice Parameters for Intravenous Analgesia and Sedation for Adult Patients in the Intensive Care Unit: An Executive Summary
Shapiro BA, Warren J, Egol AB, Greenbaum DM, Jacobi J, Nasraway SA, Schein RM, Spevetz A, Stone JR (Society of Critical Care Medicine, Anaheim, Calif)
Crit Care Med 23:1596–1600, 1995   2–1

Introduction.—The American College of Critical Care Medicine and the Society of Critical Care Medicine have published consensus practice parameters to aid in the prescription of IV sedatives and analgesics in the ICU. The specific recommendations and the fundamental information on which they were based are presented.

Methods.—The relevant literature was reviewed and consensus recommendations were formulated by a task force of more than 40 experts in various disciplines. The final recommendations and the executive summary reviewed here were approved by the Executive Council of the Society of Critical Care Medicine.

Findings.—The unabridged practice parameter document included 6 recommendations. First, morphine sulfate should be regarded as the analgesic agent of choice for critically ill patients. It should be given IV and titrated to achieve the desired effect. Second, fentanyl should be regarded as the analgesic agent of choice for critically ill patients with hemodynamic instability, those who have symptoms of histamine release while receiving morphine, and those who are allergic to morphine. This analgesic should be given B-1 continuous IV infusion. Third, hydromorphone is recognized as a suitable alternative to morphine.

Fourth, midazolam or propofol is preferred for the short-term treatment of anxiety in critically ill adults, i.e., less than 24 hours. Fifth, when prolonged treatment for anxiety is needed in a critically ill adult, lorazepam is preferred. Sixth, haloperidol should be regarded as the agent of choice for the treatment of delirium.

Discussion.—Consensus recommendations for IV analgesia and sedation in critically ill adult patients are presented. The selective information presented in the executive summary does not replace the information provided in the complete practice parameter document. Meperidine, opiate agonist-antagonists, and nonsteroidal anti-inflammatory drugs are not recommended for use as analgesics in the ICU. Etomidate, ketamine, barbiturates, chlorpromazine, and droperidol are not recommended for routine sedation in critically ill patients.

Practice Parameters for Sustained Neuromuscular Blockade in the Adult Critically Ill Patient: An Executive Summary

Shapiro BA, Warren J, Egol AB, Greenbaum DM, Jacobi J, Nasraway SA, Schein RM, Spevetz A, Stone JR (Society of Critical Care Medicine, Anaheim, Calif)

Crit Care Med 23:1601–1605, 1995   2–2

Introduction.—The American College of Critical Care Medicine and the Society of Critical Care Medicine have published consensus practice parameters for sustained neuromuscular blockade in critically ill adults. The specific recommendations and the fundamental information on which they were based are presented.

Methods.—The relevant literature was reviewed and consensus recommendations were formulated by a task force of more than 40 experts in various disciplines. The final recommendations and the executive summary reviewed here were approved by the Executive Council of the Society of Critical Care Medicine.

Findings.—The unabridged practice parameter document included 3 recommendations. First, pancuronium should be regarded as the neuromuscular blocking agent of choice for most critically ill patients. Pancuronium should probably not be used in patients with a history of asthma or atopy. Second, for patients with cardiac disease or hemodynamic instability in whom tachycardia may have adverse consequences, vecuronium should be regarded as the agent of choice. Third, appropriate assessment for the degree of blockade being sustained is required for patients receiving neuromuscular blocking agents. Monitoring should include direct observation of ventilatory efforts and peripheral nerve stimulation.

Discussion.—Consensus recommendations for sustained neuromuscular blockade in critically ill adult patients are presented. The selective information presented in the executive summary does not replace that provided in the complete practice parameter document. The nondepolarizing agents *d*- tubocurarine, atracurium, metocurine, and doxacurium are not recommended for routine use in the ICU.

▶ Practice parameters, another name for practice guidelines, have arrived and in some cases it is a good thing. These 2 articles, which outline analgesic, sedative, and neuromuscular blockade practice parameters, speak for themselves. My advise is to read them and to the extent possible adopt them. By adopting these guidelines, not only is it possible to save money, but having a well-justified uniform approach to analgesia, sedation, and neuromuscular blockade can help avoid confusion in the ICU and thereby potentially improve patient outcome.

E.A. Deitch, M.D.

Changes in Acetylcholine Receptor Number in Muscle From Critically Ill Patients Receiving Muscle Relaxants: An Investigation of the Molecular Mechanism of Prolonged Paralysis

Dodson BA, Kelly BJ, Braswell LM, Cohen NH (Univ of California, San Francisco)

Crit Care Med 23:815–821, 1995   2–3

Objective.—An autopsy study was conducted to examine the possible pathophysiologic causes for the prolonged paralysis that can occur after critically ill patients are given muscle relaxants to facilitate mechanical ventilation. There is complete lack of sensory involvement in most such cases of paralysis, which suggests that the pathology occurs along the motor pathway.

Methods.—The autopsy specimens studied were from 14 patients who required mechanical ventilatory support before death. Samples were obtained within 24 hours of death. The patients, who had a variety of diagnoses, were arbitrarily divided into 3 groups on the basis of total vecuronium dose and number of days mechanically ventilated before death. Muscle specimens were examined for nicotinic acetylcholine receptor numbers as measured by specific ^{125}I-α-bungarotoxin binding.

Results.—Three patients assigned to the control group died within 72 hours of the initiation of ventilatory support and received a total dose of less than 5 mg of vecuronium. The 6 patients in the low-dose group required ventilatory support for more than 3 days before death and received a total vecuronium dose of 200 mg or less. The remaining 5 patients, who required ventilatory support for longer than 3 days before death and were administered a total vecuronium dose of more than 200 mg, were considered the high-dose group. Nicotinic acetylcholine receptor numbers generally reflected the clinical requirements for muscle relaxation in individual cases. Thus patients with increasing requirements for muscle relaxants before death had increases in receptor numbers as compared with controls.

Conclusion.—Paralysis lasting as long as 12 months can occur after long-term administration of nondepolarizing muscle relaxants. Even short-term use of these agents has resulted in prolonged paralysis in individuals simultaneously treated with high-dose corticosteroids. Because muscle relaxants act by inhibiting acetylcholine binding to the postsynaptic nicotinic acetylcholine receptor at the neuromuscular junction, denervation-like changes in receptor function may underlie the molecular basis for prolonged paralysis.

▶ A major problem with muscle relaxants is the occasional, but not rare incidence (5%) of prolonged muscle paralysis or weakness observed after the muscle relaxants have been stopped. Treatment or prevention of this complication is hindered by the fact that it is not known why this phenomenon of prolonged paralysis occurs. Thus the importance of this study is that it provides some insight into the potential mechanism underlying this side effect of muscle relaxant use. Until more is known, the best approach is to use these agents for as short a period and at as low a dose as possible. Remember, the best approach for a patient fighting the ventilator is not paralysis but sedation and/or modification of the method of ventilatory support.

E.A. Deitch, M.D.

Survey of Critical Care Management of Comatose, Head-Injured Patients in the United States

Ghajar J, Hariri RJ, Narayan RK, Iacono LA, Firlik K, Patterson RH (Cornell Univ, New York; Baylor College of Medicine, Houston)
Crit Care Med 23:560–567, 1995   2–4

Introduction.—The use of intracranial pressure monitoring is controversial despite evidence of its efficacy in the management of increased intracranial pressure in patients with severe head injuries. A nationwide telephone survey of trauma centers in the United States was conducted to ascertain neurotrauma monitoring and treatment practices.

Methods.—Of 624 trauma centers, 227 were randomly selected for a telephone interview of neurotrauma nurses. Trauma centers from rural, suburban, and large metropolitan areas were included. A total of 261 centers (94%) participated. Of these, 219 (84%) reported that they treated patients with severe head injuries. To verify the accuracy of the survey, at 6 months 40 centers (15%) were resurveyed. The questions remained the same, but a different nurse was interviewed.

Results.—Level I, II, and III centers were represented by 49%, 32%, and 2% of the respondents, respectively. There was a designated neurologic or neurosurgical ICU in 34% of the hospitals. A neurosurgeon or neurologist headed 24% of these units. Of 219 centers, just 28% used intracranial pressure monitoring routinely in the treatment of patients with severe head injuries, and 16 centers never used intracranial pressure monitoring. There was a significant correlation between the number of patients with severe head injuries and the use of intracranial pressure monitoring. Hyperventilation and diuretics were used in 83% of the centers to reduce increased intracranial pressure. Cerebrospinal fluid drainage, barbiturates, and corticosteroids (administered more than half the time) were used in 44%, 33%, and 64% of the centers. Excessive hyperventilation ($PaCO_2 < 25$ mm Hg) was used in 29% of the centers.

Conclusion.—The care of patients with severe head injuries varies greatly. Practice guidelines are needed to improve the standard of care.

▶ The importance of this study is that it highlights the disparity between best-available care based on well-controlled clinical trials and what is actually done. Specific mistakes highlighted include the overuse of steroids and the failure of many physicians to recognize the adverse effects of hyperventilation or to appreciate the benefits of routine intracranial pressure monitoring or the use of phenobarbital coma in patients with unresponsive intracranial hypertension. The authors believe that this disparity in care is related to a lack of standardized national guidelines for the care of comatose head-injured patients. If your unit is one in which any of these mistakes occur, I strongly recommend this important article to you.

E.A. Deitch, M.D.

Physicians Do Not Have a Responsibility to Provide Futile or Unreasonable Care If a Patient or Family Insists
Luce JM (Univ of California, San Francisco)
Crit Care Med 23:760–766, 1995   2–5

Objective.—The position that physicians do not have to administer futile or unreasonable care even if a patient or patient's family insists is argued and supported by data from the literature.

Design.—Data from articles on medical ethics, concepts of futility and reasonableness in medicine, and legal and health care reform are analyzed to argue the point that physicians are not responsible for providing futile care.

Discussion.—Four moral principles of medical ethics are discussed in the context of the issue of administering futile treatment. These principles are autonomy, or respect for the patient's capacity for self-determination; nonmaleficence, or the duty to not inflict intentional harm; beneficence, or the need to provide treatment that benefits the patient; and distributive justice, or the fair and equitable distribution of appropriate medical resources to all of society. The trend in modern medicine for autonomy to rule and physicians' "single master view of medicine" result in patients or their families making medical decisions and insisting on certain types of therapy that may be futile or unreasonable. If the physician believes that a treatment is futile or unreasonable, the other 3 moral principles can be used to support the decision to deny such treatment. That is, the physician is justified in refusing to treat a patient if the treatment is not likely to benefit the patient (principle of beneficence), if the care is likely to cause more harm than good (principle of nonmaleficence), and/or if providing the treatment is neither beneficial nor harmful but would prevent a truly needy patient from receiving the treatment (principle of distributive justice).

Conclusion.—Principles of medical ethics support the view that physicians are not obligated to provide futile or unreasonable care to patients. However, no legal resolution of this issue has been accomplished to date.

Decision to Limit or Continue Life-Sustaining Treatment by Critical Care Physicians in the United States: Conflicts Between Physician's Practices and Patient's Wishes

Asch DA, Hansen-Flaschen J, Lanken PN (Univ of Pennsylvania, Philadelphia; Veterans Affairs Med Ctr, Philadelphia)
Am J Respir Crit Care Med 151:288–292, 1995   2–6

Objective.—The decision to limit or to withdraw life support by critical care physicians is, in general, accepted in the abstract. However, few studies have measured actual physician practice. This study focused on decisions by critical care physicians to withhold or withdraw life support on the basis of medical futility or to continue life support against the wishes of the patient or surrogate.

Methods.—A survey was mailed to all 1,970 members of the Critical Care Section of the American Thoracic Society to determine their attitudes and practices with regard to withholding or withdrawing life support on the basis of medical futility or continuing life support against the wishes of the patient or surrogate.

Results.—A total of 879 surveys were included in the analysis. Self-reporting results showed that 96% of the respondents had discontinued treatment with the expectation that the patient would die (Table 3). In the past year, 85% had discontinued mechanical ventilation at least once, 29% had withdrawn it 3 to 5 times, and 26% had done so more than 5 times. On the basis of medical futility, 83% had withheld life-sustaining treatment, and 73% had withdrawn it. Many had withdrawn or withheld treatment without the consent or without the knowledge of the patient or the family, and some did so over the objections of patients or family.

Conclusion.—Physicians do not automatically accept patients' or surrogates' decisions to continue or discontinue treatment, but weigh the requests along with other factors, including the possibly medical futility of continuing treatment.

▶ Being caught between the wishes of the patient, the family, the limits of medical care, the law, and society is no fun. However, it is too often a reality

TABLE 3.—Proportion of 879 Physicians Who Have Withdrawn Various Forms of Life-Sustaining Treatments

Form of Treatment	n (%)
Mechanical ventilation	786 (89%)
Intravenous vasopressors	758 (88%)
Renal dialysis	604 (71%)
Blood or blood products	687 (80%)
Artificial nutrition and/or hydration	486 (58%)
Never	31 (4%)

(Courtesy of Asch DA, Hansen-Flaschen J, Lanken PN: Decisions to limit or continue life-sustaining treatment by critical care physicians in the United States: Conflicts between physician's practices and patient's wishes. *Am J Respir Crit Care Med* 152:288–292, 1995.)

in the ICU. Unfortunately, as the social and financial pressures of health care reform and limited resources increase, the frequency of being "caught" will undoubtably increase. For that reason, the 2 abstracts above were chosen. The first by Dr. Luce discusses the ethical issues involved in futile care, while the second documents that the practice of withholding and withdrawing life-sustaining treatment is widespread nationally.

E.A. Deitch, M.D.

A Look Into the Nature and Causes of Human Errors in the Intensive Care Unit

Donchin Y, Gopher D, Olin M, Badihi Y, Bieski M, Sprung CL, Pizov R, Cotev S (Hebrew Univ, Jerusalem; Israel Institute of Technology, Jerusalem)
Crit Care Med 23:294–300, 1995   2–7

Background.—There are only a few studies on the nature of human errors in critical care. To address this deficit, a study was conducted to investigate the nature and causes of human errors in the ICU by using approaches proposed by human factors engineering. The latter focuses on studying the interface between humans and their working environment, with a particular emphasis on technology.

Setting.—A concurrent incident study was conducted in a medical-surgical ICU of a university hospital during a 4-month period. Errors reported by physicians and nurses immediately after they were discovered were recorded. In addition, activity profiles were determined from 24-hour continuous bedside observations of investigators with human engineering experience on a random sample of patients. Human error was defined as a deviation from standard conduct, including the addition or omission of actions relating to standard operational instructions or routines; medical decisions were excluded. Errors were rated for severity and classified according to the body system and type of medical activity involved.

Findings.—A total of 554 human errors were recorded, including 476 errors by physicians and nurses and 78 detected by observers during an average of 178 activities per patient per day. The estimated number of errors per patient per day was 1.7. Almost one third (29%) of the errors were graded as severe or potentially detrimental, and such errors occurred, on average, twice a day. Errors were more likely to occur with input and CNS activities.

Peak activity occurred during the late morning and early afternoon hours for both physicians and nurses. The number of activities performed by physicians decreased sharply outside this period, whereas nurses' activity remained high at all hours. Although nurses committed more errors (55%) than physicians (45%), physicians carried out only 4.7% of the daily activities vs. 84% performed by nurses. Most errors were committed in the morning, with physicians showing a distinct peak around the time of the physician's morning rounds. Errors committed by nurses peaked similarly, but with a 1-hour delay, and peaked as well during each shift change. Verbal exchanges between physicians and nurses were surprisingly high (37%) in error reports, but verbal communications constituted only 2% of the overall activity profile.

Conclusions.—A significant number of human errors occur in the ICU, and many of these errors could be attributed to problems of communication between the physicians and nurses. The tools and concepts provided by cognitive psychology and human factors engineering may be useful in the analysis of human errors in a specific ICU. The nature and causes of the errors identified in this ICU are not unique and may have general relevance for other ICUs.

▶ So someone screwed up. Take heart, evidently it's not all that uncommon, or is it? This prospective study on human error in the ICU was designed to answer that question. Based on their results, the authors' conclusion that human error is common in the ICU appears valid. One observation from this study that holds the most importance for all of us is that 37% of the errors occurred during just 2% of the overall activity profile, that involving verbal communication. Thus misunderstanding or misinterpretation of verbally transmitted information or requests appeared to be the most common cause of human error in this study. The message is clear. We should all work extra hard to be sure that we are correctly understood when giving verbal orders and instructions. This study reminded me of a sign I saw when I was a medical student doing my psychiatry rotation. It said: I know you think you know what I said, but what you don't know is that what I said is not what I meant. This appears to be true in the ICU as well as in psychiatry.

E.A. Deitch, M.D.

Right Ventricular End-Diastolic Volume as a Measure of Preload
Durham R, Neunaber K, Vogler G, Shapiro M, Mazuski J (St Louis Univ, Mo)
J Trauma 39:218–224, 1995   2–8

Objective.—Preload, defined as ventricular fiber length at end-diastole, is clinically described as end-diastolic volume. Because of changes in ventricular compliance, it is difficult to evaluate ventricular preload on the basis of measurements of end-diastolic pressure. Pulmonary capillary wedge pressure (PCWP) is commonly used as an indicator of preload because it is easy to measure at the bedside. Recent modifications of pulmonary artery thermodilution catheters permit measurement of right ventricular (RV) diastolic volume. Right ventricular end-diastolic volume index (RVEDVI), PCWP, and central venous pressure (CVP) were compared with cardiac index (CI) to determine which was the best indicator of ventricular preload.

Methods.—The study sample comprised 38 critically ill patients with modified thermodilution catheters in place. For 1 to 7 days, the patients' hemodynamic parameters were recorded at 2- to 4-hour intervals. This yielded a total of 1,008 complete data sets. For the entire group and in individual patients, PCWP, RVEDVI, and RV ejection fraction (RVEF) were compared with CI by regression analysis. Correlation between RVEDVI and CI was corrected for possible mathematic coupling.

Results.—Before correction for mathematical coupling, CI was significantly correlated with RVEDVI, $r = 0.60$; with RVEF, $r = 0.37$; and with PCWP, $r = 0.10$. Correction for mathematical coupling reduced the correlation between RVEDVI and CI only slightly to 0.56. Considered individually, 71% of the patients showed a significant uncorrected correlation between RVEDVI and CI. For the rest, there was a significant correlation between PCWP and CI. Even after correction for mathematical coupling, CI was more closely correlated with RVEDVI than with PCWP.

Conclusions.—When compared with other measures, RVEDVI as measured by a modified thermodilution catheter is a better indicator of cardiac preload. This is so when patients are considered both as a group and individually. With RVEDVI as with PCWP, there is no particular end point or range than can reliably be used to predict cardiac function in an individual patient.

▶ So you and the PCWP measurement disagree about whether the patient would benefit from more fluid. This is not surprising because ventricular pressure is not as accurate a criterion for determining preload as ventricular volume. This is especially true in our sickest patients, who may have impaired myocardial compliance or pulmonary hypertension and be receiving positive-pressure ventilation. In this situation, use of the modified Swan-Ganz catheter that measures RVEDVI (cost, $225 vs. $125 for a standard Swan-Ganz catheter) appears to provide more accurate information.

Whether one uses PCWP or RVEDVI, the take-home message is that for an individual patient there is no absolute number that indicates that cardiac output cannot be improved by more volume, although the likelihood of this occurring is low if the RVEDVI is greater than 120 mL/m². Therefore, patients with inadequate cardiac output should still be treated empirically by expanding intravascular volume while monitoring cardiac output.

E.A. Deitch, M.D.

Renal Support in Critically Ill Patients: Low-Dose Dopamine or Low-Dose Dobutamine?
Duke GJ, Briedis JH, Weaver RA (Preston & Northcote Community Hosp, Preston, Victoria, Australia)
Crit Care Med 22:1919–1925, 1994   2–9

Introduction.—Low-dose dopamine, because of its specific dopamine-receptor agonist properties, which can increase renal blood flow and diuresis, has been used to prevent renal dysfunction in critically ill patients. However, its benefit has not been clinically proved. A prospective, double-

TABLE 7.—Renal Indices (Means ± SD)

	Placebo	Dobutamine	Dopamine	p Value
Creatinine clearance (mL/min)	79 ± 38	97 ± 54	88 ± 42	<.01*, .25†
Urine volume (mL/hr)	90 ± 44	97 ± 85	145 ± 148	.05†, <.01*
Fractional excretion of sodium (%)	0.95 ± 0.72	0.73 ± 0.48	1.15 ± 0.95	.04‡

* Dobutamine vs. placebo.
† Dopamine vs. placebo.
‡ Dopamine vs. dobutamine.
(Courtesy of Duke GJ, Briedis JH, Weaver PA: Renal support in critically ill patients: Low-dose dopamine or low-dose dobutamine? *Crit Care Med* 22(12):1919–1925, 1994.)

blind, randomized trial of low-dose dopamine and low-dose dobutamine examined the renal effects of these agents in critically ill patients.

Methods.—Eighteen stable patients with a critical illness associated with a significant risk of renal dysfunction were each given 3 sequential, randomized 5-hour infusions of low-dose dopamine, low-dose dobutamine, and placebo. Hemodynamic, arterial blood gas, glucose, lactate, serum creatinine, and electrolyte measurements were taken at baseline and just before completion of each infusion. Urine samples were collected during the last 4 hours of each infusion for analysis of urine volume, sodium potassium, creatinine, creatinine clearance, and fractional excretion of sodium.

Results.—Over the course of the 3 infusions there were no changes in the serum biochemical profile. There were no changes in central venous pressure, pulmonary artery occlusion pressure, or fluid balance. Dopamine infusion was associated with a significant increase in urine output but no change in the fractional excretion of sodium or creatinine clearance (Table 7). Creatinine clearance was significantly increased during dobutamine administration, although urine output was only slightly increased. Dopamine side effects included sinus tachycardia in 6 patients, hypertension in 4, and decreased peripheral oxygenation in 10. Dobutamine side effects included sinus tachycardia in 4 patients and hypertension in 3.

Discussion.—In this group of critically ill patients, low-dose dopamine had a primary diuretic effect without improving creatinine clearance, whereas low-dose dobutamine improved creatinine clearance without changing urine output. These findings suggest that there is no benefit associated with the routine use of dopamine in critically ill patients.

▶ Another widely accepted traditional therapy appears to be flawed. Based on this prospective, controlled, double-blinded clinical trial, the routine use of prophylactic low-dose dopamine does not appear to be indicated. In contrast, the authors surprisingly found that low-dose dobutamine (2.5 µg/ kg/min), perhaps because of it inotropic effects, did improve renal function, although it did not increase urine output. Whether low-dose dobutamine will be effective in preserving renal function in high-risk patients was not addressed in this study, and thus its potential clinical benefits in this patient population must remain speculative.

A note of caution is warranted. No conclusions should be made concerning patients with incipient renal failure since the current study only examined patients with normal renal function. Furthermore, since the combination of low-dose dopamine and furosemide may have a role in converting oliguric to nonoliguric renal failure, in patients who remain oliguric despite adequate volume restitution and have a good cardiac index, the administration of low-dose dopamine (or dobutamine perhaps) in combination with furosemide may be beneficial.

E.A. Deitch, M.D.

Frequency of Mortality and Myocardial Infarction During Maximizing Oxygen Delivery: A Prospective, Randomized Trial
Yu M, Takanishi D, Myers SA, Takiguchi SA, Severino R, Hasaniya N, Levy MM, McNamara JJ (Univ of Hawaii, Honolulu)
Crit Care Med 23:1025–1032, 1995   2–10

Introduction.—Maximizing oxygen delivery (DO_2) in critically ill patients remains controversial. Whether there is a subset of patients who may benefit from this treatment is clinically relevant. A study was conducted to determine the frequency of myocardial infarction and mortality during treatment that increased DO_2 to 600 or greater and to define the characteristics of patients achieving a high DO_2 without inotropes in order to design future studies.

Study Design.—Eighty-nine patients from 2 surgical ICUs who required pulmonary artery catheter monitoring were studied. Patients with sepsis, septic shock, hypovolemic shock, or adult respiratory distress syndrome were included, but not those facing imminent death. In a random fashion, patients were assigned to a treatment group that received fluid boluses, blood products, and inotropes, as indicated, to achieve a DO_2 of 600 mL/min/m^2 or greater in the first 24 hours or a control group that received the same interventions to achieve a DO_2 of 450–550 mL/min/m^2.

Results.—Thirteen patients in the treatment group and 19 control patients achieved a DO_2 of 600 mL/min/m^2 or greater with only preload optimization with fluids and blood. These patients were classified as self-generating high DO_2 and reflected patients with better cardiac reserve and low mortality rates. These patients were excluded in the final analysis. The mortality rate was 14% among the 14 patients who achieved a DO_2 of 600 mL/min/m^2 or greater with vasopressor support as compared with 67% in 15 patients who failed to reach a high DO_2 with vasopressor support but achieved a normal DO_2 and 62% in 21 control patients who achieved a normal DO_2. Age, severity of illness, and disease process were similar in the patients who achieved the high DO_2 with inotropes and those who did not respond to inotropes. Likewise, age and severity of illness were similar in patients who received inotropes but failed to achieve the high DO_2 and in control patients, which suggests that treatment with inotropes did not lead to higher mortality rates. The frequency of new myocardial infarction was 5.6%, and this could not be attributed to catecholamine use. Logistic regression analysis indicated that by choosing patients who were older than 50 years, there was an 83% probability of not finding self-generating DO_2 values of 600 mL/min/m^2 or greater.

Summary.—A subset of patients treated with inotropes to achieve a high DO_2 has a low mortality rate with no increase in the frequency of myocardial infarction. Age older than 50 years will identify patients who will not self-generate high DO_2. Future prospective, controlled trials examining this select group may demonstrate a difference between control and treatment groups by eliminating the majority of patients who generate the high DO_2 with only preload optimization.

▶ One strength of this prospective study was the exclusion of patients in whom a DO_2 greater than 600 mL/min/m^2 developed since these self-selected patients have a good prognosis. If one believes in the concept of maximizing oxygen delivery, then one can take heart from the fact that the mortality rate of the 14 patients receiving inotropic drugs intended to raise their DO_2 to greater than 600 mL/min/m^2 was just 14% vs. 67% in the therapeutic group patients who failed to reach this oxygen delivery end point and 62% in the control patients, who received inotropic support just sufficient to maintain a normal level of oxygen delivery (DO_2 of 450–550 mL/min/m^2). Furthermore, this study indicates that there is an identifiable subset of critically ill patients (those over 50 years old) who will potentially benefit from an aggressive approach to increase oxygen delivery. On the other hand, if one does not believe in maximizing oxygen delivery, then one can quote the fact that prospective randomized trials have not documented a survival benefit from this approach.[1, 2]

Thus depending on one's bias one can argue either way. So I guess a reasonable question would be, what is my bias? My bias is to use modest but not heroic doses of inotropes to increase oxygen delivery to supranormal levels, knowing that not all patients will respond. Once I have reached a DO_2 value greater than 600–650 mL/min/m^2, I stop. The rationale behind this bias is that inotropic use is not dangerous and I believe that at least some patients will be helped by maximizing oxygen delivery. This is especially true in patients who are getting worse or not getting better.

E.A. Deitch, M.D.

References

1. Barone J: Maximization of oxygen delivery: A plea for moderation, part II *J Trauma* 37:337–338, 1994.
2. Gattinoni L, Brazzi L, Pelosi P, et al: A trial of goal oriented hemodynamic therapy in critically ill patients. *N Engl J Med* 333:1025–1032, 1995.

Hospital Survival Rates of Patients With Acute Respiratory Failure in Modern Respiratory Intensive Care Units: An International, Multicenter, Prospective Survey

Vasilyev S, Schaap RN, Mortensen JD (CardioPulmonics Inc, Salt Lake City, Utah)
Chest 107:1083–1088, 1995   2–11

Objective.—Hospital survival rates for patients with acute respiratory failure (ARF) are as low as 9%. Although the literature shows that the survival rates of ARF patients treated with intensive postive-pressure mechanical ventilation have not improved over the last 2 decades, most critical care specialists consider these reports to be outdated. Because clinical classification of ARF patients for comparative purposes has proved to be difficult, this multicenter prospective survey was conducted to evaluate hospital survival rates of ARF patients according to current treatment protocols.

Methods.—All ARF patients admitted to 11 U.S. and 14 European clinical centers within a 60-day period in 1991 and 1992 who received closed-system mechanical ventilation at an FiO_2 of 0.50 or greater for at least 24 hours were included in the study. Group A patients were hypoxemic or hypercarbic. Group B patients were neither.

Results.—There were 375 patients in group A and 1,051 patients in group B. Most group A patients had advanced lung dysfunction, and 82% had end-stage lung dysfunction. Group A patients had an overall survival rate of 33.3%. Group A ARF patients with postshock lung injury had the

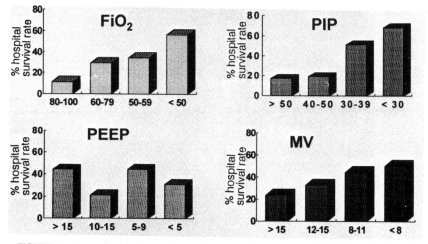

FIGURE 1.—Hospital survival rates of group A patients related to mechanical ventilation parameters at the time of entry into the survey. *Abbreviations: FiO_2,* fraction of oxygen in inspired air; *PIP,* peak inspiratory pressure; *PEEP,* positive end-expiratory pressure; *MV,* minute volume of gas delivered by the mechanical ventilator. (Courtesy of Vasilyev S, Schaap RN, Mortensen JD: Hospital survival rates of patients with acute respiratory failure in modern respiratory intensive care units: An international, multicenter, prospective survey. *Chest* 107:1083–1088, 1995.)

highest survival rates (46.4%), followed by ARF patients with sepsis (30.1%) and ARF patients with pneumonia or pneumonitis (28.5%). Group B patients had a survival rate of 63.6%. Group B ARF patients with pneumonia had a survival rate of 63%, followed by ARF patients with postshock lung injury (67%) and ARF patients with sepsis (46%). Prognostic factors included the severity of lung injury, with survival rates of 18.4% for patients with far-advanced disease to 66.7% for patients with less severe injuries; the intensity of mechanical ventilator support, with patients requiring an FIO_2 greater than 0.70, peak inspiratory pressure greater than 40 cm H_2O, and minute volume over 15 L/min; the extent of hypoxemia; duration of tracheal intubation; duration of mechanical ventilator support; and multiorgan dysfunction (Fig 1). The survival rate of patients with 2-system dysfunction was 16%, and that in patients with 3-system dysfunction was 10%.

Conclusion.—Hospital survival rates for patients with severe ARF appear to be unchanged over the past 2 decades. Major predictors of survival include severity of lung dysfunction, etiology of the ARF, intensity and duration of mechanical ventilation, severity of hypoxemia, and presence of multisystem organ failure. Additional methods of blood gas transfer need to be considered.

▶ Where do we stand in our ability to successfully treat patients with severe actue respiratory failure is a hard question to answer. Consequently, this benchmark prospective multicenter study was chosen since it provides up-to-date prognostic information on 1,426 patients treated over a short time period at 25 well-respected critical care centers. Unfortunately, this survey indicates that the survival of patients treated between 1991 and 1992 has not significantly improved in comparison to what it was 10 or 20 years earlier. Although I believe this study is unduly pessimistic, it does highlight the need for new approaches to the care of these severely ill patients.

E.A. Deitch, M.D.

Liquid Ventilation Improves Pulmonary Function, Gas Exchange, and Lung Injury in a Model of Respiratory Failure
Hirschl RB, Parent A, Tooley R, McCracken M, Johnson K, Shaffer TH, Wolfson MR, Bartlett RH (Univ of Michigan, Ann Arbor; Temple Univ, Philadelphia)
Ann Surg 221:79–88, 1995   2–12

Background.—Various interventions have been tried in attempts to resolve lung injury and improve pulmonary function and gas exchange in patients with severe acute respiratory failure (ARF). However, such "lung management" methods have had little effect on the 50% mortality rate in children and adults with ARF. Research has shown that perfluorcarbon liquid ventilation (LV) provides adequate gas exchange in full-term and premature newborn lambs and other animals, with and without lung injury. Gas exchange, pulmonary function, and lung histology were compared during perfluorocarbon LV and during gas ventilation (GV) in a model of severe respiratory failure.

Methods.—A stable model of lung injury was induced in 12 young sheep weighing a mean of 16.4 kg. Right atrial injection of 0.07 mL/kg of oleic acid was followed by saline pulmonary lavage and bijugular venovenous extracorporeal life support (ECLS). All sheep were ventilated with gas for the first 30 minutes of ECLS and then ventilated with 15 mL/kg gas or perflubron over the next 2.5 hours. Subsequently, ECLS was discontinued in 5 GV animals and 5 LV animals. Gas ventilation or LV was then continued for 1 hour or until death.

Findings.—After 3 hours of ECLS, physiologic shunt was decreased significantly in the LV sheep as compared with the GV sheep (Fig 2). Also at that point, pulmonary compliance was increased significantly in the LV group as compared with the GV group. The ECLS flow rate needed to maintain PaO_2 in the 50– to 80–mm Hg range was significantly lower in the LV group than in the GV group. All GV sheep died after ECLS was discontinued. By contrast, all LV sheep showed effective gas exchange without extracorporeal support for 1 hour. Lung biopsy light microscopy showed a marked decrease in alveolar hemorrhage, lung fluid accumulation, and inflammatory infiltration in the LV as compared with the GV group.

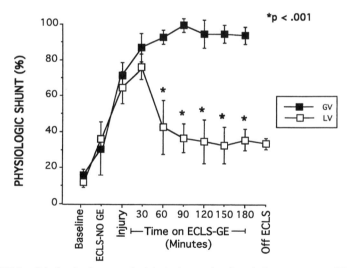

FIGURE 2.—Calculated pulmonary physiologic shunt at baseline, during extracorporeal life support but without membrane lung gas exchange *(ECLS-NO GE)*, after lung injury, for 3 hours during extracorporeal life support with membrane lung gas exchange *(ECLS-GE)*, and after discontinuation of extracorporeal life support *(ECLS)*. Animals underwent gas ventilation *(GV)* or liquid ventilation *(LV)* during ECLS and after discontinuation of ECLS, although all animals underwent GV for the first 30 minutes of ECLS-GE. *$P < 0.021$. (Courtesy of Hirschl RB, Parent A, Tooley R, et al: Liquid ventilation improves pulmonary function, gas exchange, and lung injury in a model of respiratory failure. *Ann Surg* 221:79–88, 1995.)

Conclusions.—In this model of severe respiratory failure, LV improved pulmonary gas exchange and compliance. It also decreased alveolar hemorrhage, edema, and inflammatory infiltrates.

▶ This experimental study was chosen because it adds to the accumulating experimental evidence that liquid ventilation may be of significant clinical value. Although it appears counterintuitive that drowning the lungs with perfluorocarbon solution can improve the function of injured lungs, this appears to be true. This study indicates that liquid-ventilated lungs had better compliance and a lower shunt fraction than gas-ventilated lungs. The beneficial effects of liquid ventilation on pulmonary function appear to be largely related to (1) the removal of pulmonary exudate through the lavage effect of the liquid and (2) the fact that liquid ventilation is associated with a lower alveolar surface tension and is better than gas ventilation at recruiting atelectatic or consolidated alveoli. We should shortly know whether the optimistic results of experimental studies with liquid ventilation are also observed clinically since clinical trials evaluating liquid ventilation in patients with acute respiratory failure are ongoing.

E.A. Deitch, M.D.

A Liquid Perfluorochemical Decreases the In Vitro Production of Reactive Oxygen Species by Alveolar Macrophages

Smith TM, Steinhorn DM, Thusu K, Fuhrman BP, Dandona P (State Univ of New York, Buffalo; Millard Filmore Hosp, Buffalo, NY)
Crit Care Med 23:1533–1539, 1995   2–13

Purpose.—Perfluorocarbon-associated gas exchange is being studied as an adjunctive form of therapy in animal models of acute hypoxic respiratory failure. The results thus far suggest that the reduced inflammation observed in the lungs of animals treated with partial liquid ventilation using liquid perfluorochemicals may be linked to reduced production of reactive oxygen metabolites by alveolar macrophages. A controlled experiment was performed to test this hypothesis.

Methods.—Alveolar macrophages were obtained from rabbits and piglets and divided into those exposed to perfluorooctylbromide and control groups. Production of reactive oxygen metabolites was determined by measurement of hydrogen peroxide production and by chemiluminescence after chemical stimulation.

Results.—The mean hydrogen peroxide production by alveolar macrophages exposed to perfluorooctylbromide was 1.4 nmol/10^6 cells as compared with 1.6 nmol/10^6 cells for control macrophages. Chemiluminescence activity was significantly less for the exposed than the control cells, 0.70 vs. 1.5 mV of relative activity per 3.5×10^5 cells (Fig 2).

Conclusions.—After in vitro exposure to perfluorooctylbromide, alveolar macrophages show decreased responsiveness to potent stimuli. The results may help account for the decreased lung inflammation observed

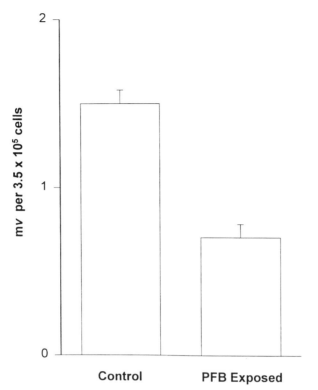

FIGURE 2.—Chemiluminescence activity as measured in millivolts (*mv*) obtained from non–perfluorooctylbromide-exposed (*Control*) and perfluorooctylbromide-exposed (*PFB Exposed*) piglet alveolar macrophages after stimulation with phorbol myristate. Perfluorooctylbromide-exposed alveolar macrophages produced significantly less peak chemiluminescence activity than did control macrophages. *Error bars* represent SE (n = 6; $P = 0.005$). (Courtesy of Smith TM, Steinhorn DM, Thusu K, et al: A liquid perfluorochemical decreases the in vitro production of reactive oxygen species by alveolar macrophages. *Crit Care Med* 23(9):1533–1539, 1995.)

after partial liquid ventilation in models of induced lung injury. The findings should be confirmed in vivo to see whether perfluorooctylbromide may have a role as a nonspecific anti-inflammatory agent.

▶ An unexplained, but consistently observed phenomenon in experimental studies evaluating liquid ventilation in lung injury models is that the liquid-ventilated animals have less histologic evidence of inflammation than the control gas-ventilated animals. The results of this study support the hypothesis that this decrease in inflammation observed with liquid ventilation is due to the ability of perfluorochemicals to reduce the production of potentially destructive reactive oxygen metabolites. These results thus suggest that perfluorochemicals may also exert a beneficial effect through their actions as anti-inflammatory agents. However, since bacterial killing is mediated by the same oxidants that injure the lung, whether this effect of perfluorochemicals will be clinically beneficial in the presence of pneumonia remains unknown.

E.A. Deitch, M.D.

Effect of Erythromycin on Gastric Motility in Mechanically Ventilated Critically Ill Patients: A Double-Blind, Randomized, Placebo-Controlled Study

Dive A, Miesse C, Galanti L, Jamart J, Evrard P, Gonzalez M, Installé E
(Mont-Godinne Hosp, Yvoir, Belgium)
Crit Care Med 23:1356–1362, 1995   2–14

Background.—Erythromycin has recently been found to be a powerful prokinetic agent that has documented efficacy against refractory gastroparesis resulting from diabetes mellitus, vagotomy, and the intestinal pseudo-obstruction syndrome. No studies have yet investigated the effects of this agent on the gastric motor function of critically ill patients. A study was therefore performed to determine the action of erythromycin on gastric emptying and motility among mechanically ventilated patients.

Patients and Methods.—Ten general ICU patients 40 to 77 years old were included in this crossover, double-blind, randomized, placebo-controlled study. All patients were mechanically ventilated and in a stable hemodynamic condition. Erythromycin, 200 mg IV over a 30-minute period, and placebo were administered in a random fashion at midmorning on 2 consecutive days. A multilumen manometric tube was used to record pressure changes in the gastric antrum. Gastric emptying was

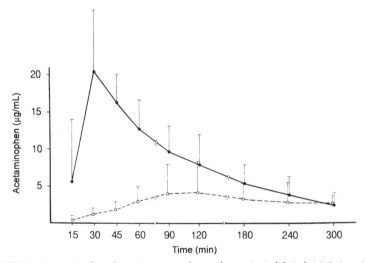

FIGURE 1.—Acetaminophen absorption curve after erythromycin (*solid circles*) infusion. Acetaminophen (1 g) was administered via the nasogastric tube when starting the erythromycin or placebo infusion. (Courtesy of Dive A, Miesse C, Galanti L, et al: Effect of erythromycin on gastric motility in mechanically ventilated critically ill patients: A double-blind, randomized, placebo-controlled study. *Crit Care Med* 23(8):1356–1362, 1995.)

concurrently evaluated by the kinetics of the absorption of acetaminophen delivered into the stomach just before the infusion.

Results.—During the first hour after erythromycin infusion, significant increases in the mean number of contractions, mean amplitude of contractions, and the motility index were noted at 104, 52 mm Hg, and 13.06 vs. 5, 20 mm Hg, and 4.45 for placebo, respectively. A shorter time to peak acetaminophen concentration, a higher maximal acetaminophen concentraction, and a marked increase in the area under the concentration-time curve at 60 minutes were also noted after erythromycin infusion (Fig 1).

Conclusions.—Intravenous erythromycin delivered at 200 mg over a 30-minute period leads to increased antral motility and accelerated gastric emptying among critically ill mechanically ventilated patients.

▶ Gastroparesis, or decreased gastric motility, is a common problem in ICU patients and complicates successful enteral feeding. Since successful enteral feeding has been shown to be associated with a number of beneficial effects in several ICU populations, it makes sense that any agent that will improve gastric motility will have a positive clinical effect. Thus the importance of this article. It clearly documents that IV erythromycin improves gastric motility and emptying in mechanically ventilated patients.

E.A. Deitch, M.D.

Are Corticosteroids Salvage Therapy for Refractory Acute Respiratory Distress Syndrome?
Biffl WL, Moore FA, Moore EE, Haenel JB, McIntyre RC Jr, Burch JM (Univ of Colorado, Denver)
Am J Surg 170:591–596, 1995   2–15

Introduction.—Interstitial fibroproliferation is the histologic hallmark of late acute respiratory distress syndrome (ARDS) and is associated with a mortality rate in excess of 80%. The primary cause of death in 15% to 40% of late ARDS nonsurvivors is dysregulated fibroproliferation. It is also a contributing factor to lethal sepsis-related multiple organ failure (MOF) in the remaining nonsurvivors. Reported is the experience of using steroids as salvage therapy for 6 patients with advanced refractory ARDS.

Methods.—None of the patients improved during ventilatory support measures. They were given IV methylprednisolone sodium succinate, 1 to 2 mg/kg every 6 hours. Bacterial cultures and bronchoalveolar lavage specimens were routinely obtained every 3–5 days.

Results.—The mean age of 4 women and 2 men was 38.5 years. At a mean of 3.0 days after a variety of insults, ARDS developed in all 6 patients. Steroid therapy was started at an average of 15.8 days of ventilatory support. All 6 patients demonstrated improvement in PaO_2FIO_2 over the first 7 days of steroid therapy. Five of 6 patients had improvement in lung injury scores. One patient undergoing lung cancer resection did not respond and died. The 5 responders showed improvements in pertinent

TABLE I.—Ventilatory Indices During Steroid Therapy for Late Acute Respiratory Distress Syndrome

Parameter	Day 0	Day 3	Day 7	P Value Versus Day 0 Day 3	Day 7
PaO_2/FiO_2	85 ± 14	127 ± 25	172 ± 23*	0.16	0.01
LIS	3.6 ± 0.1	3.3 ± 0.2	2.9 ± 0.2	0.28	0.01
V_T (mL/kg)	7.7 ± 0.6	8.0 ± .06	8.5 ± 0.4*	0.74	0.29
PEEP (cm H_2O)	14.5 ± 2.6	11.3 ± 2.0	9.3 ± 1.1	0.36	0.10
V_e (L/min)	14.4 ± 2.4	13.9 ± 2.1	12.6 ± 2.0	0.86	0.58
PAP (cm H_2O)	64.8 ± 5.6	52.0 ± 5.2	50.8 ± 6.6	0.12	0.14
C_{stat} (mL/cm H_2O)	11.9 ± 1.6	16.9 ± 2.8	18.8 ± 4.1	0.15	0.13

* Difference from index on day 0, *P* < 0.05.

Abbreviations: PaO₂/FiO₂, ratio of arterial oxygen tension to fractional inspired oxygen concentrations; *LIS*, lung injury score; *VT*, tidal volume; *PEEP*, positive end-expiratory pressure; *VE*, minute ventilation; *PAP*, peak airway pressure; *Cstat*, static lung compliance.

(Reprinted by permission of the publisher from Biffl WL, Moore FA, Moore EE, et al: Are Corticosteroids salvage therapy for refractory acute respiratory distress syndrome? *Am J Surg* 170:591–596, Copyright 1995 by Excerpta Medica Inc.)

ventilatory indices within 3 days (Table 1). The mean duration of steroid therapy was 21.3 days. The mean total number of ventilator days was 43.8 days.

Conclusion.—Steroid therapy was effective in 5 of 6 patients treated for refractory late ARDS. The optimal dose of steroids for treating late ARDS has yet to be established.

► Because the study was retrospective, covered a 5-year period, and only involved 6 patients, why was it chosen? The answer is that 5, or 83%, of their 6 steroid-treated patients survived, although the expected mortality rate of these patients exceeded 80%. This is an impressive result.

In putting this study into perspective, it is important to remember that large prospective trials have shown that steroids do *not* improve survival when given during the *early* phases of ARDS. However, this study and a few other clinical reports provide optimistic survival data on the use of steroids in patients with clinically unresponsive late ARDS (overall survival rate of 79%; 49 of 62 treated patients). The physiologic explanation for the differing effects of steroids in patients with early vs. late ARDS is that late ARDS is associated with progressive interstitial fibrosis whereas early ARDS is a neutrophil-mediated disease and steroid therapy appears to be more effective in preventing continued pulmonary fibroplasia than in limiting neutrophil-mediated lung injury.

One important caveat to keep in mind. The patients enrolled in these studies had isolated ARDS, were not in multiple organ failure, and had no evidence of active infection.

E.A. Deitch, M.D.

The Natural History of the Systemic Inflammatory Response Syndrome (SIRS)
Rangel-Frausto MS, Pittet D, Costigan M, Hwang T, Davis CS, Wenzel RP
(Univ Hosp, Geneva; Univ of Iowa Hosp and Clinics, Iowa City)
JAMA 273:117–123, 1995   2–16

Background.—Recent clarifications of sepsis and septic shock have allowed for more specific definitions of aspects of "sepsis syndrome." Currently, sepsis syndrome is subdivided into systemic inflammatory response syndrome (SIRS), sepsis, severe sepsis, and septic shock. The rates and distribution of these stages of sepsis in hospitalized patients have not been studied. The epidemiology and natural history of SIRS, sepsis, severe sepsis, and septic shock were examined in this prospective study of 2,527 hospitalized patients.

Methods.—Surveys for patients with 2 or more symptoms of SIRS were performed 5 days per week for 1 year in 3 critical care units and 3 wards in a single hospital. All patients were followed for 28 days or until discharge, the patients were rechecked 3 and 6 months later, and development of criteria of the more advanced stages of sepsis or other complication was noted.

Results.—Sepsis developed in 26% of the participating patients during the 28-day follow-up, severe sepsis in 18%, and septic shock in 4%. An additional 35% were believed to have been septic and were given antibiotics; however, no organism could be cultured. Patients in any inflammatory class and with cardiovascular disease or trauma were approximately 1.5 times more likely to have negative than positive bacterial cultures, whereas patients with sepsis and gastrointestinal or respiratory disease were 1.4–2.3 times more likely to have positive than negative cultures. The number of symptoms of SIRS was positively associated with the likelihood of progressing to more severe inflammatory stages and negatively associated with the time required to make the transition. End-organ dysfunction became more likely with meeting of increasing numbers of criteria of SIRS and with culture-positive vs. culture-negative sepsis. Similarly, the mortality rate increased with increasing numbers of SIRS criteria and with progression from SIRS (7%) or sepsis (16%) to severe sepsis (20%) and septic shock (46%).

Conclusions.—These data validate the hypothesis that the natural history of the inflammatory response to infection can be described as a continual progression from SIRS to septic shock. Although half of the patients with sepsis did not have a documented infection, it is premature to conclude different pathogeneses for culture-negative and culture-positive syndromes. It is possible, however, that cardiovascular disease and trauma may be participatory in culture-negative patients.

▶ The value of this prospective epidemiologic study is that it provides prevalence data and defines the natural history and progression of patients with SIRS, sepsis, severe sepsis, and septic shock as defined by several recent consensus conferences. Although the authors are quite optimistic about this grading system, I am not so sanguine. I believe that their data highlight the weakness of the SIRS system. That weakness is that the SIRS definition is too broad and includes too many patients. This concern is well supported by the finding that a large number of patients admitted to the *wards* of their hospital as well as the vast majority of their ICU patients met the criteria for SIRS. So what. The what is that this terminology was adopted with the hope that it would allow adequate stratification of patients for enrollment in clinical trials evaluating anti-inflammatory agents. I am concerned that just meeting the criteria for SIRS is not enough and that trials enrolling patients based on their having SIRS will lose the power to detect true effects due to the lack of sensitivity of the SIRS definition. I hope I am being too pessimistic. Time will tell.

E.A. Deitch, M.D.

Multiple Organ Dysfunction Score: A Reliable Descriptor of a Complex Clinical Outcome
Marshall JC, Cook DJ, Christou NV, Bernard GR, Sprung CL, Sibbald WJ (Univ of Toronto; McMaster Univ, Hamilton, Ont, Canada; McGill Univ, Montreal; et al)
Crit Care Med 23:1638–1652, 1995   2–17

Purpose.—In the ICU, multiple organ dysfunction syndrome represents the primary cause of patient morbidity and mortality. In this study, an objective scale for determining the severity of the multiple organ dysfunction syndrome as an outcome in critical illness was developed and evaluated.

Methods.—All patients admitted to a surgical ICU for more than 24 hours between May 1988 and March 1990 were included. Clinical studies of multiple organ failure published between 1969 and 1993 were identified by MEDLINE review. Variables from these studies were assessed for construct and content validity to determine optimal organ dysfunction descriptors. Clinical and laboratory data were obtained each day to assess the effectiveness of these variables both individually and in combination as an organ dysfunction score. Descriptors of organ dysfunction were then assessed for criterion validity (ICU mortality rate) by using the clinical database. Intervals for the most abnormal value of each variable were developed from the first half of the database (the development set). A scale of 0 to 4 was used, with 0 representing primarily normal function and an ICU mortality rate of less than 5% and 4 exemplifying distinct functional impairment and an ICU mortality rate of 50% or more. Testing of these intervals was next performed by using the second half of the data set (the validation set).

Results.—Maximal scores for each variable were totaled to determine a multiple organ dysfunction score, the maximum of which was 24 (Table 3). The score correlated in a graded fashion with the ICU mortality rate.

TABLE 3.—Multiple Organ Dysfunction Score

Organ System	Score				
	0	1	2	3	4
Respiratory* Po_2/Fio_2 ratio)	>300	226–300	151–225	76–150	≤75
Renal† (serum creatinine)	≤100	101–200	201–350	351–500	>500
Hepatic‡ (serum bilirubin)	≤20	21–60	61–120	121–240	>240
Cardio-vascular§ (PAR)	≤10.0	10.1–15.0	15.1–20.0	20.1–30.0	>30.0
Hematologic‖ (platelet count)	>120	81–120	51–80	21–50	≤20
Neurologic¶ (Glasgow Coma Score)	15	13–14	10–12	7–9	≤6

* The Po_2/Fio_2 ratio is calculated without reference to the use or mode of mechanical ventilation and without reference to use of the level of positive end-expiratory pressure.

† The serum creatinine concentration is measured in micromoles per liter without reference to the use of dialysis.

‡ The serum bilirubin concentration is measured in micromoles per liter.

§ The pressure-adjusted heart rate (PAR) is calculated as the product of the heart rate (HR) multiplied by the ratio of the right atrial (central venous) pressure (RAP) to the mean arterial pressure (MAP): PAR = HR × RAP/mean blood pressure

‖ The platelet count is measured in platelets per cubic milliliter.

¶ The Glasgow Coma Score is preferably calculated by the patient's nurse and is scored conservatively (for patients receiving sedation or muscle relaxants, normal function is assumed unless there is evidence of intrinsically altered mentation).

(Courtesy of Marshall JC, Cook DJ, Christou NV, et al: Multiple organ dysfunction score: A reliable descriptor of a complex clinical outcome. *Crit Care Med* 23(10):1638–1652, 1995.)

This occurred both when applied on day 1 of ICU admission as a prognostic indicator and when determined over the ICU stay as an outcome measure. When used as an outcome measure, the ICU mortality rate was about 25% at 9 to 12, 50% at 13 to 16, 75% at 17 to 20, and 100% at more than 20 points.

Conclusions.—The multiple organ dysfunction score, developed by using simple physiologic measures of dysfunction in 6 organ systems, is strongly associated with the ultimate risk of both ICU and hospital mortality. An instrument that can provide objective measures of organ dysfunction severity at ICU admission and that can quantify ensuing deterioration during the ICU stay may be valuable as an alternative end point for clinical studies assessing critically ill patients.

▶ The importance of developing a user-friendly, accurate, and easily quantitated multiple organ dysfunction score cannot be overstated. Lack of such a scoring system has confounded interpretation of studies at different institutions using different scoring systems and has greatly limited the conduct of outcome studies and clinical trials. The scoring system proposed by

Marshal et al., although it requires validation at other centers, is quite attractive. The scoring system has incorporated much of what is best from other scoring systems, and the individual components were chosen only after being validated in a large group of ICU patients. One particularly attractive aspect of this scoring system is that it provides a gradation of organ dysfunction, thereby allowing a potentially more accurate degree of risk stratification. Additionally, since the score can be calculated daily, it can be used to provide an up-to-date assessment of individual patients. Hopefully, if validated by further studies, this or a similar scoring system will be uniformly adopted.

E.A. Deitch, M.D.

Pretreatment of Normal Humans With Monophosphoryl Lipid A Induces Tolerance to Endotoxin: A Prospective, Double-Blind, Randomized, Controlled Trial

Astiz ME, Rackow EC, Still JG, Howell ST, Cato A, Von Eschen KB, Ulrich JT, Rudbach JA, McMahon G, Vargas R, Stern W (Cato Research, Durham, NC; Ribi ImmunoChem Research, Hamilton, Mont; Research Ctr, New Orleans, La; et al)
Crit Care Med 23:9–17, 1995   2–18

Background.—Endotoxin is an important mediator of gram-negative septic shock. In experimental animals, pretreatment with monophosphoryl lipid A, a hydrolyzed derivative of endotoxin from *Salmonella minnesota* R595, has been shown to promote endotoxin tolerance and nonspecific resistance to infection. Human response to and the ability of monophosphoryl lipid A to lessen the response to U.S. reference Ec-5 endotoxin were prospectively investigated.

Patients and Methods.—Forty-four healthy volunteers participated in this 2-part study. A double-blind dose escalation was first performed, during which 29 participants were randomly assigned to receive either IV vehicle control or monophosphoryl lipid A. In the second part of the study, 12 participants were randomly assigned to receive either 20 μg/kg monophosphoryl lipid A or vehicle control. After 24 hours, all participants were challenged with a 20-unit/kg IV bolus injection of U.S. reference Ec-5 endotoxin. The systemic response to endotoxin challenge was compared between groups.

Results.—In the first part of the study, subjective effects and increases in cytokine levels were not observed until a dose of 10 μg/kg monophosphoryl lipid A was given. Six participants experienced mild to moderate symptoms after receiving a maximum dose of 20 μg/kg, although therapy was not required. Moderate elevations in temperature, heart rate, and tumor necrosis factor α (TNF-α, interleukin-6 (IL-6), and IL-8 release were also noted. Although IL-1α and IL-1β were not observed, a significant increase in IL-1 receptor antagonist was found. In the second part of the study, pre-treatment with monophosphoryl lipid A led to a decrease in subjective complaints after endotoxin administration, with side effects reported by only 3 of 6 participants vs. 6 of 6 given vehicle control. Significant reductions in febrile and tachycardiac responses were also noted in participants pretreated with monophosphoryl lipid A. In comparison with vehicle control participants, the monophosphoryl lipid A–pretreated participants had significant reductions in TNF-α, IL-6, and IL-8 concentrations. Mean concentrations were 244 vs. 84 pg/mL, 268 vs. 100 pg/mL, and 632 vs. 136 pg/mL, respectively, in the vehicle control and monophosphoryl lipid A–pretreated participants.

Conclusions.—Monophosphoryl lipid A at a dose 10,000 times that of endotoxin is well tolerated in humans. Pretreatment with monophosphoryl lipid A also leads to significant reductions in systemic responses to bacterial endotoxin. Further clinical testing of monophosphoryl lipid A for the prevention or amelioration of the severe effects of sepsis is recommended.

▶ This article was chosen to illustrate the strategy of limiting the adverse systemic inflammatory consequences of sepsis by inducing tolerance in the host. The concept behind this approach is similar to that of prophylactic antibiotics where the drug is given prior to the insult. I am not optimistic about this approach, but since it is an area of active investigation, I have included it.

E.A. Deitch, M.D.

Progressive Magnesium Deficiency Increases Mortality From Endotoxin Challenge: Protective Effects of Acute Magnesium Replacement Therapy

Salem M, Kasinski N, Munoz R, Chernow B (George Washington Univ, Washington, DC; Massachusetts Gen Hosp, Boston; Harvard Med School, Boston; et al)
Crit Care Med 23:108–118, 1995   2–19

Rationale.—Recent experimental studies have related magnesium deficiency to a proinflammatory state in which levels of free radicals and cytokines are increased and tissue injury subsequently takes place. Sepsis itself may be associated with a state of dysregulated inflammation that is initiated by tissue injury or infection and mediated by cytokines, free radicals, and eicosanoids. It is conceivable that magnesium deficiency increases mortality after exposure to endotoxin and that magnesium administration would limit mortality.

Methods.—The effects of endotoxin on magnesium balance were studied in rats given 0.3, 3, or 30 mg/kg of endotoxin or placebo and sampled at intervals for up to 3 hours afterward. The study was repeated in animals randomized to receive a magnesium-repleted or magnesium-deficient diet for 6 weeks. In addition, groups of magnesium-deficient rats were randomized to receive 50 mmol/kg of magnesium chloride or a placebo before or after administration of 3 mg/kg of endotoxin.

Results.—Circulating magnesium levels increased significantly 2 and 3 hours after a 30-mg/kg dose of endotoxin. Ionized magnesium also increased significantly after 3 mg/kg. Magnesium deficiency correlated closely with an increased mortality risk after endotoxin challenge (Fig 3). Magnesium-deficient rats that received replacement therapy survived significantly more often than did placebo recipients after endotoxin challenge (52% vs. 17%).

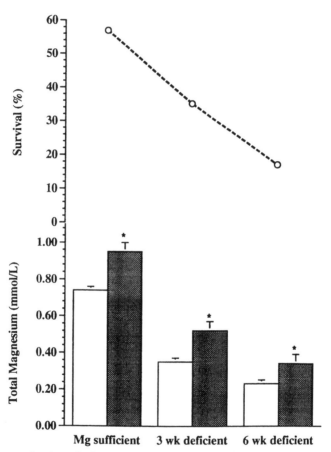

FIGURE 3.—The relationship between progressive magnesium deficiency and survival after endotoxin challenge is represented (**top**). The mean circulating baseline and 24-hour total magnesium concentrations in magnesium-sufficient and progressively deficient animals after endotoxin challenge with 3.0 mg/kg of *Escherichia coli* (**bottom**) are presented. *$P < 0.001$ vs. baseline values. All values are expressed as means ± SEM. *Open bars,* mean baseline determinations; *solid bars,* mean 24-hour determinations; *open circles,* percentage of surviving animals. (Courtesy of Salem M, Kasinski N, Munoz R, et al: Progressive magnesium deficiency increases mortality from endotoxin challenge: Protective effects of acute magnesium replacement therapy. *Crit Care Med* 23(1):108–118, 1995.)

Implications.—Hypomagnesemia is closely associated with increased mortality in this model of experimental sepsis. Replacing magnesium protects significantly against a subsequent endotoxin challenge. The findings strongly suggest that it will be advantageous to correct magnesium deficiency in septic patients.

▶ Magnesium, until recently a relatively neglected ion, is receiving increasing press. The potential clinical importance of magnesium deficiency as a risk factor was first observed in patients with myocardial infarction. More recently, clinical studies have suggested that hypomagnesemia is also a risk factor in additional ICU patient populations. This clinical information, together with experimental and biochemical information highlighting the importance of normal magnesium levels in normal and injury-related cellular homeostasis, immune and inflammatory functions, and organ function, have caused several investigators to focus on this ion. The current study documenting that magnesium deficiency potentiates the lethal effects of endotoxin provides evidence that magnesium may be important in septic states as well.

In spite of this emerging body of information, determining whether magnesium deficiency plays a causal role in the exaggerated inflammatory response and the pathogenesis of organ dysfunction seen in septic ICU patients will be difficult. The difficulty lies in the fact that sepsis or tissue injury causes an *increase* in circulating magnesium levels even when total-body magnesium (i.e., intracellular levels) are decreased. Since it is at the intracellular level that magnesium plays its greatest role and extracellular plasma levels may be misleading, studies evaluating the relationship between magnesium deficiency and outcome from sepsis will require measurement of cellular magnesium levels. Until such studies are performed, the clinical relevance of magnesium deficiency will remain interesting but speculative.

E.A. Deitch, M.D.

Failure of Prophylactic and Therapeutic Use of a Murine Anti-Tumor Necrosis Factor Monoclonal Antibody in *Escherichia coli* Sepsis in the Rabbit
Stack AM, Saladino RA, Thompson C, Sattler F, Weiner DL, Parsonnet J, Nariuchi H, Siber GR, Fleisher GR (Children's Hosp, Boston; Dana Farber Cancer Inst, Boston; Dartmouth Med School, Hanover, NH; et al)
Crit Care Med 23:1512–1518, 1995   2–20

Background.—Because an infusion of tumor necrosis factor (TNF) can induce hemodynamic collapse and end-organ injuries resembling the effects of gram-negative sepsis, TNF has been hypothesized to be a primary mediator of lethal endotoxin shock. Studies of the neutralization of TNF for the treatment of sepsis have shown variable response to TNF antibodies. The effects of a murine monoclonal antibody against TNF administered as either prophylaxis before or treatment after peritoneal endotoxic challenge were studied in an immunocompetent rabbit model.

Methods.—Rabbit pairs were divided into 2 groups. In 1 experiment, the animals were given either IV anti-TNF monoclonal antibody or albumin placebo 3 hours before peritoneal challenge with *Escherichia coli*. In the other experiment, the animals were given either IV anti-TNF monoclonal antibody or albumin placebo 1 hour after peritoneal challenge with *E. coli*. All animals were treated with IV gentamicin and ceftriaxone 1 hour after the challenge. Physiologic measurements were recorded before and 1, 2, 3, and 6 hours after the challenge. Samples of arterial blood were collected before and 1.5, 2, and 2.5 hours after challenge and were analyzed for blood culture and TNF concentration.

Results.—Within 1 hour after intraperitoneal bacterial challenge, all animals were bacteremic. There were no significant differences between the prophylaxis, treatment, and control animals in any physiologic signs of shock or in survival. The peak serum TNF concentration was significantly lower in the prophylaxis and treatment groups than in the control group.

Conclusions.—In a rabbit model, either prophylactic or post–*E. coli* challenge administration of a murine monoclonal antibody against TNF results in the neutralization of TNF in the serum but not in protection against the physiologic derangements of sepsis or in improved survival.

▶ Several recent conceptual and technical advances have led to clinical trials testing a number of biological agents, including anti-TNF monoclonal antibodies. These clinical trials have been disappointing. Why have these trials failed to show clinical benefit? Each agent tested has been proved effective in preclinical experimental models. That is the rub. The models used in which TNF antibodies or other agents were effective were almost all models in which the animals received huge doses of bacteria or endotoxin IV. These models are clearly clinically *irrelevant* models. When studies are performed in clinically *relevant* models, such as this study investigating TNF antibodies in a peritonitis model, TNF antibodies are not beneficial.

There are several morals to this story. The most important is that agents being tested for clinical use should be tested in clinically relevant experimental models. Failure to do so will continue to result in huge and expensive clinical trials with ineffective agents. So when reading about some new and improved magic bullet, remember to ask yourself whether the model used to prove that this agent is potentially great is clinically relevant. If not, exercise caution.

E.A. Deitch, M.D.

Protective Effect of Heat Shock Pretreatment With Heat Shock Protein Induction Before Hepatic Warm Ischemic Injury Caused by Pringle's Maneuver

Saad S, Kanai M, Awane M, Yamamoto Y, Morimoto T, Isselhard W, Minor T, Troidl H, Ozawa K, Yamaoka Y (Kyoto Univ, Japan; Univ of Cologne, Germany)
Surgery 118:510–516, 1995   2–21

Background.—Induction of heat shock proteins (HSPs) may have a cytoprotective effect against environmental stress and may lead to improved ischemic tolerance. The protective effect of heat exposure and HSP 72 induction before warm ischemia caused by Pringle's maneuver was investigated.

Methods.—Eighty male Wistar rats weighing on average 300 to 350 g were anesthetized, with 40 then assigned to a heat shock group. These animals were placed in a temperature-controlled water bath to raise body temperature to 42°C. The remaining 40 rats received an anesthetic but no additional treatment. A second anesthetic was administered 48 hours after heat exposure. The abdomen was opened and the liver detached from its ligaments. The portal vein, hepatic artery, and bile duct were clamped to induce liver ischemia. After 30 minutes, declamping was carried out. Liver energy metabolism and levels of standard liver enzymes were evaluated during 40 minutes of in situ reperfusion. Northern and Western blot analyses were done to determine the gene expression (messenger RNA) of HSP 72, as well as HSP 72 itself. Survival rates were evaluated after 7 postoperative days.

Results.—The HSP 72 gene was strongly expressed after heat shock exposure as compared with only slight expression in control livers. After 48 hours of recovery, a very minimal band of gene expression was noted in the liver tissue of the heat shocked rats, much less than that noted immediately after heat exposure.

Before ischemia onset, adenosine triphosphate (ATP) concentrations and the energy charge potential showed high values in each group of rats. Both parameters decreased to very low values at the end of the ischemic period. After 10 minutes of reperfusion, the ATP concentration in the heat shock animals was significantly greater than in controls, 1.23 vs. 0.57 µmol/g wet weight, respectively. Similar findings were also observed after 40 minutes, with 1.95 µmol/g wet weight noted in the heat shock group as compared with 0.97 µmol/g wet weight in controls. The heat shock group also had a significantly better energy charge recovery after 10 and 40 minutes of reperfusion: 0.62 and 0.70, respectively, vs. 0.44 and 0.58 in controls. Serum liver alanial aminotransferase (ALT) and lactate dehydrogenase (LDH) levels were low in both groups before clamping and at the end of the ischemic period. After declamping, the release of both enzymes was significantly higher in the controls than in the heat shock rats (Fig 5). The heat shock rats also had a 100% survival rate after postoperative day 7 vs. only 50% in the controls.

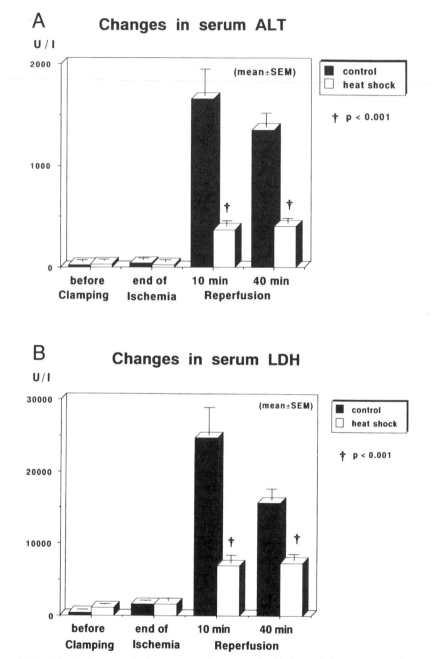

FIGURE 5.—**A**, changes in alanine aminotransferase serum level before and after 30 minutes of warm ischemia and during reperfusion. **B**, changes in lactate dehydrogenase serum level before and after 30 minutes of warm ischemia and during reperfusion. (Courtesy of Saad S, Kanai M, Awane M, et al: Protective effect of heat shock pretreatment with heat shock protein induction before hepatic warm ischemic injury caused by Pringle's maneuver. *Surgery* 118:510–516, 1995.)

Conclusions.—A significant protective effect against warm ischemic liver injury is observed after heat exposure associated with HSP induction. This effect also leads to better recovery of high-energy metabolites and decreased serum levels of ALT and LDH, as well as improved survival rates.

▶ I chose this article to acquaint you with a new and promising area of research: the field of heat shock proteins. These evolutionarily conserved intracellular proteins are found in all organisms, including man. They function to protect essential proteins and enzymes from denaturation during periods of cellular stress and injury. As shown in this study and an increasing number of other studies, the induction of a heat shock response, by preventing cellular death, can convert a lethal to a nonlethal insult. Since a heat shock response can be induced pharmacologically as well as by heat, it has potential clinical application. My guess is that once the heat shock response is understood better, it will be able to be applied in the clinical arena.

Keep your eyes open; this is likely to be a hot topic.

E. A. Deitch, M.D.

3 Burns

Introduction

In 1988, in response to the need for national outcome data on burn injury, the American Burn Association with support from the National Coalition of Burn Center Hospitals began the process of developing a burn registry. After extensive development and piloting projects, in 1992 the burn registry program and manual were offered to all burn centers in the United States and Canada. The initial report from this registry by Dr. Saffle et al. provides survival, cost, and outcome data on 6,417 burn patients treated between 1991 and 1993. Since this important article is likely to serve as a baseline upon which future economic and resource allocation decisions will be made, it is included as the lead article in this year's burn care selections. On an optimistic note, the subsequent article chosen provides evidence that the administration of pharmacologic agents directed at controlling the inflammatory response and improving anabolism leads to increased survival in patients with major thermal injury. Additionally, studies included in this year's selections also deal with the concept of the deleterious effects of excessive or uncontrolled liberation of normal endogenous factors such as glucocorticoids.

The initial resuscitation of burn patients remains an active area of investigation. The paper included by Dr. Matsuda et al. illustrates that the administration of reduced volumes of resuscitation fluid containing high doses of the antioxidant vitamin C will both maintain hemodynamic stability and reduce burn wound edema. This article is important because it illustrates the potential effectiveness of the concept of resuscitative pharmacology, where drugs are given to limit the subsequent deleterious tissue and organ effects of volume loss and tissue injury. In fact, the use of pharmacologic agents such as vitamin C to reduce the volume needed to resuscitate burn patients becomes even more attractive given the potential adverse effects of hypertonic sodium resuscitation as described in the article by Huang et al. The final article on resuscitation included in this year's selections documents that the prophylactic administration of albumin to burned children to maintain a serum albumin level between 2.5 and 3.5 g/dL does not improve outcome and is therefore not necessary. Thus at a time when the costs of medical care are coming under greater and greater scrutiny, this approach may be one safe way of containing costs.

A number of studies dealing with the burn wound are included. These studies range from the use of laser Doppler flowmetry to assess burn depth in pediatric burn patients to the biology of burn wound healing and the use of growth hormone to enhance donor site healing. Taken together, these articles highlight some of the areas of active investigation in this field at both the experimental and clinical levels.

Since the combination of an inhalation injury and a surface burn is associated with a greater mortality rate and more morbidity than would be expected based on the consequences of either one alone, studies investigating the modulatory effects of smoke on the response of burned animals remain an active area of investigation. One such study indicates that it is the degree of airway inflammation rather than alveolar dysfunction that correlates with and perhaps causes the accentuated metabolic response and increased fluid requirements observed in combined smoke and surface burn injuries. Evidence that macrophages and endothelial cells in the lung significantly contribute to the inflammatory response after thermal injury by Bankey et al. provides further support for the concept that lung inflammation can accelerate the metabolic response after thermal injury. This study, taken together with the previous study, supports the concept that the lung is an important immune organ and helps explain how pulmonary injuries can contribute to the increased metabolic and inflammatory response observed in burn patients.

Among the many other articles chosen, one shows that heliox can be used to reduce the need for reintubation in patients with postextubation stridor; still others deal with the immune consequences of thermal injury.

Edwin A. Deitch, M.D.

Recent Outcomes in the Treatment of Burn Injury in the United States: A Report From the American Burn Association Patient Registry
Saffle JR, Davis B, Williams P, The American Burn Association Registry Participant Group (Univ of Utah Health Ctr, Salt Lake City)
J Burn Care Rehabil 16:219–232, 1995   3–1

Introduction.—In 1988 the American Burn Association began distributing to its membership a computerized registry of patients with burns in order to acquire more and better data on burn care. Outcome data were analyzed for 6,417 patients attending 28 participating institutions between 1991 and 1993.

Selected Findings.—Nonsurvivors showed larger burns and suffered a much higher incidence of inhalation injury than did survivors. Patients with burn wounds covering less than 10% total body surface area constituted 53.5% of the burn population. The overall survival rate was 95.9%, and mortality rate for patients with inhalation injury was 29.4%. Survival could not be accurately predicted by any combination of factors present at the time of admission. The burn size determined (by probit analysis and survival curves) lethal to 50% of young adults was 81% of total body

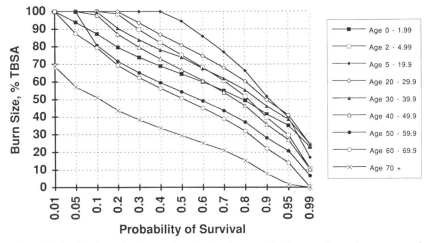

FIGURE 1.—Probit survival curves for 6,417 patients divided by age. For each age group, the probability of survival is plotted against burn size, expressed as percent total body surface area (% *TBSA*). (Courtesy of Saffle JR, Davis B, Williams P, et al: Recent outcomes in the treatment of burn injury in the United States: A report from the American Burn Association Patient registry. *J Burn Care Rehabil* 16:219–232, 1995.)

surface area (Fig 1). Patients showed a mean length of hospital stay (LOS) of 13.5 days. Length of stay and clinical comorbidity factors were linked to resource utilization; total mean charges were $39,533. Multiple regression analyses were performed, with the outcome variables of survival, LOS, and total hospital charges for inpatient treatment used as dependent variables. Patient age, LOS, total burn size, presence of inhalation injury, and total days of ventilator support were the most important variables in prediction of survival.

Discussion.—Three areas of potential inaccuracy of these data are the limitations of burn size estimation, the limits of probit analysis, and the comparability of patient populations. The values derived herein should be regarded as averaged data most valuable in the demonstration of trends; the use of such data to predict individual survival is discouraged. If collection of data is recognized by caregivers as an important part of clinical care, future data analysis on burn outcomes may be significantly improved.

► As outcome data are being used to make decisions about reimbursement, allotment of resources, managed care contracts, plus other important issues by those inside and outside medicine, it is critical that clinicians and hospital administrators have accurate, up-to-date information on the outcome and costs of burn care. This initial report from the American Burn Association registry provides this information on over 6,000 patients treated between 1991 and 1993 at 28 U.S. burn centers. Because of the depth and importance of the material contained in this article, not only should everyone who treats burn patients keep this article at hand, but it should also be actively shared with hospital administrators, interested third-party groups, and government officials. My advice: If you do not have this article, get it. If you have it, reread it and distribute it widely. No abstract can do justice to the breadth and depth of the material this article contains.

E.A. Deitch, M.D.

Increased Survival After Major Thermal Injury: The Effect of Growth Hormone Therapy in Adults

Knox J, Demling R, Wilmore D, Sarraf P, Santos A (Brigham and Women's Hosp, Boston; Harvard Med School, Boston)

J Trauma 39:526–532, 1995

3–2

Background.—Major thermal injury is considered a severe form of trauma. The generalized inflammatory response caused by such injuries results in significant catabolism leading to impaired wound healing, decreased lean body mass, and organ dysfunction. Rapid removal of burned tissue and wound closure, optimization of tissue perfusion, and nutritional support can help reduce morbidity and mortality. In addition, antioxidants, endotoxin-binding drugs, and nonsteroidal anti-inflammatory agents reportedly mitigate the inflammatory response. Human growth hormone (HGH), an anabolic agent that enhances wound healing and diminishes the protein catabolic response, has also been identified as another means of treatment for burned patients. The authors have used HGH in burn patients with estimated mortality surpassing 50%, all of whom had impaired wound healing as indicated by the rate of donor site healing. Preliminary data concerning the safety and potential efficacy of HGH administration in high-risk burn patients were reported herein.

Patients and Methods.—Sixty-nine patients with major burns, defined as patient age plus percentage of body surface area with deep second- and third-degree burns 90 or greater, were evaluated over a 4-year period. The mean patient age was 56 years, and the average body surface area burned was 58%. Thirty percent of the patients had also experienced smoke inhalation. Routine treatment consisted of anti-inflammatory pharmacotherapy, including antioxidants, an endotoxin binder, and a cyclooxygenase inhibitor. Approximately 1 week after injury, 27 of the 54 patients who survived for more than 7 days and exhibited decreased wound healing were also given HGH to facilitate healing. The average treatment time was 61 days. The remaining 27 patients with evidence of sufficient donor site healing (greater than 50% epithelization by day 5 postharvest) served as controls. Injury severity, morbidity, and mortality were compared between groups.

Results.—Predicted mortality estimated from outcome data was more than 70%. This was significantly greater than the actual mortality of 41%. Age, extent of injury, burn management, pharmacotherapy, incidence of smoke inhalation and pneumonia, and in-hospital morbidity were well matched between patients given HGH and controls. Although the HGH

TABLE 2.—Mortality in High-Risk Patients Surviving More Than 7 Days in Patients Receiving Human Growth Hormone vs. Those Without Human Growth Hormone

Group	Patients	Age (Years)	% BSA Burned	Incidence of Smoke Inhalation (%)	Mortality Rate		Actual (%)
					Predicted (%)		
					NBIE	MLR	
HGH	27	50 ± 24	62 ± 26	35	88 ± 11*	77 ± 20†	11‡§
No HGH	27	57 ± 22	49 ± 21	29	80 ± 16	62 ± 29	37‡

Data are means ± SD.
* Significantly different from no HGH, $P = 0.044$.
† Significantly different from no HGH, $P = 0.049$.
‡ Significantly different from that predicted by the NBIE and MLR ($P < 0.05$).
§ Significantly different from no HGH, $P = 0.027$.
Abbreviations: BSA, body surface area; *NBIE,* National Burn Information Exchange; *MLR,* multiple logistic regression; *HGH,* human growth hormone.
(Courtesy of Knox J, Demling R, Wilmore D, et al: Increased survival after major thermal injury: The effect of growth hormone therapy in adults. *J Trauma* 39(3):526–532, 1995.)

group had a slightly higher predicted mortality than controls, actual mortality was 11% for those given HGH vs. 37% in the control patients (Table 2). The HGH-treated patients did have greater tachycardia, required more insulin to maintain serum glucose levels below 200 mg/dL, and had greater calcium levels than the controls; however, no clinical impairment was associated with these findings. No other irregularities were observed.

Conclusions.—The improved survival noted in this patient group suggests that the use of anti-inflammatory agents is safe and may be beneficial. The HGH-treated patients had only slight drug-related complications and showed improvement in mortality rates when compared with predicted mortality rates and with well-matched, simultaneously treated controls. These findings remain to be verified in additional prospective blinded trials using larger numbers of patients.

▶ The basic premise of this clinical study is that uncontrolled inflammation contributes to morbidity and mortality by impairing wound healing, accelerating the rate of catabolism, and predisposing the patient to organ failure. If this concept is correct, then the administrations of anti-inflammatory drugs and anabolic agents (i.e., growth hormone) should improve outcome. The current clinical study tends to support this concept since the patients receiving growth hormone plus the anti-inflammatory drug regimen had a significantly improved survival rate. This pharmacologic approach fits with other clinical approaches directed at controlling the inflammatory response, such as early excision and skin grafting. So does this mean that every burn patient with a high predicted mortality should get this anti-inflammatory cocktail plus growth hormone? The answer is maybe. Because many people are actively investigating these agents, the definitive answer should be known in the next few years.

E.A. Deitch, M.D.

Chronic Pathophysiologic Elevation of Corticosterone After Thermal Injury or Thermal Injury and Burn Wound Infection Adversely Affects Body Mass, Lymphocyte Numbers, and Outcome

Hawes AS, Richardson RP, Antonacci AC, Calvano SE (Cornell Univ, New York)

J Burn Care Rehabil 16:1–15, 1995   3–3

Hypothesis.—It is proposed that the dysfunctional host immunity observed in thermally injured individuals may be related to the glucocorticoid response to injury. The finding that glucocorticoid levels are persistently increased in victims of major burn injury prompted studies in rats to determine the in vivo effects of chronically increased glucocorticoid levels on body mass and lymphocytes.

Methods.—Groups of noninjured and thermally injured rats were studied. The latter animals had 45% body surface area injuries of the dorsal and ventral surfaces. Some burn-injured animals had their burn wounds inoculated with varying concentrations of *Pseudomonas aeruginosa*.

Results.—Burn-injured rats had an acute 10-fold increase in plasma corticosterone and a 5% decrease in body weight. Lymphocytes were markedly increased in circulating blood and in lymph nodes draining the

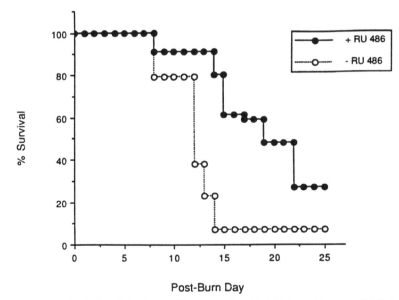

Post-Burn Day

FIGURE 10.—Survival analysis of rats subjected to a dorsal full-thickness injury superficially inoculated with 10^8 colony-forming units of live *Pseudomonas aeruginosa* immediately after injury and not treated ($-Ru$ 486) or treated ($+RU$ 486) with 5 mg/kg/day of RU 486 beginning on the day of injury. Survival curves were significantly different ($P < 0.005$) by log-rank analysis. Ultimate survival was not significantly different by chi-square analysis. (Courtesy of Hawes AS, Richardson RP, Antonacci AC, et al: Chronic pathophysiologic elevation of corticosterone after thermal injury or thermal injury and burn wound infection adversely affects body mass, lymphocyte numbers, and outcome. *J Burn Care Rehabil* 16:1–15, 1995.)

burn wound, whereas splenic lymphocytes decreased by about 60%. When nonburned rats had corticosterone pellets implanted to chronically increase circulating steroid levels, lymphocytes decreased in all tissues and body weight decreased substantially. Animals given corticosterone for 4 days before thermal injury survived for significantly shorter times. Rats subjected to burn wound infection, like uninjured rats given corticosterone, lost substantial body weight and had generalized lymphopenia. Administration of a glucocorticoid receptor antagonist (RU 486) to burned animals with wound infection significantly lengthened their survival time (Fig 10).

Implications.—An acute increase in endogenous glucocorticoid is no doubt important in the immediate postburn period, but a persistently increased level may result in skeletal muscle wasting, lymphopenia, and diminished phagocyte function. Ultimately, specific immunity may be compromised and allow microbial growth to progress.

▶ Why burn patients develop such profound impairment of their immune responses after injury has been a major focus of interest and investigation for several decades. The reason for this interest is the belief that if we understand the mechanisms leading to burn-induced immune dysfunction, then therapeutic approaches directed toward correcting these immune defects can be developed with the ultimate result of fewer infections and improved survival. Although a large amount of information has been generated by these studies, the exact triggers that lead to the development of immune dysfunction continue to be debated. In this study, the authors present evidence that chronically elevated levels of glucocorticoids are an important factor contributing to global immune depression after thermal injury.

Although their results are interesting, an analysis of why the authors decided to carry out these studies provides important insight into understanding the experimental approach and how animal experimentation can contribute to a better understanding of human disease even when the experimental animal's response is *different* from humans'. That is, the authors recognized that burned rats, in contrast to burned humans, do not have chronically elevated glucocorticoid levels or commonly developed spontaneous burn wound infections. They therefore postulated that the elevated glucocorticoid levels seen in patients after thermal injury predisposes these patients to infectious complications based on the immunosuppressive effects of steroids. The results of the experiments described in their abstract indicate that this hypothesis may be correct. Thus this experimental study is a nice example of science at work.

E.A. Deitch, M.D.

Antioxidant Therapy Using High Dose Vitamin C: Reduction of Postburn Resuscitation Fluid Volume Requirements

Matsuda T, Tanaka H, Reyes HM, Richter HM, Hanumadass MM, Shimazaki S, Matsuda H, Nyhus LM (Univ of Illinois, Chicago; Hektoen Institute for Medical Research, Chicago; Kyorin Univ, Tokyo)
World J Surg 19:287–291, 1995   3–4

Introduction.—Extensive burn injuries require a large volume of fluid resuscitation for the first 24 hours after injury because of postburn increases in microvascular permeability. Oxygen free radicals are thought to be involved in the increase in permeability. Previous studies have demonstrated a reduction in fluid requirements with the use of antioxidant therapy given 0.5 to 24 hours postburn. The minimum duration of antioxidant therapy needed to establish hemodynamic stability using reduced fluid volumes was investigated.

Methods.—After preparation for the procedure, third-degree burns covering 70% body surface area were produced on 24 adult Hartley guinea pigs. All animals received fluid resuscitation with Ringer's lactate beginning 0.5 hour postburn. One group (controls) received only Ringer's lactate. A second group (VC 4 HR) received adjuvant vitamin C until 4 hours postburn. A third group (VC 8 HR) received vitamin C until 8 hours postburn, and a fourth group (VC 24 HR) received vitamin C until 24 hours postburn. Total volume intake was the same in all 4 groups. The infusion schedule used was calculated to provide each animal with a total 24-hour fluid volume that was 30% of the Parkland formula calculation. Vitamin C was administered at a rate of 14.2 mg/kg/hr. Preburn and postburn heart rate, blood pressure, cardiac output, hematocrit, and burn skin water content were measured.

Results.—No significant differences in hematocrit were found 2 hours postburn, and all groups showed gradual increases during the first 2 hours postburn. Hematocrit was significantly higher in the control group at 3 and 4 hours postburn, possibly because of hypovolemia. Hematocrit was the same in the 3 treatment groups up until 4 hours postburn. At 6 hours postburn and after, the VC 4 HR group had a significantly higher hematocrit than the other 2 treatment groups. Hematocrit values in the VC 8 HR and VC 24 HR groups were not significantly different for the remainder of the 24 hours. At 0.5 hour postburn, all groups showed a 50% decrease from preburn cardiac output values. By 2 hours postburn, cardiac output was 68% of preburn values for all groups. The 3 treatment groups had similar cardiac output values at 3 and 4 hours postburn and were significantly higher than control values. Cardiac output was significantly higher in the VC 8 HR and VC 24 HR groups after 6 hours postburn than in controls or the VC 4 HR group. Water content in the burned skin was significantly higher in the control and VC 4 HR groups than in the other 2 treatment groups.

Conclusion.—Eight hours was found to be the minimum duration of adjuvant vitamin C administration needed to achieve optimal reduction in fluid volume requirements. The optimal duration of vitamin C administration, as well as the effects of delayed initiation of antioxidant therapy, still need to be determined.

▶ The use of vitamin C as a component of a volume resuscitative regimen is an example of the emerging concept of resuscitative pharmacology, where drugs are given to improve the effectiveness of the resuscitative fluid. In this study, vitamin C was used because of its antioxidative properties. Other agents such as desferoxamine (antioxidant) or heparin (anti-inflammatory) have also been shown to be beneficial when administered with standard resuscitative fluids in various shock, hemorrhage, or ischemia-reperfusion models. When thinking about the concept of resuscitative pharmacology, it is useful to view conditions such as hemorrhagic shock or burn injury as examples of global ischemia-reperfusion models, where during the reperfusion (i.e., volume restitution) phase, oxidant-mediated tissue or organ injury may occur. Within this context, the use of agents to prevent or limit oxidant-mediated injury during reperfusion makes eminent sense.

E.A. Deitch, M.D.

Hypertonic Sodium Resuscitation Is Associated With Renal Failure and Death

Huang PP, Stucky FS, Dimick AR, Treat RC, Bessey PQ, Rue LW (Univ of Alabama, Birmingham; Univ of Rochester, NY)
Ann Surg 221:543–557, 1995   3–5

Introduction.—One of the triumphs of modern surgical therapy has been the development of effective fluid resuscitation for burn patients, which has minimized deaths from burn shock in all but those with the most extensive burn injuries. The 2 major approaches involve either the use of an isotonic saline (lactated Ringer's solution [LR]) or a hypertonic sodium solution (HSS). Although both methods are effective, a direct comparison of the 2 approaches was the purpose of this investigation.

Methods.—A total of 109 burn patients were treated with LR-1 (the earliest portion of the study) and 65 were treated with HSS. At a later date, another 39 were treated with LR (LR-2). Lactated Ringer's solution (130 mEq/L sodium) was given at 4 mL/kg per percent surface area burned. After treatment for 24 hours, the solutions were changed to hypotonic solutions with or without a colloid suspension. The patients treated with HSS were initially treated with LR, but this was changed to the hypertonic solution given at a rate of 0.52 mEq/L per percent surface area burned on arrival at the burn unit. Demographic, clinical, and laboratory data as well as outcome were recorded for all patients.

Results.—There were no patient differences in the LR-1 and HSS groups in age (46 vs. 43.6 years), burn area (39.2% vs. 39.9%), predicted mortality (35% vs. 30%), or inhalation injury incidence (42% vs. 48%). The resuscitation volume was lower for the HSS group (3.9 mL/kg per percent

TABLE 5.—Demographic Data for Renal Failure vs. No Renal Failure Groups

	LR-1		HSS	
	No RF	RF	No RF	RF
N	98	11	39	26
Age, years	42.3 ± 2.0	55.5 ± 6.1*	40.3 ± 3.1	54.5 ± 3.6*
TBSA burn, %	37.6 ± 1.9	59.5 ± 8.0†	38.5 ± 3.6	40.4 ± 4.2
Inhalation injury frequency, % (N)	49.8 (43)	81.8 (9)†	38.5 (15)	46.2 (12)
Pneumonia frequency, % (N)	10.2 (10)	27.3 (3)	7.7 (3)	61.5 (16)†
Observed mortality, % (N)	19.4 (19)	90.9 (10)†	25.6 (10)	96.2 (25)†
Predicted mortality, %	25.0 (24)	76.8 (8)	22.8 (9)	52.3 (14)
95% CI, %	18.5–31.5	58.7–94.9	12.1–33.5	38.6–66.0

Note: Values for age and burn size are means ± SEM. P values are for No RF vs. RF subsets for each group.
Abbreviations: LR-1, lactated Ringer's solution; HSS, hypertonic sodium solution; RF, renal failure.
* $P < 0.05$.
† $P < 0.001$.
(Courtesy of Huang PP, Stucky FS, Dimick AR, et al: Hypertonic sodium resuscitation is associated with renal failure and death. Ann Surg 221:543–557, 1995.)

surface area burned) than the LR-1 group (5.3 mL/kg per percent surface area burned). After 48 hours, the cumulative sodium load was greater in the HSS group, as expected, and the cumulative fluid volumes were similar. In HSS-treated patients, serum sodium levels were marginally elevated at 153 vs. 135 mEq/L. The patients treated with HSS had a 4-fold increase in kidney failure. The mortality rate for patients treated with HSS was twice that of the LR-1 group. Patients in whom renal failure subsequently developed were significantly older than those without renal failure in both the LR-1 and HSS groups (Table 5). After these data were analyzed, the decision was made to return to the use of LR for resuscitation. On returning to LR therapy, the sodium load was less, renal failure developed in only 15%, and 33% died—results similar to the LR-1 group and significantly less than the HSS group.

Conclusion.—The expected benefit of HSS was not observed in spite of appropriate use of the therapy. The use of hypertonic sodium solutions leads to a greater incidence of renal failure and mortality. Use of the HSS did not lead to a reduced resuscitation volume. The use of HSS for burn resuscitation is discouraged.

▶ I included this article not because I am convinced that hypertonic saline resuscitation is bad, but because I am convinced it is not good. Hypertonic saline resuscitation offers no clearly documentable advantages over Ringer's lactate (Parkland formula) and is associated with a number of potential complications as outlined in this study. Therefore, if you get the urge to use hypertonic saline, wait awhile until the urge passes.

E.A. Deitch, M.D.

Maintenance of Serum Albumin Levels in Pediatric Burn Patients: A Prospective, Randomized Trial

Greenhalgh DG, Housinger TA, Kagan RJ, Rieman M, James L, Novak S, Farmer L, Warden GD (Shriners Burns Inst, Cincinnati, Ohio)

J Trauma 39:67–74, 1995   3–6

Background.—Although there are many reasons why serum albumin levels should not be permitted to drop too low in critically ill patients, there are also arguments against its unnecessary replacement. Assumptions about albumin being predictive of nutritional status during critical illness have come into question, as have the effects of albumin supplementation on morbidity and mortality. The influence of maintaining serum albumin levels on morbidity and mortality was assessed in children with burns.

Methods.—Seventy pediatric patients with burns of greater than 20% total body surface area participated in the prospective, randomized trial. After resuscitation from burn shock, the patients were assigned to either a high-albumin group, which received supplemental albumin to maintain levels of 2.5 to 3.5 g/dL, or a low-albumin group, in which supplemental albumin was given only if levels fell below 1.5 g/dL. The 2 groups were similar in terms of age, burn size, depth of injury, and inhalation injury. The patients were followed for differences in edema and other variables of morbidity such as fluid needs, nutritional supplementation, and pulmonary status.

Results.—Patients in the high-albumin group received about twice the amount of 25% human albumin solution as the low-albumin group. Predictably, there were significant differences between groups in serum albumin levels throughout hospitalization. However, there were no differences in resuscitation needs, maintenance fluid needs, urinary output, number of tube feedings, days of antibiotic treatment, or ventilatory needs. Nor were significant differences observed in the results of hematologic, electrolyte, or nutritional laboratory tests. Albumin group assignment made no difference in length of hospital stay, complication rate, or mortality. Albumin costs exceeded $50,000 for the high-albumin group as compared with less than $2,500 in the low-albumin group.

Conclusions.—Previously healthy children with large burns do not appear to need maintenance of normal serum albumin levels. Albumin supplementation does not appear to be indicated in these patients unless they have a clinical indication such as excessive edema. The results suggest that aggressive nutritional support rather than exogenous supplementation should be used to support albumin levels.

▶ The message of this article is simple. One can save money and not affect the quality of care by limiting the routine practice of prophylactic supplemental albumin administration to burn patients with albumin levels greater than 1.5 g/dL. As pressure mounts to reduce costs and maintain quality, I expect other routine, traditional, and established practices to be found less important than once thought. On the other hand, I do not believe this article should be interpreted to say that albumin supplementation may not be helpful in specific circumstances, such as in the very severely burned or elderly burn patients with hemodynamic instability.

E.A. Deitch, M.D.

Early Assessment of Pediatric Burn Wounds by Laser Doppler Flowmetry

Atiles L, Mileski W, Spann K, Purdue G, Hunt J, Baxter C (Univ of Texas, Dallas)
J Burn Care Rehabil 16:596–601, 1995   3–7

Introduction.—Laser Doppler flowmetry has been used to detect differences in microcirculatory blood flow between wounds that do and do not require grafting in adult patients with burn injuries. A flexible multichannel probe with integrated temperature control circuitry to diminish spatial variations was used to determine whether laser Doppler flowmetry could be used to help ascertain burn wound outcome in pediatric patients.

Methods.—Laser Doppler blood flow measurements were taken immediately after initial wound débridement and daily for 3 days, or until the

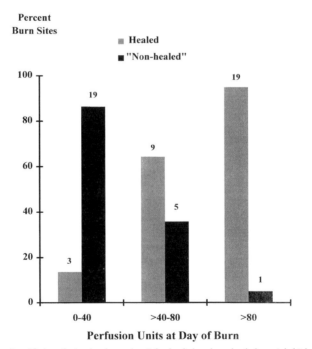

FIGURE 2.—Stratified perfusion levels on day 0 for healed and nonhealed partial-thickness burns as a percentage of measured wounds (the number of actual wounds measured is indicated by the inset data). (Courtesy of Atiles L, Mileski W, Spann K, et al: Early assessment of pediatric burn wounds by laser Doppler flowmetry. *J Burn Care Rehabil* 16:596–601, 1995.)

wounds were excised and grafted. Burn wound depth classification as partial thickness or full thickness was done independently of perfusion values. Only partial-thickness burns were evaluated. Wounds were categorized as either "healed" or "nonhealed."

Results.—Twenty-two patients with 57 separate burn wounds were measured. The mean burn size was 16% total body surface (range, 5%–45%). The age range was 7 months to 15 years (mean, 3.6 years). Thirty-two of 57 partial-thickness wounds healed within 21 days. Twenty-five wounds did not heal or necessitated grafting. The average perfusion level for healed partial-thickness wounds was significantly higher than that for nonhealed wounds at all time points. Ninety-six percent of the wounds with values greater than 80 perfusion units (PU) on day 0 healed as compared with 67% for wounds with initial perfusion values of 80 or less PU (Fig 2).

Conclusion.—These findings in pediatric patients support previous work with adult patients. Measurement of wound blood flow can be used to classify burn wounds that will or will not heal in 21 days.

▶ Perhaps we are getting there. The search for a way to predict which burn wounds will heal within 21 days has been a goal for many years since the incidence of hypertrophic scarring is much higher in burns that take 3 weeks or longer to heal than burns that heal quicker. Therefore if it were possible to accurately predict which burns will and will not heal within this 21-day grace period, it would be possible to offer immediate early surgery only to those patients who will benefit. Thus this preliminary clinical trial showing that 95% of the burns with values of 80 PU or greater healed whereas only 5.5% of the burns with PU values of 40 or less healed is both encouraging and important. Let's hope further studies will validate this approach.

E.A. Deitch, M.D.

Characterization of Growth Hormone Enhanced Donor Site Healing in Patients With Large Cutaneous Burns

Herndon DN, Hawkins HK, Nguyen TT, Pierre E, Cox R, Barrow RE (Univ of Tex, Galveston; Shriners Burns Inst, Galveston, Tex)
Ann Surg 221:649–659, 1995   3–8

Objectives.—Studies in which recombinant human growth hormone (rhGH) has been shown to increase the rate of skin graft donor site healing in massively burned patients has led to the hypothesis that growth hormone acts by increasing the production of insulin-like growth factor type 1 (IGF-1) in the liver and upregulating IGF-1 receptors. This hypothesis was tested in 10 burn patients, and the results are debated in a discussion by physicians.

Methods.—Patients with full-thickness burns covering more than 40% of their bodies were studied prospectively. Each patient served as his own control. Biopsy samples were taken from split-thickness skin graft donor sites on the thigh to determine donor site healing in 6 patients treated with rhGH (0.2 mg/kg/day) by subcutaneous injection at the time of the second split-thickness skin harvest and in 4 patients who received placebo. Biopsy specimens were prepared for histologic, electron microscopic, or cryostat study.

Results.—The time to heal at the donor site was significantly decreased by more than 2 days in patients receiving rhGH as compared with those receiving placebo. Also, IGF-1 serum concentrations increased 3-fold during rhGH treatment as compared with placebo periods. Treatment with rhGH had no significant effect on keratinocyte size or differentiation. However, the extent of basal lamina production and coverage, measured as a percentage of the total length of the dermal-epidermal junction, was much greater during treatment with growth hormone (68% coverage) than during the placebo period before rhGH treatment (26%). Treatment with rhGH also resulted in increased laminin, types IV and VII collagen, and cytokeratin-14 levels in skin.

Conclusion.—Treatment with rhGH improves wound healing time in burn patients by accelerating differentiation of the junctional mechanisms necessary for dermal-epidermal adhesion. This effect may be a direct effect of rhGH or an indirect effect of factors that are increased by rhGH treatment, such as IGF-1, laminin, collagen, and cytokeratin-14.

▶ That growth hormone increases donor site healing in burned children and reduces hospitalization time by about 25% appears well established. However, the mechanisms underlying the beneficial effects of growth hormone on donor site healing remain unclear. Thus the goal of the current study was to help elucidate how growth hormone works. The overall conclusion of the authors was that growth hormone, either directly or through secondary mediators, stimulates dermal and epidermal cells to produce structural proteins and other components needed for optimal wound healing.

With that said, why was this particular article chosen? The answer is that any therapy that speeds up donor site healing so that the donor sites can be reharvested faster will shorten the hospital stay and may improve survival. This is especially true in massively burned patients, where lack of donor sites are the limiting factor in resurfacing the burn wound.

E.A. Deitch, M.D.

Cultured Epithelial Autograft: Five Years of Clinical Experience With Twenty-Eight Patients
Williamson JS, Snelling CFT, Clugston P, MacDonald IB, Germann E (Univ of British Columbia, Vancouver, Canada)
J Trauma 39:309–319, 1995   3–9

Introduction.—Because all the materials and techniques presently used for burn wound coverage have their disadvantages, various types of cultured grafts have been suggested. Cultured epithelial autograft (CEA) was the first of these materials to be developed and thus far has been the most used in patients. At the authors' center, CEA has been available for use as an adjunct for burn wound coverage since 1988. A 5-year experience with the use of CEA is reported.

Methods.—From 1988 through 1992, CEA was used in 28 burn patients who survived long enough for assessment. There were 23 males and 5 females with a mean age of 35 years. The mean total body surface area (BSA) of the burns was 52%, and the mean total full-thickness injury was 42%. The mean BSA of the wounds in which CEA was used, after excision to fat or fascia, was 10%. Interim homograft was placed in most of these wounds. In 3 patients, an unsuccessful attempt was made to preserve the homograft dermis at the time of removal. "Take" was evaluated 14 days after CEA placement. When CEA grafting was successful, the wounds were observed for adherence, percent engraftment, blistering, and contracture. The effects of CEA on patient outcome were evaluated as well.

Results.—Mean take was 27% of the area grafted with CEA. Take was 50% or greater in 8 patients who had 1% to 19% BSA covered with CEA at discharge. Another 13% of the patients showed no take of CEA on wounds covering 2% to 16% BSA. Overall mortality among burn patients at the study center was no different in the 5 years before and after the availability of CEA. These 2 populations were comparable in total BSA burned, age, proportion with inhalation injury, and homograft availability. Comparison with a matched population of controls from the previous 5 years found that CEA had no significant influence on length of hospital stay or number of autograft harvests. Each patient with CEA did undergo about 1 more débridement without autograft harvest. Good vs. poor take was unaffected by the timing or depth of wound excision, interim coverage, the type of dressing, or the microbiologic findings of the wound. The most favorable recipient sites for CEA coverage were the anterior of the trunk and thighs. Cultured epithelial autograft had some subjective disadvantages when compared with meshed autograft, particularly in terms of adherence and stability.

Conclusions.—Five years' experience with CEA as an adjunct in burn wound coverage finds that engraftment is still unpredictable and inconsistent. Thus CEA should be limited to use as a biological dressing and an experimental adjunct to conventional split-thickness autograft coverage. The use of CEA has yielded valuable experience in mass tissue culture techniques, wound preparation, and cultured graft care, which it is hoped will serve as a foundation for the eventual production and clinical use of culture composite autologous skin.

▶ Cautious optimism in the evaluation of new therapies is good, but in the case of cultured epithelial autografts, early optimism has not been rewarded with good clinical results. As the study documents, the use of cultured epithelial autografts has not been clinically effective. Thus I concur with the authors that until more is known about how to improve long-term graft take, this exceedingly expensive technique must remain unproven. One potential solution to this problem of successful transplantation of cultured epithelial cells would be the use of composite grafts combining a dermal base onto which epithelial cells are grafted (see Abstract 3–10).

E.A. Deitch, M.D.

An Investigation Into the Mechanisms by Which Human Dermis Does Not Significantly Contribute to the Rejection of Allo-Skin Grafts

Wu J, Barisoni D, Armato U (Univ of Verona, Italy; Southwestern Hosp, Chongqing, China)

Burns 21:11–16, 1995   3–10

Background.—The dermis has been shown to play an important role in skin transplantation. It favors the taking of thin, fragile cultured epidermal sheets and accelerates keratinocyte growth. It also prevents scars from

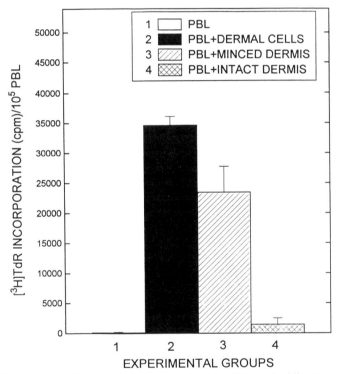

FIGURE 1.—Response of peripheral blood mononuclear cells (*PBM*) to the different components of human allodermis. DNA synthesis of the PBM was very low in the absence of allostimulators (*bar 1*). Conversely, maximal reactive proliferation of the PBM was obtained in the presence of isolated allodermal cells (*bar 2* vs. *bar 3*, P < 0.01, and vs. *bar 4*, P < 0.001). The response of the PBM to the minced pieces of dermis (*bar 3*) was also distinctly more intense than that to large pieces of intact dermis (*bar 4*; *bar 3* vs. *bar 4*, P < 0.001). (Reprinted from *Burns*, vol 21, Wu J, Barisoni D, Armato U: An investigation into the mechanisms by which human dermis does not significantly contribute to the rejection of allo-skin grafts, pp 11–16, copyright 1995, with kind permission from Butterworth-Heinemann Journals, Elsevier Science Ltd, The Boulevard, Langford Lane, Kidlington 0X5 1GB, UK.)

forming and shrinking in the wounded areas. Most important, it does not elicit any clinically detectable immune response. It is not known why the allodermis is not significantly immunogenic, even though it contains many cell types. The mechanisms underlying the inert role of the allodermis in the immune rejection of skin grafts were investigated.

Methods.—A new in vitro model was used to study the distribution of the host's lymphocytes inside the alloskin. Other parameters such as mixed lymphocyte reactions and immunohistochemistry were assessed to define the possible mechanisms of the interactions between the peripheral blood mononuclear (PBM) cells and the dermis or epidermis.

Findings.—In the alloskin/PBM coculture model, most of the PBM cells migrated slowly, yet preferentially to the alloepidermal compartment rather than remaining in the allodermis. This did not appear to be due to the fact that isolated dermal cells could not induce an immune response, but because intact dermis is immunologically inert (Fig 1). Little intercellular adhesion molecule type 1 (ICAM-1) could be detected immunohistochemically in the epidermis. Conversely, both the dermal cells and the dermal matrix were ICAM-1–positive. Most PBM cells migrating into the alloskin pieces expressed either the CD18, CD19, or CD9 molecule. However, very few of them showed lymphocyte function-associated antigen type 1 (LFA-1), which binds to ICAM-1 and none were CD4-positive.

Conclusions.—Because the migrated PBM cells were LFA-1–negative, the ICAM-1–positive allodermal cells and matrix could not trap the migrating PBM through an ICAM-1/LFA-1 mechanism. Thus the immunocompetent allodermal cells had no opportunity to get in touch and stimulate the PBM.

▶ Although the data presented may seem esoteric and somewhat complex, in reality the authors present a very important and elegantly simple set of experiments that help illustrate why human dermis can be transplanted successfully while epidermis cannot. That is, these results indicate that the immunologic inertia of intact dermis is due to factors that inhibit contact between the patient's immune cells and the transplanted allodermis and not due to the inability of dermal cells to induce an immune response. These findings help explain the paradoxical clinical observation of why cadaver dermis placed on burn wounds has been documented to survive indefinitely in some reports.

The potential implications of this observation are enormous. Because dermis decreases scarring and improves the quality of skin, the ability to transplant dermis successfully would be a major advance. These results indicate that a combination of dermal-epidermal (cultured epidermal autografts) grafts may be successful where cultured epidermal grafts fail.

E.A. Deitch, M.D.

A Study of Cytokines in Burn Blister Fluid Related to Wound Healing

Ono I, Gunji H, Zhang J-Z, Maruyama K, Kaneko F (Fukushima Med College, Japan)
Burns 21:352–355, 1995   3–11

Background.—In vitro studies have demonstrated the importance of cytokines in wound healing, and research is now focusing on the role of cytokines in the local treatment of burns. Blister fluid appears to contain various cytokines and growth factors that facilitate the wound healing process. Exudate retained in burn blisters was collected for measurement of cytokines and examination of the fluid's effect on proliferation of keratinocytes.

Methods.—Blister fluid was collected from 12 patients with a mean age of 34.5 years. All patients had come to the hospital within 48 hours of sustaining partial–skin thickness burns. Cytokines measured by enzyme-linked immunosorbent assay were interleukin-1α (IL-1α, IL-1β, IL-6, IL-8, epidermal growth factor (EGF), basic fibroblast growth factor (bFGF), platelet-derived growth factor (PDGF), transforming growth factor (TGF)-α, TGF-β₁, and TGF-β₂. Blister fluid was added to keratinocyte culture medium to evaluate its ability to stimulate growth.

Results.—Cytokines present at relatively high levels in burn blister fluid were IL-8 (10.21 ng/mL), IL-6 (2.470 ng/mL), TGF-β₁ (2.037 ng/mL), TGF-α (0.684 ng/mL), and PDGF (0.154 ng/mL). The remaining 5 cytokines were present in relatively low levels ranging from 12.69 pg/mL for bFGF to 0.063 ng/mL for IL-1α. The addition of blister fluid to keratinocyte basic medium (KBM) increased keratinocyte growth to 315.5%

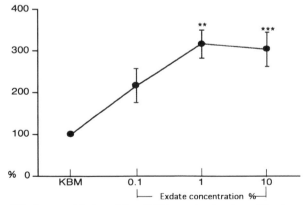

FIGURE 3.—Effectiveness of the burn blister fluid in accelerating the proliferation of keratinocytes. Results show means ± SE; n = 6. **P < 0.001; ***P < 0.005. (Reprinted from *Burns*, vol 21, Ono I, Gunji H, Zhang J-Z, et al: A study of cytokines in burn blister fluid related to wound healing, pp 352–355, copyright 1995, with kind permission from Butterworth-Heinemann Journals, Elsevier Science Ltd, The Boulevard, Langford Lane, Kidlington 0X5 1GB, UK.)

with a 1% addition, a statistically significant increase when compared with the 100% keratinocyte growth achieved by incubation with KBM alone (Fig 3).

Conclusion.—Contrary to expectations, levels of IL-8 and IL-6 were rather high and levels of IL-1α and IL-1β relatively low. The apparent coexistence of various cytokines in a balanced state in burn blister fluid suggests that a cytokine network operating on the wound surface may regulate epithelialization. A dressing that is strongly effective in retaining cytokines, particularly endogenous growth factors, is recommended for burn injuries.

▶ The message of this article is simple. Whenever possible, leave the blisters alone. It hurts less and wound healing is optimized.

E.A. Deitch, M.D.

A Study to Determine the Efficacy of Treatments for Hydrofluoric Acid Burns
Seyb ST, Noordhoek L, Botens S, Mani MM (Univ of Kansas, Kansas City)
J Burn Care Rehabil 16:253–257, 1995   3–12

Objectives.—Treatment of hydrofluoric acid burns is complicated because of the 2-fold nature of the tissue damage; that is, hydrofluoric acid causes immediate tissue damage because of a high concentration of hydrogen ions, as well as liquefaction necrosis because of the free fluoride ion in the acid. The efficacy of several methods of neutralizing the free fluoride ion is compared in this study with rats.

Methods.—Hydrofluoric acid burns were initiated on the shaved hindquarters of 84 female Sprague-Dawley rats by dispensing about 0.02 mL of a 70% hydrofluoric acid solution onto the leg. The control group was burned but not treated, and the remaining groups were treated by various methods. These methods included subcutaneous injection with 10% calcium gluconate, subcutaneous injection with 10% magnesium sulfate, topical application of 2.5% calcium gluconate burn jelly, topical application of a 50% aqueous solution of dimethyl sulfoxide containing 20% calcium gluconate, topical application of 20% calcium gluconate in sterile water, and short-term (5 minutes) topical application of gauze pads soaked with dimethyl sulfoxide (the other topical applications were continued throughout the week of the study).

Results.—Significant reduction of the damage caused by exposure to hydrofluoric acid was seen after subcutaneous injections of calcium gluconate and magnesium sulfate solutions and topical application of calcium gluconate mixed with the penetration enhancer dimethyl sulfoxide. Histologically, however, none of the treatments affected the coagulation necrosis of the skin observed 24 hours after the burn or the liquefaction necrosis of the skin.

Conclusions.—Successful treatment of hydrofluoric acid burns with subcutaneous injections of calcium gluconate or magnesium sulfate solutions or topical application of calcium gluconate with a penetration enhancer indicates that rapid neutralization of the destructive free fluoride ion in hydrofluoric acid is necessary for successful treatment of hydrofluoric acid burns.

▶ Hydrofluoric acid burns, especially to the hands, are relatively common because of the acid's widespread use in industry and its presence in certain commercial products. Because of the persistent pain and tissue destruction associated with hydrofluoric acid burns, a number of treatments have been proposed. Yet little comparative information is available on the effectiveness of these putative treatments. Thus the value of this experimental study is that it shows that of the available treatments, only the subcutaneous injection of calcium gluconate or magnesium sulfate is effective. So when a patient with a hydrofluoric burn arrives, ignore the jellies and reach for the syringe.

E.A. Deitch, M.D.

Effect of Graded Increases in Smoke Inhalation Injury on the Early Systemic Response to a Body Burn

Demling R, Lalonde C, Youn YK, Picard L (Brigham and Women's Hosp, Boston; Beth Israel Hosp, Boston; Children's Hosps, Boston; et al)
Crit Care Med 23:171–178, 1995   3–13

Objective.—In combination, body burn and smoke inhalation injury produce greater morbidity and mortality than either type of injury alone. The early effect of increasing levels of lung exposure to smoke on the hemodynamic response to body burn was studied in sheep.

Methods.—In the prospective, randomized study, an 18% body surface burn was produced in adult sheep. The animals were then exposed to 12 breaths of cotton toweling smoke at a tidal volume of 5, 10, or 20 mL/kg. After the animals were awakened and resuscitated to their baseline oxygen delivery level, they were killed at 24 hours.

Results.—At 5 mL/kg tidal volume, smoke exposure did not produce significant airway inflammation or alter the cardiopulmonary response to body burn alone. For animals in this group, oxygen consumption remained at baseline. Net 24-hour positive fluid balance was 1.5 L, similar to that produced by a burn alone. A moderate airway injury resulted when the smoke exposure was increased to 10 mL/kg tidal volume. Early fluid requirements increased significantly, with a 40% early increase in oxygen consumption, a doubling of positive fluid balance, and a striking increase in burn edema. Gas exchange was unaffected, however.

An early 100% increase in oxygen consumption was noted with the 20-mL/kg tidal volume exposure. Fluid requirements at 1 to 4 hours in-

TABLE 2.—Fluid Balance

	Intake	Output	Net Balance
Control	1.4 ± 3	1.3 ± 0.3	+0.2 ± 0.1
Burn Alone	2.9 ± 0.6*†	1.4 ± 0.3	+1.5 ± 0.4*
Burn-Smoke			
5 mL/kg	3.2 ± 0.5*	1.2 ± 0.4	+1.9 ± 0.5*
10 mL/kg	4.5 ± 0.6*†	1.6 ± 0.4*†	+2.9 ± 0.5*†
20 mL/kg	5.9 ± 0.6*†	1.4 ± 0.5	+4.4 ± 1.2*†

Note: Values are liters per 24 hours, means ± SD; n = 8.
* Significantly different from controls, $P < 0.05$.
† Significantly different from burn alone, $P < 0.05$.
(Courtesy of Demling R, Lalonde C, Youn YK, et al: Effect of graded increases in smoke inhalation injury on the early systemic response to a body burn. *Crit Care Med* 23(1):171–178, 1995.)

creased by 3-fold (Table 2). There was also severe airway inflammation with mucosal sloughing that led to impaired gas exchange.

Conclusions.—In subjects with body burns, smoke exposure severe enough to produce airway inflammation and injury will increase early systemic metabolic demands and fluid requirements when compared with body burn alone. The degree of burn edema and positive fluid balance is increased as well. The degree of airway inflammation, rather than alveolar dysfunction, is correlated with the magnitude of the accentuated response.

▶ Although it is recognized that burned patients who have a concomitant inhalation injury often require more fluid for adequate initial resuscitation than would be expected on the basis of the surface burn only, little information is available to predict how great this increased fluid need might be. The value of this study is that the authors showed that the magnitude of the increased metabolic response and the extent of fluid retention correlated with the degree of airway damage and not with gas exchange abnormalities. These results suggest that airway injury contributes to the systemic inflammatory response and that the presence of bronchorrhea and other signs of airway damage could identify patients in whom greater than predicted volumes of fluid resuscitation will be required.

E.A. Deitch, M.D.

Interleukin-6 Production After Thermal Injury: Evidence for Nonmacrophage Sources in the Lung and Liver
Bankey PE, Williams JG, Guice KS, Taylor SN (Univ of Texas, Dallas; Duke Univ, Durham, NC)
Surgery 118:431–439, 1995   3–14

Introduction.—Thermal injury leads to systemic inflammation resulting from the production of endogenous mediators, including interleukin-6 (IL-6). The main sources of IL-6 have been suggested to be the liver and lungs; however, these organs include several types of cells that could produce IL-6. The cellular sources of IL-6 after thermal injury were studied in rats.

Methods.—A 35% to 40% total body surface area scald injury was made in Wistar rats. The animals' serum, liver and lung tissue, and tissue macrophage IL-6 response to this injury were determined. Production of IL-6 by cultured pulmonary microvascular endothelial cells (PMECs) was determined after treatment with serum from the injured rats. 7TD1 cell proliferation was used to measure IL-6 bioactivity and reverse transcriptase–polymerase chain reaction was used to measure IL-6 mRNA levels. Bronchoalveolar lavage was performed to obtain alveolar macrophages, and enzyme digestion of the liver and lungs was used to obtain PMECs.

Results.—Through the third day after the burn, circulating IL-6 activity was significantly increased in the burned animals: 388 U/0.1 mL vs. 80 U/0.1 mL in controls. Animals with thermal injury showed increased lung and liver IL-6 mRNA but no corresponding increase in alveolar macrophages or Kupffer cells. In the lung, elevated IL-6 mRNA persisted after bronchoalveolar lavage. Mean IL-6 activity was 1,118 U per culture in PMECs cultured in the presence of serum from injured animals vs. 288 U per culture in PMECs cultured with sham rat serum. The PMECs cultured with postburn serum also had more readily detectable levels of IL-6 mRNA.

Conclusions.—After thermal injury, microvascular endothelium may be an important source of IL-6 in the lung and liver. Microvascular endothelial cells could be activated via serum factors generated by the tissue injury. Generalized endothelial activation may be the common pathophysiologic mechanism for systemic inflammation.

▶ This article is important for its scientific findings. That is, the observation that microvascular endothelial cells rather than macrophages are the primary producers of IL-6 is important. This study and other similar studies indicating that epithelial and endothelial cells significantly contribute to the inflammatory response after injury greatly enhances our understanding of the inflammatory response. Only by understanding the inflammatory response to injury and which cell populations contribute to this response will we be able to develop effective agents to combat the adverse consequences of excessive inflammation, such as organ dysfunction and the development of multiple organ failure syndrome.

E.A. Deitch, M.D.

Use of a Helium-Oxygen Mixture in the Treatment of Postextubation Stridor in Pediatric Patients With Burns

Rodeberg DA, Easter AJ, Washam MA, Housinger TA, Greenhalgh DG, Warden GD (Univ of Cincinnati, Ohio)
J Burn Care Rehabil 16:476–480, 1995   3–15

Objective.—Because the mixture of helium and oxygen—or "heliox"—is less dense than room air, it can flow with less turbulence past airway narrowings. As such, it decreases airway resistance while increasing gas exchange volume. More than 90% of patients requiring reintubation will have stridor as a manifestation of airway obstruction. The use of heliox for the treatment of postextubation stridor or retractions in children with burns was assessed.

Methods.—The subjects were 8 children with burns who had postextubation stridor or retractions that did not respond to treatment with nebulized racemic epinephrine. All were treated with heliox via face mask. The mean treatment time was 28 hours, and initial helium concentrations ranged from 50% to 70%. The helium concentration was adjusted downward to the lowest concentration that relieved stridor; when it declined to less than 50%, helium was discontinued.

Results.—Just 2 of the 8 children treated with heliox had respiratory distress requiring reintubation. The duration of stridor before the start of heliox therapy was 10 and 24 hours in these patients as compared with a mean of 1 hour in those who did not require reintubation. The mean respiratory distress score decreased from 6.8 to 2.0 after the start of heliox therapy.

Conclusions.—In pediatric burn patients, heliox is an effective treatment for postextubation stridor that does not respond to nebulized racemic epinephrine. Heliox treatment should be started as soon as possible after the onset of stridor. Heliox may help in preventing respiratory distress and the need for reintubation.

▶ This straightforward article speaks for itself. Heliox is a useful adjuvant in patients in whom stridor develops after extubation. When effective, it prevents the need for reintubation and the potential adverse consequences of prolonged intubation. Likewise, in immunocompromised burn patients where steroid use for upper airway edema is potentially dangerous, heliox provides an attractive option.

E.A. Deitch, M.D.

Chronic Ethanol Intake and Burn Injury: Evidence for Synergistic Alteration in Gut and Immune Integrity

Napolitano LM, Koruda MJ, Zimmerman K, McCowan K, Chang J, Meyer AA
(Univ of North Carolina, Chapel Hill)
J Trauma 38:198–207, 1995   3–16

Objective.—The combination of alcohol abuse and injury is associated with an increased susceptibility to infection. One possible explanation for this observation is that alcohol may alter immune responses and increase gastrointestinal bacterial translocation rates. The results of a rat study of the effects of chronic oral or IV ethanol intake and injury on immune and gastrointestinal changes were presented.

Methods.—Rats were randomly divided into 8 groups of 9 to 11 animals each. Rats received 20% ethanol or saline daily for 14 days either orally or IV. Four hours after the final dosing, the animals were burned over 30% of their bodies and killed 4 days later. Spleen cell mitogenesis assays were performed, and intestinal DNA content, diamine oxidase activity, protein content, and bacterial translocation were determined. Plasma endotoxin concentration was measured, and histopathologic analysis was performed on the intestinal mucosal structure.

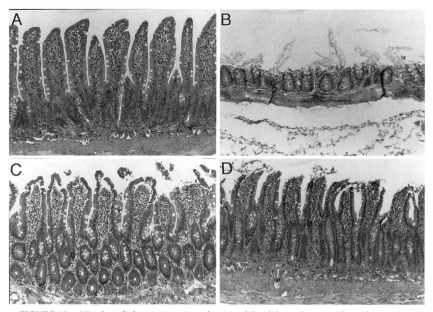

FIGURE 10.—Histologic light microscopic evaluation of distal ileum (hematoxylin and eosin; 40×) in nonburned animals. **A,** chronic oral normal saline: normal villous architecture. **B,** chronic oral ethanol: blunted and exfoliated villi. **C,** chronic IV normal saline: submucosal edema of the villi and exfoliation. **D,** chronic IV ethanol: prominent exfoliation of the villous tips. (Courtesy of Napolitano LM, Koruda MJ, Zimmerman K, et al: Chronic ethanol intake and burn injury: Evidence for synergistic alteration in gut and immune integrity. *J Trauma* 38(2):198–207, 1995.)

Results.—Oral ethanol but not IV ethanol significantly reduced the splenic mitogenic response to the T-cell mitogens concanavalin A and phytohemagglutinin. In the oral ethanol but not the IV ethanol burn group, splenic mitogenic response to the T-cell mitogens concanavalin A and phytohemagglutinin and to the B-cell mitogen lipopolysaccharide was reduced. Ileal mucosal weight was lower in both the IV and oral ethanol burn groups than in the saline burn groups. The bacterial translocation rate for oral ethanol–treated rats was 70% whereas for saline controls it was 10%. Oral ethanol significantly reduced ileal mucosal diamine oxidase activity, DNA content, and concentrations of circulating endotoxins. Oral ethanol produced significant mucosal disruption and exfoliation (Fig 10). In the burn group receiving oral ethanol, bacterial translocation rates were 80% vs. 33% for the saline-treated group, and there was a significant reduction in ileal mucosal weight, DNA content, and diamine oxidase activity.

Conclusion.—Chronic oral administration of alcohol produces changes in the immune system and in gastrointestinal function and impairs the host's ability to repair burn injuries.

▶ It is well documented that injured patients with a history of alcohol abuse have higher mortality rates and an increased incidence of infectious complications than do equally injured patients without a history of alcohol abuse. One explanation for this observation is that chronic alcohol exposure impairs intestinal barrier function and predisposes these patients to bacterial translocation and gut-origin septic states. This article was chosen because it provides experimental evidence in support of this hypothesis and indicates that the gastrointestinal tract may be a potentiator of the immune dysfunction observed after chronic alcohol ingestion.

Although the potential clinical ramifications of this study are hard to predict, it would suggest that injured patients with a history of chronic alcohol abuse would be especially likely to benefit from therapy directed at restoring intestinal barrier function, such as the institution of early enteral feeding.

E.A. Deitch, M.D.

Major Injury Leads to Predominance of the T Helper-2 Lymphocyte Phenotype and Diminished Interleukin-12 Production Associated With Decreased Resistance to Infection

O'Sullivan ST, Lederer JA, Horgan AF, Chin DHL, Mannick JA, Rodrick ML (Harvard Med School, Boston; Brigham and Women's Hosp, Boston)
Ann Surg 222:482–492, 1995 3–17

Background.—Patients with serious injuries or burns are at increased risk of infection because of impaired immune function. This impaired immunity subsequent to injury is characterized by reduced interleukin-2 (IL-2) production by T-helper (Th) lymphocytes. Naive Th cells can be induced to convert to either a Th-1 or a Th-2 phenotype. Th-1 cells produce IL-2 and interferon-γ (IFN-γ) and initiate cellular immunity. Th-2 cells secrete IL-4 and IL-10 and stimulate antibody production. Conversion to the Th-1 phenotype is stimulated by IL-12, and conversion to the Th-2 phenotype is stimulated by IL-4. It is possible that the decreased immune capability of seriously injured patients may be due to conversion of Th cells to Th-2, as opposed to generalized immune suppression. To examine this possibility, 24 trauma and burn patients were investigated along with a mouse model of burn injury with decreased resistance to infection.

Methods.—Peripheral blood mononuclear cells were examined from 16 major burn patients, 8 trauma patients, and 13 age- and sex-matched healthy controls to determine cytokine production after stimulation with phytohemagglutinin. A mouse model of 20% body surface burn injury was also examined. Splenocytes were collected from burned mice and sham-burn controls after activation with concanavalin A or bacterial antigen to determine cytokine production. Burn and control animals were treated in vivo with IL-12 and observed for response to septic challenge.

Results.—Peripheral blood mononuclear cells (PBMCs) from severely injured patients produced less IFN-γ, which is produced by Th-1–type cells, than did PBMCs from healthy controls (Fig 1) 1 to 14 days after

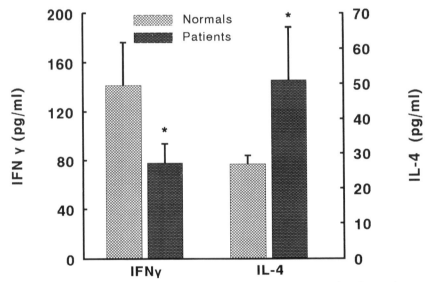

FIGURE 1.—Freshly harvested peripheral blood mononuclear cells (PBMCs) from burn and trauma patients 1 to 14 days after injury and from age- and sex-matched healthy control subjects were cultured with phytohemagglutinin and supernatants assayed for interferon-γ (IFN-γ) and interleukin-4 (IL-4). Patients' PBMCs produced significantly less IFN-γ than did PBMCs from healthy control subjects, whereas the patients' PBMCs produced significantly more IL-4 than did PBMCs from control cells (* P < 0.05). (Courtesy of O'Sullivan ST, Lederer JA, Horgan AF, et al: Major injury leads to predominance of the T helper-2 lymphocyte phenotype and diminished interleukin-12 production associated with decreased resistance to infection. *Ann Surg* 222:482–492, 1995.)

injury. However, PBMCs from severely injured patients produced increased amounts of IL-4, which is produced by Th-2–type cells, than did PBMCs from healthy controls. In the mouse model, splenocytes from burn mice had decreased IL-2 and IFN-γ production and increased IL-4 and IL-10 production than did splenocytes from controls. Splenocytes from burn mice also produced less IL-12 than did splenocytes from controls. When burn mice were treated with IL-12, mortality from sepsis was reduced 70% and IFN-γ production by splenocytes was significantly increased.

Conclusions.—Production of IL-12 is reduced and Th cells are shifted to the Th-2 phenotype, with increased production of IL-4 and IL-10, in both a mouse model of severe injury and in severely injured or burned patients. In the burn mouse model, in vivo administration of IL-12 significantly improved survival after septic challenge and restored Th-1 cytokine production. These preliminary results suggest a therapeutic role for IL-12 in the treatment of trauma and burn patients.

▶ The importance of this study is that it provides insight into the complex regulation of the immune response to thermal injury and helps explain why burn patients are immune-suppressed. Specifically, by clarifying some of the basic biology of the immune-suppressed state seen in burn patients, it provides potential avenues for therapy. The recognition that not all T lymphocytes are the same and that different T-cell subpopulations exist with different functions has helped advance our understanding of all types of injury and infection-related changes in immune function. Confusing or not, the interleukin and immune cell vocabulary is fast becoming part of our clinical vocabulary. So now it is time to add Th-1 and Th-2 cells to that vocabulary.

E.A. Deitch, M.D.

A Double-Blinded Prospective Evaluation of Recombinant Human Erythropoietin in Acutely Burned Patients
Still JM, Belcher K, Law EJ, Thompson W, Jordan M, Lewis M, Saffle J, Hunt J, Purdue GF, Waymack JP, DeClement F, Kagan R, Chen A (Augusta Regional Med Ctr, Ga; Med College of Georgia, Augusta; Washington Hospital Ctr, DC; et al)
J Trauma 38:233–236, 1995   3–18

Background.—Postburn hemolysis, surgical blood loss, disturbed metabolism, and other factors can result in severe anemia in patients with extensive burn injury. Multiple transfusions are routinely performed in such patients, but they carry the risk of disease transmission. The value of recombinant human erythropoietin (r-HuEPO) in burn victims and its capacity for reducing transfusion needs were investigated.

Methods.—Forty patients treated at 7 centers were enrolled in the double-blind, placebo-controlled, parallel group study. All had burns over

25% to 65% of their total body surface. Treatment with r-HuEPO or placebo was initiated within 72 hours of hospitalization.

Findings.—Hemoglobin, hematocrit, and reticulocyte counts did not differ between the placebo and active treatment groups. Ferritin values, serum iron measures, and total iron-binding capacity were also comparable. Treatment with r-HuEPO did not significantly reduce the need for transfusion, even though blood loss between the groups was not statistically different. Reticulocyte counts were significantly greater in patients with burns over 25% to 35% total body surface area.

Conclusions.—The administration of r-HuEPO in these acutely burned patients did not prevent postburn anemia from developing or reduce transfusion needs. Erythropoiesis was increased in smaller burns, which may warrant further research.

▶ This article was selected to illustrate that clinical trials based on a lack of basic biology but on simplistic reasoning frequently fail. If the authors had thoroughly investigated the literature prior to performing the study, they would have found evidence that erythropoietin levels are increased after thermal injury. Unfortunately, this article validates the aphorism "show me a simple answer to a complex problem and I will show you an answer that does not work."

E.A. Deitch, M.D.

4 Trauma

Introduction

This year's selections include a number of clinical articles that highlight certain concepts or support recent or changing trends in trauma care. One such topic deals with the controversy over whether the risks of a negative laparotomy are significant. This topic assumes importance because of the fact that a significant minority of laparotomies performed for blunt or penetrating trauma are nontherapeutic. The general concept of performing a laparotomy whenever one is in doubt has emerged over the past 3 decades and is based on the fact that missed injuries contribute to mortality and the assumption that a negative laparotomy is relatively benign. This latter assumption may not be fully correct based on the overall 41% perioperative complication rate reported in a prospective study of 254 trauma patients who had negative (nontherapeutic) laparotomies. The risk of postlaparotomy complications appears to persist even after discharge, as documented in a prospective study of small-bowel obstruction in the first 6 months postlaparotomy for penetrating trauma. In this study the incidence of small-bowel obstruction was 7.4% for the entire group and 2.3% in patients who underwent a nontherapeutic laparotomy. Thus these 2 studies clearly indicate that nontherapeutic laparotomies are not benign. How can the incidence of nontherapeutic laparotomies be reduced? As far as some gunshot wounds are concerned, one answer may be diagnostic laparoscopy. The next article reviewed indicates that diagnostic laparoscopy can be used successfully to decrease the rate of nontherapeutic laparotomy. In this study, 121 hemodynamically stable patients with abdominal gunshot wounds who met the study protocol (18% of all abdominal gunshot wound patients) underwent diagnostic laparoscopy. Based on the findings at laparoscopy, 79 (65%) of these 121 patients were spared a laparotomy. There were no false-negative diagnostic laparoscopies in this series, indicating that in stable patients with questionable intra-abdominal injuries, diagnostic laparoscopy is one potential method of avoiding nontherapeutic laparotomies. As illustrated in 2 articles, emergency room sonography is also an evolving diagnostic option that may ultimately aid in deciding which patients with abdominal trauma require laparotomy.

Several articles dealing with specific management issues were selected. The first article focuses on the timing of femoral fracture fixation in blunt multitrauma patients. This article questions the dogma that all femoral fractures be fixed within 24 hours of injury in all patients and stresses the importance of surgical judgment and individualized care. Although it has long been recognized that blunt trauma to the liver can be satisfactorily treated in children, the recognition that nonoperative treatment is safe in stable adult blunt trauma patients has only recently been established. For that reason, 2 articles dealing with this topic have been included. These 2 articles clearly show that in appropriately chosen patients, nonoperative therapy is the best therapy. Another area of controversy concerns the debate over ligation vs. repair of venous injuries; thus an article comparing the results of venous ligation and repair was chosen for review. The results of this large clinical series indicate that venous ligation is safe and that repair, while conceptually superior, is not mandatory to ensure limb salvage or prevent long-term extremity dysfunction. Because of their importance, an article indicating that a policy of routine vena cava filter insertion decreases the incidence of pulmonary embolism in severely injured trauma patients was chosen as well as a prospective study documenting that primary repair of colon injuries is the optimal method for treating penetrating colon injuries.

Hypotensive or deliberate under-volume resuscitation until operative control of the bleeding site can be obtained is receiving increasing attention in hypotensive patients with uncontrolled torso bleeding since this strategy appears to clinically and experimentally improve survival. For those patients with multiple injuries who survive, information on the rate of recovery and the risk of long-term disability is relatively meager. For that reason, an article providing important outcome information on multitrauma patients was included in this year's selections.

The final articles chosen deal with a potpourri of clinical and experimental topics ranging from the effect of hypotension on cytokine production to organ blood flow.

Edwin A. Deitch, M.D.

Unnecessary Laparotomies for Trauma: A Prospective Study of Morbidity

Renz BM, Feliciano DV (Grady Mem Hosp, Atlanta, Ga; Emory Univ, Atlanta, Ga)

J Trauma 38:350–356, 1995 4–1

Background.—Authorities favoring liberal indications for laparotomy in patients with penetrating trauma believe that unnecessary laparotomy is associated with minimal morbidity. Other authorities, who believe that unnecessary laparotomy is associated with substantial morbidity, feel that the incidence of such procedures can be decreased without increasing the incidence of missed injuries. To date, there are no prospective studies that provide comprehensive data on the true risks of performing unnecessary laparotomies for trauma.

Methods and Results.—Two hundred fifty-four trauma victims undergoing unnecessary laparotomy were included in a prospective case series. In 98% of the patients, a penetrating wound was the mechanism of injury. Forty-one percent of the patients had complications. These included atelectasis in 15.7%, postoperative hypertension requiring medical treatment in 11%, pleural effusion in 9.8%, pneumothorax in 5.1%, prolonged ileus in 4.3%, pneumonia in 3.9%, surgical wound infection in 3.2%, small-bowel obstruction in 2.4%, and urinary infection in 1.9%. The complication rates for the 111 patients who had an associated injury and for the 143 who did not were 61.3% and 25.9%, respectively. Complications occurred in 19.7% of the 81 patients without an associated injury and with no intraperitoneal or retroperitoneal penetration. Overall mortality was 0.8%, but mortality was unassociated with laparotomy.

Conclusions.—When complications are documented prospectively, unnecessary laparotomies for penetrating trauma are associated with significant morbidity. Current attempts to decrease the incidence of these procedures without increasing the incidence of missed injuries are appropriate.

▶ A popular surgical aphorism during my training period in the late 1970s was "never let the abdominal wall stand between you and the diagnosis." This aphorism was based on the generally held belief that a negative laparotomy was a relatively benign procedure in most patients. Like many beliefs, it was based more on remembered experience or retrospective chart reviews than on prospectively collected data. The current prospective study provides us important hard data since it is the first prospective study carried out to systematically determine the true complication rate in trauma patients undergoing nontherapeutic laparotomies. Recognition that nontherapeutic laparotomies are associated with a relatively high rate of complications (but negligible mortality) does not mean that one should necessarily operate less, but it does mean that one should consider the consequences of a negative laparotomy in deciding on the risk-benefit ratio of laparotomy in certain patients with borderline or questionable indications for laparotomy. Based on the current limitations of physical examination and the current diagnostic tests, it is clear that all surgeons will perform some nontherapeutic laparotomies, but all of us should work as hard as possible to limit these to the fewest number possible.

E.A. Deitch, M.D.

Incidence and Risk Factors for Early Small Bowel Obstruction After Celiotomy for Penetrating Abdominal Trauma
Tortella BJ, Lavery RF, Chandrakantan A, Medina D (Univ of Medicine and Dentistry of New Jersey, Newark)
Am Surg 61:956–958, 1995   4–2

Background.—Celiotomy can be complicated by early (occurring within 6 months of surgery) small-bowel obstruction (SBO), which has a reported overall incidence of 0.69%. Because peritoneal contamination has been associated with adhesions, patients experiencing penetrating abdominal trauma (PAT) may be at increased risk for SBO. The incidence of early SBO and risk factors in PAT patients were evaluated in the present report.

Patients and Methods.—Three hundred forty-one patients admitted to a level 1 trauma center between May 1991 and December 1993 were identified. All patients had undergone celiotomy for PAT. Patients surviving to discharge who were followed for at least 6 months for readmission for SBO were considered evaluable. Medical records were reviewed, and the incidence and risk factors for early SBO were analyzed.

Findings.—Two hundred ninety-eight of the 341 patients were considered evaluable. All patients undergoing celiotomy for PAT were found to be at greater risk for early SBO than were elective surgery patients. The overall incidence of early SBO in this population was 7.4%—more than 10 times the overall incidence of SBO found in general surgery patients. The lowest incidence was noted among nontherapeutic celiotomy patients (2.3%), negative celiotomy patients (4.5%), and stab wound patients (4.8%). The highest incidence was found among those with small- or large-bowel injuries (10.8%) or gunshot wounds (nearly twice the incidence of early SBO as compared with stab wounds). The risk of early SBO was not increased by a history of previous abdominal surgery, high Injury Severity Scale score, or high abdominal trauma index.

Conclusions.—Celiotomy for PAT is associated with a high incidence of early SBO. For this reason, celiotomy should be avoided among such patients whenever possible. Both surgeons and managed care managers should carefully monitor all patients undergoing celiotomy for PAT, especially those with identified risk factors. These patients may need additional medical attention should SBO be identified and would then incur higher costs. Failure to include these additional costs may result in incorrect cost and capitation estimates, thereby compromising appropriate budgeting and patient care.

▶ The message of this brief article is quite simple. Patients undergoing laparotomy for penetrating trauma have a relatively high incidence of postoperative small-bowel obstruction that greatly exceeds that observed in patients undergoing elective surgery. The importance of this study is that although all of us have had the experience of patients developing small-bowel obstruction after laparotomy for trauma, the true incidence of this complication is not well appreciated. The lesson to be learned from this study and the previous abstract is that there is no free lunch and that a laparotomy does have significant potential complications.

E.A. Deitch, M.D.

Laparoscopy in 121 Consecutive Patients With Abdominal Gunshot Wounds

Sosa JL, Arrillaga A, Puente I, Sleeman D, Ginzburg E, Martin L (Univ of Miami, Fla)
J Trauma 39:501–506, 1995   4–3

Background.—Abdominal gunshot wounds are managed by mandatory laparotomy in the United States to decrease missed intra-abdominal injuries and their associated morbidity. However, the negative laparotomy rate is high and laparotomy is associated with significant morbidity. In an effort to reduce the negative laparotomy rate, diagnostic laparoscopy (DL) has been used to examine patients with abdominal gunshot wounds. The sensitivity, specificity, and predictive value of DL were examined in a large group of stable patients with abdominal gunshot wounds.

Study Design.—Over a 2.5-year period, DL was performed in 121 consecutive abdominal gunshot wound patients who were hemodynamically stable and had no overt peritoneal penetration.

Results.—There were 42 positive and 79 negative DL findings (Fig 1). Of those with a positive DL, 39 had exploratory laparotomy. Of these, laparotomy was therapeutic in 32, nontherapeutic in 6, and negative in 1 patient. In this group the DL failure rate was less than 1%. In 3 cases with positive DL results, laparotomy was not performed because of nonbleeding liver injuries. Nontherapeutic laparotomy was avoided. There were no false-negative DL findings, delayed laparotomies, or mortality in the entire study group. The sensitivity of DL for peritoneal penetration was 100%, the specificity was 98.7%, the positive predictive value was 97.6%, and the negative predictive value was 100%. Diagnostic laparotomy had an 82% positive predictive value and a 100% negative predictive value on the need for laparotomy.

Conclusions.—In stable patients with abdominal gunshot wounds and no overt signs of peritoneal penetration, DL can be safely and effectively used to reduce the incidence of negative and nontherapeutic laparotomies.

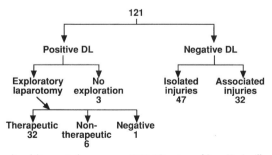

FIGURE 1.—Results of diagnostic laparoscopy (*DL*). (Courtesy of Sosa JL, Arrillaga A, Puente I, et al: Laparoscopy in 121 consecutive patients with abdominal gunshot wounds. *J Trauma* 39(3):501–506, 1995.)

A prospective, randomized study, including a cost analysis, should now be performed for this technique.

▶ This article adds more support to the argument that diagnostic laparoscopy can avoid negative and nontherapeutic laparotomies in patients with abdominal trauma, including selected patients with abdominal gunshot wounds. Because diagnostic laparoscopy is associated with a shorter hospital stay and a lower risk of early and late complications than a negative laparotomy, its use may be helpful in carefully selected patients. The term "carefully selected" is very important. In this series of gunshot patients, diagnostic laparoscopy was used only in hemodynamically stable patients with questionable abdominal injury. In the authors' series, this represented 18% of their patients with abdominal gunshot wounds. Since 65% of the patients undergoing diagnostic laparoscopy were spared a laparotomy, the use of diagnostic laparoscopy led to an overall 11% reduction in the rate of laparotomy.

Although diagnostic laparoscopy is accurate in experienced hands, caution must be exercised in patients who may have retroperitoneal injuries since these are easily missed. Thus at the current time this technique is not indicated for patients with flank or back wounds.

E.A. Deitch, M.D.

Ultrasonographic Examination of Wound Tracts
Fry WR, Smith RS, Schneider JJ, Organ CH Jr (Univ of California–Davis, East Bay)
Arch Surg 130:605–608, 1995   4–4

Introduction.—Local wound exploration to identify penetration of the peritoneum or pleura does not always yield adequate information. A pilot study was conducted to determine the feasibility of using ultrasonography as a noninvasive method of examining penetrating truncal injuries in patients with no physical or plain radiographic evidence of peritoneal or pleural violation.

Patients and Methods.—Of the 29 patients studied, 17 had gunshot wounds, 10 had stab wounds, and 2 had shotgun wounds. The abdomen was at risk for penetration in 21 cases and the thorax in 8, but physical examination and plain x-ray results suggested that the pleura or peritoneum might be intact. Wound tracts were visualized with a 7-MHz transducer, with the operator looking for soft-tissue air and/or echolucent areas consistent with blood in soft tissue. Penetration was ruled out if the entire tract was visualized or the injury appeared superficial to the deepest fascial structure in the area. For shotgun injuries, all pellets seen on x-ray films had to be identified by ultrasound in the abdominal wall.

Results.—The average time to perform wound tract exploration with ultrasonography was 2 to 3 minutes. Penetration was observed in 4 abdominal wounds (3 small-bowel injuries and a nonbleeding liver laceration) and 1 thoracic wound. The abdominal cases were confirmed at surgery and the thoracic case by chest radiography. Nonpenetration was confirmed by various means, including serial abdominal examinations over 24 hours, chest radiography, and diagnostic laparoscopy. There were no false-positive or false-negative results.

Conclusion.—Performing traditional local wound exploration by using operative techniques cannot always provide sufficient information on the extent of penetration, particularly in patients with stab wounds. Exploration of penetrating truncal injuries with ultrasound was rapidly completed with a positive and negative predictive accuracy of 100%. When used as part of the initial physical examination, ultrasound evaluation of wound tracts can be cost-effective by replacing diagnostic laparoscopy, peritoneal lavage, and repeat chest radiography.

▶ What should one do with the asymptomatic stable patient with a flank wound? This is currently a tough question because neither local exploration nor diagnostic peritoneal lavage nor CT scans are fully helpful. This small clinical series indicates that ultrasonography of the wound tract may help identify patients in whom peritoneal penetration has not occurred.

I bring this study to your attention, not because I believe that the accuracy of this approach has been established, but because I think that emergency room ultrasonography is likely to be used more frequently in the future because of its speed and relatively low cost. Thus my advice is to begin using ultrasonography, but until adequate local experience is gained with this modality, do not let it unduly influence your clinical decisions. That is, try it and see how accurate the information is compared with your current approach; then decide.

E.A. Deitch, M.D.

A Prospective Study of Emergent Abdominal Sonography After Blunt Trauma
Boulanger BR, Brenneman FD, McLellan BA, Rizoli SB, Culhane J, Hamilton P (Univ of Toronto)
J Trauma 39:325–330, 1995   4–5

Purpose.—Diagnostic evaluation of the abdomen in victims of multisystem trauma poses challenging problems. Many centers overseas use emergency abdominal ultrasonography as the initial screening test for blunt abdominal injury. In North America, however, diagnostic peritoneal lavage (DPL) and CT continue to be the gold standards. Abdominal ultrasonography was prospectively compared with DPL and CT for the evaluation of adult patients with blunt trauma.

Methods.—The study included 206 adult patients with blunt trauma who had either DPL or CT as part of their initial evaluation. Before or after these studies, the patients also underwent real-time ultrasound evaluation of the abdomen. The ultrasonographic examinations were aimed at

TABLE 2.—Comparison of Emergent Abdominal Sonography to the Gold Standard Test in the Assessment of Intraperitoneal Fluid After Blunt Trauma

| | Gold Standard (DPL or CT) | |
	(+)	(−)
US+	25	3
US−	6*	172

Note: US+, intraperitoneal fluid; US−, no intraperitoneal fluid; CT+, intraperitoneal fluid; CT−, no intraperitoneal fluid; DPL+, positive as per Advanced Trauma Life Support criteria.
* One required laparotomy.
Abbreviations: DPL, diagnostic peritoneal lavage; US, ultrasonography.
(Courtesy of Boulanger BR, Brenneman FD, McLellan BA, et al: A prospective study of emergent abdominal sonography after blunt trauma. *J Trauma* 39(2):325–330, 1995.)

the detection of intraperitoneal fluid, with no attempt to evaluate individual organs for injury.

Results.—The patients' mean Injury Severity Scale score was 24, and their mean Glasgow Coma Scale score was 12. Computed tomography was performed in two thirds of the patients and DPL in the remaining third. Abdominal ultrasonography had a positive predictive value of 90% for intraperitoneal fluid and a negative predictive value of 97%. Its sensitivity was 81%; specificity, 98%; and accuracy, 96% (Table 2). Six patients had false-negative ultrasound examinations, but only 1 of them went on to have surgery. The mean time for ultrasound examination was less than 3 minutes.

Conclusions.—For adult patients with multisystem blunt trauma, emergency abdominal untrasonography is a quick and accurate examination for the presence of intraperitoneal fluid. It may therefore be a useful screening test for abdominal injury. Emergency abdominal ultrasonography should be a routine part of the initial assessment at North American trauma centers.

▶ This prospective study indicates that the accuracy of ultrasonography is comparable to DPL and CT scanning. Ultrasonography has several attractive properties. It is fast, taking on average only 3 minutes to perform, and it can be used in unstable patients and in patients in whom DPL is contraindicated or relatively contraindicated (i.e., pregnancy, previous abdominal surgery). Other studies published in 1995, including a prospective study of 371 trauma patients,[1] support its clinical utility. With that said, what is my opinion? Cautious optimism.

E.A. Deitch, M.D.

Reference

1. Rozycki G, Ochsner, M, Schmidt A, et al: A prospective study of surgeon-performed ultrasound as the primary adjuvant modality for injured patient assessment. *J Trauma* 39:492–500, 1995.

Is the Timing of Fracture Fixation Important for the Patient With Multiple Trauma?

Reynolds MA, Richardson JD, Spain DA, Seligson D, Wilson MA, Miller FB
(Univ of Louisville, Ky)
Ann Surg 222:470–481, 1995   4–6

Background.—Multiple trauma is a major cause of death and permanent disability. In this difficult situation, the decision of which injuries must be treated immediately is of paramount importance. Prompt fixation of femoral shaft fractures has been believed to result in a reduction in pulmonary and septic complications, mortality, and length of ICU stay. Recently, evidence has accrued that immediate fracture fixation is not always optimal for these patients. The University of Louisville has permitted femoral shaft fixation to be delayed based on surgical judgment in cases of multiple trauma. The results of this variable schedule for femur fracture fixation were reviewed to determine the effect of delayed fixation on pulmonary complications and morbidity in patients with multiple trauma.

Study Design.—The outcomes of all patients hospitalized at the University of Louisville from 1983 to 1994 with a discharge diagnosis of femoral shaft fracture treated by intramedullary rod (IMR) placement were examined. Injury Severity Scale (ISS) scores were determined from discharge diagnostic codes. Of the 879 patients during this period with femur fractures, 692 had IMR placement. Of these, 424 consecutive patients were divided into 2 groups—those with an ISS score below 18 and those with an ISS score of at least 18—to determine the effect of increased injury severity and IMR placement timing on pulmonary complications, adult respiratory distress syndrome, multiple organ failure, pneumonia, severe atelectasis, mortality, sepsis, duration of mechanical ventilation, duration of ICU stay, and duration of hospital stay.

Findings.—In the group of 424 patients studied, over half the patients underwent fracture fixation within the first 24 hours. However, 40 patients had IMR placement after more than 7 days. For those patients with an ISS score below 18, there was a statistically insignificant increase in pulmonary complications with a delay in fixation. For patients with an ISS score of at least 18, there was no relationship between pulmonary complications and IMR placement. Pulmonary complications appeared to be associated with injury severity, not with timing of IMR placement. Delayed fixation was associated with a greater degree of head injury, pulmonary injury, and a higher alveolar-arteriolar gradient at admission. There was no significant association between the timing of fixation and outcome (Table 5). The only significant outcome difference was an increased length of stay in the hospital, which also appeared to be related to the severity of injury. Two deaths occurred in this group of patients. Both occurred in patients who had received IMR placement within 24 hours.

Conclusions.—Although femur fractures are an important part of the condition of multiply injured trauma patients, they are only one of many elements affecting outcome. Delays in fracture fixation did not appear to

TABLE 5.—Outcome of Patient Groups

	IMR <24 hr (n = 35)	IMR 24–48 hr (n = 13)	IMR >48 hr (n = 57)	Total (n = 105)
Age	32.7	24.7	34.6	32.8
Sex (M/F)	26/9	8/5	37/20	71/34
Mortality (%)	2(5.7)	0 (0)	0 (0)	2(1.9)
Mean hospital LOS (days)	13.7	17.3	21.9*	18.6
ICU admission (%)	62.9	38.5	73.9	65.7
ICU LOS (days)	6.7	21.9	9.4	9.4
Mechanical ventilation (%)	48.6	23.1	66.7	55.2
Ventilation days	4.9	13.0	7.1	6.7

Abbreviations: IMR, intramedullary rod placement; *LOS*, length of stay.
* $P < 0.05$ (analysis of variance) vs. IMR less than 24 hours.
(Courtesy of Reynolds MA, Richardson JD, Spain DA, et al: Is the timing of fracture fixation important for the patient with multiple trauma? *Ann Surg* 22:470–481, 1995.)

adversely affect patient outcome in severely injured patients. Outcome depended more on total injury severity than on the timing of IMR placement. Therefore, fixation of all long-bone fractures within 24 hours should not be the primary determinant of treatment for severely traumatized patients. Instead, surgical judgment should be used to determine when stabilization of the patient, treatment of other injuries, and the orthopedic reconstruction plan should be allowed to delay fracture fixation.

▶ This article stresses the underlying concept covered in some articles in last year's selections that immediate femoral fracture fixation may not be for everyone. Specifically, in some patients with severe head injury, significant pulmonary contusions, or otherwise multisystem injuries, delaying femoral fracture fixation for 2 or 3 days may be a good thing.

Although the study is retrospective and thus cannot definitely prove that delaying femoral fracture fixation of these higher-risk cases for a couple of days is good, it does provide some important information. It highlights the importance of "judgment" even when dealing with protocols. We know that weight-bearing fractures should be fixed as soon as possible. We also know that "too much" stress or surgery can be bad—witness the emergence of abbreviated damage control laparotomies in severely injured, unstable patients. Likewise, we are beginning to find out that patients with pulmonary contusions are most susceptible to the development of adult respiratory distress syndrome after internal fixation of femoral fractures. So where does that leave us? In my mind it leaves us with the concept that early fracture fixation is good, but this approach should be tempered with surgical judgment.

E.A. Deitch, M.D.

The Current Status of Nonoperative Management of Adult Blunt Hepatic Injuries

Pachter HL, Hofstetter SR (New York Univ; Bellevue Hosp, New York)
Am J Surg 169:442–454, 1995   4–7

Background.—In the last 10 years several important advances have been made in the management of hepatic injuries, including the nonsurgical treatment of selected adults with blunt hepatic trauma. Initially viewed with skepticism, this approach is now accepted as the current preferred method of management in patients meeting certain criteria. The current status of the nonoperative management of adult blunt hepatic injuries was reviewed.

Review.—Fourteen recent publications were included in this analysis. A total of 495 patients were reported. The most important inclusion criterion was hemodynamic stability. When this and other inclusion criteria were met, management was successful in 94%. There were no liver-related deaths in any of the reports. There were also no documented instances of missed enteric injuries. Delayed bleeding that resulted in laparotomy occurred in 2.8% of the patients. Mean length of hospitalization was 13 days. The mean transfusion requirement was 1.9 units of blood per patient. Computed tomography played a key role in defining the extent of the injury. With CT, other intra-abdominal injuries needing immediate laparatomy were identified. Computed tomography was also useful in following the progress of healing. Thirty-four percent of all blunt liver injuries were nonsurgically managed. As of 1993, this percentage rose to 51%.

Conclusions.—Nonsurgical management of adults with blunt hepatic injury is currently the treatment of choice for patients meeting strict inclusion criteria (Table 1). The disadvantges of this approach continue to be the possibility of a missed intra-abdominal injury or potential immediate or late hemorrhage. However, published reports indicate that bleeding complications occur in fewer than 3% of patients. Furthermore, no instances of missed bowel injury have appeared in the literature.

TABLE 1.—Criteria for Nonoperative Management of Liver Injuries
Caused by Blunt Trauma in Adults*

Hemodynamic stability
Absence of peritoneal signs
Neurologic integrity
CAT scan delineation of injury
Absence of associated intra-abdominal injuries
Need for no more than 2 hepatic-related blood transfusions
CAT scan documented improvement or stabilization with time

---

* Based on a consensus of 12 sources in the literature.
Abbreviation: CAT, computed axial tomography.
(Reprinted by permission of the publisher from Pachter HL, Hofstetter SR: The current status of nonoperative management of adult blunt hepatic injuries. *Am J Surg* 169:442–454, Copyright 1995 by Excerpta Medica Inc.)

Nonoperative Management of Blunt Hepatic Trauma Is the Treatment of Choice for Hemodynamically Stable Patients: Results of a Prospective Trial

Croce MA, Fabian TC, Menke PG, Waddle-Smith L, Minard G, Kudsk KA, Patton JH Jr, Schurr MJ, Pritchard FE (Univ of Tennessee, Memphis)
Ann Surg 221:744–755, 1995   4–8

Objectives.—The safety of nonoperative management of blunt hepatic trauma in hemodynamically stable patients was studied prospectively to determine whether severity of the injury made a difference in the success of nonoperative management and whether management failure could be predicted.

Patients and Design.—A study population of 112 hemodynamically stable patients with liver injury were compared with a control group of patients from another prospective study who had received immediate surgery for blunt liver injuries. Liver injuries were graded according to the Hepatic Injury Scale on the basis of CT scan results. Morbidity criteria included the presence of biloma, perihepatic abscess, hepatic artery pseudoaneurysm, hepatic artery–portal vein arteriovenous fistula, and length of hospitalization.

Results.—Eighty-nine percent (100 patients) of the 112 patients were successfully treated without surgery. Five of the 12 failures were liver related. Severity of the liver trauma was not a factor in the success of the nonoperative management of these patients; that is, of the 100 patients who were treated successfully without surgery, 30% had minor injuries and 70% had major injuries. The development of hemodynamic instability, but not injury grade, hemoperitoneum, or the presence of associated injuries, reliably predicted failure of nonoperative management. When compared with patients with blunt hepatic trauma who were managed with surgery, those with nonoperative management had significantly fewer blood transfusions (1.9 vs. 4.0 units) and fewer abdominal complications (3% vs. 11%). Follow-up CT scans revealed that none of the patients who were successfully treated without surgery had worsening of the liver injury and 15% had completely resolved liver injury.

Conclusions.—Nonoperative management of patients with all grades of blunt hepatic injury is feasible. These patients experience a lower incidence of abdominal complications and need fewer blood transfusions than patients with blunt hepatic trauma who are treated surgically. The ultimate development of hemodynamic instability is the only reliable predictor of failure of nonoperative management of blunt hepatic injury.

▶ As shown in Abstracts 4-7 and 4–8, the data now clearly support nonoperative treatment of selected patients with blunt trauma of the liver (see Table 1). The rationale for nonoperative therapy is based on the fact that in the majority of stable patients undergoing empirical laparotomy for hepatic injury, the laparotomy is nontherapeutic and in fact 70% or more of these liver injuries are not bleeding at the time of the laparotomy.

I chose 2 rather than 1 article for specific reasons. The first article (review of 14 retrospective studies) provides a lot of information on all facets of liver injury, including the natural history of blunt liver injuries and pitfalls in diagnosis and therapy. In fact, so much good information is contained in this first article that I recommend it highly to anyone who desires an up-to-date review of this topic. The second article was chosen because it is a prospective study and clearly documents that nonoperative management can be safely used in patients with major as well as minor liver injuries. One of the most important clinical and practical observations of this prospective study was that the development of hemodynamic instability, but *not* the CT scan appearance of the liver, was the best criterion for deciding which patients have failed nonoperative therapy and will require operative intervention.

E.A. Deitch, M.D.

Venous Injury: To Repair or Ligate. The Dilemma Revisited
Timberlake GA, Kerstein MD (West Virginia Univ, Morgantown)
Am Surg 61:139–145, 1995   4–9

Objective.—How best to manage injuries to major veins remains controversial. Accordingly, management was reviewed in 322 patients with such injuries.

Managements.—Eighty-three patients had isolated venous injuries and two thirds of them had the injured vein ligated. Of 239 patients with combined arterial and venous injuries, 71% underwent ligation. Vein injuries were repaired by either end-to-end anastomosis or lateral phlebor-rhaphy. Fasciotomy was performed as indicated. The average follow-up was 52 months.

Results.—In no patient with isolated vein injury did permanent sequelae develop, but in approximately one third of them transient limb edema developed (Table 4). Edema also occurred transiently in 36% of the patients with combined arterial and venous injuries and occurred permanently in 4 patients (2%). Whether the injured vein was ligated or repaired did not influence the occurrence of edema. No limb loss followed ligation of an injured vein.

Conclusion.—Ideally all venous injuries will be repaired, but in the civilian setting, ligation rarely leads to permanent sequelae. Vein ligation is therefore acceptable for hemodynamically unstable patients and those with extensive local injuries or associated organ injury.

▶ The debate over venous ligation vs. repair had been ongoing since the 1970s when it was shown that repair of venous injuries improved the results of arterial repair in military injuries. However, based on the present clinical series plus other smaller clinical series, it appears that this debate is more smoke than fire in civilian injuries. With the possible exception of popliteal venous injuries, vein repair is not mandatory to ensure limb salvage or

TABLE 4.—Method of Treatment and Results in 239 Patients With Combined
Venous Injury

Vein Injured	Treatment Modality*	Adjunctive Fasciotomy	None	Sequelae Transient Edema	Long Term Edema
Upper extremity (56)	Ligation (56)	0	54	2	0
	Repair (0)	0	0	0	0
Distal leg (20)	Ligation (19)	1	18	1	0
	Repair (1)	0	1	0	0
Popliteal (67)	Ligation (36)	35	1	35	4
	Repair (31)	26	15	16	0
Femoral (71)	Ligation (42)	22	21	21	0
	Repair (29)	1	18	11	0
Iliac (25)	Ligation (17)	1	13	4	0
	Repair (8)	0	8	0	0

* Ligation = 170: 59 with fasciotomy, 59 with transient edema, and 4 with permanent edema. Repair = 69; 27 with fasciotomy and 27 with transient edema.
(Courtesy of Timberlake GA, Kerstein MD: Venous injury: To repair or ligate. The dilemma revisited. *Am Surg* 61:139–145, 1995.)

prevent long-term extremity morbidity. Thus in many situations the debate over "ligation" vs. "repair" is quite similar to the famous beer debate of "less filling" vs. "more taste." So what is the take-home message? It is repair when feasible but do not hesitate to ligate when repair is not readily feasible or the patient has other injuries that require immediate or urgent attention.

E.A. Deitch, M.D.

Routine Prophylactic Vena Cava Filter Insertion in Severely Injured Trauma Patients Decreases the Incidence of Pulmonary Embolism

Rogers FB, Shackford SR, Ricci MA, Wilson JT, Parsons S (Univ of Vermont, Burlington)
J Am Coll Surg 180:641–647, 1995   4–10

Background.—Standard prophylactic measures designed to prevent pulmonary embolism are often ineffective or contraindicated in trauma patients. Patients with head injuries, spinal cord injuries, complex pelvic fractures, and hip fractures appear to be at particularly high risk for pulmonary embolism. In an attempt to decrease the incidence of this complication, physicians at the study institution have used prophylactic vena cava filters. Results were reported for 63 patients.

Methods.—Starting in July 1991, prophylactic vena cava filters were inserted percutaneously in the radiology suite in all high-risk trauma patients. Excluded were elderly patients with isolated hip fractures who could safely undergo anticoagulation if venous thromboembolism were to occur. The filters were normally inserted through the right femoral vein. Patients were followed for the development of deep vein thrombosis by weekly impedance plethysmography. Filter position and patency were checked by abdominal duplex ultrasonography 1 month after discharge, at 6 months, and then yearly.

Results.—The trauma service admitted 3,151 patients between July 1991 and July 1994. Of the 71 patients considered to be at high risk for pulmonary embolism, 63 had a prophylactic vena cava filter inserted as soon as their condition was stabilized. The mean time between admission and insertion of the filter was 4.3 days. Two cases of deep vein thrombosis developed within 48 hours of insertion and 3 cases occurred after hospital discharge. Overall, deep vein thrombosis developed in 30% of the patients with prophylactic vena cava filters, a significant reduction when compared with historical controls. There was 1 case of pulmonary embolism: an obese, 19-year-old man with a severe pelvic fracture died of a sudden, massive pulmonary embolism 10 days after fracture fixation. Five of 6 patients who did not receive the vena cava filter and in whom pulmonary embolisms developed were elderly individuals with isolated hip fractures. Patency rates for the filters were 100% at 30 days and 96.1% at 1 and 2 years.

Conclusion.—Standard prophylactic regimens do not prevent venous thromboembolism in trauma patients. The use of vena cava filters was effective in decreasing the risk of pulmonary embolism in patients at high risk for this complication, although at a high cost (approximately $5,000).

▶ The abstract of this article says it all. Nothing prevents pulmonary emboli (PEs) as well in high-risk trauma patients as prophylactic vena cava filter placement. This concept that prophylactic vena cava filter placement is the optimal way to prevent PEs is further supported by a meta-analysis of 1,102 trauma patients showing that standard deep vein thrombosis (DVT) prophylaxis does not prevent the development of DVT or PE (10% DVT/PE incidence with anticoagulation vs. 7% without anticoagulation).[1] Because PEs are found in 4% to 20% of autopsies performed on trauma patients, the prevention of fatal and nonfatal PEs is of importance. For this reason, many trauma centers, including my own, follow a liberal policy of early prophylactic vena cava insertion in high-risk trauma patients.

E.A. Deitch, M.D.

Reference

1. Upchurch G, Demling R, Davies J, et al: Efficacy of subcutaneous heparin in prevention of venous thromboembolic events in trauma patients. *Am Surg* 61:749–755, 1995.

Primary Repair of Colon Injuries: A Prospective Randomized Study

Sasaki LS, Allaben RD, Golwala R, Mittal VK (Louisiana State Univ, Shreveport; Wayne State Univ, Detroit)
J Trauma 39:895–901, 1995   4–11

Introduction.—Several retrospective investigations have indicated that primary repair may be preferable to diversion for colon injuries. A randomized prospective evaluation was performed to verify and strengthen the validity of these findings.

Methods.—Seventy-one patients with penetrating colon injuries were randomized for primary repair with or without resection and diversion. Most injuries were graded according to the Colon Organ Injury Scale (CIS). The Penetrating Abdominal Trauma Index (PATI) was used to evaluate the severity of injuries. Risk factors for adverse outcomes were measured.

Results.—Forty-three patients were treated with primary repair or resection and anastomosis and 28 patients underwent diversion. The average PATI score was 25.5 and 23.4 for the primary and diversion groups, respectively. Most injuries were CIS grades 2 or 3. There were no significant between-group differences in CIS grades. Eight patients (19%) in the primary group had colon- and non–colon-related complications (Table 8). There were 10 patients (36%) with colon-, non–colon-, and colostomy-related complications in the diversion group (see Table 8). Two patients (7%) had complications after colostomy reversal. The probability of adverse outcomes was determined to be statistically greater in the diversion group than in the primary group.

Conclusion.—Patients undergoing primary repair with and without resection had an overall lower complication rate than those in the diversion group. By adding the risk of complications associated with colostomy reversal, the complication rate for diversion is even higher. Findings indicate that primary repair can be performed on all colon injuries with a PATI score below 25 and will have a lower complication rate than diversion.

▶ Doc—will I need a bag? The answer is no because at least 5 prospective randomized trials have documented that primary repair of colon injuries is superior to fecal diversion. This is true since the risk-benefit ratio favors primary colon repair over diversion with subsequent colostomy closure even

TABLE 8.—Type of Treatment and Total Complications

Type of Treatment	Complications
Primary Repair	
Without resection (n = 31)	5 (12%)
With resection (n = 12)	3 (7%)
Diversion (n = 28)	10 (36%)

(Courtesy of Sasaki LS, Allaben RD, Golwala R, et al: Primary repair of colon injuries: A prospective randomized study. *J Trauma* 39(5):895–901, 1995.)

in the presence of gross fecal contamination and other organ system injuries. Not only is primary repair more socially humane and cost-effective, it is also associated with fewer complications. So in the absence of profound shock, coagulopathy, or hypothermia—where a damage control or abbreviated laparotomy approach may be necessary—if the colon is injured, fix it.

E.A. Deitch, M.D.

Further Experience With Transesophageal Echocardiography in the Evaluation of Thoracic Aortic Injury
Buckmaster MJ, Kearney PA, Johnson SB, Smith MD, Sapin PM (Univ of Kentucky, Lexington)
J Trauma 37:989–995, 1994   4–12

Objective.—The role of transesophageal echocardiography (TEE) in diagnosing thoracic aortic injuries was examined in a prospective series of 160 patients suspected of having blunt injury of the thoracic aorta. Transesophageal echocardiography was performed in 121 patients, most often on the basis of the chest radiographic findings alone. Thirty-nine patients had aortography.

Results.—Transesophageal echocardiography correctly identified 14 aortic injuries. Five injuries were confirmed by aortography, 7 at surgical exploration, and 2 at autopsy. In 2 other cases, the TEE findings suggested injury in patients who were found to have aortic injuries, but these findings were not diagnostic. With these exceptions, the TEE findings were 100% sensitive and specific for aortic injury. In contrast, aortography was 99% specific but had a sensitivity of only 73% because aortography had 4 false-negative studies.

Conclusions.—Aortography may no longer be the "gold standard" for diagnosing blunt injuries of the thoracic aorta. Transesophageal echocardiography is an accurate bedside method of detecting these injuries. Several patients have been operated on after TEE alone. Aortography may be done when the TEE findings are equivocal, TEE is not tolerated or is contraindicated, or other vascular injuries are suspected.

▶ Although aortography is reliable, the procedure is invasive and time-consuming and the patient must be transported from the trauma area or ICU to the x-ray department. These limitations of aortography plus the fact that only about 10% of aortograms are positive were some of the reasons for the initial evaluation of TEE. Since TEE is noninvasive and rapid and can be performed at the bedside, it has many potential advantages over aortography. Since TEE has these advantages, the next question is how accurate is TEE. Well, based on the present article and other recently published articles, at least in some hands (usually a team composed of cardiologists and trauma surgeons), TEE is very accurate for thoracic aortic injuries. However, other published studies[1] were not as positive about the accuracy of TEE as the one selected. The major difference between these 2 studies was that the incidence of indeterminate studies was much higher (17 of 114 patients vs. 2 of 160) in the study that did not find TEE to be as accurate as aortography.[1] Thus it appears that the accuracy of this test is clearly influenced by the team performing and interpreting it.

Regardless, it is important to remember that TEE cannot accurately visualize the great vessels. Thus if a subclavian or carotid artery injury is suspected, arteriography must be performed. Other contraindications to TEE are suspected esophageal injuries, severe maxillofacial injuries, and cervical spine fractures. Finally, since TEE is able to provide information on cardiac function in addition to information about aortic injury, this technique is beginning to be used in a semiroutine fashion in patients with significant blunt thoracic injury.[2]

E.A. Deitch, M.D.

References

1. Saletta S, Lederman E, Fein, S, et al: Transesophageal echocardiography for the initial evaluation of the widened mediastinum in trauma patients. *J Trauma* 39:137–142, 1995.
2. Catoire P, Orliaguet G, Liu N, et al: Systematic transesophageal echocardiography for detection of mediastinal lesions in patients with multiple injuries. *J Trauma* 38:96–102, 1995.

Improved Outcome With Fluid Restriction in Treatment of Uncontrolled Hemorrhagic Shock
Capone AC, Safar P, Stezoski W, Tisherman S, Peitzman AB (Univ of Pittsburgh, Pa)
J Am Coll Surg 180:49–56, 1995   4–13

Introduction.—Current guidelines recommend rapid infusion of crystalloid solution to quickly restore normal blood pressure in hypotensive, hemorrhaging patients before they reach the hospital. However, recent studies have challenged prehospital fluid resuscitation in treating uncontrolled hemorrhage inasmuch as fluid resuscitation or vasopressors increase bleeding and the risk of cardiac arrest or early death. The long-term effects of deliberate hypotensive treatment of uncontrolled hemorrhage were examined in this report.

Methods.—Forty rats underwent a preliminary bleed (3 mL/p100 g) followed by 75% tail amputation to produce uncontrolled hemorrhagic shock. The study had 3 phases: a "prehospital" phase comprising 90 minutes of uncontrolled bleeding with or without fluid resuscitation, followed by a "hospital" phase of 60 minutes that included treatment with lactated Ringer's (LR) solution and blood and a 3-day observation phase. The rats were divided into 4 groups: group 1 consisted of untreated controls, group 2 had no fluid resuscitation in the prehospital phase, group 3 received prehospital resuscitation to a mean arterial pressure (MAP) of

40 mm Hg, and group 4 had prehospital resuscitation to a MAP of 80 mm Hg. Groups 2, 3, and 4 all had LR and blood resuscitation to a MAP of 80 mm Hg during the hospital phase.

Results.—Untreated rats in group 1 died within 2.5 hours. In group 2, 5 rats without prehospital fluid resuscitation survived 90 minutes, but only 1 survived 3 days. All 10 rats in group 3 survived 2.5 hours and 6 were alive at 3 days. Eight rats in group 4 died within 90 minutes and all were dead at 3 days. Blood loss was 3.75 for group 1, 3.35 for group 2, 4.15 for group 3, and 8.45 mL/100 g for group 4.

Conclusions.—Data from this and other studies strongly suggest that attempting to restore normal MAP during uncontrolled hemorrhage is not possible and may actually increase mortality. Contributing factors may include acute, profound hemodilution and transient, relative hypervolemia. However, this study also suggests that patients with severe hemorrhagic shock should be given some fluid to prolong life until operative procedures can be performed. Controlled hypotension to a MAP of 40 mm Hg lessens acidemia and improves the chances for survival.

▶ This experimental study documenting that hypotensive resuscitation (i.e., resuscitation to a lower than normal MAP) results in improved long-term survival adds further support to a recent prospective clinical trial[1] and experimental studies indicating that attempts to normalize blood pressure in situations of uncontrolled hemorrhage prior to operative intervention increase blood loss, worsen acidosis, and increase mortality. The general concept behind the dangers of full-volume resuscitation before mechanical (operative) control of the bleeding site can be obtained is that the decrease in blood viscosity due to hemodilution and the increase in blood pressure and hence blood flow through the injured site will impair blood clot formation and/or disrupt any clot that has formed and result in increased blood loss.

What might this challenge to traditional aggressive volume resuscitation practices mean clinically? To me, it means that obtaining a mean arterial pressure of 50–60 mm Hg is sufficient volume resuscitation and that more aggressive volume resuscitation prior to operative control of the bleeding site may not be beneficial. Clearly, this is an area that will require further study, but for my money, the emerging data supporting the concept of hypotensive volume resuscitation seem increasingly compelling.

E.A. Deitch, M.D.

Reference

1. Bickell W, Wall M, Pepe P, et al: Immediate versus delayed fluid resuscitation for hypotensive patients with penetrating torso injuries. *N Engl J Med* 331:1105–1109, 1994.

Fatal Injuries After Cocaine Use as a Leading Cause of Death Among Young Adults in New York City

Marzuk PM, Tardiff K, Leon AC, Hirsch CS, Stajic M, Portera L, Hartwell N, Iqbal MI (Cornell Univ, New York; New York Univ)

N Engl J Med 332:1753–1757, 1995   4–14

Introduction.—Drug-related deaths include not only those from overdose but also those resulting from drug-induced altered mental states. This study examined the extent of cocaine use among New York City residents with fatal injuries.

Methods.—Of the 14,843 New York residents with fatal injuries in the period 1990–1992, 12,960 (87.3%) were tested at autopsy for the cocaine metabolite benzoylecgonine, 12,745 (85.9%) for free cocaine, and 12,976 (87.4%) for ethanol. For those aged 15 to 44, fatal injury after cocaine use was ranked with other causes of death as though it were a separate cause.

Results.—Cocaine use as measured by benzoylecgonine was found in 26.7% of the fatalities, and free cocaine was detected in 18.3%. Approximately one third of the deaths after cocaine use resulted from drug intoxication, but two thirds involved traumatic injuries resulting from homicides, suicides, traffic accidents, and falls. Among those aged 15 to 44, cocaine use ranked among the 5 leading causes of death. For those aged 15 to 24, fatal injuries after cocaine use exceeded other causes of death for all racial and ethnic groups except white women.

Discussion.—At least 1 in 4 New York City residents who died of intentional or unintentional injuries was a recent cocaine user. Cocaine itself was detected at autopsy in nearly 1 in 5 fatal injury cases. More than two thirds of those identified as cocaine users through the detection of benzoylecgonine also tested positive for active free cocaine, which suggests that most people who died shortly after using cocaine were under the influence of the drug at the time of injury.

▶ This article was chosen not just because cocaine and substance abuse is common in trauma patients, but also because cocaine use may result in severe myocardial dysfunction and hemodynamic instability. In fact, our clinical experience has incriminated cocaine use as a cause of death in some trauma patients with only moderate and theoretically survivable injuries. These patients were characterized by an inadequate hemodynamic response to volume therapy and died of refractory hypotension or myocardial failure.

E.A. Deitch, M.D.

Multiple Injuries: An Overview of the Outcome
van der Sluis CK, ten Duis HJ, Geertzen JHB (Univ Hosp, Groningen, The Netherlands)
J Trauma 38:681–686, 1995   4–15

Introduction.—Little information is available about the final functional outcome in patients with multiple injuries, how fast they recover, and how many have residual injuries. It would be helpful to have answers to these questions because many of these patients are young and their disabilities are likely to have an impact on the social security system. The functional outcome of 723 consecutive patients with multiple injuries was evaluated by measuring the degree of disability at various intervals after injury.

Methods.—The Abbreviated Injury Scale (AIS) was used to categorize each injury by body area on a severity scale of 0 to 5. This scale was used to compute the Injury Severity Scale (ISS). Data obtained from patients' records included age, sex, type of accident, mortality, AIS/ISS, length of hospital stay, discharge destination, and functional outcome at 6 weeks, 3 and 6 months, and 1 and 2 years after trauma.

Results.—The mean patient age of 545 males and 178 females was 33.4 years. The distribution of accidents was traffic, 77.2%; home, 9.3%; work, 6.2%; sports, 2.3%; and unknown causes, 4%. Of the 186 patients (25.7%) who died, 121 (65.1%) died within 48 hours of trauma. The mean ISS of nonsurvivors was 37.3 vs. 27.6 for survivors. The mean hospital stay for nonsurvivors and survivors was 6.1 and 30.4 days, respectively. Patients were discharged to home (47.1%), a rehabilitation center (29.2%), another hospital (11.2%), and a nursing home (9.7%). Patients discharged home tended to be younger and had a shorter hospital stay than those who went to a nursing home. Patients with serious injuries to the extremities or pelvic girdle were more likely to be discharged to a rehabilitation center. Patients with major head, neck, thorax, abdomen, or face injuries were more likely to be discharged home. Using the Glasgow Outcome Scale (GOS) for functional outcome, at 6 weeks after trauma, 15.6% of the survivors completely recovered (GOS 5), 36.9% had moderate disabilities (GOS 4), and 42.8% were severely disabled (GOS 3). At 6 months, these figures reflected major recuperation: GOS 5, 42.3%; GOS 4, 43.9%; and GOS 3, 10.6%. At 1 year the figures were GOS 5, 62.4%; GOS 4, 26.8%; and GOS 3, 7.6%. At 2 years the figures were GOS 5, 68.5%; GOS 4, 19.4%; and GOS 3, 7.1%. Twenty patients were comatose (GOS 2) for a mean of 87.3 days. Of these, 5 died and 15 came out of the coma but never recovered completely. Mortality was 8.2% in the elderly and 1.5% in younger patients. Surviving younger patients had more GOS 3 and 4 disabilities than elderly patients did (27.8% vs. 16.4%). The percentage of patients who recovered was similar in both age groups. At 2 years, permanent disabilities according to body area were as follows: GOS 3, 14.2% in the head and neck area, 6.5% in the thorax (spinal cord injuries), and 4.1% in the extremities; and GOS 4, 35.5% in the head and neck and 24.9% in the extremities (Fig 5).

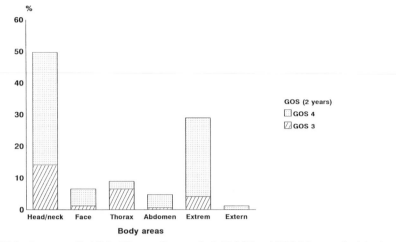

FIGURE 5.—Permanent disabilities (Glasgow Outcome Scale [*GOS*] 3 and GOS 4, 2 years after injury) of different body areas (by analogy with the Abbreviated Injury Scale). (Courtesy of van der Sluis CK, ten Duis HJ, Geertzen JHB: Multiple injuries: An overview of the outcome. *J Trauma* 38(5):681–686, 1995.)

Conclusion.—Functional outcome deteriorated linearly with increasing AIS/ISS scores in patients with multiple injuries. Two years after injury, 68% had no or mild disabilities, 19% had moderate disabilities, and 7% were severely disabled.

▶ Over the last several years, outcomes research has become a legitimate research area, even for surgeons. As the buzzwords and acronyms of business have begun to influence the daily practice of medicine, it has become more and more important for surgeons who care for trauma patients to know not just the acute but the chronic consequences of injury as well. Thus the importance of this study is that it provides some of the most complete information currently available on the rate of recovery and the long-term functional outcome of multitrauma patients.

Because of their importance, certain specific points in the article warrant repetition. First, it was not until 6 months postinjury that the majority of the patients had recovered. Second, most of the patients who recovered did so sufficiently to return to work by 1 year postinjury. Third, only 40% of the patients with an ISS score greater than 40 ever fully recovered. Finally, the authors found that the ISS was a reasonably good predictor of ultimate disability.

Knowing these few facts should allow all of us to provide better prognostic information to patients, their families, insurance companies, government agencies, and our own hospitals.

E. A. Deitch, MD

End-Diastolic Volume Versus Pulmonary Artery Wedge Pressure in Evaluating Cardiac Preload in Trauma Patients

Diebel L, Wilson RF, Heins J, Larky H, Warsow K, Wilson S (Wayne State Univ, Detroit; Detroit Receiving Hosp, Mich; Univ Health Ctr, Detroit)
J Trauma 37:950–955, 1994   4–16

Purpose.—Pulmonary artery wedge pressure (PAWP) is not always a good predictor of preload status in critically ill patients. Newer flow-directed pulmonary artery catheters with a fast-response thermistor are available for determination of right ventricular volumes and ejection fraction. The relative accuracies of right ventricular end-diastolic volume index (RVEDVI) and PAWP were compared for use in determining cardiac preload.

Methods and Results.—Thirty-two trauma patients were studied. A total of 238 measurements of RVEDVI, PAWP, and cardiac index (CI) were made with a modified pulmonary artery catheter. The initial mean values were 99 mL/m^2, 14.8 mm Hg, and 3.4 L/min/m^2, respectively. There was a better correlation between CI and RVEDVI than between CI and PAWP or CI and central venous pressure (CVP). Eighty-four studies in 19 patients showed a high PAWP despite a low or midrange RVEDVI, and another 12 studies showed a high RVEDVI with a relatively low PAWP. The information provided by PAWP was therefore different from that provided by RVEDVI in 35% of the cases. Preload was increased in 65 cases; CI responded by 20% or more in 40% of these. The PAWP did not affect the incidence of response, but the response rate became lower at increasing levels of RVEDVI: 64% at an RVEDVI of less than 90 mL/m^2, 27% at an RVEDVI of 90 to 140 mL/m^2, and 0% at an RVEDVI of greater than 140 mL/m^2 (Table 5).

Conclusions.—In critically ill patients, RVEDVI correlates better with CI and stroke volume index than does CVP or PAWP. It also provides more accurate predictions of preload recruitable increases in CI than PAWP

TABLE 5.—Incidence of an Increase of 20% or Greater in Cardiac Index After a Preload Increase at Various Pulmonary Artery Wedge Pressures and Right Ventricular End-Diastolic Volume Index Levels

PAWP	RVEDVI (mL/M^2)			
(mmHg)	< 90	90–140	>140	Totals
>18	57% (7)	50% (10)	—	53% (17)
12–18	70% (10)	22% (18)	0 (5)	33% (33)
<12	63% (8)	17% (6)	0 (1)	40% (15)
Totals	64% (25)*	27% (34)	0 (6)	40% (65)

Note: Numbers in parentheses are the numbers of times that the preload was increased from that PAWP/RVEDVI combination. Percentages are the percentages of times the cardiac index increased by 20% or more in response to the increased preload.
* $P < 0.05$.
Abbreviations: PAWP, pulmonary artery wedge pressure; RVEDVI, right ventricular end-diastolic volume index.
(Courtesy of Diebel L, Wilson RF, Heins J, et al: End-diastolic volume versus pulmonary artery wedge pressure in evaluating cardiac preload in trauma patients. *J Trauma* 37(6):955–955, 1994.)

does. Right ventricular volume monitoring data provide valuable information for hemodynamic decision making.

▶ Although in general PAWP measurements are exceedingly helpful in assessing volume status and in making clinical decisions about fluid therapy, PAWP measurements are less accurate in the critically ill. As suggested in this article, direct measurement of RVEDVI allows a more accurate assessment of volume status and hence is a better predictor than PAWP measurement of which patients will respond to fluid therapy with an increase in their cardiac output. This observation is not surprising since according to Starling's law, cardiac volume (i.e., RVEDVI) and not pressure (PAWP) is the key determinant of cardiac output.

Thus in the subgroup of critically ill patients receiving high levels of positive end-expiratory pressure or those with significant pulmonary dysfunction, RVEDVI measurements may provide better information than PAWP does on volume status.

E.A. Deitch, M.D.

Gastric Mucosal pH Oxygen Delivery and Oxygen Consumption Indices in the Assessment of Adequacy of Resuscitation After Trauma: A Prospective, Randomized Study

Ivatury RR, Simon RJ, Havriliak D, Garcia C, Greenbarg J, Stahl WM (New York Med College, Bronx)
J Trauma 39:128–136, 1995   4–17

Background.—There is controversy as to the importance of maximizing oxygen delivery during resuscitation after major trauma. Data suggest that normalization of gastric mucosal pH (pHi) may be a useful marker of the adequacy of resuscitation. The tissue-specific indicator pHi was compared with the global oxygenation indices oxygen delivery index (DO_2I) and oxygen consumption index (VO_2I) as resuscitation end points in patients with moderately severe trauma.

Methods.—The prospective, randomized study included 27 trauma patients with significant hypotension in the prehospital or early hospital phase, an Injury Severity Scale of greater than 25, an initial base deficit of worse than 5 mmol/L, or an initial lactate level of greater than 4 mmol/L. During resuscitation, 11 patients (group 1) were assigned to normalization and maintenance of pHi at or greater than 7.30. A gastrointestinal tonometer was used to estimate pHi. The remaining 17 patients (group 2) were assigned to maintenance of DO_2I at 600 and VO_2I at greater than 150. The 2 groups were similar in their indicators of trauma severity.

Results.—By 24 hours after admission, the goals of treatment were achieved in 10 of 11 patients in group 1 and in 15 of 16 patients in group 2. There was 1 death in group 1 for a mortality rate of 9%. This patient's pHi stabilized transiently at 7.3, after which mucosal acidosis developed and persisted. Nine of 10 patients whose pHi exceeded 7.3 at 24 hours survived. In group 2, the mortality rate was 31%. Four of the 5 deaths occurred in patients who met the Do_2I and Vo_2I goals but whose pHi was less than 7.3 at 24 hours.

In a comparison of the time needed to stabilize different variables, pHi and lactate were the variables that differed between survivors and non-survivors. Multiple organ dysfunction syndrome occurred in 8 patients, 6 of whom had a pHi of less than 7.3 at 24 hours. A persistently low pHi was noted at the initial sign of intra-abdominal abscess, intra-abdominal hypertension, bacteremia, small-bowel gangrene or pregangrene, and intestinal anastomotic leak. Furthermore, persistently low pHi was the initial finding in all nonsurvivors and occurred at least 72 hours before death.

Conclusions.—In trauma patients, pHi appears to be a valuable marker of the adequacy of resuscitation. Tissue-specific monitoring of pHi may provide early warning of the development of systemic complications in the period after resuscitation. It also has important prognostic implications.

▶ Based on the results of this study and other published clinical trials showing that gastric mucosal pHi is a better predictor of outcome than global oxygen delivery indices, it appears that gut mucosal pHi may be the "canary" of the body, and when it stops singing (i.e., pHi drops), trouble may be brewing. The attractiveness of measuring gut mucosal oxygen delivery, as reflected by the pHi, is that the splanchnic bed is among the first vascular beds to show hypoperfusion during shock and the last to recover to normal after resuscitation. However, there is a fly in the ointment. That is, there is a lack of data documenting that having this measurement influences outcome. Thus a decision on whether gastric mucosal pHi measurements should become a routine parameter to monitor will depend on further studies showing that having this information makes a clinical difference.

E.A. Deitch, M.D.

Transmural Gut Oxygen Gradients in Shocked Rats Resuscitated With Heparan
Zabel DD, Hopf HW, Hunt TK (Univ of California, San Francisco)
Arch Surg 130:59–63, 1995   4–18

Introduction.—A wide variety of insults including thermal injury, trauma, hemorrhagic shock, ionizing radiation, bowel obstruction, and arterial hypoxia have been shown to cause intestinal mucosal damage and translocation of bacteria. Recent data have suggested that infusion of heparan sulfate may enhance tissue oxygenation and preserve gut function. This study measured transmural gut tissue Po_2 to determine the gradient from serosa to mucosa during normovolemia and hypovolemia in an animal model.

Methods.—Sixteen adult male rats were divided into 4 groups. Fluorescent tissue oxygen sensors were attached to the serosal and mucosal surfaces of rat colon. Hemorrhagic shock was induced by using a fixed-pressure model, and the animals were resuscitated with saline solution or heparin. Temperature, mean arterial pressure, and tissue oxygen tensions were continuously monitored, and measurements were recorded at 5- or 15-minute intervals.

Results.—Serosal and mucosal tissue oxygen tensions (PO_2) were stable in control animals (64 ± 4 and 10 ± 2 mm Hg, respectively). Baseline serosal PO_2 decreased to 37 ± 2 mm Hg in shocked animals at a mean of 19 ± 7 minutes after hemorrhage was initiated, whereas mucosal values decreased to a minimum of 4 ± 2 mm Hg at 45 ± 15 minutes after hemorrhage initiation. Serosal PO_2 returned to baseline in both control and heparan-resuscitated rats; however, mucosal PO_2 baseline values were not restored in the shock/no-heparan group. Mucosal PO_2 rose above baseline (13 ± 3 mm Hg) 3 hours after completion of hemorrhage in heparan-resuscitated animals.

Conclusions.—Mucosal PO_2 is much lower than serosal PO_2 across the colon, and both values decrease during hypovolemia. The PO_2 values of the entire gut wall are in a range that impairs phagocytic killing by hypoxia. Mucosal PO_2 was improved during heparan administration. The use of heparan may restore and/or protect gut function through tissue oxygen-related mechanisms. Further research is needed to evaluate the influence of hypoxia alone on gut functions, including permeability and bacterial translocation.

▶ The value of this basic science paper on gut oxygen (PO_2) levels during shock is 2-fold. First, it shows that gut mucosal PO_2 levels drop profoundly during the shock period and that even with adequate volume resuscitation, gut mucosal PO_2 values do not return to normal. Second, it documents that mucosal PO_2 levels dropped below the critical level (i.e., 5–10 mm Hg) required for host cell aerobic energy production and bactericidal activity. Taken together, these two facts help explain why the gut is so susceptible to injury during stress states and also helps explain the phenomenon of bacterial translocation.

Additionally, the ability of the "rheologically active" substance heparan to allow mucosal PO_2 to return to normal may have important clinical implications since this agent can be administered clinically. This concept of giving adjuvant agents to limit potential organ injury during volume resuscitation is discussed in more detail in the burn article section.

E.A. Deitch, MD

Hypoxemia in the Absence of Blood Loss or Significant Hypotension Causes Inflammatory Cytokine Release

Ertel W, Morrison MH, Ayala A, Chaudry IH (Michigan State Univ, East Lansing)

Am J Physiol 269:R160–R166, 1995   4–19

Introduction.—Experimental studies of hemorrhagic shock have demonstrated a rise in circulating levels of the proinflammatory cytokines tumor necrosis factor α (TNF-α), interleukin (IL)-1β, and IL-6. It is not known, however, whether hypoxemia in the absence of blood loss leads to alterations in macrophage cytokine release and blood levels of cytokines. Researchers exposed mice to nonlethal hypoxia to assess the release of TNF-α, IL-1β, and IL-6 by different macrophage populations and to identify changes in blood levels of these mediators.

Methods.—The experiment used 6- to 8-week-old male C3H/HeN mice that were placed in a plastic box flushed with a gas mixture containing 95% N_2–5% O_2 at a flow rate of 10 L/min. The mice were returned to room air after 60 minutes. Control animals were placed in a plastic box flushed with room air. The mice were killed by ether overdose immediately after hypoxemia and at 2 or 24 hours after hypoxic exposure. Blood samples were obtained and peritoneal macrophages were harvested at these time points and both assayed for TNF-α, IL-1β, and IL-6.

Results.—When compared with the control animals, those with induced hypoxemia had elevated levels of circulating TNF—immediately and at 2 and 24 hours. Hypoxemia also induced a significant increase in circulating IL-6 (313% at 24 hours) as compared with control animals; plasma IL-6 levels did not differ significantly in the 2 groups at 0 and 2 hours (Fig 2). In addition, the release of TNF-α, IL-1β, and IL-6 by peritoneal macrophages and Kupffer cells was significantly increased after hypoxemia as compared with control conditions.

Conclusion.—In this animal model, hypoxemia itself, without severe hypotension or blood loss, induced marked synthesis and release of proinflammatory cytokines by different macrophage populations. Because this effect may contribute to systemic inflammation, lengthy periods of hypoxemia should be avoided in trauma patients. Early intubation and ventilation after traumatic injury may help reduce or eliminate additional cytokine release.

▶ This experimental study was chosen because it illustrates the important concept that limited periods of hypoxia (as well as other insults) can prime macrophages such that they have an exaggerated cytokine response upon subsequent stimulation. The clinical relevance of this basic observation is that it could help explain why some patients who sustain a modest insult may develop a much more profound systemic inflammatory response or more severe organ dysfunction after a second or subsequent insults than would otherwise be expected. This concept of a mild nonlethal insult priming the host such that an exaggerated inflammatory response occurs after a

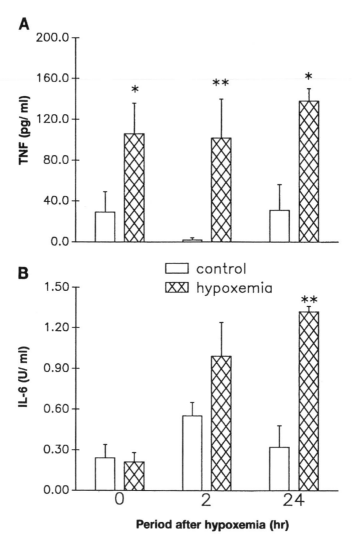

FIGURE 2.—Circulating tumor necrosis factor (*TNF*; **A**) and interleukin-6 (*IL-6*; **B**) plasma levels. Plasma was obtained from hypoxemic (n = 5) and sham (n = 5) animals at 0, 2, or 24 hours after the insult. Plasma levels of TNF were measured with an enzyme-linked immunosorbent assay, and IL-6 plasma levels were determined with a bioassay using the IL-6–specific cell line 7TD1. Data are means ± SE. *P < 0.05, **P < 0.01 for hypoxemic vs. sham control. (Courtesy of Ertel W, Morrison MG, Ayala A, et al: Hypoxemia in the absence of blood loss or significant hypotension causes inflammatory cytokine release. *Am J Physiol* 269:R160–R166, 1995.)

second insult is known as the 2-hit model of organ failure. Thus this study and others like it imply that preventing small insults in a high-risk patient may make a big difference.

E.A. Deitch, M.D.

A Monoclonal Antibody to P-Selectin Ameliorates Injury Associated With Hemorrhagic Shock in Rabbits

Winn RK, Paulson JC, Harlan JM (Univ of Washington, Seattle; Cytel Corp, San Diego, Calif)
Am J Physiol 267:H2391–H2397, 1994   4–20

Introduction.—Reperfusion injuries are leukocyte dependent and can be almost ameliorated with monoclonal antibodies (MAbs). The roles of CD62P (P-selectin) and CD18 in hemorrhagic shock and resuscitation were investigated.

Methods.—Catheters were placed in the femoral artery and femoral vein in anesthetized New Zealand White rabbits. The arterial catheter was used for thermal dilution cardiac output determinations and systemic pressure measurements. The venous catheter was used to inject drugs, fluid, and cold saline. After stabilization, cardiac output was reduced to 33% of baseline by removal of blood into syringes. After 1.5 hours, resuscitation was initiated by infusion of shed blood and warmed lactated Ringer's solution until cardiac output reached 90% of baseline. At the time of resuscitation, 6, 7, 6, and 6 animals were treated with saline, the anti-CD18 MAb 60.3, the anti-CD62P MAb PB1.3, or the isotype-matched control MAb PNB1.6, respectively.

Results.—No significant differences were noted between the saline- and MAb PNB1.6–treated groups. These 2 groups acted as controls. The MAb PB1.3– and MAb 60.3–treated groups required significantly less fluid resuscitation, than did the control groups (Fig 2).

Conclusion.—Blocking neutrophil adherence with either an anti-CD18 or anti-CD62P MAb results in protection from the injury of hemorrhagic shock. It is likely that the anti-CD18 MAb does this by preventing firm adherence to the endothelium. The anti-CD62P MAb most likely prevents leukocyte rolling. Inhibition of this adherence cascade was effective enough to reduce leukocyte-mediated vascular injury. These findings are compatible with the therapeutic benefit of anti-CD18 or anti-CD62P treatment of hypotensive trauma patients.

▶ The concepts behind this study are quite simple. First, hemorrhagic shock can be viewed as a global example of the ischemia/reperfusion syndrome; ischemia occurs during the shock period and reperfusion occurs with volume resuscitation. Second, the ischemia/reperfusion injury is mediated by leukocytes that bind to activated endothelial cells. Finally, for leukocyte-mediated endothelial cell and subsequent organ injury to occur, the leukocytes must bind to the endothelial cells, and this occurs through an increasingly well-described series of cell-cell receptor interactions. Within this context, the current study documented that monoclonal antibodies directed against leukocyte (CD18) or endothelial cell (CD62P) adhesion molecules will improve outcome in animals subjected to hemorrhagic shock. A major strength of this

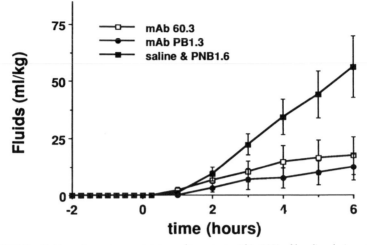

FIGURE 2.—Fluid requirements to maintain cardiac output within 90% of baseline during a 6-hour resuscitation period. The groups treated with monoclonal antibody (*MAb*) directed to functional epitopes of either CD18 or CD62P were both significantly different from the combined saline- and nonfunctional CD62P MAb PNB1.6–treated group. There were no differences between the 2 groups treated with functional MAbs. (Courtesy of Winn RK, Paulson JC, Harlan JM: A monoclonal antibody to P-selectin ameliorates injury associated with hemorrhagic shock in rabbits. *Am J Physiol* 267:H2391–H2397, 1994.)

article is that the monoclonal antibodies were given with the resuscitation fluid and *after* the 90-minute shock period. Thus the model is clinically relevant.

E. A. Deitch, M.D.

5 Infection

Introduction

Traditionally, prophylactic antibiotics are given only for clean-contaminated operations. They are therapeutic for contaminated or dirty operations, and antibiotic prophylaxis is traditionally not used for clean operations. In 1990 an article appeared that suggested using antibiotics for clean operations. A paper from McGill University, Montreal, Quebec, Canada (Abstract 5–5), also suggests using prophylactic antibiotics for clean operations, although the authors considered cholecystectomy, usually regarded as a clean-contaminated operation, to be a clean procedure. Using prophylactic antibiotics for clean operations continues to be controversial.

With over 50% of surgical procedures in the United States being done on an outpatient basis, it is difficult to obtain reliable wound infection data. A paper from Brazil (Abstract 5–6) monitors patients for wound infections in the outpatient clinic. Even with this method, wound infections might have been missed because patients failed to return for clinic visits or their wound infections might not have become evident until after their clinic visits. Wound infections are expensive when measured by either increased hospital stay or cost. Another study from Canada (Abstract 5–7) finds that postoperative wound infections increase patient stay an average of 19.5 days longer than that of control patients. Class III and class IV wounds have traditionally been left open to heal by secondary intention or by delayed primary closure. There has been a recent tendency to close some class III or class IV wounds. Primary closure is compared with leaving the wound open (Abstract 5–7). It is clear that leaving wounds open is associated with a lower wound infection rate and a shorter hospital stay.

Health care workers are at risk for hospital-acquired viral infections such as HIV, hepatitis C, and hepatitis B. Investigators from the University of Pittsburgh (Abstract 5–8) examined the prevalence of hepatitis B among their health care workers. Five of 241 tested had antibody to hepatitis C. Four of the 5 worked in the liver transplant division, where hepatitis C is common. Three of the 5 may have had hepatitis C before entering the study.

Acute pancreatitis may progress to pancreatic necrosis, which may then become infected, a problem associated with a high mortality rate. A study from the Netherlands (Abstract 5–10) demonstrates that selective bowel decontamination can lead to a lower incidence of pancreatic infection. The treatment of infected pancreatic necrosis remains controversial. One study (Abstract 5–11) compared open packing with closed drainage in patients with this condition. Open packing resulted in lower mortality than closed catheter drainage. There is a movement to treat patients with this disease by open packing.

Hepatic abscess continues to be a problem. Radiologists have an increasing role in the diagnosis and treatment of this disease (Abstract 5–12). In fact, surgeons may be entirely bypassed in the diagnosis and treatment of hepatic abscess. Only a small percentage of patients ultimately require surgical drainage. Alveolar hydatid disease frequently involves the liver. An article from Alaska (Abstract 5–13) contains the most complete description of the pathophysiology, surgical treatment, chemotherapy, and complications of infections by *Echinococcus*. While most patients in this study were Eskimos, this infection can also be seen in the central United States and, because of the importation of infected foxes into the Southeast, may be seen in this region as well.

Necrotizing soft tissue infections continue to be a challenge for the surgeon. An analysis of cases from Cleveland, Ohio (Abstract 5–14), found that only the time between admission and surgery was associated with mortality. Certainly there are numerous parameters that may affect mortality in these patients. But these authors found that only this interval was important.

Postoperative toxic shock syndrome, although exceedingly rare, can occur after surgical procedures. Twelve patients with postoperative toxic shock syndrome were identified during a 13-year period at Southern Illinois University School of Medicine (Abstract 5–1). All patients survived.

One paper (Abstract 5–2) analyzes the Gram stain and culture results of bile obtained at cholecystectomy. While organisms were cultured from 23.3% of the bile specimens, it is still not clear whether Gram staining and culturing the bile are valuable. A concern with the ever-increasing use of antibiotics is the development of bacterial resistance. Bacterial resistance was analyzed over a 12-year period in specimens obtained from patients with intraperitoneal infections (Abstract 5–3). The authors found that there was no change in the antibacterial susceptibility spectrum.

The number of patients with *Clostridium difficile* colitis has increased substantially over the past 10 years (Abstract 5–4). Most of this increase is due to the wide use of perioperative antibiotic prophylaxis, again emphasizing the need to use antibiotic prophylaxis only where indicated and for a short duration.

Richard J. Howard, M.D., Ph.D.

Postoperative Toxic Shock Syndrome

Graham DR, O'Brien M, Hayes JM, Raab MG (Springfield Orthopaedic Center, Ill; Southern Illinois Univ, Springfield)
Clin Infect Dis 20:895–899, 1995   5–1

Background.—Postoperative wound infections are rare, but they can lead to postoperative toxic shock syndrome (PTSS). The purpose of this retrospective study was to determine the risk factors for PTSS at a community hospital from 1981 to 1993.

Methods.—All patients at a community teaching hospital who had symptoms of PTSS related to postsurgical infection but not to tampon use were identified. Toxin production was evaluated in the *Staphylococcus aureus* samples of 11 patients.

Results.—Twelve patients with PTSS were found over this time period. The operations performed and the surgical teams involved varied from patient to patient. The clinical picture was classic in that all 12 had a rash. Eleven patients had a fever, 11 had desquamation, and 10 demonstrated hypotension. Nine Gram stains showed gram-positive cocci, and 11 cultures revealed the presence of *S. aureus,* but the blood cultures of all were negative. The mean time to the onset of symptoms was 4 days. The temperature peaked at 38.4°C 5 days postoperatively. The antibiotic treatment given initially was based on Gram stain results, and this was adjusted depending on susceptibility reports. After the clinical symptoms resolved, 8 patients were given 1 of the following antibiotics: dicloxacillin, erythromycin, or amoxicillin/clavulanic acid. Fluid replacement and wound débridement were also integral to the treatment of these patients.

Discussion.—Postoperative toxic shock syndrome is believed to be underreported. The signs and symptoms are easily overlooked in the early stages, and wound openings should always be cultured, especially in the presence of other symptoms. Physicians also need to be aware that because of early discharge and the potential 4-day lag period before the appearance of clinical signs and symptoms, this complication may not be manifested until after the patient is released. The very low incidence of PTSS does not warrant routine perioperative prophylaxis. Because the patients in this study had low or zero antibody titers to enterotoxin F, which is uncharacteristic of the general population, measurement of such titers may be a method of screening patients susceptible to PTSS, which then can be treated prophylactically. When PTSS is diagnosed, immunotherapy should be initiated. In summary, although the risk for PTSS is only 0.003% per operation, early recognition is essential and PTSS should be included in the differential diagnosis for any febrile postoperative patient with a surgical wound.

▶ This article was included to emphasize that although exceedingly rare, postoperative toxic shock syndrome caused by *Staphylococcus aureus* can occur after a variety of surgical procedures. Wound botulism and tetanus are other exceedingly rare, but potentially devastating infections (really, intoxications) that can occur in the postoperative period. Although all the patients in this series survived, they required vigorous fluid resuscitation and intensive support of care. Toxic shock syndrome was first described in 1978 among 7 children with infection caused by S. aureus.[1] In 1980 toxic shock syndrome received much publicity when its association with the use of tampons was identified.[2] Shortly thereafter, toxic shock syndrome was also reported in association with postoperative wound infection.

R.J. Howard, M.D., Ph.D.

References

1. Todd J, Fishaut M: Toxic-shock syndrome associated with phase-group-I staphylococci. *Lancet* 2:1116–1118, 1978.
2. Symposium: The toxic shock syndrome. *Ann Intern Med* 96:831–996, 1982.

Association of Positive Bile Cultures With the Magnitude of Surgery and the Patients' Age

Samy AK, MacBain G (Garrick Hosp, Stranraer, Scotland; Southern Gen Hosp, Glasgow, Scotland)
J R Coll Surg Edinb 40:188–191, 1995   5–2

Introduction.—A relationship between the presence of gallstones and bacteria in the bile has been suspected. Cholic and deoxycholic acids are thought to have some antimicrobial properties, with gallstone formation and infection occurring when concentrations of these bile acids are low. In previous studies, positive bile cultures have been reported in 60% of the patients who underwent cholecystectomies. However, the significance of positive bile cultures in patients undergoing elective, uncomplicated cholecystectomies has not been evaluated. The presence of positive bile cultures was evaluated in relationship to the type of surgery and patient age, and the microorganisms isolated were reviewed.

Methods.—Results of bile cultures taken from 366 patients after elective uncomplicated gallbladder surgery were reviewed and the types of organisms isolated recorded. Surgical procedures were classified as cholecystectomy only, cholecystectomy with operative cholangiography, and chole-

TABLE 1.—Positive Bacteriologic Films

Type of Organisms	Number (%)
Gram-negative bacilli	33 (49.2)
Gram-positive cocci	22 (32.8)
Mixed organisms	9 (13.4)
Gram-positive bacilli	3 (4.2)
Total positive films	67 (18.3)

(Courtesy of Samy AK, MacBain G: Association of positive bile cultures with the magnitude of surgery and the patient's age. *J R Coll Surg Edinb* 40:188–191, 1995, Blackwell Science Ltd.)

TABLE 2.—Positive Bacteriologic Cultures

Order	Organism	Occurrence	%
1	*E. coli*	33	45.2
2	Streptococci	12	16.4
3	*Cl. welchii*	11	15.1
4	Klebsiella	7	9.6
5	*Strep. faecalis*	7	9.6
6	Bacteroides	6	8.2
7	Coliform	5	6.8
8	Staphylococci	5	6.8
9	Citrobacter	4	5.5
10	Diphteroid	2	2.7
11	Enterobacter	2	2.7
12	Hafnia	2	2.7
13	*Cl. fragilis*	1	1.4
14	Salmonella	1	1.4
15	Lactobacillus	1	1.4
16	Acinetobacter	1	1.4
17	*Candida albicans*	1	1.4
	Total	73	19.9

(Courtesy of Samy AK, MacBain G: Association of positive bile cultures with the magnitude of surgery and the patients' age. *J R Coll Surg Edinb* 40:188–191, 1995, Blackwell Science Ltd.)

cystectomy with exploration of the common bile duct. Patient age and the rate of positive culture for each type of surgery were determined.

Results.—Gram staining, performed before culture, found 33 cases to have gram-negative bacilli, 22 to have gram-positive cocci, 3 with gram-positive bacilli, and 9 with mixed organisms (Table 1). Seventy-three of the 366 cases were found to have a positive culture, with a single organism isolated in 51. Two organisms were isolated in 17 and 3 or more organisms in 5. *Escherichia coli*, the most common organism isolated, was found in 33 cases (Table 2). Streptococci were found in 12 cases, followed by *Clostridium welchii* in 11 and *Klebsiella* in 7. When evaluated by the type of surgical procedure, positive cultures were found in 48 (17.5%) cholecystectomies, 17 (23.6%) cholecystectomies with cholangiography, and 8 (44.4%) cholecystectomies with exploration of the common bile duct. Positive cultures were also significantly associated with an increase in patient age, with a 6% incidence in patients between 50 and 59 years and 75% for patients 80 years or older.

Conclusion.—*Escherichia coli*, streptococci, clostridia, and *Klebsiella* were the organisms most commonly isolated. Age was found to be significantly associated with positive culture, with an increase in age more likely to result in a positive culture. Although a higher incidence of positive cultures was found in cholecystectomy with exploration of the common bile duct as compared with cholecystectomy alone or cholecystectomy with cholangiography, when adjusted for age, no significant association between positive cultures and the type of surgery was found.

▶ Culturing and obtaining a Gram stain of bile during cholecystectomy are routine practice of many surgeons. Reasons for this practice include knowing what organisms are present if postoperative infection develops or treating the patient with penicillin if gram-positive rods (*Clostridium* species) are identified on Gram stain. Others criticize this practice because only 50% of wound infections that occur after cholecystectomy are due to the organisms cultured in the bile and because Gram stain can only identify bacteria in concentrations greater than 10^5 organisms/mL. Thus *Clostridium* might be present in bile specimens but not identified by Gram staining techniques. Therefore, even if it is appropriate to give penicillin to patients who have *Clostridium* species in their bile, many (there is no evidence that routine prophylactic antibiotics are not sufficient) patients would be untreated. This paper provides some data to help answer these questions. Of the 366 patients whose bile was sampled, only 3 had gram-positive bacilli detected on Gram stain, and *Clostridium welchii* was cultured from 11. Thus surgeons whose practice it is to give penicillin to patients with gram-positive bacilli identified by Gram stain would miss most of the patients who have gram-positive bacilli in their bile. Unfortunately, the authors provided no information about wound infections in these patients.

R.J. Howard, M.D., Ph.D.

Surgical Sepsis: Constancy of Antibiotic Susceptibility of Causative Organisms
Krepel CJ, Gohr CM, Edmiston CE, Condon RE (Med College of Wisconsin, Milwaukee)
Surgery 117:505–509, 1995   5–3

Introduction.—It is well documented that antibiotic therapy can lead to bacterial resistance. There is evidence that in the intestine this resistance may be transmitted by plasmids. The purpose of this investigation was to determine the rate of antibiotic resistance in abdominal surgery.

Methods.—Wet swab specimens and abscess fluid were obtained from 255 patients with abdominal infections primarily caused by intra-abdominal abscess or gastrointestinal perforation. Patients who had been given antibiotics 3 days or sooner before surgery were excluded. The major bacterial strains used for susceptibility testing were *Escherichia, Bacteroides, Gemella, Streptococcus, Pseudomonas, Clostridium, Peptostreptococcus, Porphyromonas, Fusobacterium, Klebsiella, Enterobacter, Proteus, Prevotella, Enterococcus,* and *Klebsiella.* They were tested against the following antibiotics: all generations of the cephalosporins, animoglycosides, β-lactams, clindamycin, chloramphenicol, imipenem, and metronidazole.

Results.—A comparison of the swab and the fluid specimens showed no significant differences, except that specimens from patients with ischemic small bowels showed an increase in the number of aerobic organisms in their fluid samples. No changes in resistance or susceptibility were apparent for any of the drugs when tested against any of the antibiotics.

Discussion.—Resistant bacterial strains are found in the feces of most individuals, and one suggested method of conferring resistance is that metal ion pressure can promote plasmid acquisition. However, this study shows that the susceptibility of these endogenous strains to appropriate antimicrobial therapy is stable. Therefore, because of the low resistance, standard first-line antibiotic treatment is appropriate initial therapy for community-acquired abdominal infections.

▶ Bacterial resistance can develop in response to selective antibiotic pressure. This bacterial resistance is frequently cited as one of the reasons for avoiding antibiotic therapy except where absolutely needed and keeping the use of prophylactic antibiotics brief. This paper examines changes in antibiotic resistance occurring in specimens obtained from intra-abdominal infections over a 12-year period. There were consistent bacterial susceptibility patterns over this period. The consistency of bacterial sensitivity shows that first-line antibiotic therapy is appropriate for community-acquired infections unless antibiotic resistance can be demonstrated. Most instances of bacterial resistance are due to bacteria isolated from hospital-acquired infections. Most intra-abdominal infections are likely to have originated before the patient entered the hospital. This does not mean that we should not be careful in our use of antimicrobial agents to treat infections.

R.J. Howard, M.D., Ph.D.

Clostridium difficile Colitis: An Increasing Hospital-Acquired Illness

Jobe BA, Grasley A, Deveney KE, Deveney CW, Sheppard BC (Oregon Health Sciences Univ, Portland; VA Medical Ctr, Portland, Ore)
Am J Surg 169:480–483, 1995   5–4

Objective.—*Clostridium difficile*, found in 5% of the population at large, is present in the stool of as many as 21% of hospitalized adults and is associated with an increase in hospital-acquired colitis. The results of a study of the incidence, morbidity, mortality, and predisposing conditions of *C. difficile* colitis in hospitalized patients were presented.

Methods.—Retrospectively the charts of 201 patients (64 women) were reviewed for antibiotic use, immune status, length of time to diagnosis and treatment, symptoms, and outcomes.

Results.—The incidence of *C. difficile* colitis among hospitalized patients has increased over the past 10 years (Fig). Age at diagnosis ranged from 2 months to 93 years. Surgery patients accounted for 55% of the cases and immunocompromised patients, 20%. Diarrhea was present in 97% of the patients, with other gastrointestinal symptoms also being present. The most frequent use of antibiotics was for perioperative prophylaxis, and the antibiotics most frequently associated with the development of colitis were the cephalosporins. Ten patients required surgery, and 3 died. Overall mortality was 3.5% and was associated with delayed

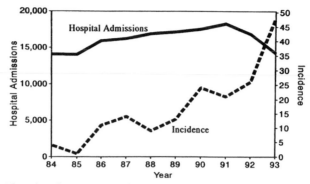

FIGURE.—The right ordinate represents the incidence (*dotted line*) of *Clostridium difficile* colitis, and the left ordinate represents the total admissions (*solid line*) to the Oregon Health Sciences University and the VA Medical Center hospitals from 1984 to 1994. (Reprinted by permission of the publisher from Jobe BA, Grasley A, Deveney KE, et al: *Clostridium difficile* colitis: An increasing hospital-acquired illness, *Am J Surg*, 169:480–483, Copyright 1995 by Excerpta Medica Inc.)

diagnosis. Survivors averaged 5.43 days from symptom onset to treatment, whereas patients who died averaged 10.7 days.

Conclusion.—Most cases of *C. difficile* colitis among hospitalized patients are associated with perioperative prophylactic antibiotic administration. Prompt diagnosis and aggressive treatment are very important.

► Despite a consistent number of hospital admissions at the Oregon Health Sciences University and Veterans Administration Medical Center, the number of cases of *Clostridium difficile* colitis has increased markedly over the past 10 years. Fifty-five percent of the patients were surgical patients, and most had perioperative antibiotic prophylaxis. Perioperative prophylaxis was the most frequent indication for antibiotics (25% of the *C. difficile* colitis cases). Virtually all patients in whom *C. difficile* colitis developed had received antibiotics for prophylaxis or to treat established infections. At several other institutions there has also been an alarming increase in the incidence of *C. difficile* colitis. Certainly some increase is due to heightened awareness of the disease and more frequent testing for *C. difficile* toxin. *Clostridium difficile* colitis is another disease that occurs as a result of modern medical therapy. It tells us that we must use antibiotics only when indicated and must not prolong their use.

R.J. Howard, M.D., Ph.D.

Should Antibiotic Prophylaxis Be Used Routinely in Clean Surgical Procedures: A Tentative Yes
Lewis RT, Weigand FM, Mamazza J, Lloyd-Smith W, Tataryn D (McGill Univ, Montreal)
Surgery 118:742–747, 1995   5–5

Background.—Antibiotic prophylaxis has not generally been given for clean surgical procedures because the reports of postoperative wound infections have been quite low. However, as hospital stays are reduced and more procedures are performed on an outpatient basis, the risk of postoperative infection is increased, even with clean surgical procedures. Therefore, the impact of preoperative antibiotic administration on surgical infection after clean procedures was evaluated in a randomized, double-blind, placebo-controlled study.

Methods.—A total of 775 patients undergoing a clean general surgery procedure or a simple elective cholecystectomy underwent a routine history, physical examination, and blood analysis. Based on these data, they were classified as high or low risk. Each risk group was then randomly assigned to receive either IV cefotaxime or placebo before surgery. Wound infection surveillance was performed at 1–2 weeks and 4–6 weeks after surgery, with a final surveillance performed by telephone.

Results.—In the low-risk group, the risk ratio was significant at 0.25, with surgical infections developing in 5 patients in the antibiotic group and 12 in the placebo group. In the high-risk group, the trend was similar, but the difference was not statistically significant, with a risk ratio of 0.48.

Conclusions.—There was a 75% reduction in postoperative wound infections associated with antibiotic prophylaxis among low-risk patients undergoing clean surgical operations. The less significant benefit of antibiotic prophylaxis among high-risk patients indicates a need for further study of this surgical population. Antibiotic prophylaxis is recommended for low-risk patients undergoing clean surgical procedures.

▶ Traditionally, prophylactic antibiotics have been given only for clean-contaminated operations. Then in 1990 Platt et al.[1] published a large series showing that prophylactic antibiotics reduced the overall incidence of infection but did not statistically decrease the wound infection rate in clean operations (hernia and breast surgery). The current authors performed a placebo-controlled trial in a variety of clean operations. However, they included cholecystectomy in the group of clean operations. Traditionally, cholecystectomy is a clean-contaminated operation; the bile is contaminated in a small proportion of these patients. They divided their patients into high-risk and low-risk groups based on criteria of the National Nosocomial Infection Surveillance System. Surprisingly, there was a reduction in surgical wounds in the low-risk group but not a statistically significant reduction in high-risk patients. They did not comment on the cost of prophylactic antibiotics and the potential cost of drug reactions. Nor did they comment on the cost of caring for patients with wound infections. In any case, the risk of wound infection, even in the group that did not have prophylactic antibiotics, was low. They used cefotaxime, a third-generation cephalosporin; first- and second-generation cephalosprins, which are less expensive, would have been as effective. It is my belief that third-generation cephalosporins should not be used for antibiotic prophylaxis. The study results are confounded by the wide variety of surgical procedures. The authors did not state whether certain surgical procedures were more likely to be associated with postoperative infection than others.

I and several of the discussants reached a different conclusion than the authors: that antibiotic prophylaxis is not warranted for clean operations. An alternative conclusion is that one can't really say for certain whether prophylactic antibiotics should be used in clean surgical procedures because of the wide variety of surgical procedures used and the lack of data about which procedures are more likely to be associated with infectious complications.

R.J. Howard, M.D., Ph.D.

Reference

1. Platt R, Zaleznik DF, Hopkins CC, et al: Perioperative antibiotic prophylaxis for herniorrhaphy and breast surgery. *N Engl J Med* 322:153–160, 1990.

Postdischarge Surveillance for Nosocomial Wound Infection: Does Judicious Monitoring Find Cases?
Ferraz EM, Ferraz AAB, D'Albuquerque Coelho HST, Viana VP, Sobral SML, Vasconcelos MDMM, Bacelar TS (Fed Univ of Pernambuco, Recife, Brazil)
Am J Infect Control 23:290–294, 1995   5–6

Introduction.—Infection is still the most serious postoperative complication. It is also an important indicator of the quality of care. Data on postoperative surgical wound infection have an important impact on hospital design, surgical technique, and infection control measures. However, it is likely that the true incidence of surgical wound infection is substantially underestimated. In an attempt to obtain more accurate infection data, an outpatient clinic for inspecting wound status after hospital discharge was set up. The accuracy of this method of surveillance for postoperative wound infection was evaluated.

Methods.—Findings regarding the detection of surgical wound infections in 6,604 patients who underwent general surgical and cesarean procedures were reviewed. An infection control practitioner examined each patient preoperatively to identify any pre-existing infections. Each operation was classified as clean, clean-contaminated, contaminated, or dirty. Postoperatively, the patient's wound status, antimicrobial use, and temperature were monitored daily while in the hospital. The patients were instructed to appear at the outpatient clinic on postoperative day 8, where the stitches were removed, dressings changed, and instructions given for return to the appropriate specialized surgical clinic.

Results.—The patients reported to the outpatient clinic at rates ranging from 68.4% to 91.2%. At the outpatient clinic, wound infections were detected at rates of 32.2% to 50% among patients undergoing general surgical procedures and 52.9% to 91.4% for patients undergoing cesarean sections. Most (87.6%) of the surgical wound infections were detected within the first 15 postoperative days, with infections occurring later after clean operations than after operations with other classifications.

Conclusions.—Postdischarge surveillance of wound infection is a cost-effective method of obtaining more accurate data on the incidence of wound infection, particularly with surgical patients who are discharged early. More accurate data are essential for the study of and hospital education about epidemiology, disease etiology, and risk factor assessment, as well as the design of effective infection control measures.

▶ With over 50% of surgical procedures in the United States being done on an outpatient basis and with the ever-increasing early discharge of hospital patients, most wound infections occur after discharge. This paper from Brazil shows that postdischarge surveillance can find some wound infections that occur following discharge. But even these authors only monitored patients who returned to the outpatient clinic, and only 68.4% to 91.2% of the patients returned, so many wound infections were likely missed. Other methods of identifying surgical wound infections after discharge include mailed questionnaires, telephone follow-up, and home visits by public health nurses. These methods are all expensive. Surgeons may be reluctant to report wound infections that are detected in their offices or clinics. Thus it is likely that in the future wound surveillance data will never be as good as that obtained in the past. The problem will likely increase as more operations are done on an outpatient basis and as more patients are discharged earlier in their posthospital courses.

R.J. Howard, M.D., Ph.D.

The Effect of Surgical Wound Infection on Postoperative Hospital Stay
Taylor GD, Kirkland TA, McKenzie MM, Sutherland B, Wiens RM (Univ of Alberta, Edmonton, Canada)
Can J Surg 38:149–153, 1995   5–7

Introduction.—Wound infections in surgical patients account for 25% of all nosocomial infections. The purpose of this case-control study was to determine the effect of surgical wound infection on the length of postoperative hospitalization.

Methods.—A cohort study of patients over a 1-year period on whom certain surgical procedures had been performed was undertaken. Patients who were hospitalized for a minimum of 48 hours were followed for either 14 days or until discharge. Patients were grouped according to the type of surgery as indicated by the National (Canadian) Nosocomial Infection Surveillance System. Fifteen surgical procedures were included in this study. Controls were patients who underwent the same procedure but in whom postoperative infections did not develop. Anesthesia risks for each procedure, as defined by the American Society of Anesthesiology, were included.

Results.—Sixty-eight cases of infection were included in the study (Table 2). There were no significant differences in anesthesia risks between the controls and the cases. Case patients remained in the hospital for 19 days longer than the controls, and "organ-space" infections resulted in longer stays than did incisional infections. Joint replacement and pancreatic-biliary-hepatic procedures involved the longest stays. Surgical or other nosocomial complications may have contributed to the prolongation of patient hospitalization.

Discussion.—Wound infection does lengthen hospitalization by 19 days. It is possible that although infection was present in all these patients, other complications contributed to the increased hospitalization inasmuch as a frequency of 44% was found for other complications in these patients. However, the wound infection rate was reduced by the transfer of patients to other hospitals for management. Because many patients are released early, this can increase the probability of infection among the remaining patients, who are more ill. It is also possible that because this was a tertiary care hospital, the wound infection results could have been different for another hospital. However, because the 68 patients studied required an extra 1,326 days of inpatient care, this is an indication that prevention of wound infection in Canadian hospitals needs to be seriously addressed.

TABLE 2.—Duration of Postoperative Hospital Stay for Wound Infection Cases and Control Cases

Procedure	No. of Cases	Mean Postoperative Length of Stay, Days		Difference, days
		Cases	Controls	
Neurosurgery				
Ventricular shunt	5	17.4	31.2	−13.8
Craniotomy	2	47	8	+39
Orthopedic surgery				
Open reduction, internal fixation	2	19	9.5	+ 9.5
Joint replacement	3	61.7	13.7	+48
General surgery				
Gastric	5	32.2	12.4	+19.8
Colonic	7	24.1	11.6	+12.5
Small-bowel	6	46.1	12.9	+33.2
Pancreatic-biliary-hepatic	4	57.3	12	+45.3
Cholecystectomy	2	26.5	6	+20.5
Vascular	3	52	57.3	− 5.3
Cardiovascular and thoracic surgery				
Coronary artery bypass grafting	11	34.6	22	+27.1
Cardiac	7	41.3	17.4	+23.9
Vascular	3	16	11.5	+ 4.5
Thoracic	3	15.7	10.6	+ 5.1
Obstetrics and gynecology				
Cesarean section	5	11.0	6.6	+ 4.4
Total	68	34.0	14.5	+19.5

(Reprinted from Taylor GD, Kirkland TA, McKenzie MM, et al: The effect of surgical wound infection on postoperative hospital stay, by permission of the publisher, *CJS*, Vol. 38, No. 2, April 1995.)

▶ By any measure—increased hospital stay or cost—wound infections are expensive. This study from Canada showed that patients with postoperative wound infections remained in the hospital 19.5 days longer than case-control patients. Unfortunately, the authors did not present data showing the increased cost of wound infections. This series was limited to patients who were hospitalized for a minimum of 48 hours postoperatively. In the United States, over 50% of operative procedures are being done on an outpatient basis or with brief hospital stays. These patients would have been excluded from this study. Because many wound infections do not occur while the patient is in the hospital, current wound infection data are not as good as they were formerly. It is more difficult to learn about wound infections that occur outside of hospitals. These authors followed patients for 14 days postoperatively. Although most wound infections occur within 14 days of surgery, many do not occur until after this time. Nevertheless, the underlying message remains: wound infections are expensive. I am not sure whether the increased length of stay demonstrated in this series (19.5 days) is representative of the situation in the United States. Even the case-control patients appear to have much longer hospital stays than found in American hospitals. For instance, the mean length of stay was 6 days following cholecystectomy and 22 days following coronary artery bypass grafting. Most operations in the United States are associated with shorter hospital stays. No doubt the increased length of stay due to wound infection is also less.

R.J. Howard, M.D., Ph.D.

Contaminated Wounds: The Effect of Initial Management on Outcome
Smilanich RP, Bonnet I, Kirkpatrick JR (Uniformed Services Univ of Health Sciences, Washington, DC)
Am Surg 61:427–430, 1995   5–8

Introduction.—The National Research Council classifies the degree of wound contamination as class I, or clean; class II, clean-contaminated; class III, contaminated; and class IV, dirty. The infection risk is related to the choice of wound closure. Some surgeons continue to use antibiotics alone in managing class III and IV wounds rather than using open wound management with or without delayed primary closure, which is considered the treatment of choice for contaminated wounds. The study determined the magnitude of this practice and its impact on the economics of health care delivery and patient safety.

Methods.—The retrospective review evaluated 918 consecutive operations performed during a 1-year period. Within each classification, the most common diagnoses were hernia, breast mass, and thyroid mass for class I; cholelithiasis, hemorrhage from diverticulosis, or peptic ulcer disease for class II; cholecystitis, appendicitis, and diverticulitis for class III; and perforated appendix, perforated diverticulum, and perforated colon carcinoma for class IV. Evaluators analyzed the degree of contamination, duration of surgery, number of transfusions, microbiology of wound and blood cultures, length of stay, mortality, and method of wound management.

Results.—Class I and class II wounds were found in 768 patients (84%), and class III or class IV wounds were found in 150 patients. Class I wounds were managed with primary closure alone and had a low infection rate (1.4%) and a short length of stay (4 ± 1 days). Class II wounds were managed with primary closure, prophylactic antibiotics were used almost without exception, and the infection rate was 4.9% and length of stay was 5 ± 2 days. Of the patients with class III or IV wounds, only 32 (21%) had their incision left open despite obvious contamination. For class III and IV wounds, the aggregate wound infection rate was 3% (1 patient). Among the 118 wounds that were managed with primary closure, 32 infections occurred. There was no difference in the length of stay of patients managed with primary closure or delayed primary closure if infection did not occur. However, if infection occurred, there was a significantly longer length of stay in the primary closure group.

Discussion.—The optimal method of management for wounds is delayed primary closure. The ideal time has been shown to be after the third or fourth day for delayed primary closure because earlier closure has had inferior results. All contaminated wounds should be left open to heal by delayed primary closure or by secondary intention. In this setting, surgeons should consider the benefits of open wound management to be equal to or greater than the benefits of antibiotics, and patients should be warned of the rationale of having an open wound.

▶ Traditionally, class III and class IV wounds have been left open to heal by secondary intention or delayed primary closure. These authors compare 150 patients who had class III or class IV wounds treated by primary closure or by leaving the wound open. There was only 1 wound infection among 32 wounds left open as compared with 32 wound infections among 118 wounds primarily closed. Wounds that were primarily closed and became infected resulted in significantly longer hospital stays. Therefore, the authors conclude that delayed primary closure is the treatment of choice for class III and class IV wounds. There are other alternatives. We place skin sutures at wide (2 to 3 in) intervals for class III and class IV wounds and put gauze dressings in between the sutures. Four to 5 days later we can close the wound easily in the clinic or at the bedside with adhesive tape because the widely placed sutures do not permit the wound to gape open.

R.J. Howard, M.D., Ph.D.

Prevalence of Hepatitis C Infection in Health Care Workers Affiliated With a Liver Transplant Center

Goetz AM, Ndimbie OK, Wagener MM, Muder RR (Veterans Affairs Med Ctr, Pittsburgh, Pa; Univ of Pittsburgh, Pa; Central Blood Bank of Pittsburgh, Pa)

Transplantation 59:990–994, 1995   5–9

Background.—Prior hepatitis C infection has been identified in 16% of the patients undergoing liver transplantation at Presbyterian-University Hospital and 50% of the patients at the Veterans Affairs Medical Center in Pittsburgh, Pennsylvania. Because of the potential occupational risk of exposure and the unknown risk of hepatitis C infection to health care workers associated with liver transplantation, a serologic survey was conducted to determine the prevalence of hepatitis C infection in hospital staff with varying degrees of exposure to infected patients.

Methods.—An occupational and health history questionnaire was completed by health care workers recruited from these 2 transplant centers; participation was voluntary and results were held confidential. Blood was donated for testing with a second-generation, enzyme-linked immunosorbent assay (EIA) and confirmed with a second-generation recombinant immunoblot assay. Samples that were indeterminate with the latter were tested by reverse transcriptase–polymerase chain reaction.

Participants.—Of the 241 health care workers, 24% were at very high risk for exposure to hepatitis C through direct care of the liver transplant patients and frequent exposure to their blood and body fluids, 66% were considered at high risk because of frequent blood and body fluid exposure, and 10.8% were in a low-risk occupation. The mean age of the participants was 38.7 years, and 59% were women. Almost half (48.5%) were nurses, 24.9% were physicians, and 17% were laboratory personnel. The mean number of years in their occupation was 13.5 years.

Results.—Five (2.1%) health care workers were reactive to hepatitis C by EIA testing (Table 1). Of these, 3 were RT-PCR–positive, but none had a history of hepatitis or transfusion. All 3 were among the 57 health care workers in the very-high-risk category (5.3%; 95% confidence interval, 1.3%–15.5%), whereas none of the other 184 workers in the other risk categories was infected.

Conclusion.—Health care workers who are directly involved in the care of hospitalized liver transplant patients may be at substantial risk of acquiring hepatitis C. The risk appears to be low for other health care workers, including those with frequent blood and body fluid exposure.

▶ Human immunodeficiency virus, hepatitis C, and hepatitis B are the most common blood-borne pathogens that can be acquired by health care workers. This report from the University of Pittsburgh hospitals, where patients with hepatitis C make up 16% to 50% of the patients undergoing liver transplantation, examined the prevalence of hepatitis C infection among health care workers at risk for exposure to hepatitis C.

TABLE 1.—Hepatitis C Antibody Results and Background of 5 Health Care Workers Associated With 2 Liver Transplant Centers

HCW	Age	Race	Sex	Hospital*	Profession	History of		Area working	Years since graduation	Years in current position	Hepatitis C		
						Transfusion	Hepatitis				EIA	RIBA	PCR
1	40	?*	F	PUH	RN	No	No	Liver transplant ICU	8	8	+	+	+
2	37	W	F	VAMC	RN	No	No	Liver transplant surgical ward	15	6	+	Ind	Neg
3	42	Other†	M	VAMC	Anesthesia technician‡	No	No§	Liver transplant operating room	17	4	+	Ind	+
4	38	W	M	VAMC	RN	No	No||	Liver transplant operating room	3.5	15 mo	+	+	+
5	35	W	M	VAMC	Surgeon	No	Yes¶	General surgery	9	4	+	Ind	Neg

* No response.
† Not white, black, Hispanic, or Asian.
‡ Formerly a laboratory technician.
§ History of elevated liver function studies.
|| Found to be baseline hepatitis C antibody–positive after a needlestick injury. This occurred at the same time as participation in the study.
¶ Hepatitis C history.

Abbreviations: HCW, health care worker; EIA, enzyme immunosorbent assay; RIBA, recombinant immunoblot assay; PCR, polymerase chain reaction; PUH, Presbyterian-University-Hospital; RN, registered nurse; VAMC, Veterans Affairs Medical Center; Ind, indeterminate; Neg, negative.
(Courtesy of Goetz AM, Ndimbie OK, Wagener MM, et al: Prevalence of hepatitis C infection in health care workers affiliated with a liver transplant center. Transplantation 59(7):990–994, 1995.)

Five had evidence of hepatitis C infection, but the authors could not state whether the infection occurred as a result of occupational blood and body fluid exposure. Three of the 5 infected health care workers were nurses, 1 was a surgeon, and 1 was an anesthesia technician. The surgeon performed general surgery, not liver transplantation, at the Veterans Administration Medical Center and had a history of hepatitis C. The anesthesia technician had a history of elevated liver function studies, and 1 nurse at the Veterans Administration Medical Center had hepatitis C antibody in a baseline blood sample obtained right after a needlestick injury. Four of the 5 individuals were at the Veterans Administration Medical Center. One nurse was in the liver transplant ICU at Pittsburgh University Hospital.

Because a high percentage of individuals undergoing liver transplantation at many transplant centers have hepatitis C, health care workers involved in the care of these patients are at increased risk of infection. Blood-borne infections can affect any health care worker, however. Postexposure infection rates for hepatitis C are approximately 3% (for HIV it is approximately 0.3% and for hepatitis B it is 30%). Approximately 3 million individuals in the United States are estimated to be chronically infected with hepatitis C. Because most patients who have infections with blood-borne viruses are not identified, it is important that health care workers continue to practice universal precautions to minimize the risk of acquiring infection.

R.J. Howard, M.D., Ph.D.

Controlled Clinical Trial of Selective Decontamination for the Treatment of Severe Acute Pancreatitis
Luiten EJT, Hop WCJ, Lange JF, Bruining HA (Univ Hosp Rotterdam Dijkzigt, The Netherlands; Erasmus Univ, Rotterdam, The Netherlands; St Clara Hosp, Rotterdam, The Netherlands)
Ann Surg 222:57–65, 1995   5–10

Introduction.—Mortality from acute necrotizing pancreatitis is high, ranging from 20% to 70%. Although infected pancreatic necrosis has been implicated as a cause of mortality, the value of prophylactic antibiotics has not been demonstrated, partly because parenteral antibiotics penetrate necrotic nonperfused pancreatic tissue poorly. Translocation of digestive tract bacteria has been proposed as a source of infection of pancreatic necrosis. Eradication of gram-negative organisms in the digestive tract would prevent translocation of bacteria and may prevent infection of pancreatic necrosis. The efficacy of selective decontamination of the digestive tract in reducing mortality in patients with severe acute pancreatitis was evaluated.

Methods.—One hundred two patients with severe acute pancreatitis were randomized to receive either standard treatment (control) or standard treatment plus selective decontamination. Colistin sulfate, 200 mg, amphotericin, 500 mg, and norfloxacin, 50 mg, were administered every 6 hours for selective decontamination. The antibiotic combination was applied as a 2% paste to the upper and lower gums every 6 hours and to the tracheostomy site. The combination was also administered as a rectal enema daily. Cefotaxime, 500 mg every 6 hours, was given parenterally until the oral cavity and rectum were free of gram-negative bacteria. Selective decontamination was continued until the patient was no longer at risk for infection.

Results.—The mortality rates between the control and the selective decontamination groups were not significantly different; 18 patients (35%) in the control group and 11 patients (22%) in the selective decontamination group died. However, when adjusted for Imrie score and Balthazar grade, the difference in mortality between the 2 groups was found to be significant. Mortality was found to increase with increasing Imrie score and with increasing Balthazar grade; the correlation between mortality and Imrie score was found to be significant. Gram-negative pancreatic infections developed in significantly fewer patients who received selective decontamination than control group patients (8% vs. 33%). For both groups, digestive tract colonization preceded the development of gram-negative pancreatic infections.

Conclusion.—Use of selective decontamination of the digestive tract was successful in reducing the rate of mortality from pancreatic infection in patients with acute necrotizing pancreatitis. Additionally, the Imrie scoring system was found to be valuable in identifying patients at risk for mortality.

▶ Acute pancreatitis may progress to necrotizing pancreatitis, which subsequently becomes infected and leads to infected pancreatic necrosis. The mortality rate of necrotizing pancreatitis is extremely high (20% to 70%), and the cause of late mortality is frequently infection. Trials of prophylactic antibiotics in patients with severe acute pancreatitis have not been beneficial in reducing mortality. These authors try another approach: selective bowel decontamination. This study suggests that a reduction in gram-negative colonization of the digestive tract can reduce patient morbidity and mortality in severe acute pancreatitis. The rationale is that bacteria find their way to the pancreatic necrosis by bacterial translocation. By decreasing the number of bacteria in the intestine, the likelihood of translocation and infection is decreased. Even though the overall mortality rate was not decreased, this regimen was statistically successful in preventing secondary pancreatic infection. Certainly the only goal of selective decontamination is to reduce the likelihood of infection. Mortality involves additional factors. Thus decreasing the risk of infection itself may be sufficient to warrant the use of selective bowel decontamination even though the overall mortality rate is not affected.

R.J. Howard, M.D., Ph.D.

Closed Drainage Versus Open Packing of Infected Pancreatic Necrosis
Harris JA, Jury RP, Catto J, Glover JL (William Beaumon Hosp, Royal Oak, Mich)
Am Surg 61:612–618, 1995   5–11

Introduction.—Despite improvements in the detection and treatment of infected pancreatic necrosis, mortality remains high. Early and complete removal of infected necrotic tissue is important in the treatment of this infection. The use of open packing was compared with closed drainage after surgical débridement of infected pancreatic necrosis.

Patients.—Twenty patients with severe acute pancreatitis complicated with infected pancreatic necrosis were included in the study. Pancreatic or peripancreatic necrosis infection was documented by either Gram stain or culture in all patients. Infection was diagnosed either by using a combination of CT and fine-needle aspiration or by the presence of extraluminal gas alone. Monomicrobial infections were present in 13 patients and polymicrobial infections in 7.

Procedure and Results.—Nine patients underwent surgical débridement followed by closed catheter drainage as the initial treatment (Table 2). Repeat of surgical débridement or use of percutaneous drainage was required in 7 patients because of persistent infected necrosis and abscess. Four of these patients died, 3 of sepsis and 1 because of multisystem organ failure. Both patients who did not require a reoperation or redrainage survived. The overall mortality rate after this procedure was 44% (4 of 9 patients died). Eleven patients underwent surgical débridement followed by open packing as the initial treatment (Table 3). Redébridement and

TABLE 2.—Closed Catheter Drainage

Patient	Age	Days Until Surgery	Drains	Reoperation or Redrainage	Outcome
1	63	28	4 sumps 2 Tenckhoff	POD 7, 26	Survived, d/c POD 79
2	59	20	5 penrose	POD 24	Survived, d/c POD 137
3	39	19	3 penrose 2 sumps 2 Tenckhoff	None	Survived, d/c POD 26
4	70	35	2 penrose 2 sumps	None	Survived, d/c POD 82
5	52	25	8 penrose 3 sumps	POD 8, 12	Died POD 31, sepsis
6	58	8	2 Tenckhoff 3 sumps	POD 8	Died POD 35, MSOF
7	49	8	2 sumps 2 Tenckhoff	POD 12	Died POD 15, sepsis
8	62	19	3 sumps	Perc. dr. POD 21, 28, and OR 80	Died POD 307, sepsis
9	18	14	2 Tenckhoff	Perc. dr. POD 12, 28, and OR 80	Survived, d/c POD 57

Abbreviations: POD, postoperative day; *d/c*, discharge from the hospital; *MSOF*, multisystem organ failure; *Perc. dr.*, percutaneous drainage.
(Courtesy of Harris JA, Jury RP, Catto J, et al: Closed drainage versus open packing of infected pancreatic necrosis. *Am Surg* 61:612–618, 1995.)

TABLE 3.—Open Packing

Patient	Age	Days Until Surgery	Redébridements	Outcomes
1	36	26	20 times, 40 days	Survived, d/c POD #47
2	38	35	8 times, 11 days	Survived, d/c POD #72
3	66	37	12 times, 39 days	Survived, d/c POD #47
4	71	35	17 times, 21 days	Survived, d/c POD #55
5	68	19	none	Died POD #2, cardiac failure
6	29	18	one time in O.R.	Survived, d/c POD #109
7	72	13	7 times, 15 days	Died POD #21, MSOF
8	71	33	7 times, 14 days	Survived, d/c POD #75
9	60	10	5 times, 12 days	Survived, d/c POD #35
10	52	14	12 times, 25 days	Survived, d/c POD #36
11	55	38	10 times, 20 days	Survived, d/c POD #54

Abbreviations: d/c, discharge from the hospital; *POD*, postoperative day; *O.R.*, operating room.
(Courtesy of Harris JA, Jury RP, Catto J, et al: Closed drainage versus open packing of infected pancreatic necrosis. *Am Surg* 61:612–618, 1995.)

repacking were repeated at 1- to 3-day intervals and performed an average of 10 times (range rate 1–20). Two of 11 patients who underwent open packing died for an overall mortality rate of 18% for this procedure. One patient died of multisystem organ failure and 1 patient because of cardiac failure and ventricular arrhythmia.

Conclusion.—Surgical débridement followed by open packing was found to result in a lower mortality than closed catheter drainage for the treatment of infected pancreatic necrosis. Based on this series of patients, open packing may be needed in patients with such characteristics as early infection of necrotizing pancreatitis, no encapsulation, the presence of thick infected debris, and the reaccumulation of infected debris.

▶ Infected pancreatic necrosis continues to be one of the most challenging surgical infections. Despite a variety of treatment alternatives, patients with this disease have a high mortality rate. Treatment of surgical infection is adequate drainage, and the treatment of necrosis is adequate débridement. It is clear that percutaneous drainage is inadequate in the treatment of infected pancreatic necrosis and should be abandoned, although needle aspiration can be useful in determining whether pancreatic necrosis is associated with infection. Surgical débridement followed by closed catheter drainage has a high failure rate because adequate débridement cannot always be carried out at the initial operation and the necrotic, infected tissue will not drain through most closed drainage systems. Many surgeons currently favor surgical débridement and open packing.

In the current series a mortality rate of 44% with surgical débridement and closed catheter drainage was reduced to 18% by using surgical débridement and open packing. Open packing allows better drainage and also permits repeated further débridement in the operating room or even the ICU. Repeat surgery should be a planned part of treatment and should not be thought of as a defeat or having performed an inadequate initial procedure. Open packing is usually done anteriorly, but that requires traversing the uncontaminated peritoneal cavity with the possibility of peritonitis or intraperitoneal abscess. The peritoneal cavity can be excluded by dividing the gastro-colic omentum and suturing the stomach end of the omentum to the superior portion of the wound and the colonic end of the omentum to the inferior portion of the wound, thus providing access directly to the lesser sac. Some have advocated a retroperitoneal approach,[1] but that approach does not result in a lower mortality rate.

R.J. Howard, M.D., Ph.D.

Reference

1. Villazón SA, Villazón DO, Terrasez EF, et al: *World J Surg* 15:103–108, 1991 (1993 YEAR BOOK OF SURGERY, p 116).

Pyogenic Hepatic Abscess: Results of Current Management
Hashimoto L, Hermann R, Grundfest-Broniatowski S (Cleveland Clinic Found, Ohio)
Am Surg 61:407–411, 1995   5–12

Introduction.—Previously, hepatic abscesses have been treated with operative drainage. However, CT-guided percutaneous catheter drainage has become the treatment of choice. The treatment and outcome of pyogenic liver abscesses was reviewed in a retrospective analysis.

Methods.—Treatment of pyogenic liver abscesses in 56 patients was retrospectively reviewed. Clinical features, laboratory parameters, disease characteristics, microorganisms isolated, and type of treatment were assessed.

Results.—Fever, chills, and abdominal pain were the most common symptoms, with abdominal tenderness and hepatomegaly present on physical examination. Computed tomography was used in the diagnosis for 47 patients, with abscesses observed in 46. Twenty-eight patients had a single abscess and 28 patients had multiple or loculated lesions. Bacterial cultures were positive in 44 patients. Treatment of hepatic abscess consisted of surgical drainage, nonsurgical treatment (percutaneous drainage or aspiration), or no drainage (Fig 2). Surgical drainage was initially performed on 6 patients, with 1 death and 5 cures. Thirty-eight patients underwent CT-guided percutaneous drainage as initial treatment. Twenty-seven patients were considered cured, 4 patients died, and 8 patients either failed or had a recurrence. Patients who failed percutaneous drainage underwent surgical drainage and were cured. Patients who had a recurrence underwent either repeat drainage or aspiration. Ten patients had aspiration as the initial treatment, with 6 cures, 1 repeat aspiration, and 3 deaths. One patient with advanced pancreatic cancer received antibiotics only without drainage and subsequently died.

Conclusion.—The use of CT permitted a diagnosis of hepatic abscess within 4 days. The 77% success rate of CT-guided percutaneous catheter drainage makes it the preferred method of treatment in patients with hepatic abscesses.

TREATMENT OF HEPATIC ABSCESS

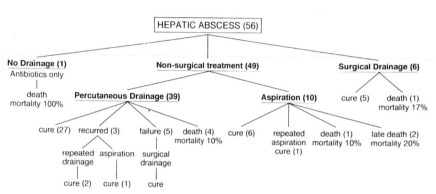

FIGURE 2.—Treatment outcome in 56 cases of pyogenic liver abscesses. (Courtesy of Hashimoto L, Hermann R, Grundfest-Broniatowski S: Pyogenic hepatic abscess: Results of current management. *Am Surg* 61:407–411, 1995.)

▶ The findings of this recent 11-year review of hepatic abscess at the Cleveland Clinic confirms the increasing role of the radiologist in the diagnosis and treatment of this disease. Ultrasonography and CT have revolutionized the diagnosis and treatment of this disease, which was once treated only by surgical drainage and antibiotic therapy. In this series of 56 patients, 49 initially had either aspiration or percutaneous drainage. Only 6 had surgical therapy as the initial treatment. Only 5 of 39 percutaneously drained abscesses ultimately required surgical drainage. Patients with hepatic abscesses frequently come to their nonsurgical physician, and diagnosis and treatment are rendered by the radiologist. Thus the surgeon may not be involved in many cases of hepatic abscess, only being called for those patients who fail percutaneous drainage or aspiration. Involving the surgeon in the treatment of these patients may help determine earlier whether percutaneous drainage or aspiration is achieving its goal or if surgical drainage is necessary.

R.J. Howard, M.D., Ph.D.

Alveolar Hydatid Disease: Review of the Surgical Experience in 42 Cases of Active Disease Among Alaskan Eskimos
Wilson JF, Rausch RL, Wilson FR (Alaska Native Med Ctr, Anchorage; Univ of Washington, Seattle)
Ann Surg 221:315–323, 1995   5–13

Introduction.—Alveolar hydatid disease (ADH) is a zoonosis caused by *Echinococcus multilocularis* in the larval stage. It is perpetuated in nature by a cycle that involves foxes and rodents in northern climates. With the exception of 1 case in rural Minnesota and 1 in Manitoba, 42 of 44 cases of active, locally acquired ADH have occurred in Eskimos from western Alaska. A retrospective review of the 42 Eskimos in whom AHD was diagnosed or treated was presented.

Methods.—The medical records of all patients in whom AHD was diagnosed or treated from 1951 to 1993 at the Alaska Native Medical Center were reviewed for information about physical examination, laboratory and imaging results, and treatment approaches.

Results.—Ages at diagnosis were 12–82 years, with a median of 53 years. Sixteen patients were asymptomatic at the time of diagnosis. The most common findings or complaints at diagnosis were right upper quadrant pain, palpable mass, and enlarged liver. Jaundice and CNS symptoms were less commonly noted. Positive serologic findings gave collaborative evidence of the diagnosis in 44% of the patients. Nine patients underwent resection for cure and had good results. Eight of these patients converted their serologic status to negative after surgery. The average survival time since diagnosis is currently 22 years. Six are still living. Postoperative recurrences developed in 3 patients, 2 of whom were treated successfully with resection and 1 with chemotherapy. Two other patients underwent incomplete resections, with recurrent disease and death in 3 and 2.3 years, respectively. The majority of patients were not resectable at the time of diagnosis. The following palliative procedures were performed: marsupialization of hepatic abscesses in 2 patients, partial resection in 1, and drainage procedures in 5 patients. Five patients with metastases to the brain survived an average of 1 year after diagnosis. Six patients with active disease did not require surgery. Twenty patients underwent abdominal surgery and 2 had thoracic procedures for diagnosis or staging. Chemotherapeutic treatment of 12 patients with mebendazole and 1 with albendazole failed to kill the larval cestode.

Conclusion.—Although alveolar hydatid disease is rare in most areas of North America, there is concern about the release of thousands of illegally imported foxes into the southeastern seaboard over the last 20 years. Physicians must be aware of the possibility of this infection when making differential diagnoses in patients with hepatic lesions.

▶ This article describes one of the largest series of locally acquired alveolar hydatid disease. Forty-two of the 44 cases described since the mid 1940s were treated at the Alaska Navy Medical Center by these authors. They likely have the most thorough knowledge of this disease that exists today. This is one of the most thorough reviews of the pathophysiology, surgical treatment, chemotherapy, and late complications of infection by *Echinococcus*. Although all of their cases occurred in Alaskan Eskimos, this zoonotic disease is also found in central North America. Because of the illegal importation of foxes from Alaska into the southeastern United States, there is a possibility that physicians in the Southeast may also encounter these infections.

R.J. Howard, M.D., Ph.D.

Determinants of Mortality for Necrotizing Soft-Tissue Infections

McHenry CR, Piotrowski JJ, Petrinic D, Malangoni MA (Case Western Reserve Univ, Cleveland, Ohio; MetroHealth Med Ctr, Cleveland, Ohio)

Ann Surg 221:558–565, 1995   5–14

Objective.—Necrotizing soft tissue infections (NSTIs) carry a mortality rate as high as 76%. Although a variety of factors can increase mortality, no studies have identified definitive risk factors. The results of a retrospective study examining the incidence and evaluating risk factors for mortality in a large group of patients with NSTI were presented.

Methods.—A total of 65 patients aged 15–87 years were treated for NSTI.

Results.—There were 51 patients with necrotizing fasciitis, 12 with necrotizing fasciitis and associated myonecrosis, and 2 with necrosis confined to the skin and subcutaneous tissues. Causes of NSTI were necrotizing fasciitis in 18 patients, trauma in 15, cutaneous infections in 15, idiopathic infections in 10, perirectal abscesses in 3, strangulated hernias in 3, and subcutaneous infections in 2. Polymicrobial infections were found in 45 patients with necrotizing soft tissue infections (Table 2). Polymicrobial infections were detected in 82% of postoperative infections. *Streptococcus pyogenes* caused 10 of 19 monomicrobial infections and carried a mortality rate of 18% (Table 3). Eight of 10 idiopathic infections

TABLE 2.—Causative Organisms for 45 Polymicrobic Necrotizing Soft Tissue Infections (N = 127)

Aerobes (gram-positive)	51(40%)
Enterococci	21
Streptococcal species*	11
Coagulase-negative staphylococci	10
Staphylococcus aureus	6
Bacillus species	3
Aerobes (gram-negative)	54(43%)
Escherichia coli	15
Pseudomonas aeruginosa	13
Enterobacter cloacae	5
Klebsiella species	5
Proteus species	4
Serratia species	4
Acinetobacter calcoaceticus	3
Others†	4
Anaerobes	19(15%)
Bacteroides species	12
Clostridium species	4
Others‡	5
Fungi§	3(2%)

* Includes group B streptococci (3), gamma-streptococci (non-*faecalis*) (3), alpha-streptococci (2), S. *milleri* (1), and S. *pyogenes* (2).
† Includes *Citrobacter freundi* (2), *Xanthomonas maltophila* (1), *Eikenella corrodens* (1), and *Aeromonas hydrophila* (1).
‡ Includes *Peptostreptococcus* (2) and diphtheroids (1).
§ Includes *Candida tropicalis* (2) and *Candida albicans* (1).
(Courtesy of McHenry CR, Piotrowski JJ, Petrinic D, et al: Determinants of mortality for necrotizing soft-tissue infections. *Ann Surg* 221:558–565, 1995.)

TABLE 3.—Causative Organisms for the 19 Monomicrobic Necrotizing
Soft Tissue Infections (N = 127)

Streptococcus pyogenes	10
Clostridium perfringens	2
Staphylococcus aureus	2
Pseudomonas aeruginosa	1
Escherichia coli	1
Serratia marscesans	1
Gamma-streptococci, not enterococci	1
Candida glabrata	1

(Courtesy of McHenry CR, Piotrowski JJ, Petrinic D, et al: Determinants of mortality for necrotizing soft-tissue infections. *Ann Surg* 221:558–565, 1995.)

were monomicrobial. Patients had an average of 3.3 débridements, and 12 patients had amputations. Nineteen patients (29%) died, 6 within 10 days after débridement. Survival was significantly increased for patients operated on within 25 hours vs. those operated on within 90 hours.

Conclusion.—Prompt recognition and treatment of NSTIs reduces mortality. Other factors previously suspected of influencing mortality did not affect clinical outcome in this study.

▶ The only factor associated with mortality was the time from admission to surgery (90 hours in nonsurvivors vs. 25 hours in survivors). I assume the delay in treatment was not because the authors didn't know these infections should be promptly operated on but rather because diagnosis was difficult. Determining the presence of necrotizing soft tissue infections can be extremely difficult because the necrosis can occur at levels deep to the skin and may not be readily apparent. The physician must be prepared to operate on patients with minimal clinical evidence because of the high mortality rate in untreated patients. Not all papers find such a strong correlation of the time between admission and surgery and the mortality rate.

I feel patients should not be sent for hyperbaric oxygen treatment before débridement is carried out. The necrotizing infection can advance to the point of death during transportation to receive hyperbaric oxygen. Débridement should be promptly carried out and hyperbaric oxygen considered as an adjunctive measure afterward. The patients can then be sent to a center that has a hyperbaric oxygen chamber. There is little evidence that hyperbaric oxygen adds much to decreasing mortality rates in patients with necrotizing soft tissue infections.

Patients in this series required an average of 3.3 débridements. Patients should be told that the initial débridement is only the first stage in the operative treatment. Re-examination in the operating room is mandatory for virtually all patients. Because dressing changes can be so painful, general anesthesia may be required. Inspection of the wound can be done during anesthesia for dressing changes, and the operating room provides the best place for adequate visibility and treatment.

R.J. Howard, M.D., Ph.D.

Randomised Comparison of Ganciclovir and High-Dose Acyclovir for Long-Term Cytomegalovirus Prophylaxis in Liver-Transplant Recipients

Winston DJ, Wirin D, Shaked A, Busuttil RW (Univ of California, Los Angeles)
Lancet 346:69–74, 1995   5–15

Background.—Cytomegalovirus (CMV) is a frequent cause of infection in recipients of liver and other solid organ transplants. Relatively few liver transplant cases have been included in previous trials of prophylaxis, and

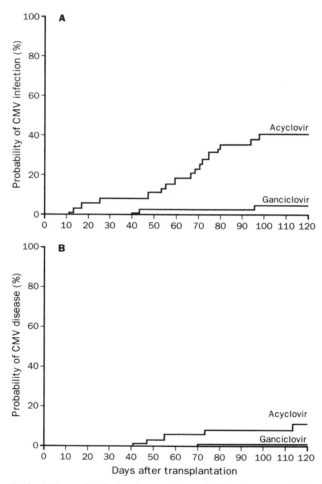

FIGURE.—Kaplan-Meier product limit estimates of the probability of cytomegalovirus (*CMV*) infection (**A**) or disease (**B**) during the first 120 days after transplantation among acyclovir- and ganciclovir-treated patients. The probabilities of CMV infection and disease were significantly different between groups (*P* < 0.0001 and *P* = 0.002, respectively). (Courtesy of Winston DJ, Wirin D, Shaked A, et al: Randomised comparison of ganciclovir and high-dose acyclovir for long-term cytomegalovirus prophylaxis in liver-transplant recipients, 346(1):69–74, copyright by *The Lancet* Ltd., 1995.)

despite a number of preventive regimens, CMV infection and disease continue to occur in a significant number of recipients.

Objective.—A randomized trial was carried out in liver transplant recipients aged 12 years and older to compare long-term ganciclovir, extending over 100 days, with a standard regimen of high-dose acyclovir prophylaxis.

Study Plan.—The 126 patients assigned to receive acyclovir were given a dose of 10 mg/kg IV every 8 hours from the first postoperative day to the time of discharge and then 800 mg orally 4 times a day up to day 100. The other 124 patients received ganciclovir IV in a daily dose of 6 mg/kg for 30 days postoperatively and then the same dose 5 days a week up to day 100. The 2 treatment groups were similar demographically and clinically. Median follow-up approached 2 years for both groups.

Efficacy.—Patients given ganciclovir had significantly fewer episodes of CMV infection and CMV-related illness than those given acyclovir (Fig). Ten percent of the latter patients and fewer than 1% of the ganciclovir recipients had symptomatic CMV disease, and the only related death was in a patient given acyclovir in whom CMV pneumonia developed. Both patients with and those without CMV antibody benefited more from ganciclovir. On multivariate analysis, the use of ganciclovir was the most significant factor preventing CMV infection and disease. Both regimens protected against herpes simplex virus infection. Among patients who were initially negative for CMV antibody, bacterial and fungal infections developed in fewer of those given ganciclovir.

Safety.—Both regimens were generally well tolerated. Severe leukopenia developed in 6% of the ganciclovir-treated patients and 3% of those given acyclovir. Thrombocytopenia developed in nearly half of both groups and was severe in 6% to 7% of patients. A majority of patients in both groups had elevated serum creatinine levels, but renal failure did not develop in any of them. Survival 4 months and 1 year after transplantation was comparable in the 2 groups.

Conclusion.—The prophylactic use of ganciclovir for 100 days after liver transplantation can virtually eliminate serious CMV-related infection. When compared with what is seen in bone marrow recipients and AIDS patients, toxicity from ganciclovir is minimal.

▶ Ganciclovir led to a significant reduction in the probability of CMV infection and CMV disease as compared with acyclovir, although the likelihood of CMV disease in both groups was low. The regimen was expensive. The acquisition cost of ganciclovir and acyclovir was $2,300 and $4,000, respectively, and the estimated patient charges (drug costs and administration fees) were $13,000 and $16,500, respectively. Antiviral prophylaxis adds substantially to the cost of liver transplantation. But the cost of CMV disease is also expensive. If patients required hospitalization, the authors estimated the cost to range from $10,000 to $50,000. The serologic status of the donor or the recipient did not seem to influence the incidence of CMV infection or disease. Thus one could not select certain donor-recipient combinations to receive prophylaxis. Whether antiviral prophylaxis is required for 100 days is unclear. Perhaps pursuing these studies with shorter duration of prophylaxis might lead to equal efficacy and yet achieve lower cost.

R.J. Howard, M.D., Ph.D.

6 Transplantation

Introduction

This past year's articles about transplantation continued to better define appropriate donors for transplantation, to study the results of transplantation, and to better define indications for transplantation. Finally, a new immunosuppressive drug, mycophenolate mofetil, was approved by the Food and Drug Administration for use in the United States. Two large randomized trials (Abstracts 6–1 and 6–2) reported that mycophenolate mofetil resulted in fewer rejection episodes than did azathioprine. It was disappointing, however, that the reduced number of graft rejection episodes did not translate into improved graft survival. Furthermore, mycophenolate mofetil was associated with a larger number of complications, and its greatly increased cost (approximately 5 times that of azathioprine) may limit its use.

With the ever-widening disparity between the number of patients on the waiting list for cadaveric organs and the number of organs available, attempts are continuing to increase the number of organs that might previously have been thought unsuitable for transplantation. A paper from the United Network for Organ Sharing (Abstract 6–3) demonstrates that using spousal and living unrelated donors results in high graft survival rates, comparable to that of living related donors. On a genetic basis one might think that living unrelated donors have no logical advantage over cadaveric grafts. Yet the avoidance of delayed graft function, for which there is a price to be paid in terms of graft survival, might explain much of the increased survival of living unrelated donors. The literature is inconsistent on whether kidneys from hepatitis C–positive donors should be used. Some have advocated using these infected kidneys in recipients who themselves are hepatitis C–positive. A study from Sweden (Abstract 6–4) establishes that in some transplant recipients who have hepatitis C and who receive kidneys from hepatitis C–positive donors, the infecting donor strain of hepatitis C can either replace or coexist with the recipient's own strain of hepatitis C (there are numerous genotypes of hepatitis C). The infecting donor strain virus might be more virulent than the recipient's own strain of hepatitis C and may possibly lead to substantial liver disease, but that was not established in this paper.

Many transplant centers have avoided organ sharing. Their rationale has been that the increased cold ischemia time of shared organs results in poor graft survival and more than offsets any advantage of tissue matching. A study from the South-Eastern Organ Procurement Foundation (Abstract 6–5) finds that cold ischemia time does not affect graft survival. Therefore, presumably, organ sharing could be done for any benefit tissue matching might provide without paying the price of increased cold ischemia times. On the other hand, a study by Troppmann (Abstract 6–6) finds that preservation times longer than 24 hours do lead to significantly reduced graft survival as compared with preservation times less than 24 hours. This study finds that delayed graft function when combined with acute rejection leads to a particularly low rate of graft survival when compared with either delayed graft function alone or rejection alone.

While virtually all transplant surgeons accept the use of living donors for kidney transplantation, the use of related donors for liver transplantation is much more controversial. Related parental donors have been used in certain transplant centers for liver transplantation in children. A study from Japan (Abstract 6–7) reports on 100 parental liver donors. The paper finds that related transplantation can be done safely and that grafts from parental donors enjoy high survival rates. Several attempts have been made to reduce immunosuppression, especially steroids. Many attempts have been abandoned because of the high rate of rejection with graft loss. A study from the University of Pittsburgh (Abstract 6–8) reports that in highly selected liver transplant recipients who have had stable function for at least 5 years, all immunosuppression can be safely withdrawn. These patients will have to be followed for a long time, however, to determine whether slowly progressive chronic rejection might occur.

A goal of transplantation is to save life and improve the quality of life. Certainly with heart, liver, and lung transplants the lifesaving effects of transplantation are paramount. The quality of life is also increased after liver transplantation (Abstract 6–10). Improvement in quality of life is seen 1 year after transplantation and does not improve markedly thereafter.

The results of pancreas transplantation have improved substantially in the last several years. An article summarizing the experience at the University of Nebraska details the current excellent graft survival (Abstract 6–11). These authors are accumulating a series of patients who are undergoing transplantation before renal failure develops. Presumably these patients might also receive transplants early enough in the course of retinopathy that pancreas transplantation might result in decreased eye problems over the long term.

Two articles (Abstracts 6–12 and 6–13) discuss multivisceral transplants. These procedures are still associated with a high mortality rate. Seven surviving patients with intestinal transplants are maintained solely on oral alimentation (Abstract 6–12). This is the latest report of the University of Pittsburgh experience.

A summary article on lung transplantation from Duke University and Washington University, St. Louis, review the indications, techniques, and results of lung transplantation. As experience with lung transplantation has increased, results have improved.

Finally, coronary artery disease is accelerated in cardiac transplant recipients. This coronary disease can be successfully treated by standard techniques, including angioplasty and coronary artery bypass grafting (Abstract 6–15).

Richard J. Howard, M.D., Ph.D.

Placebo-Controlled Study of Mycophenolate Mofetil Combined With Cyclosporin and Corticosteroids for Prevention of Acute Rejection
European Mycophenolate Mofetil Cooperative Study Group (Klinik für Abdominal und Transplantationschirurgie, Hannover, Germany)
Lancet 345:1321–1325, 1995   6–1

Objective.—Mycophenolate mofetil (MMF) is an immunosuppressant that was developed to prevent the important clinical problem of acute allograft rejection seen in 60% of renal transplant recipients. The efficacy of MMF when given with cyclosporine and corticosteroids was studied in this 1-year, multicenter, double-blind, placebo-controlled study.

Patients and Study Design.—Four hundred ninety-one male and female recipients of first or second cadaveric renal allografts were divided into 3 groups: placebo (166 patients), MMF at 2 g/day (165 patients), and MMF at 3 g/day (160 patients). Daily doses of cyclosporine and corticosteroids were adjusted as needed. For 1 year the patients were observed for allograft rejection or treatment failure and all adverse effects.

Results.—Significantly fewer patients in the 2 MMF treatment groups withdrew prematurely from the study or had biopsy-proven rejection (Table 2). The frequency of acute rejection episodes was reduced 60% to 70% by the addition of MMF to corticosteroid and cyclosporine therapy. The relative risk of treatment failure was reduced to 0.535 and 0.658 for MMF, 2 g, and MMF, 3 g, respectively, as compared with placebo. Fewer patients in the MMF treatment groups required a full course of immunosuppressive treatment for rejection: 86 patients in the placebo group, 47 in the 2-g MMF group, and 39 in the 3-g MMF group. Also, there were fewer courses of treatment with antilymphocyte preparations, lower serum creatinine concentrations, and lower percentages of patients needing dialysis in the MMF treatment groups as compared with the placebo group. Gastrointestinal adverse events, leukopenia, anemia, and cytomegalovirus tissue-invasive disease were more common in the MMF treatment groups than the control group.

Conclusions.—The number of patients with a biopsy-proven rejection episode or treatment failure was significantly lower in the MMF treatment groups than in the placebo group. Although there was a greater frequency of gastrointestinal adverse effects and leukopenia in the MMF treatment groups, a clear clinical advantage of reduced need for antilymphocyte therapy for corticosteroid-resistant rejection with MMF treatment was noted.

TABLE 2.—Biopsy-Proven Rejection, Treatment Failure, and Graft and Patient Survival by 6 Months

	Placebo	MMF 2 g	MMF 3 g
Biopsy-proven rejection, graft loss or death, or other treatment failure	93 (56.0%)	50 (30.3%)*	62 (38.8%)*
Biopsy-proven rejection	77 (46.4%)	28 (17.0%)	22 (13.8%)
Grade I	29/77 (37.7%)	12/28 (42.9%)	14/22 (63.6%)
Grade II	39/77 (50.6%)	12/28 (42.9%)	7/22 (31.8%)
Grade III	9/77 (11.7%)	4/28 (14.3%)	1/22 (4.5%)
Other treatment failure	16 (9.6%)	22 (13.3%)	40 (25.0%)
Graft loss/death	4 (2.4%)	3 (1.8%)	4 (2.5%)
Unsatisfactory therapeutic response	0	0	1 (0.6%)
Adverse event	6 (3.6%)	14 (8.5%)	29 (18.1%)
Non-compliance	3 (1.8%)	3 (1.8%)	5 (3.1%)
Other remaining reasons	3 (1.8)	2 (1.2%)	1 (0.6%)
Presumed or biopsy-proven rejection or treatment failure	104 (62.7%)	68 (41.2%)*	72 (45.0%)*
Presumed or biopsy-proven rejection	91 (54.8%)	50 (30.3%)	42 (26.3%)
Other treatment failure	13 (7.8%)	18 (10.9%)	30 (18.8%)
Graft loss/death†	2 (1.2%)	2 (1.2%)	3 (1.9%)
Unsatisfactory therapeutic response	0	0	0
Adverse event	5 (3.0%)	12 (7.3%)	22 (13.8%)
Non-compliance	3 (1.8%)	2 (1.2%)	4 (2.5%)
All remaining reasons	3 (1.8%)	2 (1.2%)	1 (0.6%)
All graft loss or death‡	17 (10.2%)	11 (6.7%)	14 (8.8%)
All graft losses	15 (9.0%)	7 (4.3%)	10 (6.3%)
Deaths with functioning kidney	2 (1.2%)	4 (2.4%)	4 (2.5%)

* $P \leq 0.001$ for difference from placebo.

† On study; graft loss or death as a cause of treatment failure (without previous presumed or biopsy-proven rejection).

‡ On study drug and after end of study.

Abbreviation: MMF, mycophenolate mofetil.

(Courtesy of European Mycophenolate Mofetil Cooperative Study Group: Placebo-controlled study of mycophenolate mofetil combined with cyclosporin and corticosteroids for prevention of acute rejection. *Lancet*, 345(5):1321–1325, copyright by *The Lancet* Ltd., 1995.)

Mycophenolate Mofetil for the Prevention of Acute Rejection in Primary Cadaveric Renal Allograft Recipients

Sollinger HW, for the U.S. Renal Transplant Mycophenolate Mofetil Study Group (Boston Univ; Univ of California, Los Angeles; Univ of Alabama, Birmingham; et al)
Transplantation 60:225–232, 1995   6–2

Introduction.—Mycophenolate mofetil (MMF) inhibits the synthesis of eukaryotic inosine monophosphate dehydrogenases, thereby inhibiting the proliferation of T and B lymphocytes, the formation of antibodies, and the generation of cytotoxic T cells. In animal models, treatment with MMF has prolonged the survival of various allografts. The safety and efficacy of MMF was evaluated in patients undergoing primary cadaveric renal transplantation in a randomized, double-blind study.

Methods.—A total of 499 adult patients scheduled to receive a primary cadaveric renal allograft as their first transplant were randomly assigned to treatment with either MMF at a dose of 2 or 3 g/day or azathioprine at a dose of 1–2 mg/kg/day for the prevention of allograft rejection. All patients were also given other immunosuppressive drugs, including cyclosporine A, corticosteroids, and antithymocyte globulin induction therapy. Efficacy was determined primarily on the basis of the occurrence of biopsy-proven acute rejection or treatment failure (defined as graft loss, death, or premature termination from the study within 6 months of receiving the transplant) and secondarily by comparing the use of corticosteroids and antilymphocyte preparations, the time to the first episode of acute rejection, graft and patient survival, and renal function. Adverse events, opportunistic infections, and malignancies were noted.

Results.—There was a premature withdrawal rate of 22.6% in the azathioprine group, 21.2% in the 2-g MMF group, and 25.9% in the 3-g MMF group. The incidence of a first biopsy-proven acute rejection episode was 47.7% in the azathioprine group, 31.1% in the 2-g MMF group, and 31.3% in the 3-g MMF group (Fig 1). The patients treated with MMF at either dosage had significantly fewer and less severe rejection episodes than did the patients treated with azathioprine. The time to the first rejection episode was significantly longer with MMF at either dosage than with azathioprine. Graft loss or death occurred in 10.4% of the azathioprine group, 5.5% of the 2-g MMF group, and 8.5% of the 3-g MMF group. There were no significant differences between the groups in the use of corticosteroids, but the patients in the azathioprine group were significantly more likely to require at least 1 full course of antirejection immunosuppressive therapy and antilymphocyte agents. The mean serum creatinine level was significantly higher at 28 days and tended to be higher at

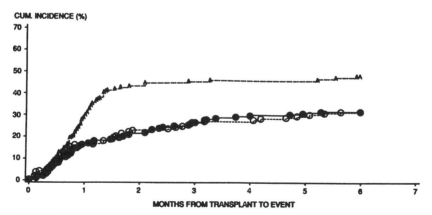

FIGURE 1.—Cumulative incidence of the first biopsy-proven rejection or treatment failure during months 0–6. *Abbreviations: A,* azathioprine, 1–2 mg/kg (n = 166); *open circles,* mycophenolate mofetil, 1.0 g twice daily (n = 167), P = 0.0036; *filled circles,* mycophenolate mofetil, 1.5 g twice daily (n = 166), P = 0.0006. Note: Kaplan-Meier estimates. (Courtesy of Sollinger HW, for the U.S. Renal Transplant Mycophenolate Mofetil Study Group: Mycophenolate mofetil for the prevention of acute rejection in primary cadaveric renal allograft recipients. *Transplantation* 60(3):225–232, 1995.)

6 months in the azathioprine group than in the other 2 groups. Nearly all patients experienced adverse events. Opportunistic infections tended to occur more frequently in the MMF groups than in the azathioprine group. All malignancies occurred in the MMF groups. The 3-g MMF group tended to have a higher incidence of severe anemia and clinically important thrombocytopenia than the other 2 treatment groups.

Conclusions.—Mycophenolate mofetil is highly effective in preventing acute rejection of a primary cadaveric renal allograft and has an acceptable side effect profile. Further study should evaluate its effectiveness in improving long-term graft survival.

▶ These 2 large controlled trials, 1 from the United States and 1 from Europe, used similar protocols, had similar numbers of patients, and came up with similar findings. Substituting mycophenolate mofetil for azathioprine after transplantation is associated with fewer graft rejection episodes. There is a price to pay, however. In both studies there was an increased number of complications. It is disappointing that the decreased number of rejection episodes did not translate into improved graft survival. Perhaps as these patients are followed longer, improved graft survival may be detected since early rejection is a determinant of long-term graft survival. Mycophenolate mofetil is approximately 5 times as expensive as azathioprine. Is it worth it? When patients are already struggling to pay for their immunosuppressive drugs, adding a more expensive drug that does not increase the likelihood of graft survival and is associated with a higher incidence of complications may be difficult to justify. Each transplant center will have to come up with its own conclusions.

R.J. Howard, M.D., Ph.D.

High Survival Rates of Kidney Transplants From Spousal and Living Unrelated Donors
Terasaki PI, Cecka JM, Gjertson DW, Takemoto S (Univ of California, Los Angeles)
N Engl J Med 333:333–336, 1995   6–3

Introduction.—There is increasing evidence of high rates of kidney graft survival from spouses and other living unrelated donors when compared with cadaveric graft survival despite substantial mismatch for HLA antigens. Factors contributing to the success rate of grafts from unrelated living donors were investigated.

Methods.—Data from the United Network for Organ Sharing Renal Transplant Registry were obtained to compare the survival rates of grafts from 368 spouses, 129 living unrelated donors, 3,368 parents, 1,984 HLA-identical siblings, and 43,341 cadavers. The relationships between donor kidney characteristics and graft survival were analyzed.

Results.—The 3-year graft survival rates for kidneys were 91% from HLA-matched siblings, 85% from spouses, 81% from living unrelated donors, 82% from parents, and 70% from cadavers. After stratification for age, survival rates were consistently higher with grafts from living than from cadaveric donors. Graft survival rates were equally high from husbands or wives (87%) if the wife had had no children but were nonsignificantly reduced (76%) if the wife had been pregnant. The survival rate for grafts from parents and from living unrelated donors was similar even though there was more HLA mismatching with the latter group. However, the number of HLA mismatches did affect the survival of spousal grafts. Delayed graft function was significantly associated with a lower survival rate regardless of the degree of HLA matching. Cadaveric grafts that functioned immediately had a survival rate similar to that of grafts from living unrelated donors. Graft survival was not significantly influenced by the duration of cold ischemia. Preoperative recipient transfusions were associated with an increased survival rate of spousal grafts.

Conclusions.—When compared with cadaveric donors, kidney grafts from living unrelated donors have higher survival rates regardless of the degree of HLA matching. The most important factor predicting graft survival is immediate graft functioning, thus suggesting that the lower rate of survival of cadaveric grafts is explained by damage to the kidney before removal.

▶ This large series taken from the renal transplant registry of the United Network for Organ Sharing demonstrates in a large series of patients what others have previously shown; that is, graft survival using spousal and living unrelated donors is extremely high. One might believe that living unrelated kidney donors would offer no advantage over cadaveric grafts. In fact, the survival rates are much better than that of cadaveric grafts. Variables normally thought to play an important role in graft survival such as HLA matching, length of cold ischemia, race, and donor age could not explain the differences. The authors believe that the crucial difference might be that 10% of cadaveric grafts are damaged before removal as indicated by a 10% difference in graft survival rates. Certainly, cadaveric grafts are more likely to have delayed graft function than spousal and living unrelated donors. Patients who have delayed graft function have significantly lower graft survival than kidney recipients who do not have delayed graft function. Living unrelated donors are another way of alleviating the organ shortage; the number of cadaveric grafts has not nearly kept pace with the demand. Because of the excellent graft survival and the extremely low risk to the donor, using spousal and unrelated donors is ethically justified.

R.J. Howard, M.D., Ph.D.

Hepatitis C Superinfection in Hepatitis C Virus (HCV)-Infected Patients Transplanted With an HCV-Infected Kidney

Widell A, Månsson S, Persson NH, Thysell H, Hermodsson S, Blohme I
(Malmö Univ Hosp, Sweden; Lund Univ Hosp, Sweden; Sahlgrenska Univ Hosp, Göteborg, Sweden)

Transplantation 60:642–647, 1995

6–4

Introduction.—Occasionally, hepatitis C virus (HCV)-infected kidneys may be transplanted into already HCV-infected recipients. Data on outcome are meager and conflicting, partly because until recently it was difficult to determine whether infection was caused by the donor or the recipient strain. The virologic course and clinical data were studied in HCV-positive recipients of HCV-positive kidneys by polymerase chain reaction (PCR).

Methods.—Three transplant patients were studied retrospectively and 2 were studied prospectively. In all cases, the recipient and the donor had HCV infections with different genotypes. Hepatitis C virus RNA extracted from serum or plasma was genotyped by nested PCR with type-specific primers. Levels of serum alanine aminotransferase (ALT) were monitored before and after transplantation.

Results.—Recipient 1 had HCV genotype 2b infection and received a kidney with HCV genotype 3a. By 6 months after transplantation, only the donor genotype was present. His liver function tests revealed a slow increase in ALT beginning at 4 months and reaching a maximal level at 1 year and then stabilizing. Recipient 2 also had HCV genotype 2b and the donor kidney had genotype 3a. A mixed genotype infection developed by 6 months posttransplantation and persisted. Beginning at 3 months after surgery, liver enzymes increased gradually. Recipient 3 had HCV genotype 2b infection and the donor kidney had an HCV genotype 3a infection. This patient had an unchanging type 2b infection only and demonstrated periodic transient asymptomatic increases in serum ALT levels thought to be caused by azathioprine treatment. Recipient 4 had a genotype 1b infection before transplantation with a genotype 1a–infected kidney. All posttransplantation blood samples had only the recipient's original genotype. Liver enzyme levels remained normal throughout follow-up except for 2 transient ALT increases. Recipient 5 was originally infected with HCV genotype 3a and received a genotype 1a–infected kidney. Beginning at 3 weeks after transplantation, the donor genotype became detectable, and the recipient genotype was completely replaced by 2 months after surgery. Beginning at 3.5 months after surgery, ALT values doubled for 1.5 months and then returned to pretransplantation levels.

Conclusions.—Transplantation of an HCV-infected kidney into an HCV-infected patient can result in 3 different virologic courses: persistence of the recipient's genotype only, replacement by the donor's genotype, or a mixed-genotype superinfection. Although the patients will usually have a short-term benefit, superinfected patients may experience increased and unpredictable liver damage.

▶ One strategy to increase the number of organ donors suitable for transplantation is to redefine "suitable." The use of kidneys from hepatitis C–positive donors has long been controversial, with some studies finding that recipients of hepatitis C–positive kidneys did as well as recipients of kidneys from hepatitis C–negative donors and other reports finding that using kidneys from hepatitis C–positive donors resulted in worse outcomes. Still, a third course is to use hepatitis C–positive kidneys only in hepatitis C–positive recipients. A concern in this latter strategy is that the recipients could become infected with a different strain of hepatitis. The current paper addresses this issue (all 5 recipients of hepatitis C–infected kidneys were already infected with hepatitis C virus). The authors studied only a small number of patients but found that in some cases the donor strain replaced the recipient strain. In 1 other case the recipient had infection with both the donor strain and her own strain of hepatitis C. Since some strains are thought to be more likely to cause severe liver damage than others, it is possible that even a hepatitis C–positive recipient could be disadvantaged by receiving a transplant from a donor with a more virulent hepatitis C strain. This study clearly shows that liver function decreases after infection with donor-strain hepatitis C virus. Although there may be little difference if patients are studied early after their posttransplant course, significant liver disease may be encountered later.

R.J. Howard, M.D., Ph.D.

Cold Ischemia and Outcome in 17,937 Cadaveric Kidney Transplants
Peters TG, Shaver TR, Ames JE, Santiago-Delpin EA, Jones KW, Blanton JW
(The South-Eastern Organ Procurement Foundation, Richmond, Va; Univ of Florida, Jacksonville; Walter Reed Army Med Ctr, Washington, DC; et al)
Transplantation 59:191–196, 1995   6–5

Introduction.—With the increasing need of kidneys for transplantation, it is important that no available kidneys be wasted unless sound reasons are evident. Questions remain about the ultimate outcome in organ transplantation and varying cold ischemic times. Thus the presence or absence of adverse effects was analyzed in 17,937 cadaveric renal transplants performed with varying cold preservation times.

Methods.—Information about the organ donor, the kidney, the transplant recipient, and periodic posttransplant follow-up was prospectively gathered from 1982 to 1991. Separate analyses were performed for patients who received kidneys preserved for 1–16, 16–32, 32–48, and over 48 hours. The University of Wisconsin solution became widespread after 1989, so a separate analysis was done for the 13,800 kidneys transplanted before January 1, 1990, and the 4,137 subsequent kidneys transplanted through 1991. AN HLA match at 3 or more loci occurred in 6,067 (34%) transplants.

Results.—Before 1990, graft functional survival was significantly better for kidneys stored for 1–16 hours than those preserved for longer periods.

Graft functional survival was similar in kidneys stored 16–32, 32–48, and more than 48 hours in the years from 1982 to 1989. However, there was no significant difference in preservation times and allograft survival in 1990–1991. One-year actuarial graft survival rates were 74%, 83%, and 76%, respectively, for grafts transplanted from 1982 to 1989, 1990 to 1991, and overall. Before 1990, the strongest outcome factors were delayed graft function, degree of match, retransplanted recipient, black race, and previous transfusion for all kidneys. During 1990–1991, the most significant outcome factors were delayed graft function and degree of match. Poorer outcomes were observed overall in older patients regardless of the date of transplantation. Delayed graft function occurred significantly more frequently in all kidneys preserved beyond 16 hours. However, 1-year allograft survival was not related to the duration of organ preservation in the event of delayed graft function.

Conclusion.—Functional viability of kidneys preserved 48 hours or longer may be expected with current preservation methods. Prolonged cold ischemic time is no longer a major factor in discarding organs.

▶ Organ sharing in order to achieve a more favorable crossmatch frequently means sending kidneys from 1 transplant center to another, something that increases graft preservation time. This study from the South-Eastern Organ Procurement Foundation demonstrates that with the use of University of Wisconsin solution, prolonged cold ischemia does not lead to decreased graft function. It suggests that organ sharing, which may prolong cold ischemia, in order to achieve better tissue matching does not disadvantage patients. They show as others have shown that delayed graft function does lead to worse graft outcome. In the study by Troppmann et al. (Abstract 140-96-6–6), however, graft preservation times greater than 24 hours were associated with decreased graft survival. Whether these different findings are due to this being a multi-institutional study and Troppmann and colleagues' study being from a single institution where presumably other variables were more constant cannot be determined. In any case, the finding that delayed graft function leads to lower graft survival is consistent with several other reports. Measures to lower the rate of delayed graft function will likely lead to increased graft survival.

R.J. Howard, M.D., Ph.D.

Delayed Graft Function, Acute Rejection, and Outcome After Cadaver Renal Transplantation: A Multivariate Analysis
Troppmann C, Gillingham KJ, Benedetti E, Almond PS, Gruessner RWG, Najarian JS, Matas AJ (Univ of Minnesota, Minneapolis)
Transplantation 59:962–968, 1995   6–6

Goal.—The results of studies on the effects of delayed graft function (DGF) after renal transplantation have been inconsistent because factors such as acute rejection have not been considered. Therefore, the effect of

DGF and several variables (e.g., acute rejection, preservation time and mode, gender) on outcome in cyclosporine-treated primary cadaver renal allograft recipients was assessed by multivariate analysis.

Methods.—A homogeneous patient population of 457 primary cadaver allograft recipients was studied. The transplant procedure was routine. Immunosuppression therapy consisted of a prednisone taper, a 7-day course of Minnesota antilymphocyte globulin or antithymocyte globulin, and cyclosporine administration. The graft was monitored by imaging and biopsy in cases of DGF (defined as the need for at least 1 session of dialysis within 7 days of receiving the transplant) or when rejection was suspected.

Results.—Delayed graft function was noted in 23% of the patients and was significantly associated with a cold ischemia time of greater than 24 hours and with the occurrence of acute rejection episodes. Graft survival rates after cold ischemia preservation times of less than 24 hours were 94% at 1 year and 84% at 5 years as compared with 85% and 63%, respectively, after cold ischemia of greater than 24 hours. Univariate analysis of the 200 patients who had at least 1 biopsy-proven and treated rejection episode revealed that 57% of them had DGF as compared with only 40% without DGF. Multivariate analysis of graft survival rates (87% at 1 year and 67% at 5 years) indicated that DGF in combination with rejection, rejection alone, and cold ischemia of greater than 24 hours were associated with significantly decreased graft survival. Delayed graft function alone and other parameters such as HLA match, preservation mode, diabetic status, age, and gender were not associated with a significant risk for graft loss. During the follow-up period, 18% of the patients died. Patient survival was significantly affected by the combination of DGF and rejection and by age at transplantation.

Conclusions.—Both cold ischemia time of greater than 24 hours and acute rejection episodes are significantly associated with DGF in adult, primary cadaver kidney recipients. The risk of poor graft survival is highest in patients with both DGF and rejection and after cold ischemia of greater than 24 hours.

▶ As demonstrated in the previous study by Peters et al. (Abstract 6–5), delayed graft function is a determinant of late graft survival. The authors found that only the combination of delayed graft function and rejection led to a significant reduction in late graft survival. Early events, either rejection, delayed graft function, or both together, can result in lower short-term and long-term graft survival. Early events have very long-term consequences. Univariate analysis showed an association between cold ischemic time greater than 24 hours and decreased graft survival. But by multivariate analysis there was not a significant relationship. The only relationship was between delayed graft function combined with rejection and lower graft survival. The incidence of delayed graft function in this series was 23%. Surprisingly, there was no relationship between the incidence of delayed function and the method of storage: pulsatile perfusion vs. cold storage on ice. Other studies have demonstrated that pulsatile perfusion leads to a low incidence of delayed graft function, between 5% and 10%, a main argument for using pulsatile perfusion, which is certainly more cumbersome and more expensive. This study suggests that pulsatile perfusion does not lead to low graft survival, although the authors do not state what proportion of kidneys were preserved by pulsatile perfusion and what proportion by cold preservation on ice, nor do they discuss the relationship between preservation method and delayed graft function.

R.J. Howard, M.D., Ph.D.

Safety of the Donor in Living-Related Liver Transplantation: An Analysis of 100 Parental Donors
Yamaoka Y, Morimoto T, Inamoto T, Tanaka A, Honda K, Ikai I, Tanaka K, Ichimiya M, Ueda M, Shimahara Y (Kyoto Univ, Japan)
Transplantation 59:224–226, 1995   6–7

Introduction.—The use of living related liver transplantation (LRLTx) has always been criticized because it exposes the donor to surgical risks. Cadaveric liver grafting is not a consideration in Japan, so it is important to determine the risk to the donor of LRLTx. The safety and lack of undue operative stress were analyzed in 100 parental donors whose children received LRLTx.

Methods.—One hundred parental donors were selected on the basis of willingness, liver function, suitable volumetry, and ABO compatibility. The age range of the donors was 19–51 years, and weights ranged from 44 to 80 kg. Twenty-four, 75, and 1 donor, respectively, underwent left lobectomy (L group), left lateral segumentectomy (S group), and right lobectomy (R group) to provide a liver graft. Operative stress was evaluated by the amount of blood loss, operative time, postoperative complications, alterations in arterial ketone body ratio (AKBR), and alterations in conventional laboratory testing.

Results.—Intraoperative blood loss ranged from 50 to 2,300 g, with a mean of 597 g in the L group, 368 g in the S group, and 2,300 g in the patient who underwent right lobectomy (and subsequent autologous transfusion for the blood loss). Mean operative times for the L, S, and R groups, respectively, were 7.2, 6.2, and 10.1 hours. No significant differences between groups were noted in the AKBR. Bilirubin increased significantly and red blood cells decreased significantly in the patients with right lobectomy; this necessitated hospitalization of 17 days as compared with 11 days for the L and S groups. All instances of esophagitis (1), gastritis (7), gastroduodenal ulcer (3), and bile leakage (4) required therapy, and all patients recovered within 4 weeks.

Conclusion.—Blood loss was acceptable for all patients except the patient with the right lobectomy, who required autologous blood transfusion. Findings indicate that safety and lack of undue operative stress on the donor are likely when the left lateral segment or left lobe is used for LRLTx.

▶ Virtually all transplant surgeons accept the use of living related donors for kidney transplantation. More controversial is the use of living related donors for liver transplantation because of the increased risk of removing part of an unpaired organ. This report from Japan, which does not have brain death laws, analyzes 100 parental donors whose children required liver transplantation. It demonstrates that the procedure can be done safely and that recipients of livers obtained from related donors have excellent long-term survival.

R.J. Howard, M.D., Ph.D.

Weaning of Immunosuppresion in Long-Term Liver Transplant Recipients
Ramos HC, Reyes JR, Abu-Elmagd K, Zeevi A, Reinsmoen N, Tzakis A, Demetric AJ, Fung JJ, Flynn B, McMichael J, Ebert F, Starzl TE (Univ of Pittsburgh, Pa; Veterans Administration Med Ctr, Pittsburgh, Pa)
Transplantation 59:212–217, 1995   6–8

Introduction.—Successful weaning from immunosuppressant agents in noncompliant recipients of liver transplants has raised the possibility of therapeutic drug weaning. A prospective trial of drug weaning in 59 long-surviving liver recipients with complications of chronic immunosuppression is described.

Methods.—The drug regimens patients were weaned from were azathioprine (AZA) and prednisone (PRED) in 10 patients, cyclosporine (CsA) and PRED in 19, CsA/AZA in 3, CsA/AZA/PRED in 12, CsA alone in 9, and tacrolimus in 6. When AZA was a part of triple therapy, it was weaned first. Otherwise, weaning began with a 25% to 50% reduction of prednisone, followed by further decrements at 1-month intervals. Corticotropin stimulation was done before complete steroid withdrawal. Reductions for baseline CsA, AZA, and tacrolimus were also considered each month. In patients receiving CsA, there was a 10% to 25% reduction per month until blood levels reached less than 50 ng/mL for 3 months and then a 50% reduction per month until cessation. The protocol for tacrolimus was similar. Baseline and weekly or biweekly enzyme measurements of aspartate aminotransferase, alanine aminotransferase, γ-glutamyltranspeptidase, and serum bilirubin and CsA and tacrolimus trough levels were performed.

Results.—At a mean follow-up of 15 months, 15 patients (25.1%) failed weaning without graft loss or demonstrable loss of graft function from the rejections. All liver functions eventually returned to their preweaning values, and 2 patients were subsequently placed back on the weaning protocol. At follow-up, 16 patients (27.1%) had stopped taking immunosuppressants at 3–19 months and the other 28 (47.4%) were at various stages of weaning. A high rate of weaning failure was noted in patients previously treated with triple- or double-drug CsA-based immunosuppression. Seven of 13 patients with donor leukocyte chimerism were successfully weaned.

Conclusion.—A significant number of appropriately selected patients with long-surviving liver transplants can achieve drug-free graft acceptance. Patients must be selected carefully and followed closely, with resumption of immunosuppression when needed.

▶ Many posttransplant complications are related to chronic immunosuppressive therapy. The management of posttransplant patients requires minimizing the use of immunosuppressive drugs to reduce these complications but not reducing them so much that rejection occurs. A promise of new immunosuppressive drugs such as cyclosporine and tacrolimus was that other immunosuppressive drugs, especially steroids, might be safely withdrawn. Several studies attempted steroid withdrawal after cyclosporine became available, but the rate of rejection and graft loss was high. This study from the University of Pittsburgh shows that in certain selected patients with liver transplants, all immunosuppression can be successfully withdrawn. The authors carefully chose their patients. All patients were more than 5 years posttransplant and more than 2 years without rejection episodes. They also had a history of medical compliance and evidence of complications related to chronic immunosuppressive therapy. The primary physician had to cooperate and baseline liver biopsy had to show no evidence of rejection. During weaning from immunosuppressive drugs, 25% had a diagnosis of rejection. No patients lost their graft. Although withdrawal from immunosuppression is desirable and can be accomplished in some patients, we will have to await the long-term results to determine whether long-term problems such as chronic rejection occur.

R.J. Howard, M.D., Ph.D.

The Predictive Value of Four Scoring Systems in Liver Transplant Recipients
Bein T, Fröhlich D, Pömsl J, Forst H, Pratschke E (Klinikum der Universität, Regensburg, Germany; Ludwig-Maximilians-Univ, Munich)
Intensive Care Med 21:32–37, 1995   6–9

Objective.—The ability of 4 different scoring systems to predict mortality in liver transplant recipients was compared in this retrospective study.

Methods/Patients.—The 4 scoring systems that were compared were (1) the Mortality Prediction Model at admission (MPM admission) and 24 hours after admission (MPH-24h) to the ICU, (2) the Simplified Acute Physiology Score (SAPS), (3) the Acute Physiology and Chronic Health Evaluation (APACHE II), and (4) the Acute Organ Systems Failure (OSF) score. The variables used for calculating the 4 scoring systems in 123 liver transplant recipients were available retrospectively. Receiver operating characteristics (ROC) for all 4 systems were plotted, and the areas under the curves of these plots were calculated.

Results.—The average age of the patients was 47.6 years, and the average length of stay in the ICU was 24.7 days. Three of the 4 scoring systems, MPM-24h, SAPS, and APACHE II satisfactorily predicted mortality in the 123 patients with liver transplants. In all 3 of these systems, the risk of death between survivors and nonsurvivors was significantly different. The highest sensitivity (83%) and best performance, that is, an area under the ROC curve of 0.829, were obtained with the MPM-24h. Similar sensitivities of 72% and 71% and similar areas under the ROC curves of 0.737 and 0.702 were obtained with the SAPS and APACHE II, respectively. The specificities of MPM-24h, SAPS, and APACHE II were 65%, 59%, and 59%, respectively. The OFS system of scoring failed to predict mortality in these patients.

Conclusions.—The general disease classification systems MPM-24h, SAPS, and APACHE II are adequate mortality predictors in liver transplant recipients. There is no need for an improved, specialized scoring system for these patients. The MPM-24h system is the most sensitive and specific of the systems studied, probably because it combines variables of both the physiologic disorder being assessed and therapeutic application.

▶ Predicting mortality 24 hours after liver transplantation is probably not very helpful since the operation is already done. It would be much more helpful to be able to reliably predict mortality pretransplant as a guide to whether or not patients should undergo transplantation in the first place. Scoring systems such as used here were not helpful at admission for transplantation and are unlikely to be useful in the future because many determinants of mortality occur during surgery (development of renal failure, blood loss, primary graft nonfunction). This study does demonstrate that some scoring systems such as the MPM-24h and SAPS were highly significant in predicting mortality, but only after transplantation. It's unclear what the authors would have us do with the data. If any scoring system predicts that a patient has a high likelihood of mortality after transplantation, how would that change one's behavior? Probably not at all.

R.J. Howard, M.D., Ph.D.

Quality of Life Improvements at One, Two, and Five Years After Liver Transplantation

Levy MF, Jennings L, Abouljoud MS, Mulligan DC, Godlstein RM, Husberg BS, Gonwa TA, Klintmalm GB (Baylor Univ, Dallas)
Transplantation 59:515–518, 1995   6–10

Objective.—A prospective study was conducted to evaluate the effect on quality of life (QOL) of orthotopic liver transplantation (OLTX) in adults.

Study Design.—Over an 8-year period, all adult patients undergoing OLTX voluntarily completed a psychological questionnaire that probed broad facets of QOL ranging from patient demographics and occupation to symptom distress/frequency, activities of daily living, and impact of

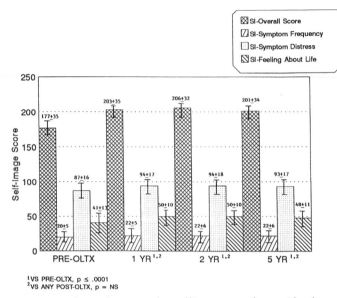

FIGURE 1.—Pretransplant and posttransplant self-image score, shown with subscores to 5 years posttransplant. *Abbreviation: OLTX*, orthotopic liver transplantation. (Courtesy of Levy MF, Jennings L, Aboujoud MS, et al: Quality of life improvements at one, two, and five years after liver transplantation. *Transplantation* 59(4):515–518, 1995.)

health on daily life. Questions were grouped by categories highlighting self-image, health perception, ability to function, and ability to work. Numerical scores were assigned to each question and added to derive global scores; higher scores reflected better QOL.

Findings.—A total of 573 questionnaires were completed, including 210 pretransplant, 150 at 1 year, 131 at 2 years, and 79 at 5 or more years posttransplant. After OLTX, there were striking improvements in self-image, functioning ability, and perception of health status as soon as 1 year after OLTX. These improvements remained nearly constant at all time points but were sustained beyond 5 years (Fig 1). Although only half the patients were working for pay 1 year post-OLTX, when compared with pre-OLTX, employment levels were regained by the second year and continued to increase thereafter.

Conclusions.—In adult recipients, OLTX appears to be quite successful in restoring QOL, in returning people to stable self-perceived health and activity levels, and in allowing their return to the workforce. Ill health interference in daily life in terms of overall function and relation to work activities continues to decrease as OLTX becomes more remote. Employment suffers early after OLTX but recovers by the second posttransplant year and continues to increase long-term.

▶ Transplantation has 2 goals: to save life and to improve the quality of life. For patients with renal disease, dialysis provides an alternative to transplantation. Patients requiring liver, heart, or lung transplants have no alternative other than medical management and, frequently, early death. Transplantation can improve the length of life after transplantation. This study demonstrates it can also improve the quality of life. The increase in quality-of-life assessment was evident a year after liver transplantation but did not change thereafter. Although self-assessment tests showed that quality of life did improve, only 39.2% of the patients were working for pay 1 year following transplantation as compared with 62.2% who were working pretransplant. The number of individuals who worked increased, however. Two years after transplantation 57.5% worked, and the number increased to 69.7% 5 years posttransplant.

R.J. Howard, M.D., Ph.D.

Surgical Treatment of Diabetes Mellitus With Pancreas Transplantation
Stratta RJ, Taylor RJ, Bynon S, Lowell JA, Sindhi R, Wahl TO, Knight TF, Weide LG, Duckworth WC (Univ of Nebraska, Omaha; Clarkson Hospital, Omaha, Neb)
Ann Surg 220:809–817, 1994   6–11

Background.—Diabetes mellitus is the third most common disease in the United States. It is the leading cause of kidney failure and blindness in adults and the leading disease cause of amputations and impotence. It is associated with accelerated atherosclerosis, abnormal lipid metabolism, and cardiovascular disease. Vascularized pancreas transplantation can normalize glycosylated hemoglobin levels, but this is counterbalanced by the operative risks and the need for chronic immunosuppression. Combined pancreas-kidney transplantation is the best treatment option for some patients with insulin-dependent diabetes mellitus who need or will need dialysis. Preemptive transplantation is the use of transplantation before the need for dialysis or transplantation. The safety and efficacy of preemptive pancreas-kidney transplantation and solitary pancreas transplantation performed earlier in the course of insulin-dependent diabetes mellitus were compared.

Methods.—During the 4-year study period, patient data were collected prospectively and analyzed retrospectively. Three groups participated: (1) 38 patients with insulin-dependent diabetes mellitus who were dialysis dependent and undergoing pancreas-kidney transplantation, (2) 44 patients with insulin-dependent diabetes mellitus undergoing preemptive pancreas-kidney transplantation before beginning dialysis, and (3) 20 patients with insulin-dependent diabetes mellitus undergoing solitary pancreas transplantation. All patients were treated with quadruple immunosuppression.

Results.—At 1 year, the patient survival rate was 100% for group 1, 98% for group 2, and 93% for group 3. The overall survival rate was 97% for group 1, 95% for group 2, and 95% for group 3. Actuarial pancreas graft survival up to 4 years is depicted in Figure 4. For all groups, the rate of rejection, infection, surgical complications, readmissions, and total days

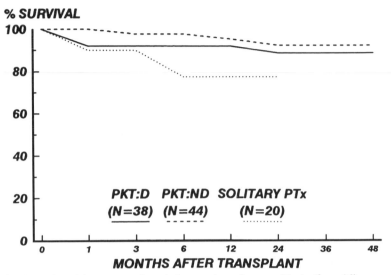

FIGURE 4.—Actuarial pancreas graft survival among the study groups. No significant differences were noted. *Abbreviations: PKT:D,* dialysis-dependent patients with insulin-dependent diabetes mellitus (IDDM) undergoing pancreas-kidney transplantation (PKT); *PKT:ND,* concurrent IDDM patients undergoing preemptive PKT before dialysis; *PTx,* pancreas transplantation. (Courtesy of Stratta RJ, Taylor RJ, Bynon S, et al: Surgical treatment of diabetes mellitus with pancreas transplantation. *Ann Surg* 220:809–817, 1994.)

in the hospital was similar. Also, long-term renal and pancreas allograft function and quality of life were similar for all groups.

Discussion.—In carefully selected patients with insulin-dependent diabetes mellitus, pancreas transplantation or preemptive pancreas-kidney transplantation can be effective. After increased waiting times for organs and the variable progression of complications of diabetes mellitus are considered, these treatments need not be regarded preemptive.

▶ Pancreas transplantation has certainly come a long way in the last decade. Graft survival rates are now high, especially when pancreas transplantation is combined with kidney transplantation. The inability of pancreas transplantation to slow the progression of other complications associated with long-standing diabetes, especially retinopathy, has been disappointing. The 20 patients with pancreas transplants who did not have renal failure and therefore did not receive kidney transplants can provide information on whether the development of secondary complications of diabetes is reduced (one would certainly hope so in this group if pancreas transplantation is going to meet its desired goals). For some patients who have very difficult-to-control blood glucose levels, pancreas transplantation may provide substantial benefits. But if it cannot be demonstrated to ameliorate the secondary complications of diabetes, it will be hard to justify over the long term in many patients. Although early pancreas transplantation may prevent the secondary complications of diabetes mellitus, not all diabetics will develop severe complications.

R.J. Howard, M.D., Ph.D.

Abdominal Multivisceral Transplantation

Todo S, Tzakis A, Abu-Elmagd K, Reyes J, Furukawa H, Nour B, Fung J, Demetris A, Starzl TE (Pittsburgh Transplantation Inst, Pa; Univ of Pittsburgh, Pa)
Transplantation 59:234–240, 1995   6–12

Objectives.—Abdominal multivisceral transplantation has been tried in very few patients and has not been very successful. Encouraging results with a new immunosuppressive agent, FK 506, in clinical trials of intestinal transplantation led to this study of 13 patients who received abdominal multivisceral transplants with FK 506 immunosuppression.

Patients/Procedures.—Thirteen patients (6 children, 7 adults) with short-bowel syndrome with or without total parenteral nutrition–related liver failure, mesenteric venous thrombosis with end-stage liver failure, juvenile polyposes, and malignant endocrine tumor were the recipients of multivisceral grafts obtained from cadavers. The multivisceral transplantation operation (Fig 1) was similar to that used in early clinical cases and included arterial reconstruction; reconstruction of the proximal gastrointestinal continuity; anastomosis of the terminal ileum or ascending, transverse, or descending colon of the grafts; and cholecystectomy. Tube jejunostomies were made for enteral feeding and endoscopic examination. Postoperative management of the patients included immunosuppression with FK 506, steroids, and prostaglandin E_1. Intestinal graft rejection and function were monitored.

Results.—The actual patient survival rate was 53.8% (7/13). These patients are alive with well-functioning grafts after 9–31 months. There was no evidence of graft-vs.-host disease (GVHD) in any of the cases. The trend in the survivors after 1 year is recovery of normal gastric emptying and intestinal transit, maintenance of body weight, and normal liver function. The 6 deaths occurred within 7 months of surgery and were due to posttransplant lymphoproliferative disease (PTLD), respiratory failure, rejection, and sepsis. Rejection was noted in 84.6% (11/13) of the recipients; the pancreas and liver were rejected in 30.1% (4/13) and 46.2% (6/13) of the recipients, respectively. Significant complications in all but 1 recipient included PTLD, intra-abdominal abscess, renal failure, and infection.

Conclusions.—Over half of the multivisceral transplant recipients in this study were restored to near-normal health and all cases were free from GVHD. Multivisceral transplantation with FK 506–based immunosuppression is not ready for widespread use, however, because of the high mortality and serious complications involved.

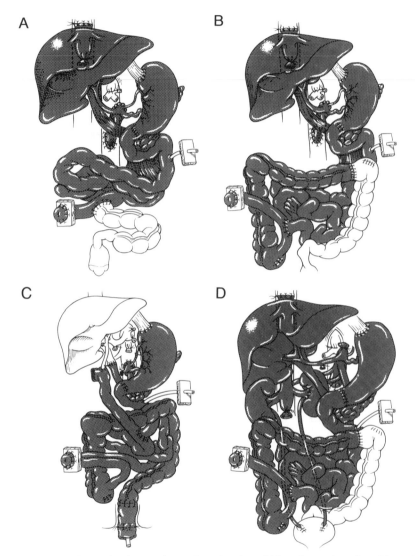

FIGURE 1.—Scheme of multivisceral transplantation. **A,** multivisceral transplantation without the colon. **B,** multivisceral transplantation with the colon. **C,** multivisceral transplantation without the liver and with rectal reconstruction by a pull-through technique. **D,** multivisceral transplantation with bilateral kidneys. (Courtesy of Todo S, Tzakis A, Abu-Elmagd K, et al: Abdominal multivisceral transplantation. *Transplantation* 59(2):234–240, 1995.)

▶ Intestinal transplantation with or without the liver is a formidable undertaking. The University of Pittsburgh group reports on 13 patients with intestinal grafts with liver (12 patients), stomach, kidney (1 patient), and colon (10 patients). All 7 surviving patients had nutrition maintained solely with an oral diet and did not need supplemental IV nutrition. Nevertheless, half the patients died and there were numerous life-threatening complications. This is a follow-up to the 23 patients reported in the 1993 and 1995 YEAR BOOK OF SURGERY.[1, 2]

R.J. Howard, M.D., Ph.D.

References

1. Todo S, et al: *Ann Surg* 216:223–234, 1992 (1993 YEAR BOOK OF SURGERY, p 151).
2. Abu-Elmagd K, Todo S, Tzakis A, et al: Intestinal transplantation: Three years experience. *J Am Coll Surg* 179:385–400, 1994 (1995 YEAR BOOK OF SURGERY, p 169).

Assessment of Five-Year Experience With Abdominal Organ Cluster Transplantation

Alessiani M, Tzakis A, Todo S, Demetris AJ, Fung JJ, Starzl TE (Univ of Pittsburgh, Pa)
J Am Coll Surg 180:1–9, 1995   6–13

Objective.—Otherwise unresectable neoplastic disease involving the upper abdominal organs may be managed by so-called cluster exenteration entailing resection of the liver, stomach, spleen, panceaticoduodenal complex, and part of the colon. The results of this procedure were reviewed in 57 patients who were operated on between mid-1988 and mid-1992 and were followed to the end of 1993.

Patients.—The patients ranged in age from 8 to 59 years. The most common malignancies were cholangiocarcinoma and hepatocellular carcinoma, present in 20 and 12 patients, respectively. Fourteen patients had endocrine tumors of pancreatic, enteric, or gastric origin, and 6 had gastrointestinal sarcomas. Lymph nodes were involved in 31 patients, and 18 had metastases to other whole organs in addition to liver involvement. Gross vascular invasion was present in the liver in 33 cases. Thirty patients had had conventional surgery, and 19 had received chemotherapy and/or radiotherapy.

Management.—A total of 61 transplant operations were performed. There were 23 conventional composite graft procedures consisting of the liver, pancreas, duodenum, and some of the proximal jejunum (Fig 1). Twenty-seven modified cluster operations were done in which only the liver was replaced. Eleven patients had donor islets injected into the portal vein of the transplanted liver.

Results.—All patients survived surgery, but 4 required retransplantation. Survival rates were 81% at 3 months, 56% 1 year postoperatively, and 30% at 5 years. Presently 18 patients (31.5%) are living 42 months postoperatively. One-year survival was improved in the group having modified transplantation, but 3-year survival was not. Eleven patients lacking node involvement and vascular invasion and in whom metastasis was limited to the liver had 1- and 3-year survival rates of 64% and 45%, respectively.

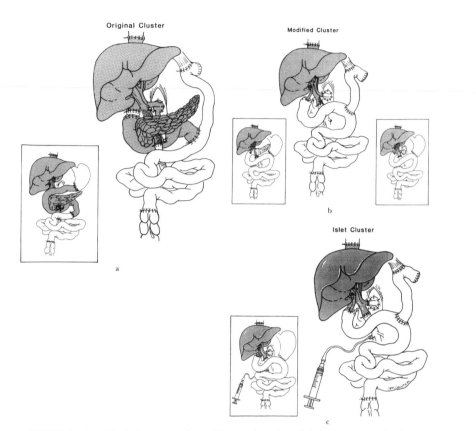

FIGURE 1.—A, original cluster procedure with transplantation of the liver-pancreas-duodenum en bloc. In 2 cases, part of the stomach was preserved and the transplanted duodenum was placed in continuity with the stomach and jejunum of the patient (*inset*). **B,** modified cluster procedure with transplantation of the liver only. In 8 patients one third or more of the recipient stomach was preserved (*inset, right*), including 3 patients in whom the body and the tail of the pancreas were also retained (*inset, left*). **C,** islet cluster procedure with transplantation of the liver and pancreatic islets injected into the portal vein of the transplanted liver. In 2 patients, part of the recipient stomach was preserved (*inset*). (Courtesy of Alessiani M, Tzakis A, Todo S, et al: Assessment of five-year experience with abdominal organ cluster transplantation. *J Am Coll Surg* 180:1–9, 1995. By permission of the *Journal of the American College of Surgeons.*)

Conclusion.—Many patients whose upper abdominal neoplasms are unresectable by conventional techniques will benefit from cluster transplantation.

▶ Cluster transplants involving multiple intra-abdominal organs are a *tour de force.* These procedures are expensive and the mortality of the patients is high. Nevertheless, for certain patients this procedure might be indicated. It probably should remain confined to selected transplant centers so that they will be able to get adequate experience to solve the numerous technical problems.

R.J. Howard, M.D., Ph.D.

Pulmonary Transplantation

Davis RD, Pasque MK (Duke Univ, Durham, NC; Washington Univ, St Louis, Mo)

Ann Surg 221:14–28, 1995   6–14

Background.—Lung transplantation today is an effective approach to end-stage pulmonary failure of varying origin. More than 2,700 procedures have been done since the initial successful cases in 1983. Improvements in lung preservation, operative methods, and immunosuppressive management have increased survival and limited morbidity. An increasingly wide spectrum of diseases are amenable to lung transplantation, but at the same time the shortage of suitable donors has become more of a problem. In general, lung transplantation is indicated for patients with irreversible end-stage lung disease who are becoming progressively disabled despite appropriate management and who are expected to live for less than 12–18 months. Single lung transplantation is appropriate for most pulmonary disorders.

Outcome.—Reports from a number of transplant centers demonstrate progressively improving actuarial 1- and 2-year survival rates after lung transplantation (Table 6). Current 1-year survival rates for single lung recipients exceed 90% at some centers, and the actuarial 1-year survival rate after bilateral lung transplantation is approaching 80%. Lung function is markedly improved in surviving patients. Decreasing pulmonary vascular impedance correlates with significantly enhanced right ventricular function. The most serious problem now is chronic allograft dysfunction, manifested as bronchiolitis obliterans with progressively limited airflow. Some patients have undergone retransplantation, but the results are far poorer than those of the initial transplantation.

▶ As with transplantation of other organs, lung transplantation went through an evolutionary phase that was characterized by improved surgical techniques, improved understanding of indications for transplantation, and improved immunosuppression. With continuing improvements in these and

TABLE 6.—Actuarial Survival After Single and Bilateral Lung Transplantation

	Years	Single Lung Transplant		Bilateral Lung Transplant	
		1 Yr	2 Yr	1 Yr	2 Yr
International Heart Lung Registry	1983–1993	70%	60%	70%	60%
St. Louis International Lung Transplant Registry	1983–1992	69%	60%	68%	60%
		n = 324	n = 129	n = 100	n = 39
Barnes lung transplant group	1988–1992	87%	87%	76%	73%
		n = 49	n = 26	n = 31	n = 19
Pittsburg lung transplant group	1988–1992	60%	60%	63%	63%
Duke lung transplant group	1991–1994	100%	100%	82%	82%

(Courtesy of Davis RD, Pasque MK: Pulmonary transplantation. *Ann Surg* 221:14–28, 1995.)

other areas, the results of lung transplantation have gotten better. This review article summarizes the state of the art of current lung transplantation.

R.J. Howard, M.D., Ph.D.

Coronary Angioplasty, Atherectomy and Bypass Surgery in Cardiac Transplant Recipients
Halle AA III, DiSciascio G, Massin EK, Wilson RF, Johnson MR, Sullivan HJ, Bourge RC, Kleiman NS, Miller LW, Aversano TR, Wray RB, Hunt SA, Weston MW, Davies RA, Rincon G, Crandall CC, Cowley MJ, Kubo SH, Fisher SG, Vetrovec GW (Virginia Commonwealth Univ, Richmond)
J Am Coll Cardiol 26:120–128, 1995   6–15

Introduction.—Coronary artery disease is a prominent cause of death in heart transplant recipients, with a prevalence of 40% to 50% 5 years after transplantation. Coronary angiography is currently considered the method of choice for diagnosing allograft coronary artery disease. However, there is currently no standard for treatment or prevention. Coronary artery revascularization (using either percutaneous transluminal coronary angioplasty, coronary atherectomy, or coronary artery bypass surgery) was evaluated in the treatment of allograft coronary artery disease.

Methods.—The medical records of cardiac transplant recipients from 13 medical centers who underwent coronary artery revascularization were retrospectively reviewed. Clinical characteristics, angiographic features, results from the procedure, and long-term outcomes were recorded. Angiographic success was considered to be a lumen diameter stenosis of less than 50%; restenosis was considered to be a return of greater than 50% lumen diameter stenosis.

Results.—A total of 3,710 cardiac transplant recipients were identified at the 13 medical centers. Sixty-six patients underwent balloon angioplasty for a total of 162 lesions. Angiographic success was found in 94% (153/162) of the lesions. For late outcome survival, 61% (40/66) of the patients were alive at a mean of 19 ± 14 months after angioplasty. Retransplantation was performed in 8 patients, with 5 patients surviving. At a mean of 8 ± 5 months after angioplasty, restenosis was present in 55% (42/76) of the lesions. Eleven patients underwent coronary atherectomy. The procedure was considered successful in 82% (9/11) of the lesions. Two patients died as a result of unsuccessful atherectomy procedures. A mean clinical follow-up of 7 ± 4 months was available for the 9 surviving patients. Two patients underwent subsequent angioplasty for restenoses or new lesion formation. Twelve patients underwent coronary artery bypass graft surgery. The procedure was considered successful, with hospital discharge for 67% (8/12) of the patients. The remaining 4 patients died after the procedure. A mean follow-up of 9 ± 7 months was available for the 8 surviving patients. One patient died 2 months after surgery, and in 1 patient angina developed and was eventually treated with an intracoronary stent.

Conclusion.—Coronary revascularization appears to be effective in the treatment of allograft coronary artery disease. In patients without angiographic distal arteriopathy, balloon angioplasty was found to result in an acceptable survival rate. Because of the small number of patients who underwent coronary atherectomy or coronary artery bypass graft surgery, evaluation of these procedures for coronary revascularization in transplant recipients is limited.

▶ This collected series from 13 medical centers examined 66 patients in whom coronary vascular disease developed and required intervention. They all had coronary angioplasty. An additional 12 patients had coronary artery bypass surgery. Coronary artery lesions in transplanted hearts are amenable to corrective procedures.

R.J. Howard, M.D., Ph.D.

7 Endocrinology

Introduction

Surgery of the thyroid and parathyroid glands continues to be the focus of most articles on surgical endocrinology. While surgery is not the first-line treatment for patients with hyperthyroidism—that is usually done by thyroid suppression and/or radioactive iodine—some patients whose hyperthyroidism is not relieved by nonsurgical treatment require operative intervention. One study (Abstract 7–1) discusses total thyroidectomy in 33 patients who previously failed thyroid suppression. A small percentage of these also had the ophthalmopathy associated with Graves' disease relieved by surgery.

Thyroid cancers are of continuing concern for endocrine surgeons. A study from New South Wales, Australia (Abstract 7–2), finds that the incidence of newly diagnosed thyroid cancer increased substantially between 1963 and 1992. The apparent increase in incidence was due in part to a decrease in benign lesions being operated on because of the wider application of fine-needle aspiration biopsy. But there was an absolute as well as a relative increase in the number of thyroid cancers in this part of the world, which the authors attributed to exposure to low levels of radiation due to nuclear weapons testing in the South Pacific.

Follicular cancer is not as common and does not enjoy as successful a long-term outcome as does papillary cancer. A paper from the University of Chicago (Abstract 7–3) reviews the experience of that institution with follicular carcinoma over a 25-year period. The authors were unable to demonstrate that the extent of the operation had any role in affecting long-term outcome, although there is a tendency for surgeons to do more extensive resections, including total thyroidectomy. While papillary and follicular cancers of the thyroid gland are associated with high long-term survival rates, anaplastic thyroid carcinoma can be a devastating tumor with a poor prognosis. Nevertheless, long-term survival can be achieved. A small series of 5 patients is presented (Abstract 7–4), 3 of whom underwent complete resection and had long-term survival. Two patients died more than 10 years after extensive resection, 1 of whom died of unrelated causes. One was alive 26 months after surgery. Extensive surgical resection with radiation can lead to long-term survival in some patients with anaplastic thyroid cancer.

Locally invasive cancer can also be successfully resected. Two papers described surgical techniques for dealing with thyroid cancer involving the trachea (Abstracts 7–5 and 7–6). These methods include either partial resection of the trachea or complete resection of the trachea along with the involved thyroid gland and reconstruction of the trachea. Application of these techniques might permit resection of some advanced thyroid cancers.

Patients with parathyroid disease have been diagnosed earlier in their clinical courses ever since routine serum calcium and parathyroid hormone testing became available. Some authors claim that it is possible to diagnose hyperparathyroidism before clinical symptoms or conditions associated with excessive secretion of parathyroid hormone develop. Others claim that if carefully questioned, all patients with hyperparathyroidism are symptomatic. A study from the University of California, San Francisco (Abstract 7–7), seeks to answer this question by comparing 152 patients with hyperparathyroidism with patients having surgery for nontoxic thyroid disorders. The authors found that only 1 of the 152 patients with hyperparathyroidism was without symptoms or associated conditions as compared with 12.9% of the group with nontoxic thyroid disorders, thus leading credence to the claim that virtually all patients with hyperparathyroidism are symptomatic or have associated conditions. These symptoms can be extremely subtle and may be found in healthy individuals, so ascribing them to the hyperparathyroid condition may at times be difficult. Subtle clinical manifestations can be especially common in the elderly population. In this population, neurologic and psychiatric disorders may be attributed to age or senile dementia and yet may be due to hyperparathyroidism. One study analyzed parathyroidectomy in patients at least 75 years old (Abstract 7–8) and found that following parathyroidectomy, neurologic and psychotic symptoms improved in most patients. Perhaps no one should be thought of as being too old to undergo parathyroidectomy if there is no medical contraindication to surgery.

Patients with renal failure have increased parathyroid hormone secretion. These patients may require parathyroidectomy for this condition. Three papers (Abstracts 7–9 to 7–11) discuss parathyroidectomy in patients with renal disease. All patients had either total parathyroidectomy with reimplantation of parathyroid tissue into the forearm or removal of 3 glands and reduction of the fourth gland to a normal-sized parathyroid gland. Hyperparathyroidism can be relieved by either of these techniques.

In previous editions of YEAR BOOK OF SURGERY we have discussed radiologic and nuclear medicine techniques for localizing parathyroid glands. The comments about these papers maintained that knowledgeable endocrine surgeons have localization rates that are higher than any radiologic test and that these tests are not required for patients having an initial parathyroidectomy. One paper (Abstract 7–12) demonstrates that preoperative localization studies of unoperated glands are not required. Parathyroid cancer can be difficult to diagnose (Abstract 7–13). The histologic and clinical criteria for diagnosing parathyroid cancer are not clear. In this paper only 7 of 16 patients had a definitive diagnosis of parathyroid cancer, and the other 9 had a likely diagnosis. Nevertheless, in patients having an equivocal diagnosis as well as patients with a definitive diagnosis, survival was extremely high.

The Mayo Clinic's experience with adrenal surgery for hypercortisolism presents clinical findings in 91 patients over an 11-year period (Abstract 7–14). There was a rather high prevalence of hypercortisolism caused by adrenocorticotropic hormone–producing tumors. Laparoscopic adrenalectomy can be done safely even for large adrenal tumors up to 12 cm in diameter (Abstract 7–15). This method of removing adrenal tumors may now be preferred over open methods. Nevertheless, morbidity and hospital stay did not seem to be reduced in patients having laparoscopic adrenalectomy.

Richard J. Howard, M.D., Ph.D.

Total Thyroidectomy in Therapy-Resistant Graves' Disease
Winsa B, Rastad J, Larsson E, Mandahl A, Westermark K, Johansson H, Juhlin C, Karlsson A, Åkerström G (Univ Hosp, Uppsala, Sweden)
Surgery 116:1068–1075, 1994   7–1

Introduction.—Although subtotal thyroid resection is generally effective in correcting the hyperthyroid state associated with diffuse thyrotoxicosis and has few complications, recurrent thryotoxicosis can occur. Persistent elevations in thyrotropin receptor antibody (TRAb) levels and ophthalmopathy are risk factors for recurrent thyrotoxicosis. Therefore the safety and efficacy of total thyroidectomy were evaluated in patients with Graves' disease who had persistent endocrine ophthalmopathy and TRAb titer elevation refractory to thyrostatic therapy.

Methods.—Thirty-three patients with Graves' disease underwent total thyroidectomy. All patients had received high-dose thyrostatic treatment for a mean of 2 years. In addition, 4 patients had undergone subtotal thyroid resection and 6 had received radioiodine treatment. Of the 33 patients, 28 had persistent ophthalmopathy and 25 had persistently elevated TRAb titers. The intraoperative, perioperative, and follow-up findings were reviewed.

Results.—Operative time for a primary total thyroidectomy procedure was 1.3–4.3 hours. The average perioperative blood loss was 200 mL, although blood loss was significantly higher in patients with substantial goiters. The thyroid specimens weighed an average of 19 g in primary procedures and 7 g or less for removal of residual thyroid lobes. Histopathologic findings included signs of weak to moderate thyroid hyperfunction, nodular hyperplasia, regressive changes including interstitial fibrosis, and leukocytic infiltration in most specimens, as well as the formation of germinal centers, oncocytic differentiation, nuclear pleomorphism, and papillary thyroid carcinoma in some. Eleven patients required postoperative injections of analgesia. There was no need for transfusion or re-exploration for hemorrhage. Hospitalization lasted an average of 3.7 days. Postoperative complications included transient hypocalcemia requiring vitamin D supplementation lasting 4–6 months in 3 patients (10%) and transient vocal cord paralysis lasting 2–5 months in 2 patients (7%). Of the 25 patients with preoperative elevated TRAb levels, the levels were normalized in 86% of those without radioiodine exposure and 33% of those with radioiodine exposure. Of the 28 patients with endocrine ophthalmopathy, 27 had subjective and objective improvement or nonprogression.

Conclusions.—Total thyroidectomy can be performed safely to achieve normalization of refractory elevated TRAb titers in patients with complicated Graves' disease. However, subtotal resection may be adequate treatment for patients with uncomplicated Graves' disease. Further research should focus on identifying the indications for total and subtotal thyroidectomy in these patients.

▶ Most patients with hyperthyroidism (Graves' disease) can be treated successfully with thyroid suppression and/or radioactive iodine. All patients in this series had previously received these treatments. When surgery is required, most surgeons perform a subtotal thyroidectomy. This series of 33 patients previously treated with thyroid suppression, some of whom had received radioactive iodine or subtotal thyroid resection, underwent total thyroidectomy. The authors comment on the difficulty of thyroidectomy in these patients because of perithyroid fibrosis and neovascularization, which were unusually prominent in patients who had received radioactive iodine treatment. The average blood lost (200 mL) was greater than that in most patients who require thyroidectomy for other diseases. Twenty-eight of the 33 patients had ophthalmopathy. Proptosis substantially improved in 3 of 21 patients followed at least 6 months after thyroidectomy. Five of 15 had improvement in conjunctival injection and periocular edema, and 2 of 12 had improvement in ocular mobility. Thus total thyroidectomy may help selected patients with ocular problems associated with Graves' disease. Others find that the ophthalmopathy of Graves' disease is not improved by thyroidectomy.

R.J. Howard, M.D., Ph.D.

Increasing Incidence and Changing Presentation of Thyroid Cancer Over a 30-Year Period
Fahey TJ III, Reeve TS, Delbridge L (Royal North Shore Hosp, St Leonards, New South Wales, Australia)
Br J Surg 82:518–520, 1995   7–2

Background.—Since the development of fine-needle aspiration biopsy, the number of thyroidectomies performed has fallen but the proportion of cancerous glands at surgery has risen. Thirty years' experience at a referral endocrinology service were reviewed to study how the incidence and manifestation of thyroid cancer have changed.

Methods.—A 30-year-long database was reviewed, with 8,561 thyroidectomies performed and 660 new cancers diagnosed. Patients not undergoing a primary procedure were excluded. The Central Cancer Registry of New South Wales provided regional epidemiologic data.

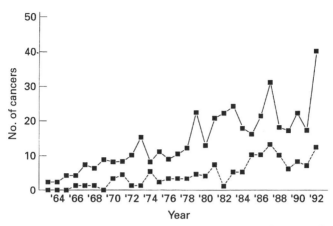

FIGURE 2.—Annual incidence of newly diagnosed differentiated thyroid cancer in clinical nodules (*solid line*) and occult papillary cancer (*broken line*) from 1963 to 1992. (Courtesy of Fahey TJ III, Reeve TS, Delbridge L: Increasing incidence and changing presentation of thyroid cancer over a 30-year period. *Br J Surg* 82:518–520, 1995, Blackwell Science Ltd.)

Results.—The percentage of primary thyroid operations for cancer rose from 2% to 17% over 30 years. The incidence of both differentiated thyroid cancer in clinical nodules and occult papillary cancer rose steadily, especially the former (Fig 2). The rate of rise for both was most noticeable over the last 10 years. The incidence of miscellaneous (lymphoma and anaplastic or medullary cancer) tumors remained stable, with a decrease in anaplastic lesions balanced by an increase in medullary ones. Epidemiology revealed an absolute increase in the incidence of thyroid cancer in New South Wales from 1972 to 1989.

Conclusions.—The increased number of thyroid cancers seen yearly reflects a true rise in the incidence of this tumor, especially in clinically significant nodules, and not a change in the surgical rate or referral patterns. Of concern is the increased rate of thyroid cancer in Pacific populations exposed to nuclear testing, such as Marshall Islanders, Polynesians born on Pacific islands (but not New Zealand Maoris), and New Guineans. Further studies are needed to explain the increase shown here.

▶ This report from a New South Wales, Australia, referral hospital documents that the incidence of newly diagnosed thyroid cancer increased substantially between 1963 and 1992 and that cancer as a reason for thyroidectomy increased from 2% to 17% of operations. Some authors have shown an increase in the incidence of thyroid cancer while others have noted a gradual decline. Thyroid cancer, a relatively rare neoplasm, has an incidence that varies geographically and ethnically around the world. The authors attribute the increase in thyroid cancer in part to the use of fine-needle aspiration biopsy resulting in a decrease in the number of benign tumors that are operated on. The absolute number of thyroid cancers increased substantially over the study period. Referral patterns may also account for the increased incidence of thyroid cancers, but the authors don't state how their referral patterns have changed. They suggest that there is an increase in thyroid cancer in populations exposed to low levels of radiation. Radiation exposure may have increased as a result of nuclear weapons testing in the South Pacific. The authors do not state whether this factor was likely to have played a role in the increased incidence of thyroid cancer in New South Wales. With a 25% decline being reported between 1973 and 1990 in the United States,[1] regional differences such as radiation exposure or other factors may play an important role in the varying incidence of thyroid cancer.

R.J. Howard, M.D., Ph.D.

Reference

1. National Cancer Institute: *Evaluating the National Cancer Program: An Ongoing Process.* Bethesda, Md, National Cancer Institute, 1994.

Morbidity and Mortality in Follicular Thyroid Cancer
DeGroot LJ, Kaplan EL, Shukla MS, Salti G, Straus FH (Univ of Chicago)
J Clin Endocrinol Metab 80:2946–2953, 1995   7–3

Introduction.—Follicular carcinoma of the thyroid is a more rare tumor than papillary carcinoma and is believed to be more aggressive. A 25-year experience with patients with follicular cancer was reviewed.

Methods.—A total of 49 patients treated for follicular thyroid carcinoma were studied. The pathologic specimens were reviewed for determination of the extent of vascular and capsular invasion, differentiation, and the presence of Hürthle cell tumors. The extent of disease at the time of diagnosis was classified. The patients were followed for an average of 10.7 years (range, 1–36 years).

Results.—Of the 49 patients, 74% had class I tumors (intrathyroidal disease only), 8.2% had class II tumors (positive cervical nodes), 10.2% had class III disease (locally invasive), and 8.2% had class IV disease (distant metastasis) at diagnosis. The mortality rate was 16% and the recurrence rate was 18%. Eight of the 9 patients with recurrent or persistent disease died. The deaths all occurred within 13 years of diagnosis. A poorer prognosis was associated with age older than 45 years, tumors larger than 3 cm, the presence of Hürthle cells, or distant metastasis at diagnosis. The risk of death or recurrence was not affected by gender, radiation exposure, thyroiditis, multifocality of the lesion, the extent of vascular or capsular invasion, the degree of differentiation, positive neck nodes, or the extent of surgery. In addition, the risk of death or recurrence in class I or II patients was not affected by the use of postsurgical radio-iodine ablation.

Discussion.—There are several differences in the characteristics and course of follicular and papillary thyroid cancers. The average age is older at diagnosis and younger at death with follicular than with papillary tumors. The mortality rate of follicular cancer is twice that of papillary cancer. However, patients with follicular cancer appear to remain disease free after approximately 13 years, whereas patients with papillary cancer can have persistent or recurrent disease and die long after the initial diagnosis. The significant mortality among patients with only intrathyroidal follicular tumors suggests that this more aggressive carcinoma may require more extensive initial therapy, possibly including larger radioiodine doses, prophylactic neck radiotherapy, or prophylactic chemotherapy in selected patients.

▶ The authors review their experience with follicular carcinoma over a 25-year period. Patients in this series underwent a variety of surgical procedures (lobectomy and subtotal thyroidectomy, total thyroidectomy with and without modified radical neck dissection) and, in some patients, the use of postoperative [131]I. It is unclear what the indications for various surgical procedures were and what the indications were for the use of radioactive iodine. Nevertheless, in their analysis the authors were unable to find any relation between the extent of the surgical procedure or the use of radioactive iodine and recurrence or mortality from cancer. Failure to find any relation may have been due to the low power of the analysis because of the small number of patients, especially when stratified by the extent of disease. There are no data that clearly define the correct surgical procedure for patients with follicular thyroid cancer. There is a tendency, however, to use more extensive surgical procedures, especially total thyroidectomy.

R.J. Howard, M.D., Ph.D.

Anaplastic Carcinoma of the Thyroid: A 24-Year Experience
Tan RK, Finley RK, Driscoll D, Bakamjian V, Hicks WL, Shedd DP (Albany Med College, NY; Wright State Univ, Dayton, Ohio; Roswell Park Cancer Institute, Buffalo, NY)
Head Neck 17:41–48, 1995   7–4

Objective.—Anaplastic carcinoma of the thyroid gland is a relatively rare but lethal neoplasm. The experience of 1 cancer institute with anaplastic carcinoma of the thyroid gland was retrospectively reviewed to evaluate outcome with regard to prognostic factors and response to treatment.

Patients.—Between 1968 and 1992, 21 patients with anaplastic carcinoma of the thyroid gland were seen; these patients represented 2.7% of 771 patients with thyroid cancer. Their mean age was 65.1 years, and the male-to-female ratio was 1:1.1. The most common complaint was a rapidly enlarging neck mass that was often associated with dysphagia, dyspnea, or dysphonia. Nine (43%) patients had a history of prior thyroid disease.

Treatment.—Complete resection was accomplished in only 5 patients. Tumor size ranged from 3.0 to 20.0 cm. The most common site of direct extension was the perithyroidal fat and strap muscles adjacent to the thyroid gland. All but 3 patients underwent radiation therapy, and 6 received chemotherapy.

Findings.—Overall median survival was 4.5 months, and the estimated 5-year survival rate was 10%. Analysis of the survival curve showed a sharp decline in the first 24 months after diagnosis in which 85.6% of the patients died; the decline then leveled off at periods beyond 60 months (Fig 1). This latter period was represented by 2 patients who died without evidence of recurrent disease at 131 and 171 months. A third patient remains alive at 26 months after diagnosis. Tumor size less than 6.0 cm and female sex were significant prognostic factors. All 5 patients who underwent complete resection had a median survival of 131.4 months and an estimated 5-year survival rate of 60%. Four of these patients had postoperative radiotherapy, with or without sequential chemotherapy, and included the 2 patients who survived more than 10 years after the diagnosis and a third who remains alive without disease at 26 months.

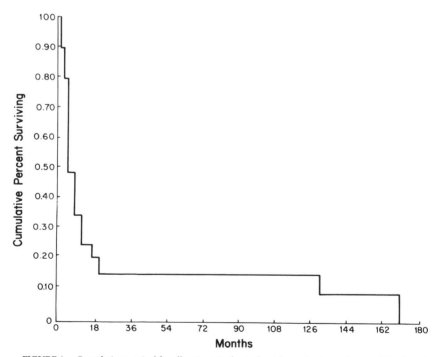

FIGURE 1.—Cumulative survival for all patients in the study with anaplastic carcinoma of the thyroid. (From Anaplastic carcinoma of the thyroid: A 24-year experience, by Tan RK, Finley RK, Driscoll D, et al: *Head Neck* 17:41–48, copyright 1995. Reprinted by permission of John Wiley & Sons, Inc.)

Conclusions.—Anaplastic carcinoma of the thyroid gland is a swiftly fatal disease, but long-term survival may be possible in a subgroup of patients who undergo complete resection and multimodality treatment. Tumor diameter less than 6.0 cm, female gender, and complete resection indicate the best prognosis. All patients, particularly those older than 60 years, with pre-existing thyroid disease should be advised to seek evaluation for any increase in size of a mass in the thyroid area. In patients with anaplastic cancer, complete resection should be attempted by total thyroidectomy and removal of adjacent lymph nodes if it can be performed without undue morbidity.

▶ Anaplastic thyroid carcinoma is a devastating tumor with a dismal prognosis. Nevertheless, 3 of 5 patients who underwent complete resection had long-term survival. Two patients died of unrelated causes more than 10 years after resection, and 1 patient was alive 26 months after surgery. The authors recommend radiation therapy with or without chemotherapy. A thorough evaluation of these patients is required preoperatively with CT scan of the neck and a search for distant metastasis to determine whether curative resection can be carried out.

R.J. Howard, M.D., Ph.D.

Management of Tracheal Wall Resection for Thyroid Carcinoma by Tracheocutaneous Fenestration and Delayed Closure Using Auricular Cartilage
Sugenoya A, Matsuo K, Asanuma K, Shingu K, Shimizu T, Masuda H, Kobayashi S, Lida F (Shinshu Univ, Japan)
Head Neck 17:339–342, 1995   7–5

Introduction.—Although the prognosis of differentiated thyroid carcinoma is usually good, surgery with resection is sometimes required when the malignancy is advanced and has infiltrated the surrounding tissues. Depending on the degree of tumor infiltration, different surgical procedures may be performed. One procedure used, tracheocutaneous fenestration, is safe and has a low rate of complications. After tracheocutaneous fenestration, a tracheostoma is needed and is maintained until it is certain that neither local recurrence nor dyspnea is present. For small tracheal wall defects, a skin flap can be used to close the tracheostoma. However, simple closures cannot be used for larger defects. The use of a free auricular cartilage autograft in the closure of large tracheocutaneous fenestration is described.

Methods.—Tracheocutaneous fenestration was performed on 5 patients with advanced thyroid carcinoma. For closure of the tracheostoma, a hinge skin flap is prepared, with undermining between the subcutaneous layer and the strap muscle (Fig 1); the skin flap is then sutured. A section of the conchal cartilage is removed from the auricle. The conchal cartilage is then positioned over the sutured skin flap.

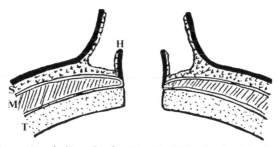

FIGURE 1.—Preparation of a hinge skin flap (*H*) with additional undermining between the subcutaneous layer (*S*) and the strap muscles (*M*). *Abbreviation: T*, trachea. (From Management of tracheal wall resection for thyroid carcinoma by tracheocutaneous fenestration and delayed closure using auricular cartilage, by Sugenoya A, Matsuo K, Asanuma K, et al: *Head Neck* 17:339–342, copyright 1995. Reprinted by permission of John Wiley & Sons, Inc.)

Results.—Tracheal wall defects were greater than one third of the tracheal circumference in all patients, with tracheostomas 12–15 mm in diameter. Four of the 5 patients who underwent tracheostoma closure remain in satisfactory condition 2 years after surgery. The remaining patient experienced increasing dyspnea after tracheostoma closure, and the closed tracheal fenestration had to be reopened the second day after surgery. Edema and redness of the larynx had been observed on tracheofiberscopic examination but did not respond to conservative treatment.

Conclusion.—Use of an auricular cartilage free graft was found to be successful for the closure of large tracheostomas. This technique is a simple procedure and provides the necessary tracheal wall skeletal support for closure of large tracheal wall defects after tracheocutaneous fenestration. The long-term outcome of patients who undergo this procedure, however, needs to be investigated further.

▶ This article presents another method for dealing with tracheal invasion by thyroid carcinoma. These authors initially resected the part of the anterior wall of the trachea that was invaded by cancer and then constructed a tracheocutaneous fenestration. Later it was closed by using skin flaps and auricular cartilage. This paper and the next one by Ozaki et al. demonstrate methods for dealing with advanced thyroid cancer.

R. J. Howard, M.D., Ph.D.

Surgery for Patients With Thyroid Carcinoma Invading the Trachea: Circumferential Sleeve Resection Followed By End-to-End Anastomosis
Ozaki O, Sugino K, Mimura T, Ito K (Ito Hosp, Tokyo)
Surgery 117:268–271, 1995   7–6

Objective.—Patients with thyroid carcinoma invading the trachea can be cured with tracheal resection. The authors prefer circumferential sleeve

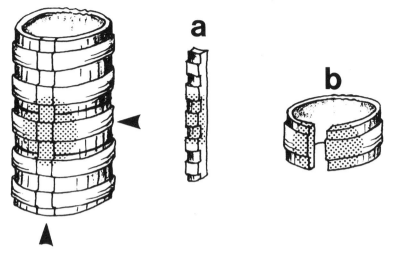

FIGURE 1.—Longitudinal (**A**) and circumferential (**B**) specimens of resected trachea for histologic examination. (Courtesy of Ozaki O, Sugino K, Mimura T, et al: Surgery for patients with thyroid carcinoma invading the trachea: Circumferential sleeve resection followed by end-to-end anastomosis. *Surgery* 117:268–271, 1995.)

resection to partial wedge resection, which can leave some carcinoma tissue behind. The results of histologic examination to determine the mode of tracheal invasion are discussed.

Methods.—Histologic examination of resected trachea performed in 21 patients (4 men) aged 29 to 75 showed papillary carcinoma in 18 patients, follicular carcinoma in 2, and medullary carcinoma in 1. Three to 9 tracheal rings were resected. One longitudinal and 1 circumferential tracheal specimen were examined (Fig 1). Patients were followed from 1 year 5 months to 10 years 1 month.

Results.—One patient required a postoperative tracheostomy. Sixteen patients were disease free at follow-up, and 4 had distant metastases. One patient died of an unrelated cause. Wall invasion was limited to the adventitia in 3 patients, was present between the rings in 2, was located in the submucosal space in 10, and protruded into the lumen in 6. Examination of longitudinal spread showed adventitial invasion in 1 to 6 rings but mucosal invasion in 0 to 4 rings. Assessment of circumferential spread demonstrated greater invasion on the adventitial side in 11 patients, similar invasion on both sides in 5 patients, and greater invasion on the mucosal side in 5 patients.

Conclusion.—Circumferential sleeve resection followed by end-to-end anastomosis of the trachea is preferable to partial wedge resection in patients with thyroid carcinoma invading the trachea. Partial wedge resection may leave carcinoma tissue behind on the mucosal side of the trachea.

▶ Aggressive surgical intervention in patients with thyroid carcinoma involving the trachea can lead to long-term survival. During the 8-year, 8-month period, the authors treated 21 patients with thyroid carcinoma invading the trachea at the Ito Hospital in Tokyo. The authors were able to achieve sufficient mobilization of the trachea by blunt dissection proximally to the larynx and distally to the carina. After this mobilization they were able to reapproximate the resection margins and perform an end-to-end anastomosis. Using this technique, the authors believed they did not have to compromise on the resection margins when cancer invaded the trachea.

R.J. Howard, M.D., Ph.D.

Clinical Manifestations of Primary Hyperparathyroidism Before and After Parathyroidectomy: A Case-Control Study

Chan AK, Duh Q-Y, Katz MH, Siperstein AE, Clark OH (Mount Zion Med Ctr, San Francisco; Veterans Affairs Med Ctr, San Francisco; Univ of California, San Francisco)
Ann Surg 222:402–414, 1995   7–7

Background.—Although there is general agreement that symptomatic patients with hyperparathyroidism or asymptomatic patients with severe hypercalcemia should be treated with parathyroidectomy, there is no agreement regarding the optimal management of asymptomatic hyperparathyroidism. It is likely that this disagreement is caused by a lack of consensus regarding the symptoms of hyperparathyroidism. Therefore, the prevalence of a predetermined set of symptoms and conditions associated with primary hyperparathyroidism was compared in groups of patients with either hyperparathyroidism or nontoxic thyroid disorders. In addition, the rate of symptom resolution after surgical treatment was compared in the 2 groups.

Methods.—The study population included 152 consecutive patients with primary hyperparathyroidism who underwent parathyroidectomy and 132 control patients with nontoxic thyroid disorders who underwent thyroidectomy during the same period. All patients were asked to complete a questionnaire asking about their experience with a list of symptoms and associated conditions of parathyroid or thyroid disease before and after surgery. They were also asked about their overall improvement after surgery. Their laboratory test results were reviewed. The 2 groups were compared for preoperative prevalence of symptoms and postoperative improvement in symptoms. Among the hyperparathyroid group, laboratory values were correlated with symptoms and associated conditions.

Results.—Among the patients with primary hyperparathyroidism, only 4.6% had none of the listed symptoms, 17.1% had none of the associated conditions, and only 1 patient (0.66%) was asymptomatic. Among the patients with nontoxic thyroid disorders, 23.5% had no symptoms, 19.7% had no associated conditions, and 12.9% were asymptomatic. The hyperparathyroid group had a greater prevalence of all 17 symptoms: fatigue, exhaustion, weakness, polydipsia, polyuria, nocturia, bone pain, back pain, constipation, increasing constipation, depression, memory loss, joint pain, loss of appetite, nausea, heartburn, and pruritus. There were statistically significant differences in the prevalence of 14 of the symptoms with or without adjustment for age. There was also a greater prevalence among the hyperparathyroid group of all 10 associated conditions: neophrolithiasis, hematuria, bone fracture, gout, joint swelling, weight loss, duodenal ulcer, gastric ulcer, pancreatitis, and hypertension. Two conditions were significantly more prevalent with or without adjustment for age. There were significant correlations between higher serum calcium levels and fatigue, polydipsia, gout, joint swelling, weight loss, duodenal ulcer, pancreatitis, and hypertension, although patients with lower but still elevated calcium levels had bone pain, memory loss, joint pain, and heartburn. After surgery there was a decrease in the frequency of all symptoms after parathyroidectomy, a decrease in 7 of 17 symptoms after thyroidectomy, a decrease in 7 of 10 conditions after parathyroidectomy, and a decrease in the frequency of 6 conditions after thyroidectomy. In addition, the degree of improvement was significantly greater after parathyroidectomy than after thyroidectomy. Overall improvement was reported by 57% of the parathyroid patients and 30% of the thyroid patients.

Conclusions.—Even in the absence of severe hypercalcemia, most patients with primary hyperparathyroidism have evidence of symptoms and/or conditions associated with hyperparathyroidism. Only 8 of the study patients with hyperparathyroidism did not experience any improvement in symptoms or associated conditions, thus supporting treatment with parathyroidectomy for these patients.

▶ A dilemma for physicians is whether to refer patients for parathyroidectomy with slightly elevated calcium levels and elevated parathyroid hormone concentrations who are otherwise "asymptomatic." This paper partially answers that question by reviewing patients with primary hyperthyroidism and using patients with nontoxic thyroid disease as controls. In fact, the authors found that only 1 of 152 hyperparathyroid patients had no symptoms or conditions preoperatively as compared with 12.9% of patients in the group with nontoxic thyroid disorders. The symptoms of hyperparathyroidism include fatigue, exhaustion, weakness, depression, loss of appetite, back pain, constipation, and nausea. These symptoms are present in many individuals without hyperparathyroidism. One might question whether operating for these symptoms, which are present in a substantial proportion of the general population, might really improve after parathyroidectomy. After surgery there was a decrease in the prevalence of all symptoms in the patients in the parathyroid group but not in the group with thyroid disorders. Nevertheless, even in the parathyroid group, in which all symptoms decreased, the data suggest that many patients continued to have symptoms after parathyroidectomy. Surprisingly, the incidence of nephrolithiasis did not decrease after parathyroidectomy. The majority of the patients said they felt better. Ninety-seven percent said they would have the operation again.

As pointed out in the discussion, these patients frequently have neuropsychiatric disorders and may enjoy substantial improvement after parathyroidectomy. This latter finding is also a suggestion of the paper by Chigot et al. (see the next abstract). One of the discussants pointed out that the spouse of the patients should really be questioned about whether or not the patient was improved because irritability is frequent and is not necessarily noticed by the patient but is noticed by the spouse.

R.J. Howard, M.D., Ph.D.

Should Primary Hyperparathyroidism Be Treated Surgically in Elderly Patients Older Than 75 Years?

Chigot JP, Menegaux F, Achrafi H (Hôpital de la Pitié, Paris)
Surgery 117:397–401, 1995   7–8

Purpose.—The detection of an unusual hypercalcemia on routine serum calcium measurement has led to an increasing number of older patients with a suspected diagnosis of primary hyperparathyroidism (PHPT). Even for elderly patients with their frequent concomitant diseases, early neck exploration with excision of the adenoma is still considered the optimal treatment of PHPT. A 15-year experience with neck exploration in elderly patients with PHPT is reviewed.

Patients.—From 1978 through 1992, 14% of the patients undergoing surgery for PHPT at the study hospital were 75 years or older. Sixty-four of these 78 patients were women; their mean age was 79 years. Forty-seven percent of the patients had neurologic and psychiatric symptoms, especially fatigue. Seventy-two patients underwent preoperative localization studies; these were successful in 47 cases for a sensitivity of 58%. Ninety-five percent of the patients were found at surgery to have a single adenoma; 3 had double adenomas and 1 had hyperplasia.

Outcomes.—Three patients died for an overall postoperative mortality rate of 4%; however, none of the deaths occurred after 1984. Significant complications occurred at a rate of 4%, including 1 myocardial infarction, 1 pulmonary embolism, and 1 cerebral hemorrhage. The patients stayed in the hospital an average of 4 days after surgery. Sixty-five patients were followed for a mean of 3 years. Ninety-four percent of them reported improvement in their symptoms, particularly in fatigue and intellectual function.

Conclusions.—For elderly patients with PHPT, exploratory neck surgery with excision of the parathyroid adenoma yields marked symptomatic improvement in the great majority of cases. Patient and family reports confirm a marked improvement in fatigue and intellectual function, with many patients describing a renewed sense of well-being. Even for patients over 75 years of age, early parathyroid surgery is the treatment of choice for PHPT.

▶ When are patients too old to undergo parathyroidectomy? Evidently, they are never too old according to this paper from Paris. A rather large percentage (14) of patients undergoing parathyroidectomy were at least 75 years old. Clinical findings were frequently subtle and included fatigue, depression, psychiatric disorders, and neurologic disorders. Since this older population often has these symptoms in the absence of hyperparathyroidism, it can be difficult to attribute these symptoms to parathyroid disease. The authors noted a marked improvement in neurologic and psychiatric disorders and osteoarticular pain in 57 of 65 patients who could be followed. The operation can be done safely in these older patients. Three patients died. One who died of pulmonary embolism was found to have a tumor of the inferior vena cava extending into the right atrium.

R.J. Howard, M.D., Ph.D.

Subtotal Parathyroidectomy in Dialysis-Dependent and Post–Renal Transplant Patients: A 25-Year Single-Center Experience
Punch JD, Thompson NW, Merion RM (Univ of Michigan, Ann Arbor)
Arch Surg 130:538–543, 1995   7–9

Introduction.—Hyperparathyroidism is known to occur in patients with renal failure. In spite of improvements in dialysis techniques, symptomatic hyperparathyroidism still occurs. Additionally, the persistence or recurrence of hyperparathyroidism in some renal transplant recipients necessitates parathyroidectomy. The outcomes of patients with hyperparathyroidism secondary to renal failure after parathyroidectomy were reviewed.

Methods.—Review of medical records identified 91 patients who had undergone parathyroid exploration secondary to renal failure–associated hyperparathyroidism. Patient characteristics, dialysis and renal transplant status, signs and symptoms, laboratory values, diagnostic tests, intraoperative findings, and outcomes were recorded and assessed.

Results.—Eighty patients were undergoing dialysis and 11 were renal transplant recipients at the time of surgery. A median of 52 months of dialysis and 34 months after renal transplantation elapsed before parathyroid surgery. Bone pain was more prominent in dialysis patients than in renal transplant recipients. The incidence of muscular weakness was similar in both groups. Hypercalcemia was an indication for surgery in 10 (91%) transplant recipients as compared with 26 (33%) patients maintained on dialysis. Transplant recipients had significantly higher serum calcium concentrations than did dialysis patients. Radiographic findings were consistent with hyperparathyroidism in 89 patients. Seventy-nine of 87 patients who underwent initial parathyroid exploration had 4 parathyroid glands. Sixty-two patients underwent subtotal excision. Complete alleviation of symptoms was achieved in 91% (10/11) of the renal transplant recipients and in 95% (86/91) of the patients overall. Recurrence of symptoms necessitating additional surgery was observed in 5 patients (6%).

Conclusion.—Parathyroidectomy was found to be effective for the treatment of renal failure–associated hyperparathyroidism in dialysis patients and renal transplant recipients. Recurrence was uncommon and was treated easily.

Results of Surgical Treatment of Renal Hyperparathyroidism

Neonakis E, Wheeler MH, Krishnan H, Coles GA, Davies F, Woodhead JS
(Univ Hosp of Wales, Cardiff)
Arch Surg 130:643–648, 1995   7–10

Introduction.—Hyperparathyroidism and persistent hypercalcemia are frequent complications of renal failure for patients undergoing hemodialysis as well as renal transplant recipients. The outcome of hemodialysis patients and renal transplant recipients after parathyroidectomy was evaluated retrospectively.

Methods.—A case series of 67 patients who had undergone parathyroidectomy for renal failure–associated hyperparathyroidism were reviewed retrospectively. Thirty-five patients were undergoing hemodialysis and 32 were renal transplant recipients at the time of surgery. Mean follow-up was 4.34 years. Fifty-two patients had a total parathyroidectomy with autotransplantation and 15 had a subtotal parathyroidectomy. Improvement in symptoms and biochemical parameters and the rate of recurrence of hyperparathyroidism were evaluated.

Results.—Preoperative symptoms included myopathy, pruritus, and skeletal pain. Symptomatic hypercalcemia was the most common indication for parathyroidectomy, and both dialysis and transplant patients had elevated parathyroid hormone concentrations. At surgery, 86.6% of the patients were found to have 4 glands (Fig 2), 5.9% had 5 glands, and 7.5% had 3 glands, for a total of 267 glands. Thirty-seven ectopic locations were found, including intrathyroidal and thymic horns. One patient died postoperatively and 14 patients died within 3.5 years of the procedure. Most of the 14 deaths were from cardiovascular causes unrelated to the surgery. Improvement in symptoms was found in 81% of the patients maintained on hemodialysis and in 72% of the renal transplant recipients. Symptomatic improvement between the 2 surgical procedures was similar; improvement was seen in 77.4% of the patients who underwent total parathyroidectomy and in 82% who underwent subtotal resection. Postoperative

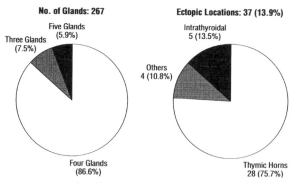

FIGURE 2.—Intraoperative findings in 67 patients undergoing parathyroidectomy. A fifth gland was found in 4 subjects (5.9%). (Courtesy of *Archives of Surgery*, June 1995, 130:643–648, Copyright 1995, American Medical Association.)

severe symptomatic hypocalcemia occurred more often after total parathyroidectomy. Preoperative serum alkaline phosphatase levels were found to correlate well with the development of postoperative hypocalcemia and with improvement in skeletal pain. Recurrent hyperparathyroidism developed in 4 of 38 patients who underwent total parathyroidectomy and 1 of 14 surviving patients who underwent a subtotal procedure.

Conclusion.—Both dialysis patients and renal transplant recipients experienced symptomatic improvement of skeletal pain and pruritus after surgery. Only patients who were maintained on dialysis at the time of surgery had recurrent hypercalcemia. Both procedures, total parathyroidectomy with autotransplantation and subtotal parathyroidectomy, resulted in symptomatic improvement and control of renal failure–associated hyperparathyroidism.

Parathyroidectomy in Chronic Renal Failure

Koonsman M, Dickerman R, Brinker K, Dunn E (Methodist Med Ctr, Dallas)
Am J Surg 168:631–635, 1994   7–11

Introduction.—The majority of patients with hyperplasia of the parathyroid glands secondary to chronic renal failure can be managed medically. For those requiring surgical intervention, there is controversy over whether subtotal parathyroidectomy or total parathyroidectomy with autotransplantation of parathyroid tissue into the forearm or neck is the best approach. Morbidity, mortality, and clinical outcomes were compared retrospectively in 77 patients with renal failure who underwent parathyroid surgery.

Methods.—All patients had significant metabolic bone disease. Fifty-nine patients had been maintained on dialysis for an average of 5.5 years at the time of surgery. Eighteen patients had previously undergone successful renal transplantation. Of 77 patients, 53 (69%) underwent subtotal parathyroidectomy and 24 (31%) underwent total parathyroidectomy with autotransplantation. During surgery, the following glands were identified in the neck: 4 glands in 63 patients, 3 glands in 11 patients, 5 glands in 2 patients, and 2 glands in 1 patient. There was no postoperative mortality or significant morbidity.

Results.—Follow-up lasted an average of 4.5 years after surgery. In the postoperative period, 53% of the patients in both groups had bone disease requiring calcium replacement. Recurrence of hyperparathyroidism was found in 3 of 24 patients who underwent total parathyroidectomy and autotransplantation. All had 4 glands at the original operation. All 3 patients underwent re-exploration of the forearm under local anesthesia at 2, 3, and 5 years, respectively. Resection resulted in control of hypercalcemia, with no morbidity or mortality. No recurrence of hyperparathyroidism was experienced in any patient who underwent subtotal parathyroidectomy.

Conclusion.—Subtotal parathyroidectomy in patients with renal failure gave good control of secondary hyperthyroidism. Total parathyroidectomy with autotransplantation gave no additional benefit.

▶ Most patients with hyperparathyroidism have a single adenoma. In most hospitals, surgery for secondary hyperparathyroidism represents only a small fraction of the patients who require parathyroidectomy. These 3 articles reporting large series of patients with secondary hyperparathyroidism all come from academic medical centers that have renal transplant programs; that is where these patients tend to accumulate. The majority of patients on dialysis can be managed medically with the use of oral phosphate binders, calcium supplementation, and vitamin D supplementation. Because oral phosphate binders cause severe constipation, compliance with this medication is not always good. Despite medical management, complications of secondary hyperparathyroidism will develop in some 5% to 15% of renal failure patients and necessitate operative intervention. These papers show that a majority (90% to 95%) of patients will have relief of their symptoms following parathyroidectomy. The operation depends on surgical preference. Some patients in each series had total parathyroidectomy with reimplantation into the forearm of enough tissue to maintain the euparathyroid state. Surgeons at 1 of the centers removed 3 glands and the fourth gland was reduced in size so that approximately 60 mg of parathyroid tissue was left. The majority of patients with recurrent hyperparathyroidism were those who had reimplantation into the forearm. The number of patients with recurrent disease was too small, however, to lead one to conclude that reimplantation should not be done. If recurrent hyperparathyroidism occurs (because renal failure persists and the drive to secrete parathyroid hormone continues), enlarged glands in the forearm can be easily removed.

R.J. Howard, M.D., Ph.D.

Parathyroidectomy in Primary Hyperparathyroidism: Preoperative Localization and Routine Biopsy of Unaltered Glands Are Not Necessary
Oerteli D, Richter M, Kraenzlin M, Staub JJ, Oberholzer M, Haas HG, Harder F (Univ Hosital, Basel, Switzerland; Washington Univ, St Louis, Mo)
Surgery 117:392–396, 1995   7–12

Objective.—The purpose of surgery for hyperparathyroidism is to remove enough hyperfunctional tissue. In patients with multiglandular disease, the incidence of persistent or recurrent disease is 3.5% to 13%. The results of a retrospective analysis of primary neck exploration for hyperparathyroidism are presented.

Methods.—A total of 173 patients (43 men) aged 17 to 88 were treated for hyperparathyroidism. Indications were nephrolithiasis in 36.4% of the patients, hypertension in 34.1%, bone disease in 22.5%, fatigue and depression in 21.4%, and gastrointestinal symptoms in 2.3%. The remainder were asymptomatic. Twenty patients had previously had neck surgery. No preoperative localization was done for primary explorations.

Results.—Uniglandular pathology was found in 142 patients, multiglandular pathology in 25, and carcinoma in 6. Location of the glands was normal in 136 and ectopic in 37 (Fig 1). A fifth gland was found in 3 patients. One enlarged gland was removed in 127 patients, 2 enlarged glands in 36, and 3½ glands in 10. Thyroid pathology was detected in 51 patients. One patient died postoperatively of myocardial decompensation, and 1 died 4 years postoperatively of coronary heart disease. Large wound hematomas developed in 3 patients. On follow-up, 163 of 171 patients were normocalcemic, 2 patients had persistent hypercalcemia, and 6 had recurrent hypercalcemia. In 7 patients who had hypoparathyroidism, 6 had undergone subtotal parathyroidectomy.

Conclusion.—Preoperative localization and routine biopsy of unaltered glands are unnecessary in patients undergoing parathyroidectomy in pri-

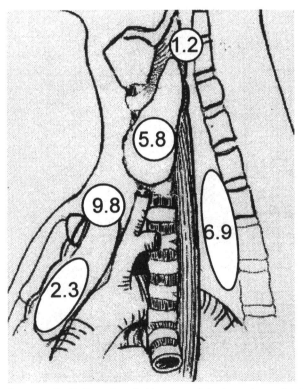

FIGURE 1.—Intraoperative findings of atypical locations of glands are shown. A total of 54 glands were found in atypical anatomic positions: cervical, intrathyroidal, retroesophageal and paraesophageal, upper mediastinum, and deep mediastinum. *Numbers* are given in percentages of the total of 173 patients. (Courtesy of Oerteli D, Richter M, Kraenzlin M, et al: Parathyroidectomy in primary hyperparathyroidism: Preoperative localization and routine biopsy of unaltered glands are not necessary. *Surgery* 117:392–396, 1995.)

mary hyperparathyroidism. Operative morbidity and mortality rates were 2.3% and 0.6%. Routine biopsy in normal-sized glands may increase the risk of hypoparathyroidism.

▶ We have previously reviewed articles dealing with the localization of parathyroid glands by radiologic and nuclear medicine techniques.[1–5] This article demonstrates that a skilled endocrine surgeon can successfully locate diseased glands at the operating table without preoperative localization studies. The authors had a favorable outcome in more than 95% of their patients. Skilled surgeons have a localization rate higher than that found in virtually all radiologic localization studies. Nevertheless, radiologic localization studies may be useful for surgeons who do not regularly perform parathyroidectomy and certainly in all patients in whom adenomas cannot be found at the initial operation.

R.J. Howard, M.D., Ph.D.

References

1. Silver CE, Velez FJ: Parathyroid re-exploration. *Am J Surg* 164:606-609, 1992 (1994 YEAR BOOK OF SURGERY, p 147).
2. Shara AR, LaRosa CA, Jaffe BM: Parathyroid localization prior to primary exploration. *Am J Surg* 166:289–293, 1993 (1994 YEAR BOOK OF SURGERY, p 165).
3. Heller KS, Attie JN, Dubner S: Parathyroid localization: Inability to predict multiple gland involvement. *Am J Surg* 166:357–359, 1993 (1994 YEAR BOOK OF SURGERY, p 167).
4. Wei JP, et al: *Ann Surg* 216:568–573, 1994 (1995 YEAR BOOK OF SURGERY, p 178).
5. Roe SN, et al: *Ann Surg* 219:582–586, 1994 (1995 YEAR BOOK OF SURGERY, p 180).

Parathyroid Cancer: Clinical Variations and Relationship to Autotransplantation
Rosen IB, Young JEM, Archibald SD, Walfish PG, Vale J (Univ of Toronto; McMaster Univ, Hamilton, Ont, Canada)
Can J Surg 37:465–469, 1994   7–13

Background.—Involving no more than 3% of patients undergoing parathyroid surgery, parathyroid cancer may be difficult to diagnose histologically. Sometimes the biological course is all that suggests malignancy despite a benign appearance. Sixteen cases, 9 with equivocal and 7 with definite parathyroid cancer, were reviewed.

Methods and Findings.—The 16 medical records, accumulated over 20 years, were reviewed for clinical features, pathologic description, therapy, and outcome. Multiple sites of parathyroid tissue in the neck after surgery developed in 3 of the 9 patients with an equivocal diagnosis. Repeat surgery did not provide relief. The other 6 demonstrated thyroid infiltration with parathyroid tissue at surgery. After en bloc removal of the thyroid and parathyroids, there has been no recurrence for up to 12 years. For the 7 patients with definite cancer, tissue samples met the stringent criteria of Castleman and Rath. Three had neck masses, 3 had symptomatic hypercalcemia, and 1 had secondary hyperparathyroidism. Six underwent en bloc removal of the thyroid, parathyroids, and adjacent involved neck structures. The seventh patient, who had secondary hyperparathyroidism, was treated by total parathyroidectomy and autotransplantation of parathyroid tissue to the forearm. Lung metastases developed and he died 1 year later. The other 6 have survived, 1 with spinal metastases 20 years after diagnosis.

Conclusions.—En bloc removal of the thyroid, parathyroids, and locally invaded soft tissue is the preferred treatment of parathyroid cancer, with regional neck dissection in node-positive cases. All 4 parathyroids must be identified and examined histologically. Microscopic diagnosis is difficult. Local tissue invasion, metastasis, or postoperative recurrence may be the first sign of malignancy. Parathyroid autotransplantation is risky because of the difficulty in diagnosing malignancy.

▶ Parathyroid cancer can be difficult to diagnose. Despite what the authors state are the "stringent" criteria of Castleman and Rath[1]—myotoses (the most important criteria), systemic and lymphatic metastases, a trabecular pattern of cell formation, fibrous-band formation, nuclear palisading, and invasion of the capsule, adjacent structures, and blood vessels—only 7 of their 16 patients had a definitive diagnosis of parathyroid cancer. In most patients the diagnosis was equivocal. All patients with equivocal diagnoses survived. Even among the 7 patients with a definitive diagnosis of cancer, only 1 died and 1 had evidence of metastatic disease. As with some other endocrine tumors, it can be difficult to make a diagnosis of cancer histologically. The diagnosis is ultimately based on their biological behavior; that is, does it metastasize, invade adjacent structures, or recur after excision? In a recent review, a definitive diagnosis of parathyroid cancer could only be established histologically in 41 of 95 patients.[2] The reader must be cognizant of the criteria used by the authors of papers like this to define parathyroid cancer. The much lower recurrence rate and higher survival rate in this paper than in published reports may reflect different criteria used for diagnosis and/or a more aggressive surgical approach. The authors try to do an en bloc resection of the parathyroid glands as well as locally invaded tissues, and they were willing to sacrifice the recurrent laryngeal nerve and other invaded structures.

R.J. Howard, M.D., Ph.D.

References

1. Castleman B, Rath S: *Tumors of the Parathyroid Glands: Carcinoma.* Washington, DC, Armed Forces Institute of Pathology, 1977, pp 74–79.
2. Sandelin K, Auer G, Bondesin L, et al: Prognostic factors in parathyroid cancer: A review of 95 cases. *World J Surg* 16:724–731, 1992.

Adrenal Surgery for Hypercortisolism: Surgical Aspects

van Heerden JA, Young WF Jr, Grant CS, Carpenter PC (Mayo Clinic and Mayo Found, Rochester, Minn)
Surgery 117:466–472, 1995   7–14

Background.—Endogenous hypercortisolism, or Cushing syndrome, may occur in response to elevated adrenocorticotropic hormone (ACTH) from the pituitary or ectopic tumors (ACTH dependent) or be autonomous within the adrenal gland (ACTH independent). Hypercortisolism causes poor wound healing and increased risk of infection, which is believed to place such patients at high risk for any surgery. An 11-year experience with adrenal surgery was reviewed to study the indications, results, and complications of the procedure.

Methods and Results.—The charts of 91 patients undergoing adrenal resection for endogenous hypercortisolism were reviewed. Females were in the majority in each group when patients were classified by etiology. Patients with adrenal-dependent and therefore ACTH-independent Cushing syndrome represented 51% of the total (46 patients). Thirty-three of these had benign adrenocortical adenoma, 4 had adrenocortical carcinoma, and 9 had bilateral nodular adrenal hyperplasia. For 24 patients in whom the diagnosis was Cushing's disease (ACTH dependent with a pituitary source of ACTH), transsphenoidal surgery was unsuccessful and led to bilateral adrenalectomy. These 24 patients represented 11% of the total undergoing transsphenoidal surgery for hypercortisolism during the 11 years. Twenty-one patients had ectopic ACTH-producing tumors, 5 of whom had undergone transsphenoidal hypophysectomy before the etiology was clear. Eleven (52%) of these patients died, 8 because of the tumor. For the full series, the posterior surgical approach in 72 patients (80%) entailed a mean length of stay of 6.0 days for unilateral or bilateral surgery. The anterior approach was associated with a mean stay of 8.0 days for unilateral and 11.0 days for bilateral surgery. Only 2 deaths (2.2%) occurred in the first 30 postoperative days, neither directly resulting from the surgery. Only 1 patient suffered significant postoperative morbidity, a subphrenic abscess. Three patients reported slow wound healing.

Conclusions.—Adrenalectomy patients are no longer at high risk for morbidity or mortality after surgery. The posterior approach is preferred. Before laparoscopic adrenalectomy becomes standard, it must meet this success rate.

▶ This is a review of the Mayo Clinic's experience with adrenal surgery for hypercortisolism. There are few institutions that can accumulate such a large experience in a relatively brief period. There was a rather high (23%) prevalence of hypercortisolism caused by ectopic ACTH-producing tumors. The authors treated ectopic ACTH-secreting tumors by bilateral adrenalectomy. Twenty-seven percent of the patients had Cushing's disease as a result of excessive ACTH production caused by pituitary pathology. All these patients had failed transsphenoidal procedures. This article does not provide information about the number of patients with hypercortisolism who had successful transsphenoidal operations. Therefore, patients with Cushing's disease likely represent a greater percentage of patients with hypercortisolism than this paper suggests.

R.J. Howard, M.D., Ph.D.

Laparoscopic Adrenalectomy
Deans GT, Kappadia R, Wedgewod K, Royston CMS, Brough WA (Stepping Hill Hosps, Stockport, England; Airedale Hosp, Keighley, England; Castle Hill Hosp, Hull, England; et al)
Br J Surg 82:994–995, 1995   7–15

Introduction.—The outcomes of 8 patients who underwent laparoscopic adrenalectomy are described.

Methods.—Laparoscopic adrenalectomy was performed on 8 patients for the removal of a tumor. The diagnoses included pheochromocytoma (2 patients), Conn's syndrome (4 patients), cystic hemangioma (1 patient), and lymphangiomatous tumor (1 patient).

Results.—The procedure was considered successful in all patients, with a median operating time of 105 minutes and a median hospital stay of 4 days. Two patients experienced complications after surgery. A splenectomy was performed 20 hours after the adrenalectomy on the patient with a lymphangiomatous tumor. Another patient with pheochromocytoma required a blood transfusion. The size of the glands removed ranged from 1 to 12 cm, with a median of 6 cm. Patients were able to return to normal activity in 10 to 25 days.

Conclusion.—Laparoscopic adrenalectomy appears to compare favorably with the open procedure in regard to hospital stay and the patient's return to normal activity. Operating time with the laparoscopic approach was longer than with the open procedure, and bleeding occurred because of difficult dissection. The laparoscopic approach does offer the advantage of less tumor handling, good access, and smaller surgical wounds.

▶ This brief article demonstrates that laparoscopic adrenalectomy can be done safely even for large tumors up to 12 cm in diameter. Hospital stay and inactivity from work do not seem to be less than with open methods.

R.J. Howard, M.D., Ph.D.

8 Nutrition and Metabolism

Introduction*

DETERMINANTS OF THE MAGNITUDE OF CATABOLIC RESPONSE IN SURGICAL PATIENTS

The catabolic response to elective surgery, injury, sepsis, and cancer invariably results in erosion of lean body mass. At some point, weight loss has a negative impact on outcome. The nature, intensity, and duration of the stress are fundamental determinants of both the host mediators activated and the physiologic changes observed. The responses that follow a minor elective operation are similar to those observed during a comparable, brief period of fasting and bed rest. On the other hand, major thermal injury results in a prolonged period of hypermetabolism and a severe drain on the body's energy and protein stores, resolving only with wound closure and resolution of the sepsis that may have developed.

Body composition is a major determinant of the metabolic responses observed during surgical illness, and posttraumatic nitrogen excretion is directly related to the size of the body protein mass. It is the muscular young man in whom nitrogen losses are most marked after injury, and it is the elderly, sedentary woman in whom they are least marked. Observed differences between the metabolic responses of men and women in general reflect differences in body composition.

Major elective surgery in patients with pre-existing nutritional depletion is associated with diminished nitrogen losses as compared with normally nourished patients, although endocrine responses are similar. A strong relationship between protein depletion and postoperative complications has been demonstrated in nonseptic, nonimmunocompromised patients undergoing elective major gastrointestinal surgery. Protein-depleted patients have significantly lower preoperative respiratory muscle strength and vital capacity, an increased incidence of postoperative pneumonia, and a longer postoperative hospital stay. Impaired wound healing and respi-

---

* Comments modified from Souba WW: Nutrition support (parenteral/enteral nutrition). *N Engl J Med,* in review; and Souba WW, Austen WG Jr: Nutrition and metabolism, in Greenfield L (ed): *Surgery, Scientific Principles and Practice.* Philadelphia, Lippincott, in press.

ratory, hepatic, and muscle function in protein-depleted patients awaiting surgery have also been reported.

The capacity of muscle to serve as a substrate source may be limited during prolonged illness in elderly patients, and muscle strength may rapidly become inadequate for respiratory and other vital muscle function. The changes in resting energy expenditure that occur with aging can be accounted for in large part by changes in body composition, specifically, decreases in muscle mass. The physiology of aging, in general terms, is marked by a diminished sensitivity to perturbations of homeostasis and diminished effectiveness of the mechanisms to restore and maintain homeostasis.

Rationale for the Use of Nutrition Support

The rationale for providing nutrition support to patients has been an attempt to prevent or reverse host tissue wasting, broaden the spectrum of therapeutic options, improve the clinical course, and prolong survival. Nutritional therapy as a component of patient care is based on two different rationales: therapy to prevent death from malnutrition as opposed to the administration of nutrients to have a favorable impact on the natural history or treatment of a specific disease process. The former situation includes patients who in the absence of nutrition support would die of starvation because they cannot eat. The second rationale is based on knowledge of existing nutritional/metabolic abnormalities arising from the disease and is directed toward correcting these abnormalities with the intent that outcome will improve. The role of nutritional support in this latter scenario is more controversial, and definitive indications for the use of nutrition support in many patients are unclear. Nonetheless, the use of such nutritional therapy is widespread for multiple reasons: (1) malnutrition is commonly observed in patients with injury, sepsis, AIDS, cancer, and debilitating gastrointestinal disease; (2) there is an association between malnutrition and increased morbidity and mortality; (3) nutrition support can now be provided safely to most patients; (4) several randomized prospective clinical trials suggest that nutrition support is beneficial in selected patients; and (5) it seems intuitive that a well-nourished patient will respond more favorably to therapeutic intervention than will a malnourished patient.

The Difficulty in Defining (Proving) a Role for Nutrition Support

Protein-calorie malnutrition (PCM), a state of undernutrition resulting in a reduction in body cell mass, is common in hospitalized patients. Although its evolution during illness frequently reflects the severity of the underlying disease or toxicity associated with certain therapies, a cause-and-effect relationship between malnutrition and a poorer outcome has not been definitively established. To date no single measurement of nutritional status is of value in an individual patient, and it has been shown that global clinical assessment is a more reproducible technique for evaluating nutritional status. Multivariate analysis using serum albumin and weight loss as predictor variables has been used by some investigators in an effort to define malnutrition, but these formulas are not perfect. Thus despite evidence of an association between malnutrition and increased morbidity, methods of identifying malnourished patients who are at risk are not entirely satisfactory. At present, unintentional weight loss is the cheapest, simplest, and most common measurement used to screen for nutritional risk.

A second reason that it has been difficult to define the role of nutrition support has been the paucity of well-designed clinical trials. Hundreds of trials have evaluated the use of nutrition support in hospitalized patients, but the results are conflicting because of the lack of rigorous studies. Published trials suffer from problems with study design, heterogeneous study populations, small sample size, and/or inappropriate end points or are retrospective in nature. Many of these studies have included well-nourished or minimally malnourished patients who were unlikely to benefit from nutritional intervention, introducing the possibility of masking therapeutic efficacy. Finally, studies that evaluate the efficacy of nutrition support require large numbers of patients and are expensive. It has been difficult to obtain funding to support them.

In surgical patients it is fairly well established that the patient's metabolic stress will influence the amount and rate of weight loss, which will have a negative impact on outcome. For example, short-term undernutrition is well tolerated in minimally stressed postoperative patients, while aggressive early feeding of a previously well nourished patient who sustains a severe catabolic insult has been shown to be beneficial. Thus the factors determining nutritional risk are multiple and interrelated and include pre-existing nutritional status, the magnitude and anticipated length of associated catabolic stresses, and current nutritional therapy.

Specialized nutrition support is an expensive technology that has been used extensively in patient care over the past 2 decades. Prior to recommending its routine use, its therapeutic benefits must be established. At the present time the most reliable method for evaluating clinical efficacy is the prospective randomized clinical trial. Unfortunately, the decision to begin nutrition support is often based on empiricism rather than scientific evidence. Predictably, there are no clear-cut answers for several key questions: Which patients should receive nutrition support and for how long? What is the optimal route of delivery and composition of nutritional formulations? Does nutrition support improve outcome and reduce costs?

Wiley W. Souba, M.D., Sc.D.

Nutrition and Organ Function

Efficacy of Glutamine-Enriched Enteral Nutrition in an Experimental Model of Mucosal Ulcerative Colitis

Fujita T, Sakurai K (Jikei Univ, Tokyo)
Br J Surg 82:749–751, 1995   8–1

Objective.—The intestine becomes permeable to bacteria and endotoxins in response to stress. Many systemic inflammatory responses such as inflammatory bowel disease may be the result of bacterial translocation and endotoxemia. Because glutamine provides energy for rapidly dividing cells such as lymphocytes and enterocytes, the authors investigated the effect of dietary supplementation with glutamine on ornithine decarboxylase activity and prevention of portal vein endotoxemia in guinea pigs.

Methods.—Gut mucosal ornithine carboxylase activity and endotoxin levels in portal vein blood were determined in 3 groups of 7 Hartley guinea pigs with ulcerative colitis that had been fed standard chow (group 1), 1.5% degraded λ-carrageenan (to induce mucosal ulcerative colitis) and standard chow (group 2), or λ-carrageenan and standard chow plus 2% glutamine (group 3).

Results.—The control group gained significantly more weight than did the other 2 groups. There were no significant histologic differences between the mucosae of groups 2 and 3. There were no significant differences in the ileal mucosal ornithine decarboxylase activity between groups, but decarboxylase activity in the cecal mucosa of the 2 treatment groups was significantly lower than for the control group. Although glutamine supplementation did not induce decarboxylase activity in the cecum, the endotoxin level in group 3 portal vein blood was significantly lower than that for group 2 (Table 3).

Conclusion.—Dietary supplementation with 2% glutamine did not induce ornithine decarboxylase activity in the mucosa of guinea pigs with mucosal ulcerative colitis but did reduce endotoxin levels in portal vein blood. This information may have dietary implications for patients with inflammatory bowel disease.

▶ This study corroborates the findings of several other animal studies demonstrating that supplemental glutamine in the diet can improve gut

TABLE 3.—Level of Endotoxin in Portal Vein Blood

	Endotoxin level (pg/ml)
Group 1 (*n* = 7)	4·1 (2·0)
Group 2 (*n* = 7)	71·2 (21·0)*
Group 3 (*n* = 7)	25·3 (10·8)

Note: Values are means (SD).
* $P < 0.01$ vs. groups 1 and 3 (Student's *t* test).
(Courtesy of Fujita T, Sakurai K: Efficacy of glutamine-enriched enteral nutrition in an experimental model of mucosal ulcerative colitis. *Br J Surg* 82:749–751, 1995, Blackwell Science Ltd.)

barrier function. Glutamine has also been shown to preserve barrier function (permeability) in humans.[1] The mechanism by which glutamine is beneficial to the gut mucosa and its function as a barrier remains unclear. Although glutamine is an important fuel for enterocytes, it also plays an important role as a precursor for nucleotide biosynthesis and in glutathione biosynthesis. In the colitis model studied by Fujita and Sakurai, glutathione metabolism was not evaluated, but one might suspect an increase in oxygen radical formation in the bowel. In other models of oxidant stress, glutamine has been shown to be beneficial.[2-4]

W.W. Souba, M.D., Sc.D.

References

1. Van der Hulst R, Van Kreel BK, Von Meyenfeldt MF, et al: Glutamine and the preservation of gut integrity. *Lancet* 341:1363–1365, 1993.
2. Hinshaw DB, Burger JM: Protective effect of glutamine on endothelial cell ATP in oxidant injury. *J Surg Res* 49:222–227, 1990.
3. Austgen TR, Dudrick PS, Sitren HS, et al: The effects of glutamine-enriched total parenteral nutrition on tumor growth and host tissues. *Ann Surg* 215:107–113, 1992.
4. Hong R, Helton W, Rounds J, et al: Glutamine-supplemented TPN preserves hepatic glutathione and improves survival following chemotherapy. *Surg Forum* 41:9–11, 1990.

Fiber: Effect on Bacterial Translocation and Intestinal Mucin Content
Frankel W, Zhang W, Singh A, Bain A, Satchithanandam S, Klurfeld D, Rombeau J (Univ of Pennsylvania, Philadelphia; Food and Drug Administration, Laurel, Md; Wayne State Univ, Detroit)
World J Surg 19:144–149, 1995   8–2

Objective.—Stress increases bacterial translocation (BT) in critically ill patients, particularly those with intestinal dysfunction receiving total parenteral nutrition (TPN) or an elemental diet (ED). Bacterial translocation to mesenteric lymph nodes is an early indication of intestinal epithelial dysfunction. Because the increased rate of BT can be due to the lack of an important nutrient and because fiber is known to decrease BT, this trial was conducted to compare the rate of BT in rats provided with TPN, ED, or chow; to examine whether BT decreases when dietary fiber is added to TPN or ED; and to study the association between fiber and decreasing BT and changes in the jejunal mucosal structure and/or mucin content.

Methods.—A total of 56 male Sprague-Dawley rats were fitted with jugular catheters and randomized into 4 groups of 11 rats that received either chow, TPN, TPN with 2 g/day oral oat fiber, or ED (oral TPN) and 1 group of 12 rats that received ED with 2 g/day oral oat fiber. After 7 days, the rats were killed, blood was drawn for culture, and the proximal jejunum was excised. The total mucosal surface area, mucin surface area, and mucin content were determined.

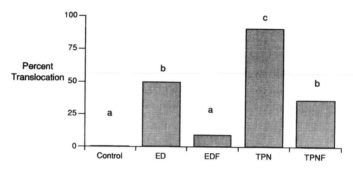

FIGURE 1.—Percent bacterial translocation to mesenteric lymph nodes observed in groups after 7 days of diet. Significant differences are indicated by different letters (*a, b, c*). *P* < 0.05 for unlike letters by chi-square analysis. *Abbreviations: ED*, elemental diet; *EDF*, ED plus oral oat fiber; *TPN*, total parenteral nutrition; *TPNF*, TPN plus oral oat fiber. (Courtesy of *World Journal of Surgery*, Fiber: Effect on bacterial translocation and intestinal mucin content, by Frankel W, Zhang W, Singh A, et al, vol 19, p 146, Fig 1, copyright 1955 by Springer-Verlag.)

Results.—Animals with positive cultures were excluded. Bacterial translocation to mesenteric lymph nodes was increased significantly in TPN and ED rats as compared with controls and increased significantly in TPN vs. ED rats (Fig 1). Oral fiber significantly decreased BT in both TPN and ED rats. When compared with controls, TPN and ED rats had significantly decreased mucosal weight, mucosal DNA, and mucosal alkaline phosphatase levels. Fiber significantly increased mucosal DNA in TPN and ED rats and maintained alkaline phosphatase levels in ED rats. Mucosal maltase was significantly decreased in TPN rats with or without fiber. The percent mucin surface area and mucin content were similar in all groups.

Conclusion.—Bacterial translocation was significantly increased in rats by TPN and ED and significantly more for TPN than for ED. Fiber significantly reduced BT in TPN and ED rats. The mucin surface area, mucin content, and mucosal alkaline phosphatase levels were not consistently affected by BT changes. Fiber-induced reduction in BT is mediated through means other than those associated with mucosal structural changes.

▶ Frankel and colleagues have shown that fiber, like glutamine, is an important nutrient for the gut mucosa. Although fiber has been shown to be an important stimulus for mucosal growth and barrier function, it is not routinely provided to many critically ill patients. In particular, patients nourished with TPN or elemental diets receive no dietary fiber. Although fiber exerts beneficial effects on the gut through its fermentation in the gut lumen to short-chain fatty acid products such as butyrate, the mechanism(s) by which fiber reduces the incidence of bacterial translocation remains unclear. It is likely the several players (nutrients, growth factors) work coordinately to preserve proper gut structure and function and that multiple derangements in this normal physiology occur in critically ill patients. Understanding these derangements and their clinical significance will hopefully lead to improved nutritional formulations.

W.W. Souba, M.D., Sc.D.

Food Deprivation Increases Bacterial Translocation After Non-Lethal Haemorrhage in Rats
Bark T, Katouli M, Svenberg T, Ljungqvist O (Karolinska Hosp and Inst, Stockholm)
Eur J Surg 161:67–71, 1995   8–3

Objective.—Complications from infection after major surgery or trauma are common. Rat studies show that enteric bacterial translocation to lymph nodes after hemorrhage may contribute to the development of postoperative infection and that mortality is increased in animals that have been fasted for 24 hours, primarily because of loss of hepatic glycogen. Pretreatment with glucose infusion increased survival. The results of an investigation of the effect in rats of brief fasting before nonlethal hemorrhage on induction of translocation of enteric bacteria to lymph nodes or blood are presented.

Methods.—Twenty Sprague-Dawley male rats were fasted 24 hours before being subjected to femoral artery hemorrhage for 60 minutes that lowered blood pressure to 55 mm Hg. Nineteen control rats were given food and water ad libitum before hemorrhage. On the morning after, blood and mesenteric lymph nodes were removed and analyzed.

Results.—When compared with fasting rats, fed rats lost significantly more blood (20%), had significantly lower reductions in packed cell volumes (11.3% vs. 16.5%), and had significantly lower increases in glucose levels (7.0 vs. 21.0 mmol/L). Lymph nodes from 6 of 19 fed rats and 14 of 20 fasting rats contained enteric bacteria. The number of pathogens found in the lymph nodes of fasting rats was significantly higher than that in fed rats. Blood cultures from 4 fasted rats but no fed rats grew pathogens.

Conclusion.—Bacterial translocation was significantly enhanced by fasting before hemorrhagic hypotension. Higher glucose levels and plasma volume may have conferred a protective effect in fed animals.

▶ Fasting for 24 hours prior to experimental hemorrhage in rats was associated with a poorer outcome that appeared to be related to an increased rate of bacterial translocation from the gut lumen. While there is no evidence for a negative surgical outcome in patients undergoing short-term preoperative fasting, there is evidence that significant preoperative weight loss or long-term (>14 days) postoperative undernutrition has an adverse impact on outcome after major elective surgery.[1, 2]

W.W. Souba, M.D., Sc.D.

References

1. The Veterans Affairs Total Parenteral Nutrition Cooperative Study Group: Perioperative total parenteral nutrition in surgical patients. *N Engl J Med* 325:525–532, 1991.
2. Sandstrom R, Drott A, Hyltander A, et al: The effect of postoperative intravenous feeding (TPN) on outcome following major surgery evaluated in a randomized study. *Ann Surg* 217:185–195, 1993.

Enteral Nutrition During Multimodality Therapy in Upper Gastrointestinal Cancer Patients

Daly JM, Weintraub FN, Shou J, Rosato EF, Lucia M (Univ of Pennsylvania, Philadelphia)
Ann Surg 221:327–338, 1995   8–4

Background.—Multimodality treatment of surgical patients with upper gastrointestinal malignancies of the esophagus, stomach, and pancreas appears to improve survival but often results in substantial malnutrition, immunosuppression, and morbidity. It has been suggested that supplementation with specific nutrients may improve immunologic function. This study investigates the long-term effects of a diet supplemented with arginine, RNA, and ω-3 fatty acids administered to patients who had undergone major surgery for upper gastrointestinal malignancies.

Method.—Sixty patients with esophageal (22), gastric (16), and pancreatic (22) lesions were randomized into 1 of 4 groups: 1 group received an enteral supplemented diet both in the hospital and as outpatients, the second group received a supplemental diet only as inpatients, group 3 received a standard enteral diet during hospitalization and as outpatients, and the fourth group received the standard enteral diet only as inpatients. Patients randomized to receive enteral feedings after discharge were scheduled to continue this for 12–16 weeks during the recovery and radiation/chemotherapy periods. Plasma and peripheral white blood cells were obtained to determine fatty acid levels and prostaglandin E_2 production.

Results.—In the supplemented-diet groups, mean plasma and cellular ω-3/ω-6 fatty acid levels (percent composition) increased significantly ($P \leq 0.05$) by postoperative day 7 (0.30 vs. 0.13 and 0.29 vs 0.14) and continued to increase over time. Mean prostaglandin E_2 production decreased significantly ($P \leq 0.05$) from 2,760 to 1,600 ng/10^6 cell/mL at day 7 in the supplemented groups, whereas no change was seen in the standard group. Infectious/wound complications were seen in 10% of those in the supplemented groups as compared with 43% of those in the standard diet groups ($P < .05$), and the mean length of hospital stay was 16 vs. 22 days, respectively. Of the patients who were randomized to the outpatient feeding group, only 1 of 18 did not continue, whereas 8 of the 13 patients not randomized to outpatient tube feedings required crossover to jejunostomy nutritional support because of complications.

Conclusion.—Supplementing enteral feeding with arginine, RNA, and ω-3 fatty acids significantly increased plasma and peripheral white blood cell ω-3/ω-6 ratios and significantly decreased prostaglandin E$_2$ production and postoperative infectious/wound complications when compared with standard enteral feeding.

▶ In an effort to improve the metabolic and clinical efficacy of nutritional formulations, several new strategies are under investigation. In this study, a diet enriched with arginine, ω-3 fatty acids, and RNA was studied in cancer patients undergoing major upper abdominal surgery. Others have reported benefits with "immune-enhancing" diets,[1, 2] but additional randomized prospective trials are necessary to better define the role of these diets in clinical medicine.

W.W. Souba, M.D., Sc.D.

References

1. Daly JM, Lieberman MD, Goldfine J, et al: Enteral nutrition with supplemental arginine, RNA, and omega-3 fatty acids in patients after operation: Immunologic, metabolic, and clinical outcome. *Surgery* 112:56–67, 1992.
2. Bower R, Cerra F, Bershadsky B, et al: Early enteral administration of a formula supplemented with arginine, nucleotides, and fish oil in intensive care unit patients: Results of a multicenter, prospective, randomized clinical trial. *Crit Care Med* 23:436–449, 1995.

Effects of TPN on Brain, Liver, and Food Intake in Rats
Meguid MM, Kubota A, Yang ZJ, Montante A, Gleason JR (State Univ of New York, Syracuse; Syracuse Univ, NY)
J Surg Res 58:367–372, 1995   8–5

Background.—The observation that total parenteral nutrition (TPN) suppresses food intake in patients led to a study of this phenomenon in more detail in laboratory rats. Postulating that TPN has a direct metabolic effect in the brain that may be similar to that in the liver, the experiment investigated the effect of TPN on brain glycogen and triglyceride levels in rats.

Method.—Forty-eight adult male rats received either normal saline via jugular catheter for 18 days (control group) or normal saline for 10 days followed by TPN-100 for 4 days and then normal saline for 4 more days (TPN group). One hundred percent of the rats' daily caloric needs was provided by TPN-100 (caloric ratio, glucose:fat:amino acid = 50:30:20). Unlimited chow and water were available during the study. Eight rats from each group were sacrificed after 1 and 4 days of TPN-100 and 4 days after stopping TPN-100. Brain glycogen, liver glycogen, triglyceride, and glycogen synthetase and phosphorylase levels were analyzed along with plasma glucose and insulin.

Results.—The TPN group showed an 85% decrease in spontaneous food intake along with an elevated plasma glucose concentration, a 3- to

5-fold increase in plasma insulin, a 23% increase in whole-brain glycogen, but a 22% to 33% decrease in liver glycogen. No change was seen in liver glycogen synthetase and phosphorylase activity, whereas whole-brain glycogen synthetase activity decreased by 27% and phosphorylase activity increased by 10% to 16%. Whole-brain triglyceride content did not change; however, there was a 155% to 241% increase in liver triglyceride levels. When TPN was stopped, an increase and normalization of food intake was seen along with a reversal of the biochemical changes that did not significantly differ to those of the control rats on day 18.

Conclusion.—This study demonstrates that TPN has a direct metabolic effect on the brain by increasing whole-brain glycogen storage, but this is temporary and persists only during TPN. This is an opposite effect to that of TPN on the liver, which causes a decrease in liver glycogen content. The brain cannot store triglycerides; however, during TPN a marked increase in liver triglyceride storage occurs that only persists during TPN.

▶ Meguid and associates have made significant contributions to our understanding of the relationship between parenteral feeding, oral food intake, and brain regulation of these events. Their work is consistent with the hypothesis that metabolic events within specific brain areas are altered by feeding and by alteration in peripheral metabolic events. The brain appears to use metabolic information from the periphery to regulate long-term energy balance through food intake control via endocrine and autonomic activity. Since catabolic responses to injury are mediated in large part via CNS efferent pathways, these data suggest that nutrients and nutritional status will modulate these responses. Indeed, there are published data suggesting that specific nutrients can improve brain function.[1]

W.W. Souba, M.D., Sc.D.

Reference

1. Young L, Bye R, Scheltinga M, et al: Patients receiving glutamine-supplemented intravenous feeding report an improvement in mood. *JPEN J Parenter Enteral Nutr* 17:422–427, 1993.

Effects of Parenteral and Enteral Nutrition on Gut-Associated Lymphoid Tissue
Li J, Kudsk KA, Gocinski B, Dent D, Glezer J, Langkamp-Henken B (Univ of Tennessee, Memphis)
J Trauma 39:44–52, 1995   8–6

Introduction.—Protection against microbial flora and infectious pathogens as well as against distant mucosal sites is provided by the gut-associated lymphatic tissue (GALT). Both affector (lymphatic follicles) and effector (lamina propria, T and B lymphocytes that control and produce IgA) sites are found in GALT. Intraepithelia (IE) lymphocytes may also have a controlling function in the effector limb. Total parenteral nutrition (TPN) has a negative influence on function of the gut barrier and can result

TABLE 10.—Absolute Number of CD4+ and CD8+ Lymphocytes (×10^6)

Experiment	Group	PP		IE		LP	
		CD4+	CD8+	CD4+	CD8+	CD4+	CD8+
1	Chow	1.24 ± 0.17	0.28 ± 0.04	0.14 ± 0.03	0.40 ± 0.07	0.92 ± 0.12	0.59 ± 0.10
	IG-TPN	0.90 ± 0.08	0.19 ± 0.02	0.09 ± 0.02	0.29 ± 0.05*	0.48 ± 0.05*	0.47 ± 0.07
	IV-TPN	0.80 ± 0.12*	0.20 ± 0.04	0.06 ± 0.01*	0.25 ± 0.05*	0.41 ± 0.09*	0.41 ± 0.07
2	Chow	1.52 ± 0.26	0.30 ± 0.06	0.15 ± 0.03	0.31 ± 0.06	0.77 ± 0.05	1.02 ± 0.19
	IG-TPN	0.81 ± 0.17*†	0.16 ± 0.04*†	0.06 ± 0.01*†	0.28 ± 0.05	0.36 ± 0.02*	0.53 ± 0.08*
	NUTREN	1.41 ± 0.17	0.46 ± 0.17	0.15 ± 0.06	0.36 ± 0.05	0.49 ± 0.05*	0.43 ± 0.11*

Note: Values are means ± SE.
* $P < 0.05$ vs. Chow.
† $P < 0.05$ vs. Nutren.
Abbreviations: PP, Peyer's patch; *IE,* intraepithelial lymphocyte; *LP,* lamina propria.
(Courtesy of Li J, Kudsk KA, Gocinski B, et al: Effects of parenteral and enteral nutrition on gut-associated lymphoid tissue. *J Trauma* 39(1):44–52, 1995.)

in intestinal bacterial growth and translocation, which then suppresses IgA levels. This study was designed to look at the effect of 3 diets on GALT in mice. The lamina propria, Peyer's patches (PPs), mesenteric lymph nodes, and IE lymphocytes were studied.

Methods.—Male mice were fed commercial chow (experiment 1) or Nutren (experiment 2) for 2 weeks before surgery. Total parenteral nutrition was administered IV, as an elemental diet, or enterally through surgically inserted catheters. The 8 control group mice were fed commercial chow. The 7 IV-TPN mice were fed a standard TPN formula (1,538 kcal/L). The mice that received intragastric feeding (IG-TPN) were given the same formula. Infusion rates after surgery were increased to 10–15 mL/day. Peyer's patches, IE lymphocytes, and lamina propria were isolated. $CD4^+$ and $CD8^+$ subtypes of lymphocytes were determined by flow cytometry. Immunoglobulin A was determined by enzyme-linked immunosorbent assay.

Results.—Mice fed commercial chow gained more weight than mice fed by TPN. Serum, not gallbladder or total intestinal IgA was lower in mice fed via TPN. Mesenteric lymph node cells were similar in all groups. Peyer's patches, IE lymphocytes, and lamina propria cell numbers were less in the IV- and IG-TPN groups when compared with controls. T cells outnumbered B cells. In the PPs, the total number of T cells dropped in the mice fed via TPN. The absolute number of $CD4^+$ cells in PPs were lower in both TPN groups (Table 10). In IE lymphocytes, both $CD4^+$ and $CD8^+$ cells dropped in response to TPN feeding. Similar trends were found for cells in the lamina propria.

Conclusion.—Gut-associated lymphotic tissue populations are altered by either of the TPN methods studied. This causes atrophy of the T- and B-cell populations of PPs, IE lymphocytes, and lamina propria, as well as decreased levels of intestinal IgA. Diet complexity (chow vs. Nutren) was not associated with the significant changes.

▶ The effects of TPN on the human gastrointestinal tract include a decrease in brush border hydrolase activity, a reduction in amino acid transporter activity, an increase in mucosal permeability, and a slight decrease in villus height. The most conclusive data demonstrating the superiority of enteral nutrition over parenteral nutrition are derived from studies done in critically injured patients.[1-4] Enteral nutrition was initiated within 24 hours of injury, was well tolerated, and resulted in a statistically significantly lower incidence of postoperative pneumonia, intra-abdominal abscess, and catheter sepsis.

Unless use of the gut is contraindicated (bowel obstruction, intractable diarrhea, high-output enterocutaneous fistula, very low birth weight infant, severe acute pancreatitis, severe enteritis, inadequate luminal surface area, feeding intolerance), enteral nutrition is always the initial route of choice for nutrient administration.

W.W. Souba, M.D., Sc.D.

References

1. Kudsk KA, Croce MA, Fabian TA, et al: Enteral vs. parenteral feeding: Effects on septic morbidity following blunt and penetrating trauma. *Ann Surg* 217:503–508, 1992.
2. Moore EE, Jones TN: Benefits of immediate jejunostomy feeding after major abdominal trauma—a prospective, randomized study. *J Trauma* 26:874–881, 1986.
3. Moore FA, Moore EE, Jones TN, et al: TEN versus TPN following major abdominal trauma—reduced septic morbidity. *J Trauma* 29:916–923, 1989.
4. Moore FA, Feliciano DV, Andrassy RJ, et al: Early enteral feeding, compared with parenteral, reduces postoperative septic complications. *Ann Surg* 216:172–183, 1992.

Enhanced Intra-Anastomotic Healing by Operative Lavage With Nutrient Solutions in Experimental Left-Sided Colonic Obstruction
Aguilar-Nascimento JE, Mathie RT, Man WK, Williamson RCN (Royal Postgraduate Med School, London)
Br J Surg 82:461–464, 1995   8–7

Introduction.—Left-sided colonic obstruction is more often being managed with a single operation using intraoperative colonic lavage rather than with traditional 2- or 3-stage procedures. The healing of anastomoses may be enhanced if nutritional solutions (short-chain fatty acids [SCFAs] or hypertonic glucose) are used in the lavage solution. The healing of left-sided colonic anastomoses with the use of intraoperative colonic lavage containing nutritional solutions was investigated in animal models.

Methods.—Colonic obstruction was induced in 108 male Wistar rats by the placement of a ligature 2.5 cm above the peritoneal reflexion. An end-to-end anastomosis without lavage was performed in 1 group of animals as a control. Antegrade colonic lavage was performed in the remaining animals with 1 of 4 randomly assigned lavage fluids: saline, 10% povidone-iodine, 10% hypertonic glucose, or an SCFA solution. The SCFA solution contained sodium acetate, 60 mmol/L, sodium propionate, 30 mmol/L, and sodium-N-butyrate, 40 mmol/L. Three or 6 days after surgery, the anastomic segment was excised and bursting pressure, bowel wall tension, and hydroxyproline concentrations determined.

Results.—In none of the animals that received SCFA lavage did dehiscence of the anastomosis develop, although there was no significant difference in the incidence of dehiscence between the groups. Bursting occurred only at the anastomotic site on day 3; at day 6, bursting sites were mostly located outside the anastomotic site. Bursting pressure at day 3 was higher in all animals that received lavage than in control animals, but it was significantly higher only in those animals that received SCFA lavage (Fig 1). Bursting pressure at day 6 was significantly higher in all lavage groups than in controls. At day 3, animals that received SCFA and hypertonic glucose lavage had significantly higher bowel wall tension than did controls. At day 6, bowel wall tension was significantly higher in all lavage groups than controls. Proximal colon hydroxyproline concentrations were

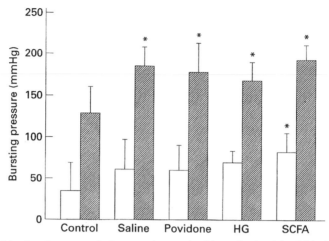

FIGURE 1.—Bursting pressure in 5 groups of rats at day 3 (*open bars*) and day 6 (*shaded bars*) after colonic anastomosis. *Abbreviations: HG*, hypertonic glucose; *SCFA*, short-chain fatty acids. Values are means (SD). *$P < 0.05$ vs. controls on the equivalent day. (Courtesy of Aguilar-Nascimento JE, Mathie RT, Man WK, et al: Enhanced intra-anastomotic healing by operative lavage with nutrient solutions in experimental left-sided colonic obstruction. *Br J Surg* 82:461–464, 1995, Blackwell Science Ltd.)

significantly increased in animals receiving SCFA lavage. At day 3, hydroxyproline concentrations at the site of anastomosis were increased in all groups and reached significance with povidone-iodine, hypertonic glucose, and SCFA lavage. Significantly higher hydroxyproline concentrations were found in animals treated with SCFA lavage at day 6 than in controls and animals treated with saline lavage, as well as higher concentrations in animals receiving hypertonic glucose than in controls.

Conclusion.—Colonic anastomosis performed in the presence of an acute obstruction was found to have improved healing with SCFA or hypertonic glucose intraoperative lavage. Bursting pressures and wall tension were greater in these animals, and bursting occurred more frequently away from the suture line. Collagen synthesis was also found to be greater at day 6 in these animals. Saline lavage showed no benefit in the first 3 days, but at 6 days all lavage solutions provided some benefit to anastomotic strength.

Acute Pouchitis and Deficiencies of Fuel

Sagar PM, Taylor BA, Goodwin P, Holdsworth PJ, Johnston D, Lewis W, Miller A, Quirke P, Williamson M (Royal Liverpool Univ Hosp, England; General Infirmary at Leeds, England)
Dis Colon Rectum 38:488–493, 1995   8–8

Objective.—In patients who undergo restorative proctocolectomy for ulcerative colitis, acute pouchitis is a troublesome complication that has many similarities with ulcerative colitis itself. Previous reports have suggested that both ulcerative and diversion colitis may involve a deficiency of fuel—especially short chain fatty acids (SCFAs)—produced by anaerobic bacterial fermentation of saccharides. A study was conducted to determine whether SCFA deficiency occurs in acute pouchitis and whether correcting SCFA deficiency corrects the pouchitis.

Methods.—The study included 32 patients who had undergone restorative proctocolectomy with a stapled ileoanal anastomosis at the top of the anal canal. Ten had acute pouchitis, as confirmed by histologic examination, and 22 did not. Gas-liquid chromatography was performed to measure the stool concentrations of SCFAs—namely, acetic, propionic, butyric, and valeric acids—and quantitative stool bacteriologic studies were performed. In addition, 4-quadrant pouch biopsies were pathologically assessed in blinded fashion. Patients in the pouchitis group received 6 weeks of metronidazole treatment, 400 mg 3 times a day, and were advised to increase their intake of dietary fermentable saccharides.

Results.—The mean stool total SCFA concentration was 340 µmol/g in the pouchitis group vs. 93 µmol/g in the patients with healthy pouches. The 2 groups were no different in either anaerobic or aerobic counts. All cases of pouchitis responded to treatment. The total SCFA concentration increased to 333 µmol/g, although anaerobic counts fell.

Conclusions.—For patients with restorative proctocolectomy, SCFA deficiency appears to play a role in acute pouchitis. With successful treatment of acute pouchitis, stool SCFA concentrations increase. This does not prove a cause and effect, however, because deficiencies of fuel may represent an epiphenomenon.

▶ Aguilar-Nascimento et al. showed an increase in bowel anastomotic strength when the lumen was irrigated with SCFAs prior to performing the colonic anastomosis. Sagar and colleagues indicate that SCFA deficiency plays a role in acute pouchitis in patients undergoing restorative proctocolectomy for ulcerative colitis. These studies are consistent with the primary role of SCFAs as energy sources for the colonic mucosa. Acetic, propionic, and butyric acids account for 83% of the SCFAs formed in the gastrointestinal tract of mammals by microbial fermentation of carbohydrates in a nearly constant molar ratio, 60:25:15. Supplementation of total parenteral nutrition (TPN) with SCFAs has been shown to support mucosal growth. In one study using normal rats, the use of SCFAs resulted in significantly greater jejunal and ileal mucosal weights and DNA content than a standard TPN control group.[1] Similar effects on small-bowel mucosa were seen with SCFA-supplemented TPN in rats with massive small-bowel resection.[2] Short-chain fatty acid irrigation has been used to treat diversion colitis.[3]

W.W. Souba, M.D., Sc.D.

References

1. Koruda MJ, Rolandelli RH, Settle RG, et al: Effect of parenteral nutrition supplemented with short-chain fatty acids on adaption to massive small bowel resection. *Gastroenterology* 95:715–720, 1988.
2. Koruda MJ, Rolandelli RH, Zimmaro-Bliss DM, et al: Parenteral nutrition supple-

mented with short-chain fatty acids: Effect on the small-bowel mucosa in normal rats. *Am J Clin Nutr* 51:685–689, 1990.

3. Harig JM, Soergel KH, Komorowski RA, et al: Treatment of diversion colitis with short chain fatty acid irrigation. *N Engl J Med* 320:23–28, 1989.

Influence of Glutamine on the Phenotype and Function of Human Monocytes

Spittler A, Winkler S, Götzinger P, Oehler R, Willheim M, Tempfer C, Weigel G, Függer R, Boltz-Nitulescu G, Roth E (Univ of Vienna)

Blood 86:1564–1569, 1995

8–9

Background.—Glutamine (GLN), a very abundant amino acid, is delivered from skeletal muscle to the bowel, liver, and kidneys, as well as to immune cells after trauma or surgery and during sepsis and some malignant states. Glutamine serves as an energy substrate in the gut, as a glucose precursor in the gut and liver, and as a counter to acidosis in the kidneys. Low levels of GLN inhibit mitogen-induced T-cell proliferation and render murine macrophages less able to phagocytose opsonized particles. Reduced expression of HLA-DR is also a prognostic factor in sepsis.

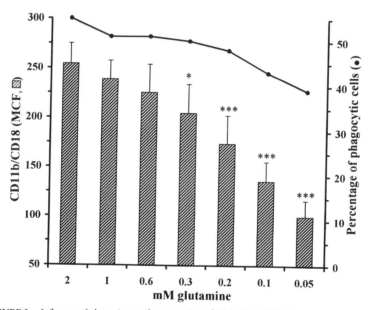

FIGURE 3.—Influence of glutamine on the expression of CR3 (CD11b/CD18) and on phagocytosis of opsonized *Escherichia coli*. Monocytes were cultured for 7 days with the indicated concentrations of glutamine, and expression of CD11b/CD18 (mean channel fluorescence [*MCF*]) as well as the percentage of cells ingesting fluorescein isothiocyanate were determined by FACScan analysis. Data on monocytes from 4 apparently healthy donors represent means ± SD. There was a statistically significant decrease in comparision to 2 mmol/L glutamine, Student's *t* test. *$P < 0.05$. ***$P < 0.001$. (Courtesy of Spittler A, Winkler S, Götzinger P, et al: Influence of glutamine on the phenotype and function of human monocytes. *Blood* 86:1564–1569, 1995.)

Objective.—A study was planned to learn whether GLN modulates the expression of cell surface markers and the function of normal human monocytes in vitro.

Findings.—Reducing the GLN concentration in the culture medium from 2 mmol/L to 200 µmol/L decreased the expression of HLA-DR on monocyte-derived macrophages by 40%. It also significantly decreased the ability of these cells to present tetanus toxoid to helper T lymphocytes. A low level of GLN downregulated the expression of intercellular adhesion molecule type 1 as well as the Fc receptor for IgG and complement receptors types 3 and 4 (Fig 3). These changes correlated with the ability of cells to phagocytose IgG-sensitized ox red blood cells and opsonized *Escherichia coli*. The ability to phagocytose latex beads was unaffected. Depletion of GLN correlated with a significant decrease in cellular levels of adenosine triphosphate.

Conclusions.—A reduced concentration of GLN impairs the phagocytic ability of normal human monocytes and may relate to the decreased expression of certain cell surface antigens on these cells. Whether these observations are relevant to clinical sepsis remains to be determined.

▶ L-Glutamine is now commercially available in Europe for clinical use. In recent years at least 10 randomized prospective clinical trials have evaluated the potential benefits of glutamine-supplemented parenteral nutrition in transplant patients,[1-3] premature infants,[4] postoperative patients,[5-7] adults with the short-gut syndrome,[8] and patients with gastrointestinal disorders.[9] These studies have shown that glutamine, when provided in pharmacologic amounts (0.2–0.5 g/kg/day), is safe and inexpensive and results in an improvement in nitrogen balance[2, 5, 7] and gut barrier function,[9] an enhanced T-cell response,[6] a decrease in infections[2] and number of days of ventilator support,[4] and a reduction in hospital stay[2, 3] and expenses.[2-4, 8]

W.W. Souba, M.D., Sc.D.

References

1. Scheltinga MR, Young LS, Benfell K, et al: Glutamine-enriched intravenous feedings attenuate extracellular fluid expansion after standard stress. *Ann Surg* 214:385–395, 1991.
2. Ziegler TR, Young LS, Benfell K, et al: Clinical and metabolic efficacy of glutamine-supplemented parenteral nutrition after bone marrow transplantation. *Ann Intern Med* 116:821–828, 1992.
3. Schloerb PR, Amare M: Total parenteral nutrition with glutamine in bone marrow transplantation and other clinical applications. *JPEN J Parenter Enteral Nutr* 17:407–413, 1993.
4. Lacey JM, Crouce J, Benfell K, et al: The effects of glutamine-supplemented parenteral nutrition in premature infants. *JPEN J Parenter Enteral Nutr* 20:75–81, 1996.
5. Stehle P, Zander J, Mertes N, et al: Effect of parenteral glutamine peptide supplements on muscle glutamine loss and nitrogen balance after major surgery. *Lancet* 1:231–233, 1989.
6. O'Riordain MG, Fearon KCH, Ross JA, et al: Glutamine-supplemented total parenteral nutrition enhances T-lymphocyte response in surgical patients undergoing colorectal resection. *Ann Surg* 220:212–221, 1994.

7. Hammarqvist F, Wernerman J, Ali R, et al: Addition of glutamine to total parenteral nutrition after elective abdominal surgery spares free glutamine in muscle,
   counteracts the fall in muscle protein synthesis, and improves nitrogen balance.
   Ann Surg 209:455–461, 1989.
8. Byrne TA, Persinger RL, Young LS, et al: A new treatment for patients with
   short-bowel syndrome. *Ann Surg* 222:243–245, 1995.
9. van der Hulst RRWJ, van Kreel BK, von Meyenfeldt MF, et al: Glutamine and the
   preservation of gut integrity. *Lancet* 341:1363–1365, 1993.

Metabolic Abnormalities and Regulation in Catabolic States

Glucocorticoids Mediate Macrophage Dysfunction in Protein Calorie Malnutrition

Hill ADK, Naama HA, Gallagher HJ, Shou J, Calvano SE, Daly JM (New York Hosp/Cornell Univ Med Ctr)
Surgery 118:130–137, 1995

8–10

Introduction.—One of the most significant worldwide public health problems is protein-calorie malnutrition. The problem can be either primary, as in underdeveloped countries, or secondary, as can occur in up to 50% of hospitalized patients. In either case, but particularly in hospitalized patients, the malnutrition can lead to infection and death. The severely depressed function of macrophages in malnutrition may lead to an increased susceptibility to infection. Stress may lead to immunosuppression by the hypothalamic-pituitary-adrenocortical axis because of excess

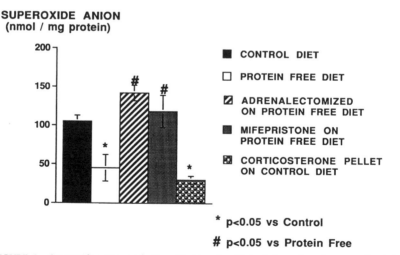

FIGURE 5.—Superoxide anion production. Blocking the effect of elevated corticosterone levels by either adrenalectomy or mifepristone restored superoxide anion production to control levels. Implanting a 50-mg corticosterone pellet into normally fed mice reproduced the impairment in superoxide production seen in protein-free mice. (Courtesy of Hill ADK, Naama HA, Gallagher HJ, et al: Glucocorticoids mediate macrophage dysfunction in protein calorie malnutrition. *Surgery* 118:130–137, 1995.)

INTERLEUKIN-6
(ng / ml)

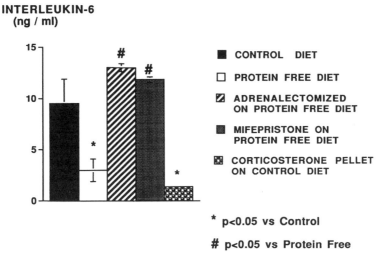

■ CONTROL   DIET

□ PROTEIN FREE DIET

▨ ADRENALECTOMIZED
   ON PROTEIN FREE DIET

▥ MIFEPRISTONE ON
   PROTEIN FREE DIET

▦ CORTICOSTERONE PELLET
   ON CONTROL DIET

* p<0.05 vs Control

\# p<0.05 vs Protein Free

FIGURE 6.—Interleukin-6 (IL-6) production. Abrogating the effect of corticosterone by either adrenalectomy or mifepristone restored IL-6 production to control levels. Implanting a 50-mg corticosterone pellet into normally fed mice reproduced the impairment in IL-6 seen in protein-free mice. (Courtesy of Hill ADK, Naama HA, Gallagher HJ, et al: Glucocorticoids mediate macrophage dysfunction in protein calorie malnutrition. *Surgery* 118:130–137, 1995.)

secretion of corticosterone, a proven immunosuppressive agent. Logically, it is possible that corticosterone may lead to decreased macrophage function.

Methods.—Virus-free female mice between 6 and 8 weeks of age were studied. They were all maintained on a 12-hour day-night cycle and fed diets with a caloric value of 4.25 kcal/g. The mice were randomized to groups: control (24% casein diet), protein-free diet (PFD), adrenalectomized and PFD, PFD plus a glucocorticoid receptor antagonist (RU 486, 10 mg/kg), or the control diet plus a 50-mg corticosterone pellet that had been implanted under the skin. The study period was 7 days, after which the mice were sacrificed by CO_2 asphyxiation. Serum corticosterone, body weight serum albumin, macrophage function, and macrophage production of interleukin-6 (IL-6) were determined.

Results.—Data for the mice fed the control diets were pooled. One week on the PFD resulted in over a 3-fold increase in corticosterone. Administration of RU 486 had no effect on corticosterone. Implantation of the corticosterone pellet also elevated corticosterone levels. Adrenalectomized mice on the PFD had a 20% mortality rate. Regardless of the experimental group, mice fed the 24% casein diet increased their body weight 7% to 9% whereas mice on the PFD lost 10% to 18% of their body weight. Serum albumin was maintained while on the casein diet, whereas mice fed the PFD experienced a decrease in albumin. There was a significant correlation between elevated corticosterone and depressed macrophage function as evidenced by superoxide anion production (Fig 5) and IL-6 (Fig 6).

Conclusion.—Elevation of corticosterone levels via the stress of a PFD or subcutaneous pellet resulted in depressed macrophage function. Minimizing corticosterone by adrenalectomy or the glucocorticoid blocker RU 486 did not reduce macrophage function. These data indicate that the neuroendocrine system, in response to a PFD, raises serum corticosteroid levels and depresses macrophage function.

▶ Hill and colleagues show that protein-calorie malnutrition impairs macrophage function via elevated levels of glucocorticoids. Blocking the stress glucocorticoid response prevented the impairment in macrophage function. It is important to recognize that the adrenocorticoid response to injury and other catabolic diseases imparts a number of beneficial responses such as mobilization of amino acid and glucose stores. Adrenalectomized animals fare much worse after major injury than do animals with intact adrenal glands. Thus although this study indicates that a significant component of the immunosuppression seen after protein-calorie malnutrition is mediated by elevated serum glucocorticoid concentrations, modulation of this derangement in an attempt to improve macrophage function would have to be very selective in its approach.

W.W. Souba, M.D., Sc.D.

Protein Metabolism in Human Colon Carcinomas: In Vivo Investigations Using a Modified Tracer Technique With L-[1-13C]Leucine
Hagmüller E, Kollmar HB, Günther HJ, Holm E, Trede M (Heidelberg Univ, Manheim, Germany; Euro-Med-Clinic, Fürth, Germany)
Cancer Res 55:1160–1167, 1995   8–11

Background.—Tumors have been repeatedly described as "nitrogen traps." Quantification of protein synthesis only does not reflect the extent of tumor anabolism; the decisive factor is the net balance. An attempt was made to analyze protein kinetics, particularly net protein balance, in human tumors in vivo during surgery.

Methods.—Intraoperative tumor leucine/protein metabolism was studied in 15 patients with resectable malignant colon tumors by using a balance model and L-[1-13C]leucine as the tracer substance. The quantitative exchange rates of 20 amino acids were studied in tumoral tissue and compared with those in peripheral (forearm) tissue. In addition, the protein kinetics of the whole body was studied by using a 2-pool model with the same tracer.

Results.—In tumors, essential and branched-chain amino acid uptakes were 1.68 and 1.52 µmol/100 g tissue/per minute, respectively, whereas an overall amino acid release was observed in peripheral tissue. The mean protein retention value for the tumors was 8.941 g/kg/24 hr, which was significantly different from the peripheral protein loss of -0.557 g/kg/24 hr and the whole-body protein loss of -0.363 g/kg/24 hr (Fig 4). The

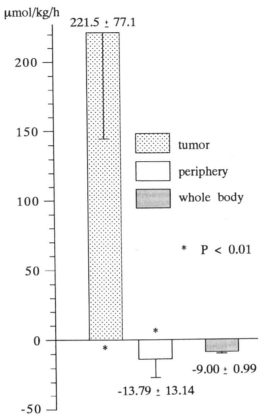

μmol/kg/h

221.5 ± 77.1

tumor

periphery

whole body

* P < 0.01

-9.00 ± 0.99

-13.79 ± 13.14

FIGURE 4.—Comparison of leucine retention rates for the tumor, peripheral compartments, and whole body. Column values are means ± SE. (Courtesy of Hagmüller E, Kollmar HB, Günther HJ, et al: Protein metabolism in human colon carcinomas: In vivo investigations using a modified tracer technique with L-[1-¹³C]leucine. *Cancer Res* 55:1160–1167, 1995.)

tumors were divided into 2 prognostic groups based on their histology. The 2 groups differed significantly in terms of the net retention rate for 10 amino acids, including leucine. Tumors with an unfavorable prognosis (mucinous histology) had a higher retention rate.

Conclusions.—These findings support the designation of tumors as "nitrogen traps." The protein balance model used here provides a satisfactory measurement of the net protein balance in tumors as well as peripheral and whole-body metabolism. The model could also be used to directly evaluate dietary measures such as adjuvant parenteral nutrition in connection with chemotherapy.

▶ Although tumors grow to large size in rodents, in humans a tumor volume exceeding 1% of body weight is uncommon. Nonetheless, malignant cells require increased amounts of amino acids, in particular, glutamine and leucine, to support DNA and protein biosynthesis. Wasa and colleagues[1] have provided insight into how malignant cells in the center of solid tumor survive despite low amino acid levels. They studied amino acid transport in hepatomas cultured in normal and amino acid–deprived media. Growth was dependent on the concentration of glutamine and leucine. In leucine-deprived cells, leucine uptake increased 2-fold due to a change attributable to enhanced transporter capacity. Decreased extracellular amino acid levels encountered by tumors *in vivo* may elicit similar adaptive responses that contribute to the maintenance of cytoplasmic levels of amino acids essential for growth.

W.W. Souba, M.D., Sc.D.

Reference

1. Wasa M, Bode B, Souba WW: Adaptive regulation of amino acid transport in nutrient-deprived human hepatomas. *Am J Surg* 171:163–169, 1996.

TNF-Stimulated Arginine Transport by Human Vascular Endothelium Requires Activation of Protein Kinase C

Pan M, Wasa M, Lind S, Gertler J, Abbott W, Souba WW (Massachusetts Gen Hosp, Harvard Med School, Boston; Univ of Florida, Gainesville)
Ann Surg 221:590–601, 1995   8–12

Background.—L-Arginine is the exclusive precursor of the short-lived bioregulatory molecule nitric oxide (NO). Enhanced NO production by the endothelium may be dependent on accelerated uptake of circulating arginine, but the mechanism that regulates arginine transport across the endothelial membrane is not known. Given that activation of protein kinase C (PKC) can modulate amino acid transport and given the potential link between arginine transport and NO production, a study was conducted to determine the endothelial arginine transport mechanism and the potential role of tumor necrosis factor α (TNF-α)-mediated transduction pathway involving PKC in regulating this transport in cultured endothelial cells.

Methods/Results.—Arginine transport was assayed in confluent human umbilical vein endothelial cells. Carrier-mediated arginine uptake was mediated by 2 Na^+-independent transporters. System y^+, which has an exclusive preference for the cationic amino acids arginine, lysine, and ornithine, accounted for 80% of the total transport, and system $b^{0,+}$ accounted for 20% of the transport. When cells were incubated with TNF, system y^+-mediated arginine transport increased in a time- and dose-dependent fashion by increasing system y^+ transport maximal capacity without affecting transporter affinity. The TNF-induced increase in arginine transport activity was abrogated by both actinomycin D and cycloheximide (Fig 4), which is consistent with DNA transcription and de novo protein synthesis. Furthermore, the specific PKC inhibitor chelerythrine chloride also blocked the TNF-mediated increase in arginine transport, thus indicating the involvement of PKC activation in the TNF-induced

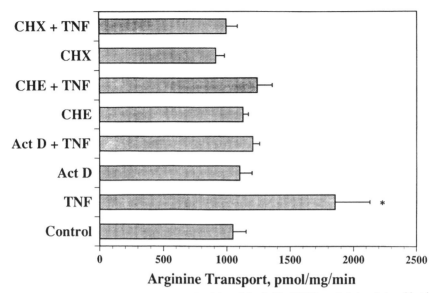

Arginine Transport, pmol/mg/min

FIGURE 4.—Effects of actinomycin D (*Act D*), cycloheximide (*CHX*), and chelerythrine chloride (*CHE*) on tumor necrosis factor (*TNF*) stimulation of system y^+-mediated arginine transport. Human umbilical venous endothelial cells were incubated with TNF (1 ng/mL) with or without Act D (1 µmol/L), CHX (20 µmol/L), or CHE (6.5 µmol/L) for 8 hours before measurements were made. Transport values are means ± SD (n = 6). *$P < 0.01$ vs. control. (Courtesy of Pan M, Wasa M, Lind S, et al: TNF-stimulated arginine transport by human vascular endothelium requires activation of protein kinase C. *Ann Surg* 221:590–601, 1995.)

response. Similar findings obtained when cells were incubated with the direct PKC activator tissue-type plasminogen activator (TPA; phorbol ester 12-myristate-13-acetate) indicated that PKC activation was involved in arginine transport. In contrast, TNF and TPA only slightly increased system $b^{0,+}$-mediated arginine transport. Incubation of cells with the protein kinase A (PKA) activator dibutyryl cyclic adenosine monophosphate failed to affect arginine transport, thus indicating that PKA was not involved in TNF-induced arginine transport. Two NO synthase inhibitors, the L-arginine analogues N-ω-nitro-L-arginine (L-NA) and N-ω-nitro-L-arginine methyl ester (L-NAME), failed to block arginine transport, which suggests that the arginine transporter and the NO synthase system may in part be independently regulated.

Summary.—Tumor necrosis factor stimulates arginine transport in human umbilical vein endothelial cells via a process that requires activation of the intracellular messenger PKC. In turn, the latter signals de novo protein synthesis, possibly of the y^+ arginine transporter protein itself.

▶ In recent years, attention has focused on arginine as a critical regulator of vascular endothelial NO production. Besides being the exclusive precursor of NO biosynthesis, the uptake of extracellular arginine is essential for both constitutive and inducible NO biosynthesis in physiologic and pathologic states. Increasing the circulating arginine concentration has been shown to correct salt-induced hypertension,[1] and arginine depletion has been shown to correct hypotension in endotoxemic rats.[2]

Endothelial cells obtain L-arginine from 2 sources: uptake of free arginine from the extracellular milieu (plasma or interstitial fluid) and intracellular regeneration of arginine. The L-arginine analogues L-NA and L-NAME are widely used as NO synthase inhibitors and compete with L-arginine for the active site on NO synthetase, thereby inhibiting NO production. The use of inhaled NO now has clinical applicability.

W. W. Souba, M.D., Sc.D.

References

1. Chen PY, Sanders PW: L-Arginine abrogates salt-sensitive hypertension in Dahl/ Rapp rats. *J Clin Invest* 88:1559–1567, 1991.
2. Palmer RMJ, Ashton DS, Moncada A: Vascular endothelial cells synthesize nitric oxide from L-arginine. *Nature* 333:664–666, 1988.

Effect of Cortisol on Energy Expenditure and Amino Acid Metabolism in Humans
Brillon DJ, Zheng B, Campbell RG, Matthews DE (Cornell Univ, New York)
Am J Physiol 268:E501–E513, 1995   8–13

Background.—Catabolic injury and stress are marked by increased energy expenditure, accelerated breakdown of skeletal muscle protein, glucose intolerance, and insulin resistance. Whereas insulin has significant anabolic effects, cortisol has catabolic effects. Because there have been no in-depth studies of cortisol's effects on energy expenditure in humans, the effects of acute hypercortisolemia on energy expenditure were studied.

Methods.—Nine normal healthy adults were studied on 3 different occasions. They received overnight hydrocortisone infusions of 0, 80, and 200 µg/kg/hr to produce plasma cortisol concentrations of 10.6, 34.0, and 64.9 µg/dL, respectively. Amino acid kinetics were measured by means of L-[1-^{13}C]leucine, L-[phenyl-^{2} H$_5$]phenylalanine, and L-[2-^{15}N]glutamine infusion during the last 7 hours of hypercortisolemia. Somatostatin, glucagon, and insulin infusions were given during the last 3.5 hours to return the cortisol-induced rise in plasma insulin to normal levels.

Results.—Plasma glucose, free fatty acid (FFA), and insulin concentrations all increased during hypercortisolemia. Although insulin returned to basal levels with the somatostatin clamp, glucose and FFA increased. The increase in leucine and phenylalanine appearance rates suggests that acute hypercortisolemia increased protein breakdown by 5% to 20%. The increase in leucine appearance rate when insulin was normalized during hypercortisolemia, suggests that insulin was affecting leucine metabolism.

Hypercortisolemia did not increase the fraction of leucine flux that was oxidized, although it did increase disposal by the nonoxidative route of leucine uptake. Protein breakdown and synthesis increased, thus increasing cycling of amino acids; however, this could have increased resting

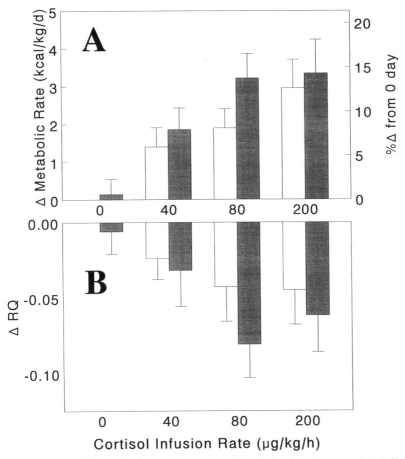

FIGURE 3.—Metabolic rate (resting energy expenditure [REE]) (**A**) and respiratory quotient (*RQ*) (**B**) as a function of cortisol infusion and somatostatin clamp. *Open bars,* before somatostatin clamp; *filled bars,* during somatostatin clamp. Values are presented as change in REE or RQ from saline infusion the day before the somatostatin clamp (23.5 ± 0.7 kcal/kg/day and 0.820 ± 0.022, respectively). The right y-axis in **A** shows the percent change in REE from the saline infusion day. Infusion of cortisol significantly increased REE (*P* < 0.01). The increase was significant when REE at an 80-µg/kg/hr infusion rate was compared with the control day but not the 40-µg/kg/hr day. Somatostatin clamp did not significantly affect REE. Infusion of cortisol did not significantly decrease RQ, but RQ decreased during the somatostatin clamp. (Courtesy of Brillon DJ, Zheng B, Campbell RG, et al: Effect of cortisol on energy expenditure and amino acid metabolism in humans. *Am J Physiol* 268:E501–E513, 1995.)

energy expenditure (REE) by no more than 1% to 2%. Glutamine flux increased in a dose-dependent manner during hypercortisolemia, apparently because of increased release from skeletal muscle. During hypercortisolemia, REE was increased by 9% to 15% at the 80- and 200-µg/kg/hr infusion rates (Fig 3). The increased REE appeared to involve increased fat oxidation since the respiratory rate tended to decrease during cortisol infusion.

Conclusions.—Hypercortisolemia appears to increase the metabolic rate in normal healthy humans. This phenomenon may play a role in the hypermetabolic state following injury. Cortisol increases amino acid cycling via protein, although it remains to be seen whether the cycling occurs within tissues or represents shifting of body protein from one tissue to another.

Protein Metabolism Kinetics in Neonates: Effect of Intravenous Carbohydrate and Fat

Jones MO, Pierro A, Garlick PJ, McNurlan MA, Donnell SC, Lloyd DA (Univ of Liverpool, England; Rowett Research Inst, Aberdeen, Scotland; State Univ of New York, Stony Brook)
J Pediatr Surg 30:458–462, 1995   8–14

Background.—Protein metabolism is dependent on both protein and energy intake. Increased protein intake is known to enhance protein synthesis, reduce endogenous protein breakdown, and enhance net protein retention. However, the influence of nonprotein energy intake on protein metabolism is less clear. The aim of this study was to determine the relative effects of glucose and fat on nitrogen balance and protein metabolism kinetics in stable newborn infants receiving total parenteral nutrition (TPN).

Method.—Fourteen infants were randomly allocated into one of 2 groups. Group A received 10.0 g/kg/day of dextrose and 4.0 g/kg/day of fat; group B received 19.0 g/kg/day of dextrose and 0.5 g/kg/day of fat. The volume of TPN varied from 120 to 180 ml/kg/day according to need. Caloric intake (86 kcal/kg/day) and amino acid intake (2.5 g/kg/day) were the same in the 2 groups. Eighteen metabolic studies were carried out on the infants. Timed urinary nitrogen excretion was determined. On the third day of the study the infants received a priming dose of 15 µmol/kg of [^{13}C]leucine, followed by a 6-hour infusion at 6 µmol/kg/hr. Plasma and breath samples were taken at hourly intervals, and carbon dioxide production was measured by indirect calorimetry. Plateau levels of plasma [^{13}C]α-ketoisocaproic acid (KIC) enrichment and expired $^{13}CO_2$ enrichment were determined by gas chromatograph mass spectrometry. Protein metabolism kinetics were also evaluated.

Results.—There were no significant differences between the 2 groups for gestational age, postnatal age, weight, days postsurgery, heart rate, and respiratory rate. Achievement of satisfactory plateau levels for plasma ^{13}C-KIC enrichment and expired $^{13}CO_2$ enrichment enabled the calculation of leucine flux and oxidation. The respective indices of energy and protein metabolism for each group were as follows: nitrogen balance, 0.27 g/kg/day; total protein flux, 10.38 g/kg/day; total protein synthesis, 9.64 g/kg/day; total protein breakdown, 7.86 g/kg/day; and total protein oxidation/excretion, 0.92 g/kg/day. The nonprotein respiratory quotient and carbohydrate utilization were higher in group B ($P = 0.0001$), and fat utilization was higher in group A ($P < 0.0001$). There was no significant difference between the 2 groups with respect to any of the components of protein metabolism.

Conclusion.—This study provides the following conclusions: infants receiving TPN have high rates of protein turnover, infants avidly retain nitrogen, and glucose and fat have an equivalent effect on protein metabolism kinetics in newborn infants receiving TPN.

▶ In catabolic patients, glucocorticoids are generally thought of as substrate-mobilizing hormones—historically the catecholamines have been viewed as the primary mediators of hypermetabolism (an increase in resting energy expenditure). The study by Brillon and associates demonstrates that hypercortisolemia also induces hypermetabolism. The accompanying decrease in respiratory quotient is consistent with a shift toward fat oxidation. The authors suggest that the increase in glutamine biosynthesis they noted was most likely to occur in muscle, but recent studies suggest that the lungs also participate in this response.[1-3]

Jones et al. studied protein metabolism in infants by using radiolabeled leucine. In contrast to healthy adults who exist in a state of nitrogen equilibrium and the subjects studied by Brillon et al., who were protein catabolic, healthy infants remain in positive nitrogen balance in order to achieve growth and development.

W.W. Souba, M.D., Sc.D.

References

1. Souba WW, Plumley DA, Salloum RM, et al: Effects of glucocorticoids on lung glutamine and alanine metabolism. *Surgery* 108:213–219, 1990.
2. Abcouwer S, Lukaszewicz G, Ryan U, et al: Molecular regulation of lung endothelial glutamine synthetase expression. *Surgery* 118:325–335, 1995.
3. Abcouwer S, Lukaszewicz G, Lustig R, et al: Glucocorticoids regulate glutamine synthetase expression in lung epithelial cells. *Am J Physiol* 270:L141–L151, 1996.

Negative Impact of Cancer Chemotherapy on Protein Metabolism in Healthy and Tumor-Bearing Rats
Le Bricon T, Gugins S, Cyober L, Baracos VE (Univ of Alberta, Edmonton, Canada; Centre Hospitalière Universitaire St-Antoine, Paris)
Metabolism 44:1340–1348, 1995   8–15

Background.—Chemotherapeutic agents are commonly used in the treatment of cancer; however, very little consideration has been given to the effects of these agents on protein metabolism. The effects of 4 chemotherapeutic agents frequently used to treat various types of human cancer were therefore investigated in healthy and tumor-bearing rats, based on their different biochemical mechanisms of action.

Methods.—Agents studied included cyclophosphamide (CYP), 120 mg/kg; 5-fluorouracil (5-FU), 50 mg/kg; cisplatin (CDDP), 5 mg/kg; or meth-

TABLE 1.—Cumulative Food Intake and Body Weight Gain After Drug Injection in
Healthy and Tumor-Bearing Rats

Parameter	Healthy	MH7777 Bearing
Cumulative body weight gain (g/6 day)		
Control (sham)	6 ± 1	−1 ± 1*
CYP	1 ± 1†	−6 ± 2*
5-FU	1 ± 1†	−2 ± 1
CDDP	−23 ± 4†	−33 ± 3†
MTX	−5 ± 2†	−12 ± 3†
Cumulative food intake (g/100 g body weight/6 day)		
Control (sham)	42 ± 1	36 ± 1*
CYP	40 ± 2	31 ± 1*†
5-FU	39 ± 1†	30 ± 1*†
CDDP	18 ± 5†	11 ± 1†
MTX	30 ± 2†	23 ± 2*†

Note: Data for food intake are expressed per unit of body weight at the time of drug injection. Healthy rats (n = 40) and rats bearing MH7777 (n = 40) were randomized to 5 treatment groups (n = 8 per group). Drugs were delivered as a single intraperitoneal injection, and the rats were studied for 6 days posttreatment.
* Significantly different from healthy animals for each drug treatment group ($P < 0.05$).
† Significantly different from control for each parameter ($P < 0.05$).
Abbreviations: MH7777, Morris hepatoma 7777; CYP, cyclophosphamide; 5-FU, 5-fluorouracil; CDDP, cisplatin; MTX, methotrexate.
(Courtesy of Le Bricon T, Gugins S, Cyober L, et al: Negative impact of cancer chemotherapy on protein metabolism in healthy and tumor-bearing rats. *Metabolism* 44:1340–1348, 1995.)

otrexate (MTX), 30 mg/kg. Single intraperitoneal (IP) injections were administered to 40 healthy rats and 40 rats with evidence of Morris hepatoma 7777 (MH7777) in a situation similar to human cancer (tumor burden less than 0.2% of body weight, moderate anorexia, and weight loss. The effects of these agents on host nitrogen metabolism were evaluated 6 days after the administration of chemotherapy.

Results.—With the exception of CDDP-treated rats, all animals had resumed normal feed intake and positive nitrogen balance 6 days posttreatment. Conversely, continued weight loss and inferior nitrogen balance were noted in animals receiving CDDP (Table 1). Antitumor activity was observed with CDDP and MTX treatment, although CDDP led to diarrhea in 6 of the 8 tumor-bearing animals. The MH7777-bearing rats also had more severe drug-induced anorexia in comparison with healthy rats. At postinjection days 3 to 4, the tumor-bearing rats had more severely decreased nitrogen balance than healthy animals did in response to 5-FU and MTX: 159 vs. 273 mg nitrogen after 2 days and -66 vs. 153 mg nitrogen after 2 days with each agent, respectively.

Conclusions.—These findings support the presence of drug-specific effects on host nitrogen balance. There is also evidence of a drug-tumor interaction for nitrogen metabolism in the tumor-bearing host. Further investigations of the mechanism and treatment of cancer-related cachexia must consider the effects of both disease and treatment.

▶ Several animal studies have documented negative nitrogen balance and impaired wound healing with the administration of chemotherapy. Intuitively, these findings would suggest that nutrition support of patients receiving chemotherapy would be advantageous. This, however, has been difficult to prove. Many randomized prospective clinical trials have evaluated the use of nutrition support in cancer patients undergoing chemotherapy, but they are flawed for one or more of the following reasons: (1) the type and duration of antineoplastic therapy varied among the patients; (2) the statistical power of the studies was poor because of small sample size; (3) in many trials, well-nourished patients, those least likely to benefit from nutritional intervention, were studied; (4) the impact of nutrition support on quality of life was rarely evaluated; (5) the patient populations studied were heterogeneous, comprised of patients with different tumors and different stages of disease; and (6) the timing and duration of nutrition support and the composition of the diets delivered make it difficult to evaluate efficacy. A role for aggressive nutrition support is more clear in patients undergoing bone marrow transplantation.[1,2]

W.W. Souba, M.D., Sc.D.

References

1. Szeluga D, Stuart, RK, Utermohlen V, et al: Nutritional support of bone marrow transplant recipients: A prospective, randomized clinical trial comparing total parenteral nutrition and an enteral feeding program. *Cancer Res* 47:3309–3316, 1987.
2. Weisdorf SA, Lysne J, Wind D, et al: Positive effect of prophylactic total parenteral nutrition on long term outcome of bone marrow transplantation. *Transplantation* 43:833–838, 1987.

Complications of Nutrition Support

Total Parenteral Nutrition–Associated Cholestasis in Surgical Neonates May Be Reversed by Intravenous Cholecystokinin: A Preliminary Report
Rintala RJ, Lindahl H, Pohjavuori M (Univ of Helsinki)
J Pediatr Surg 30:827–830, 1995   8–16

Objective.—Premature infants receiving total parenteral nutrition (TPN) are prone to TPN-associated cholestasis (TPNAC). If the cholestasis does not resolve when the child begins enteral nutrition, irreversible liver damage or death can occur. Because the peptide hormone cholecystokinin increases bile flow and promotes gallbladder emptying, a preliminary study was conducted to determine whether the hormone could reverse TPNAC in infants.

Methods.—Unresolved cholestasis developed in 8 of 780 operated infants, who were infused 3 times a day for 3 to 5 days with 2 to 4 Ivy dog units (IVD)/kg. Three infants were operated for necrotizing enterocolitis, 1 for midgut volvulus, 1 for gastroschisis, 1 for diaphragmatic hernia, 1 for necrosis of the stomach, and 1 for a cardiac anomaly. Four infants were premature. Seven infants were weaned from TPN, which averaged 35

TABLE 2.—Laboratory Data

	Normal	Pretreatment	Posttreatment (1 wk)	Posttreatment (2 wk)	Posttreatment (6 mo)
Conjugated bilirubin (mmol/L)	<5	124 (57–286)	30 (19–43)	9 (5–11)	5 (1–8)
SGOT (U/l)	<40	203 (76–958)	139 (53–272)	72 (48–165)	40 (32–69)
SGPT (U/l)	8–40	100 (60–478)	75 (40–309)	58 (40–148)	43 (30–68)

Note: Laboratory data concern the 7 patients who responded to treatment. Laboratory values are given as medians and range.
Abbreviations: SGOT, serum glutamic oxaloacetic transaminase; SGPT, serum glutamic pyruvic transaminase.
(Courtesy of Rintala RJ, Lindahl H, Pohjavuori M: Total parenteral nutrition–associated cholestasis in surgical neonates may be reversed by intravenous cholecystokinin: A preliminary report. J Pediatr Surg 30:827–830, 1995.)

days, before cholecystokinin treatment. One with short-gut syndrome could not be completely weaned. Three patients had biliary sludge or gallstones.

Results.—Bile flow was restored in 7 of 8 patients within 1 to 3 days, and jaundice resolved within 2 weeks. Two patients required the larger dose. Bilirubin normalized within 2 weeks, but liver enzyme levels declined slowly (Table 2). Jaundice resolved in the patients with short-gut syndrome in 6 weeks. No biliary sludge or stones were seen. At 3 months, biliary excretion was normal in 7 patients. One required operative irrigation of the biliary tree. At follow-up, all patients were anicteric.

Conclusion.—Intravenous cholecystokinin can reverse TPNAC in the majority of infants.

Complications of Needle Catheter Jejunostomy in 2,022 Consecutive Applications

Myers JG, Page CP, Stewart RM, Schwesinger WH, Sirinek KR, Aust JB (Univ of Texas Health Sciences Ctr, San Antonio)
Am J Surg 170:547–551, 1995   8–17

Background.—Needle catheter jejunostomy (NCJ) is a frequently used adjunct to intra-abdominal surgery in patients who require long-term enteral access because they are not able to promptly resume an adequate oral intake. Its acceptance has, however, been limited by concern over its reliability and potential for causing serious complications, including bowel necrosis.

Study Population.—Experience with NCJ was reviewed in 28,121 laparotomies performed in the past 16 years. A total of 2,022 jejunostomies were performed in 1,938 adult patients. These patients were a relatively high-risk group. Most of the catheters were placed at the time of laparotomy for reasons other than feeding access—most often the performance of a complex upper abdominal operation.

Complications.—Twenty-nine patients (1.5%) suffered a total of 34 NCJ-related complications, 3 of which were fatal. Eighteen re-explorations were necessary. Dislodgment was most often the result of inadequately securing the catheter. Occlusion usually correlated with the delivery of inappropriate medication such as a thick syrup or high-viscosity enteral formula. Subcutaneous abscesses were associated with poor skin site care. Pneumatosis intestinalis and major abdominal wall infection necessitating extensive debridement developed in 3 patients each. Two patients had late bowel obstruction, and severe bowel ischemia developed in 3 in relation to enteral feeding. Twenty-two of the 34 complications were preventable.

Literature Review.—In 11 reported series totaling 1,788 NCJ procedures, complications occurred in 4.1% of the cases. A lost catheter accounted for one third of all complications as compared with 45.5% of those in the present series.

Conclusion.—Needle catheter jejunostomy and enteral feeding are, in general, safe procedures, but they are invasive and not free of risk.

A Cross-Sectional Study of Catheter-Related Thrombosis in Children Receiving Total Parenteral Nutrition at Home

Andrew M, Marzinotto V, Pencharz P, Zlotkin S, Burrows P, Ingram J, Adams M, Filler R (Hosp for Sick Children, Toronto)
J Pediatr 126:358–363, 1995   8–18

Background.—The management of patients needing prolonged venous access has been revolutionized by cuffed, tunneled silicone rubber central venous lines. However, risks include sepsis and thrombotic occlusion. All children in a home total parenteral nutrition program were examined to establish the frequency of central venous line–related thrombosis.

Methods.—Twelve children receiving home parenteral nutrition were evaluated clinically and by venography. Central venous lines were flushed with saline and 200 U of heparin each day.

Results.—Of 49 central venous lines placed in 12 children, 39 were removed and 27 were blocked. There was clinical evidence of superficial collateral circulation in the upper portion of the chest and upper extremities in 8 patients; 5 of these had symptoms of superior vena cava obstruction. Venography showed bilateral, large-vessel thrombosis in 6 children; unilateral disease was present in 2 patients. Patients with bilateral disease had complete replacement of the upper system large vessels; small collateral vessels drained into the azygous system through the paravertebral vessels. After therapy with warfarin, 0.12 to 0.28 mg/kg/day, 5 children achieved an international normalized ratio of 1.4 to 1.8.

Discussion.—Delays in diagnosing the extent of thrombotic disease after venograms were obtained reflected the misconception that central venous lines are blocked at the tip only. Magnetic resonance imaging has recently been used to diagnose deep vein thrombosis, but there are no comparative data of MRI and venography in children. The risk of symptomatic and asymptomatic central venous line–related deep vein thrombosis is unknown, but it cannot be assumed that either is benign. Complications include pulmonary embolism, chylothorax, superior vena cava syndrome, postphlebitic syndrome, and death. The risk of having central venous line–related deep vein thrombosis that compromises venous access is high for children receiving long-term home parenteral nutrition.

Small Bowel Necrosis Associated With Postoperative Jejunal Tube Feeding

Schunn CDG, Daly JM (Univ of Pennsylvania, Philadelphia)
J Am Coll Surg 180:410–416, 1995   8–19

Background.—Postoperative enteral nutrition via jejunal tube is a widely established method of providing necessary calories and is usually well tolerated. Occasionally, however, nonspecific signs of intestinal disturbance result in a syndrome of abdominal distension, hypotension, and hypovolemic shock that causes extensive small-bowel necrosis. This complication is described in a small number of patients who received jejunal tube feeding.

>   *Case Report 1.*—Man, 38, underwent total gastrectomy for gastric adenocarcinoma. An esophagojejunostomy was created and a 12 F red rubber jejunal feeding tube was inserted. On postoperative day 4 he had hiccoughs and was mildly distended. By day 6 he became hypotensive with a heart rate of 180 and massive abdominal distension. Roentgenographs of the abdomen showed a large collection of mottled-appearing intraluminal intestinal debris in the left side. Abdominal exploration revealed gross distension of the entire small bowel and multiple areas of partial and complete circumferential transmural necrosis in the afferent limb proceeding cephalad to the Hunt-Lawrence pouch, as well as distal to the site of the jejunostomy tube insertion site. Multiple areas of intestinal necrosis required resection resulting in the removal of 130 cm of small bowel. Postoperatively the patient did well and was discharged 11 days later.

Results.—Woman, 61, required an en bloc resection of the distal portion of the stomach and transverse colon. Reconstruction was carried out with an antecolic Roux-en-Y gastrojejunostomy, and a 14 F red rubber feeding tube was placed. Seven days postoperatively the patient had abdominal distension, decreased bowel sounds, and tenderness. Roentgenograms showed dilated distal small bowel and cecum and large amounts of fecal material in the rectosigmoid colon. On postoperative day 9, she became hypotensive, with a white blood cell count of 9,800 cells/mm³ and 64% bands. During surgery, areas of normal bowel wall were found to be interspersed with areas of full-thickness necrosis. The small bowel was markedly distended. A total of 100 cm of small bowel was resected, within which were large amounts of inspissated tube feeding formula. Postoperative recovery was complicated by an intra-abdominal abscess that required prolonged parenteral nutritional support before resolution.

> *Case report 3.*—Woman, 71, underwent a pancreaticoduodenectomy and a segmental transverse colon resection for a carcinoma of the duodenum. A feeding jejunostomy was established by using a 12 F red rubber tube. Two days postoperatively she noted crampy abdominal pain and watery diarrhea, followed by distension. Her temperature and white blood cell count increased in the next 24 hours. At emergency laparotomy, ischemic intestine was found to involve the small bowel beginning at the jejunostomy tube insertion site and continuing for approximately 150 cm distally. The entire right colon was ischemic and partially necrotic. She underwent resection of the necrotic small bowel and right colon with end ileostomy and colonic mucous fistula. Pathology showed mucosal autolysis, edema, and necrosis with numerous fibrin thrombi. The patient died.

Conclusion.—Although cases such as these are rare, they demonstrate that tube feeding should be discontinued immediately and that parenteral nutrition be considered in patients with symptoms of abdominal pain, abdominal distention, increased nasogastric drainage, and signs of intestinal ileus.

Stroke Caused by Inadvertent Intra-Arterial Parenteral Nutrition
Lynch JC, Shehabi Y (Prince Henry Hosp, Sydney, NSW, Australia)
Anaesth Intensive Care 23:358–360, 1995   8–20

Introduction.—Misplacement of central venous catheters is uncommon, but serious consequences can occur if the mistake is unrecognized. The patient reported here experienced a major hemispheric stroke after inadvertent arterial administration of total parenteral nutrition (TPN).

> *Case Report.*—Woman, 65, was scheduled for nutritional support after undergoing palliative esophagectomy and gastric transposition for poorly differentiated squamous cell carcinoma of the esophagus. The patient was malnourished and cachectic preoperatively and had moderately severe chronic airflow limitation. She was successfully extubated the day after the palliative procedure. After a right internal jugular line was placed for TPN, a routine chest radiograph showed the tip of the catheter running centrally with a slight deviation to the left and ending in the region of the superior vena cava. Dark, venous-looking blood had been aspirated at catheter placement. The patient started to receive Synthamin 17 solution in 25% dextrose and maintenance fluids via the

central catheter. Within 30 minutes, complete aphasia and left-sided hemiplegia developed.

The catheter was removed after angiography revealed the puncture site in the right vertebral artery and the catheter tip in the right brachiocephalic artery. A CT scan demonstrated right anterior and middle cerebral artery infarction with minimal reactionary cerebral edema. The patient did not respond to a short course of systemic corticosteroids, a dense left hemiplegia and aphasia persisted, and tracheostomy and jejunostomy tubes were required. She died approximately 4 months later after a chest infection and aspiration.

Discussion.—Although the placement of this catheter for TPN appeared unremarkable, the misplaced line might have been detected by routine use of central venous pressure monitoring with waveform display. The high osmolar content of the TPN probably caused cerebral vasospasm leading to microthrombosis in the distal microcirculation.

Intra-Abdominal Extravasation Complicating Parenteral Nutrition in Infants
Nour S, Puntis JWL, Stringer MD (Leeds Gen Infirmary, England)
Arch Dis Child 72:F207–F208, 1995   8–21

Objective.—Two infants described in this study had intra-abdominal extravasation as a complication of parenteral nutrition delivered via central venous catheters. Although many problems have been reported in association with parenteral nutrition, intra-abdominal extravasation has rarely occurred in infants.

Findings.—The patients were a 30-week gestational age boy weighing 1 kg and a 6-month-old boy with the VATER complex (vertebral defects, imperforate anus, tracheoesophageal fistula with esophageal atresia, radial and renal dysplasia). The neonate required ventilatory support for respiratory distress syndrome and was fed parenterally from day 3 with a standard nutritional regimen. Abdominal distension and bile-stained gastric aspirates developed after a pulmonary hemorrhage. The infant had a tender indurated mass in the right iliac fossa and increasing abdominal distension by day 17. Broad-spectrum antibiotics were given when a provisional diagnosis of necrotizing enterocolitis was made. When the infant continued to deteriorate, a laparotomy was performed. About 100 mL of sterile chylous peritoneal fluid was found, identical in appearance to the parenteral nutrition solution, together with an edematous retroperitoneal mass in the right iliac fossa. The ascites was aspirated, the catheter was removed, and the infant made a rapid recovery.

The 6-month-old infant received parenteral nutrition while undergoing diagnosis and treatment of severe tracheomalacia and gastroesophageal reflux. Abdominal distension and acute respiratory distress developed within 2 days. Abdominal ultrasonography revealed a large amount of peritoneal fluid. The infant recovered after draining the chylous ascites and removing the femoral catheter.

Discussion.—Both infants were receiving parenteral nutrition via lower limb catheters, and the catheter tip in each case was positioned in the lower inferior vena cava. Abdominal distension and respiratory distress developed as the result of intra-abdominal parenteral nutrition extravasation. Drainage and removal of the catheter led to recovery in both cases. This complication can be prevented by placing the tip of the catheter in the midright portion of the atrium.

▶ Complications from both parenteral and enteral nutrition occur, and some of these can be life-threatening. Each of the preceding 6 articles addresses a serious but fortunately rather uncommon complication of nutritional support. A list of complications from both parenteral nutrition and enteral nutrition is shown below (Table 1). Many others have been reported.

W.W. Souba, M.D., Sc.D.

TABLE 1.—Complications

Complications Associated With the Use of Total Parenteral Nutrition	Complications Associated With the Use of Enteral Nutrition
Mechanical	
Pneumothorax, hemothorax	Tube dislodgment
Subclavian artery injury	Nasal erosions
Air embolism	Bowel perforation/obstruction
Catheter embolization	Catheter blockage
Venous thrombosis	Tube misplacement
Metabolic	
Hyperglycemia	Hyperglycemia
Hypoglycemia	Constipation
Electrolyte abnormalities	Electrolyte abnormalities
Fatty liver	Diarrhea/dehydration
Carbon dioxide retention	Liver function abnormalities
Fatty acid deficiency	Azotemia
Trace mineral deficiency	Hypoalbuminemia
Azotemia	Lactose intolerance
Hyperchloremic acidosis	
Bleeding (vitamin K deficiency)	
Septic	
Line sepsis	Wound infection at tube skin site
Infection at catheter entry site	Peritonitis from bowel perforation

Nutrition, Growth Hormone, and Other Anabolic Agents

Anabolic Impact of Cimaterol in Conjunction With Enteral Nutrition Following Burn Trauma

Nelson JL, Chalk CL, Warden GD (Shriner's Burns Institute, Cincinnati, Ohio)
J Trauma 38:237–241, 1995   8–22

Background.—Increased energy expenditure, weight loss, and muscle protein wasting are common manifestations of burn injury. Past studies have shown that β_2-adrenergic agonists have anabolic properties in the presence of increased metabolism. This study investigates the effects of the β_2-agonist cimaterol with enteral nutrition in the burned guinea pig model.

Method.—Sixteen adult guinea pigs with gastrostomies were given a 30% total-body full-thickness flame burn on the back area. They were then randomly divided into 2 groups receiving a daily injection of either saline or cimaterol (0.30 mg/kg). The animals were fed for 14 days. Energy expenditure was measured before burn and on postburn days 3, 6, 9, and 12. On day 14, the soleus, gastrocnemius muscles, and heart were removed and weighed as a measure of muscle catabolism and anabolism. Carcass weight was also evaluated to measure muscle catabolism.

Results.—Although all the animals lost weight after burn trauma, there were no significant differences in overall body weight loss between the animals that received saline and those that received cimaterol. However, examination of the gastrocnemius muscle weight indicated a significant anabolic effect in the animals that received daily cimaterol ($P \leq 0.05$). The mean muscle protein content of the gastrocnemius muscle and the mean carcass weight were significantly higher in the group of animals that received cimaterol than in those that received saline. No significant differences were seen in soleus muscle or heart weights or in resting metabolic rates between the 2 groups.

Conclusion.—Early enteral nutrition and daily administration of the β_2-agonist cimaterol increased muscle anabolism and protein content and did not result in an increase in resting energy expenditure. These results indicate that specific β_2-agonists may be highly beneficial as an adjunct to early enteral nutrition in restoring muscle mass after burn trauma.

▶ Cimaterol is a β_2-adrenergic agonist. Earlier studies showed that β_2-adrenergic agonists can increase muscle mass and protein concentrations in tumor-bearing rodents.[1] A previous study in thermally injured animals demonstrated that another β_2-adrenergic agonist, clenbutarol, increased weight gain, muscle mass, and muscle protein content in animals allowed to eat freely.[2] The study by Nelson et al. evaluated a combination of cimaterol and early aggressive feeding after burn injury. Although benefits from the combination therapy were reported, the use of β_2-adrenergic agonists as anabolic agents in protein catabolic states is not a component of clinical practice.

W.W. Souba, M.D., Sc.D.

References

1. Chance WT, Cao L, Zhang F, et al: Muscle-sparing effect of clenbutarol in tumor-bearing rats maintained on total parenteral nutrition. *Surg Forum* 40:411–413, 1989.
2. Chance WT, Von Allman D, Benson D, et al: Clenbutarol decreases catabolism and increases hypermetabolism in burned rats. *J Trauma* 31:365–370, 1991.

Growth Hormone and Insulinlike Growth Factor I Enhance Host Defense in a Murine Sepsis Model

Inoue T, Saito H, Fukushima R, Inaba T, Lin M-T, Fukatsu K, Muto T (Univ of Tokyo)

Arch Surg 130:1115–1122, 1995   8–23

Introduction.—Growth hormone (GH) stimulates the production of insulin-like growth factor type I (IGF-I) by various tissues. The latter mediates the anabolic effects of GH on protein metabolism. In addition, these hormones—particularly GH—have significant immunoregulatory actions.

Objective.—The effects of exogenous GH and IGF-I on host defenses and survival were examined in a murine model of *Escherichia coli* sepsis.

Methods.—Female BALB/c mice 9 weeks of age received daily subcutaneous injections of 0.48 or 4.8 mg/kg of GH, 2.4 or 24 mg/kg of IGF-I, or normal saline solution for 6 days. The animals were then challenged intraperitoneally with 10^8 colony-forming units of *E. coli*. Cytokine levels were estimated in plasma, peritoneal lavage fluid, and peritoneal exudative cells (PECs) sampled 4 or 6 hours after bacterial challenge.

Findings.—Both doses of GH and the higher dose of IGF-I significantly prolonged survival after bacterial challenge. Both GH and IGF-I significantly increased the number of PECs and lowered counts of viable bacterial in lavage fluid and the liver. Excessive systemic cytokine production was significantly suppressed by both hormones (Table 3). The in vitro production of interleukin-1 by PECs was greater in hormone-treated than

TABLE 3.—Cytokine Levels in Peritoneal Lavage Fluid and Plasma*

Group	TNF, U/mL		IL-1, ×10 pg/mL		IL-6, ×10² pg/mL	
	PLF	Plasma	PLF	Plasma	PLF	Plasma
			0 h			
Control	ND	10.6±1.3	ND	0.71±0.46	ND	0.63±0.19
GH	ND	7.0±1.9	ND	0.05±0.05	ND	0.13±0.09
IGF-I	ND	12.0±2.4	ND	1.53±0.87	ND	0.50±0.19
			4h			
Control	3.1±0.6	81.9±31.3	7.7±0.9	22.9±8.7	153±39	2512±516
GH	3.4±0.7	43.6±10.1	6.4±1.0	5.4±0.9§‖	89±18	673±142‡
IGF-I	3.7±0.6	64.4±28.9	10.4±2.0	24.6±5.3	166±49	1643±421
			6 h			
Control	14.2±1.2	64.1±12.9	25.5±2.6	46.6±11.6	670±143	6407±1090
GH	13.8±1.5	34.7±7.1§	24.1±3.0	20.1±2.5¶	409±73	2154±283†
IGF-I	12.4±1.8	26.0±5.2§	19.1±4.9	27.2±8.6	453±146	2051±745†

* Values are means ± SEM.
† $P < 0.001$ vs. the control group.
‡ $P < 0.01$ vs. the control group.
§ $P < 0.05$ vs. the control group.
‖ $P < 0.05$ vs the IGF-I group.
¶ $P < 0.08$ vs the control group.
Abbreviations: TNF, tumor necrosis factor; *PLF,* peritoneal lavage fluid; *IL-1,* interleukin-1; *ND,* not done; *GH,* growth hormone; *IGF-I,* insulin-like growth factor type I.
(Courtesy of *Archives of Surgery,* Oct 1995, 130:1115–1122, Copyright 1995, American Medical Association.)

control animals 4 and 6 hours after bacterial challenge. Production of interleukin-6 by PECs was greater in GH-treated than control animals 4 hours after challenge.

Conclusion.—Provision of either GH or IGF-I reduces bacterial counts in peritoneal lavage fluid and the liver and prolongs survival in septic mice, as well as modulates cytokine production both locally and systemically.

The Effect of Insulin-Like Growth Factor-1 on Protein Metabolism and Hepatic Response to Endotoxemia in Parenterally Fed Rats
Dickerson RN, Manzo CB, Charland SL, Settle RG, Stein TP, Kuhl DA, Rajter JJ (Univ of Tennessee, Memphis; Philadelphia College of Pharmacy and Science; Philadelphia Veterans Affairs Med Ctr; et al)
J Surg Res 58:260–266, 1995   8–24

Introduction.—Because of the limited success of conventional nutritional support during critical illness, alternative techniques for modulating the metabolic response to critical illness have been sought. Plasma levels of insulin-like growth factor type 1 (IGF-1) are depressed and its response to growth hormone blunted during critical illness. This study examined the adjuvant use of recombinant human IGF-1 (rhIGF-1) with parenteral nutrition (PN) during endotoxemia. The influence of IGF-1 on nitrogen loss and the hepatic response to endotoxemia were examined in parenterally fed rats.

Methods.—Thirty-four male Sprague-Dawley rats underwent IV cannulation, followed by 48 hours of recovery postcannulation and 28 hours of adaptation to continuous isocaloric and isonitrogenous PN. In a random fashion, the animals then received PN only (control), PN plus continuous infusion of *Escherichia coli* 026:B6 lipopolysaccharide (LPS), or PN plus LPS plus rhIGF-1 at 3 mg/kg/day for 48 hours (IGF-1). During the last 10 hours of the study, the animals received [^{15}N]glycine for determination of liver fractional synthetic rate.

Results.—Cumulative nitrogen balance during endotoxemia differed significantly between groups. The control group was in positive balance, whereas the LPS and IGF-1 groups were in negative balance. However, the markedly negative nitrogen balance during endotoxemia was halved by the administration of IGF-1 (Fig 1). Endotoxin infusion significantly increased proteolysis, as evidenced by a 130% increase in the urinary 3-methylhistidine/creatinine ratio above control; however, rhIGF-1 therapy did not significantly reduce the ratio. When compared with control, infusion of endotoxin doubled the liver fractional synthetic rate and reduced the cytochrome P-450 concentration and ethoxycoumarin O-deethylase activity by 60% to 80%. Treatment with rhIGF-1 did not significantly alter these markers of hepatic function during endotoxemia.

Conclusions.—Exogenous administration of rhIGF-1 significantly improves nitrogen balance during endotoxemia without compromising the

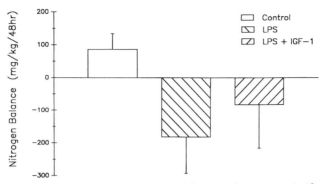

FIGURE 1.—Forty-eight-hour cumulative nitrogen balance. Each group was significantly different from each other. *Abbreviations: LPS,* lipopolysaccharide; *IGF-1,* insulin-like growth factor type 1. (Courtesy of Dickerson RN, Manzo CB, Charland SL, et al: The effect of insulin-like growth factor-1 on protein metabolism and hepatic response to endotoxemia in parenterally fed rats. *J Surg Res* 58:260–266, 1995.)

hepatic response. The adjuvant use of rhIGF-1 appears to be a promising avenue for pharmacologic modulation of the metabolic response to critical illness.

Effects of Insulin-Like Growth Factor-I and Growth Hormone on the Net Flux of Amino Acids Across the Hind Limbs in the Surgically Traumatized Pig

Malmlöf K, Cortova Z, Saxerholt H, Karlsson E, Arrhenius-Nyberg V, Skottner A (Pharmacia, Kabi Peptide Hormones, Stockholm)
Clin Sci 88:285–292, 1995   8–25

Introduction.—Of the changes in protein, carbohydrate, and fat metabolism that occur during critical illnesses, the release of large amounts of amino acid from the periphery is the most prominent. This amino acid release is thought to be an adaptive response to preserve immune function and glucose homeostasis. However, this catabolic action can have a deleterious or fatal outcome. Growth hormone (GH) has shown some promise in improving various metabolic indices during catabolic states. The effect of GH and insulin-like growth factor type I (IGF-I), a mediator of GH effects, on peripheral amino acid balance was evaluated in the presence of postsurgical trauma.

Methods.—After surgery, 18 female pigs were given total parenteral nutrition for 2 days. In addition to parenteral nutrition, 6 animals received an infusion of recombinant human IGF-I (rhIGF-I), 6 received recombinant human GH (rhGH), and 6 received vehicle only (controls). Plasma concentrations of free amino acids, urea, and hormones (cortisol, human GH, IGF-I, and insulin) were measured for each postoperative day (POD1 and POD2). The mean flux of amino acids from the hind limb was calculated.

Results.—On POD1 and POD2, plasma values of IGF-I were significantly higher in animals receiving rhIGF-1 than in the other 2 groups. Circulating insulin levels were significantly decreased with infusions of rhIGF-I but not with rhGH as compared with controls. Plasma values of GH were significantly higher in animals receiving rhGH infusion, but no GH was detected in the other 2 groups. Cortisol levels decreased on POD2 in all groups, but not significantly. Circulating levels of total essential, nonessential, and branched-chain amino acids were significantly lower with rhIGF-I than with rhGH. Urea concentrations were similar in all groups on POD1 and were significantly decreased on POD2 with rhGH as compared with controls. The influence of rhIGF-I and rhGH on hind limb net total amino acid balance was similar on POD1. The hind limb net total amino acid balance was −44.2, 69.5, and 100.9 µmol/min for controls, rhIGF-I, and rhGH, respectively (Fig 4). The values for rhIGF-I and rhGH were significantly greater than for controls, with the value for rhGH significantly different from zero. On POD2, no significant differences were found between the 3 groups. For net balance of nonessential amino acids on POD1, both treatment groups were significantly greater than controls, but not significantly greater than zero. No differences were found on POD2. The negative net balance of alanine was decreased significantly with both rhIGF-I and rhGH as compared with controls on POD1 but not on POD2. The net balance of glutamine was significantly increased with rhGH on POD2.

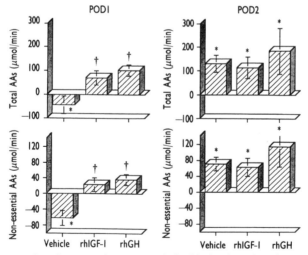

FIGURE 4.—Net flux of amino acids (*AAs*) over the hind limbs of pigs that after surgery were given IV infusions of total parenteral nutrition together with either vehicle, recombinant human insulin-like growth factor type I (*rhIGF-I*), or recombinant human growth factor (*rhGF*) for 10 hours during 2 successive days. Data represent means of 6 observations with their unpooled SEM. Values with no superscript (*, +) in common differ significantly ($P < 0.05$). *Abbreviation: POD,* postoperative day. (Courtesy of Malmlöf K, Cortova Z, Saxerholt H, et al: Effects of insulin-like growth factor-I and growth hormone on the net flux of amino acids across the hind limbs in the surgically traumatized pig. *Clin Sci* 88:285–292, 1995.)

Conclusion.—The efficacy of parenteral nutrition in postsurgical trauma was improved with both rhIGF-I and rhGH. The net uptake of most amino acids into skeletal muscle was increased, and the net efflux of nitrogen carriers such as alanine was decreased.

Insulin-Like Growth Factor–I and Insulin Reduce Leucine Flux and Oxidation in Conscious Tumor Necrosis Factor–Infused Dogs
Sajurai Y, Zhang XJ, Wolfe RR (Univ of Texas, Galveston)
Surgery 117:305–313, 1995   8–26

Introduction.—The anabolic effects observed with growth hormone are thought to be mediated by insulin-like growth factor type I (IGF-I). Plasma IGF-I serum concentrations have been shown to be increased by growth hormone. In comparison to insulin, IGF-I has been reported to have both similar and different metabolic effects. Tumor necrosis factor (TNF) has catabolic effects and is released during critical illnesses. The ability of IGF-I and insulin to prevent the catabolic effects of TNF was assessed.

Methods.—Mongrel dogs were surgically prepared and a central venous catheter inserted. Tracer infusions were begun and continued at a constant rate during the 6-hour study. Tracer infusions were administered alone for the first 2 hours (period 1); blood and expired breath samples were obtained and used as basal values. Infusion of TNF was begun after 2 hours of tracer infusion and continued for 4 hours. After 2 hours of TNF infusion (period 2), an infusion of either IGF-I or insulin was begun and continued for 2 hours with concurrent TNF infusion (period 3). A control group of animals received only saline solution along with the tracer infusion; another group received only TNF in addition to the tracer infusion. Blood and expired breath samples were collected at regular intervals. Plasma glucose, lactate, and free fatty acid (FFA) concentrations were determined. Glucose kinetics, nonoxidative leucine disappearance (NOLD), and net protein breakdown were calculated.

Results.—Infusion of TNF alone resulted in a significant decrease in plasma FFA concentrations. No further reduction in FFA concentrations occurred with the addition of IGF-I, but FFA concentrations decreased further with the addition of insulin. A significant increase in glucose production and clearance was found with TNF infusion. The addition of IGF-I or insulin increased glucose uptake but did not significantly affect plasma glucose concentrations. Insulin infusion suppressed endogenous glucose production. Later in the study period, however, IGF-I also resulted in suppression of endogenous glucose production. Plasma lactate concentrations were increased by TNF alone and by the addition of IGF-I and insulin. Whole-body protein synthesis, as indicated by NOLD, was decreased significantly by TNF, but no effect was seen with IGF-I or insulin. Tumor necrosis factor significantly impaired whole-body protein synthesis, although whole-body protein breakdown was not significantly affected. Net protein breakdown (the net balance between protein synthesis and

TABLE 4.—Indexes of Net Protein Breakdown

	TNF alone (n = 5)	Group TNF + IGF-I (n = 5)	TNF + insulin
Net protein breakdown* mg · kg⁻¹ · min⁻¹			
Period 1 (basal)	1.97 ± 0.26	1.74 ± 0.19	2.21 ± 0.25
Period 2 (210–240 min)	2.73 ± 0.24†	2.53 ± 0.17†	3.53 ± 0.26†
Period 3 (330–360 min)	2.94 ± 0.28†	1.58 ± 0.16‡	1.54 ± 0.19†‡
Ra urea (μmol · kg⁻¹ · min⁻¹)			
Period 1 (basal)	7.59 ± 0.59	7.03 ± 1.09	7.05 ± 0.74
Period 2 (210–240 min)	8.32 ± 0.64	7.59 ± 0.89	7.66 ± 0.43
Period 3 (330–360 min)	10.84 ± 0.92†	7.68 ± 0.84	8.22 ± 0.70

Note: All values presented are means ± SEM.
* Net protein breakdown was extrapolated from leucine data with the assumption that 590 μmol leucine exists in 1 g of protein (Waterlow JC, Garlick RJ, Millward DJ: *Protein Turnover in Mammalian Tissues and in the Whole Body.* Amsterdam, North-Holland, 1978, pp 225–300).
† Significantly different from the basal (period 1) value (P < 0.05).
‡ Significantly different from the value in period 2 (P < 0.05).
Abbreviations: TNF, tumor necrosis factor; *IGF-I,* insulin-like growth factor type I.
(Courtesy of Sajurai Y, Zhang XJ, Wolfe RR: Insulin-like growth factor–I and insulin reduce leucine flux and oxidation in conscious tumor necrosis factor–infused dogs. *Surgery* 117:305–313, 1995.)

breakdown) changed significantly from 1.97 mg/kg/min in the basal state to 2.94 mg/kg/min during TNF infusion (Table 4). The addition of IGF-I and insulin both resulted in significant improvements in net protein breakdown. Urea production was also increased with TNF infusion alone and was significantly different from basal values during period 3. Although the addition of IGF-I and insulin both resulted in further increases in urea production from basal values, these increases were not as pronounced as the increases seen with TNF alone and were not significantly different from basal values.

Conclusion.—Net protein balance was impaired by TNF infusion, primarily through inhibition of protein synthesis; net protein breakdown was not affected. The addition of IGF-I and insulin both improved net protein balance through inhibition of protein breakdown; however, protein synthesis was not improved. The glucose response to TNF was also modified by the addition of IGF-I and insulin.

Simultaneous Treatment With IGF-I and GH Additively Increases Anabolism in Parenterally Fed Rats

Lo H-C, Hinton PS, Peterson CA, Ney DM (Univ of Wisconsin, Madison)
Am J Physiol 269:E368–E376, 1995   8–27

Introduction.—The anabolic response to total parenteral nutrition (TPN) in patients with malnutrition and tissue wasting may be enhanced by treatment with both insulin-like growth factor type I (IGF-I) and growth hormone (GH). In combination, these hormones appear to have complementary anabolic and metabolic effects. An animal model of surgical stress and controlled hypocaloric infusion of TPN solution was used

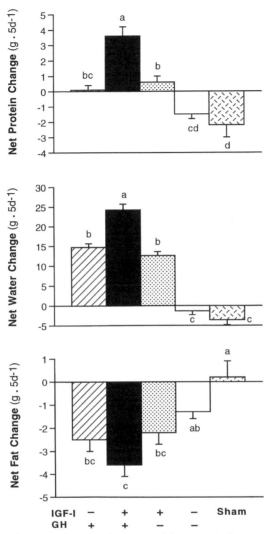

FIGURE 6.—Net changes in carcass protein, water, and fat content in sham rats and rats maintained with total parenteral nutrition and given 800 µg/day recombinant human insulin growth factor type I (*IGF-I*) and/or recombinant human growth hormone (*GH*) for 5 days after surgical stress. Values are means ± SE, n = 8–10; means with different superscripts are significantly different ($P < 0.05$). (Courtesy of Lo H-C, Hinton PS, Peterson CA, et al: Simultaneous treatment with IGF-I and GH additively increases anabolism in parenterally fed rats. *Am J Physiol* 269:E368–E376, 1995.)

to evaluate the relative anabolic and metabolic effects associated with the administration of IGF-I and GH and their combination during TPN.

Methods.—Male Sprague-Dawley rats were used in experiments to evaluate the effects of TPN coinfused with recombinant human IGF-I (rhIGF-I) or with rhGH and during simultaneous treatment with rhIGF-I and rhGH. The animals were subjected to surgical stress and maintained with TPN. The dosage for each hormone was 800 µg/day; rhGH was administered twice a day as a subcutaneous injection. Growth factors were given for 5 days after surgery, during which time TPN was the sole source of nutrition.

Results.—Animals treated with rhIGF-I or rhGH had serum concentrations of IGF-I that were about 2-fold greater than those of animals orally fed and given a sham saline infusion or given TPN without growth factors. Significantly greater concentrations of total and free IGF-I were found in animals treated simultaneously with the 2 growth factors than in those receiving a single growth factor. Weight gain induced by the combination of growth factors was double that shown by IGF-I or GH alone. Growth hormone selectively increased gastrocnemius muscle mass, whereas IGF-I increased heart, kidney, thymus, spleen, and small intestine mass. The GH-induced increase in serum insulin was reversed when IGF-I was given with GH. Carcass protein and water were increased and fat decreased by treatment with IGF-I and/or GH (Fig 6).

Conclusion.—In this animal model of surgical stress, simultaneous treatment with IGF-I and GH was confirmed to be more anabolic than treatment with either hormone alone. Administration of these growth factors during TPN produced an additive whole-body growth response that may have clinical applications in patients with tissue wasting.

Effect of Growth Hormone and Protein Intake on Tumor Growth and Host Cachexia

Bartlett DL, Stein TP, Torosian MH (Univ of Pennsylvania, Philadelphia; New Jersey Univ of Medicine and Dentistry, Camden)
Surgery 117:260–267, 1995   8–28

Introduction.—Cancer cachexia occurs as a result of host tissue catabolization to supply tumors with substrates for energy and protein synthesis. The use of nutritional support in cancer patients is controversial. Parenteral and enteral nutrition is thought to selectively stimulate tumor growth over host tissue growth without providing any beneficial effects to the patient. Growth hormone has been shown to improve some nutritional parameters and improve wound healing in some catabolic states and has not been shown to promote tumor growth in models. The effect of exogenous growth hormone in rats with metastatic adenocarcinoma was assessed.

Methods.—Four groups of Lewis rats that had been inoculated 10 days previously with MAC-33 cells were divided into 4 groups. Groups I and III were control groups and received either a protein-fed or a protein-depleted diet and placebo saline injected intraperitoneally daily. Groups II and IV received either a protein-fed or a protein-depleted diet and 1 IU/kg of growth hormone injected intraperitoneally daily. Body weight and tumor

TABLE 1.—Host and Tumor Parameters

Group	Carcass wt (g)	Tumor wt (g)	Tumor/Carcass Ratio	No. of Metastases
PD	110 ± 2.2^c	$34 \pm 2.8^{a,\ c}$	0.30 ± 0.03^a	3.1 ± 1.9^c
PD + GH	110 ± 2.2^d	$26 \pm 2.5^{a,\ d}$	0.23 ± 0.02^a	5.6 ± 2.0^d
RD	$171 \pm 2.8^{b,\ c}$	54 ± 6.6^c	0.30 ± 0.04^b	20.9 ± 10.8^c
RD +GH	$189 \pm 4.7^{b,\ d}$	47 ± 5.7^d	0.24 ± 0.03^b	11.4 ± 2.2^d

Note: For *a* vs. *a*, *b* vs. *b*, *c* vs. *c*, and *d* vs. *d*, $P < 0.05$.
Abbreviations: PD, protein-deprived diet; GH, growth hormone; RD, regular diet.
(Courtesy of Bartlett DL, Stein TP, Torosian MH: Effect of growth hormone and protein intake on tumor growth and host cachexia. *Surgery* 117:260–267, 1995.)

volume measurement were taken twice weekly and DNA, RNA, and protein content determined for tumor, liver, and muscle tissue. Amino acid analyses were also performed.

Results.—Significantly lower final carcass weights were found in rats fed protein-depleted diets with or without growth hormone as compared with all protein-fed rats. Administration of growth hormone with a protein diet resulted in significant increases in weight when compared with protein-diet alone, protein-depleted diet, or protein-depleted diet plus growth hormone (Table 1). Final tumor weight was significantly lower in rats fed protein-depleted diets with or without growth hormone than in all protein-fed rats. Rats fed protein-depleted diets with growth hormone had significantly lower tumor weight than did rats fed protein-depleted diets without growth hormone. No significant difference in tumor weight was found between protein-fed rats with or without growth hormone. The tumor/carcass ratio was significantly lower in both protein-fed and protein-depleted rats given growth hormone than in controls. No difference in tumor/carcass ratio was found between the 2 control groups. A protein-depleted diet resulted in significantly fewer metastases as compared with protein diets. Protein depletion also resulted in significantly decreased tumor and liver weight and decreased tumor, muscle, and liver DNA, RNA, and protein content. Growth hormone administration with protein-depleted diets showed significant increases in muscle protein content and decreases in tumor weight and in RNA and protein content. Threonine and tyrosine were significantly decreased in protein-depleted rats as compared with protein-fed rats. Growth hormone had no effect on amino acid content in protein-fed rats and resulted in decreases in glycine and histidine levels in protein-depleted rats.

Conclusion.—The effect of growth hormone differed between protein-depleted and protein-fed rats. Tumor growth and protein content were inhibited in protein-depleted rats given growth hormone, whereas little effect was seen on host muscle. Administration of growth hormone to protein-fed animals improved muscle weight and protein content, with little effect on the tumor. Inhibition of tumor growth and nutritional support of the host may be possible with depletion of specific amino acids from the diet and growth hormone supplementation.

▶ Growth hormone is a 191–amino acid peptide that exerts its anabolic effects via the production of IGF-1. Recombinant human growth hormone as an adjunct to nutritional support has been shown to improve donor site healing in burned children,[1] enhance intestinal amino acid uptake,[2] and improve nitrogen retention in patients with end-stage renal disease,[3] in patients with chronic obstructive lung disease,[4] in postoperative patients,[5] and in critically ill patients.[6] It remains unestablished whether these biochemical changes are associated with an improvement in outcome. Byrne et al.[7] demonstrated that the requirement for parenteral nutrition could be reduced in TPN-dependent short-gut patients by providing a nutritional regimen consisting of oral and IV glutamine, growth hormone, and a modified high-carbohydrate, low-fat diet. There was a marked improvement in the absorption of nutrients and a decrease in stool output with combination therapy. The decrease in TPN requirements resulted in considerable cost savings. In most patients who underwent successful gut rehabilitation, discontinuation of the growth hormone after 4 weeks of therapy did not increase TPN requirements. Growth hormone is associated with few side effects (hyperglycemia is one) and is likely to be used in clinical medicine as an anabolic agent in the not too distant future.

W.W. Souba, M.D., Sc.D.

References

1. Herndon DN, Barrow RE, Kunkel KR, et al: Effects of recombinant growth hormone on donor-site healing in severely burned children. *Ann Surg* 212:424–431, 1990.
2. Inoue Y, Copeland EM, Souba WW: Growth hormone enhances amino acid transport by the human small intestine. *Ann Surg* 219:715–724, 1994.
3. Ziegler TR, Lazarus JM, Young LS, et al: Effects of recombinant human growth hormone in adults receiving maintenance hemodialysis. *J Am Soc Nephrol* 2:1130–1135, 1991.
4. Suchner U, Rothkop MM, Stanislaus G, et al: Growth hormone and pulmonary disease. Metabolic effects in patients receiving parenteral nutrition. *Arch Intern Med* 150:1225–1230, 1990.
5. Vara-Thorbeck R, Guerrero JA, Rosel J, et al: Exogenous growth hormone effects on the catabolic response to a surgically produced acute stress and on postoperative immune function. *World J Surg* 17:530–538, 1993.
6. Voerman HJ, Van Schijndel RJ, Groeneveld AJ, et al: Effects of recombinant human growth hormone in patients with severe sepsis. *Ann Surg* 216:648–655, 1992.
7. Byrne TA, Persinger RL, Young LS, et al: A new treatment for patients with short-bowel syndrome. *Ann Surg* 222:243–255, 1995.

Clinical Aspects of Nutrition Support

Management of Premature Infants With Extensive Bowel Resection With High Volume Enteral Infusates

Alkalay AL, Fleisher DR, Pomerance JJ, Rosenthal P (Univ of California, Los Angeles)
Isr J Med Sci 31:298–302, 1995   8–29

Background.—The major cause of mortality among infants with short-bowel syndrome is end-stage liver disease caused by long-term parenteral nutrition. A feeding regimen of high-volume enteral infusates was used to avoid long-term parenteral nutrition in infants. This feeding regimen is described and discussed as an alternative to long-term parenteral nutrition.

Methods.—Three premature infants with extensive bowel resection were fed a high-volume enteral infusate regimen. An elemental hypo-osmolar gastric infusate was begun after surgery, and then the infants were weaned from parenteral nutrition and maintained on high-volume enteral infusate feeding. Instead of using the volume of ileostomy output or the presence of reducing substances as guides for adjusting enteral intake, a large ileostomy output was tolerated and focus was placed on the hydration, serum electrolytes, and acid-base status of the patients.

Results.—During feeding with high-volume enteral infusates, patients sustained weight gain (Fig 1); mean (± SD) enteral intakes were 373 ± 67, 689 ± 132, and 415 ± 108 mL/kg/day; the osmolarity of the enteral infusates was 250 ± 25, 225 ± 40, and 228 ± 27 mOsm/L; caloric intakes were 163 ± 29, 258 ± 54, and 153 ± 44 kcal/kg/day; and ileostomy outputs were 113 ± 47, 228 ± 59, and 175 ± 69 mL/kg/day. Gut adaptation lasted 122, 141, and 205 days for the 3 infants. At the age of 8 months, 78

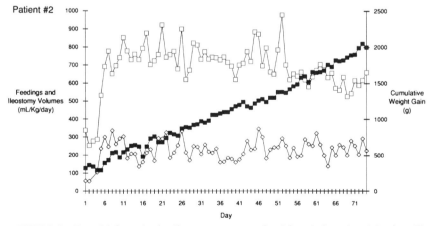

FIGURE 1.—Enteral infusate intake, ileostomy output, and weight gain in patient 2 in phase III. (Courtesy of Alkalay AL, Fleisher DR, Pomerance JJ, et al: Management of premature infants with extensive bowel resection with high volume enteral infusates. *Isr J Med Sci* 31:298–302, 1995.)

months, and 36 months, reanastomoses of the intestines were performed. At 18 months, 108 months, and 58 months, the infants' weights were in the 50th, 20th, and 5th percentiles. There were no cases of cirrhosis.

Conclusions.—High-volume enteral infusate feeding should only be used in carefully selected situations. This feeding method may help achieve gut adaptation in infants with extensive bowel resection. Patients' hydration and homeostasis must be carefully monitored because the gut is pushed to its maximum absorptive capacities and has large ileostomy losses. High-volume enteral infusate feeding may be an alternative for patients with extensive bowel resection who require parenteral nutrition for more than 4 months; for these patients, the risks and benefits should be calculated on a case-by-case basis.

▶ High-volume enteral feedings in these 3 premature infants with massive small-bowel resection was associated with significant weight gain despite high-output ileostomies (~200 mL/day). All patients developed cholestatic liver disease. I was surprised that fluid and electrolyte problems were not more severe than reported.

W.W. Souba, M.D., Sc.D.

Therapeutic Use of Albumin
de Gaudio AR (Inst of Anesthesiology, Firenze, Italy; Univ of Florence, Firenze, Italy)
Int J Artif Organs 18:216–224, 1995   8–30

Introduction.—The clinical use of albumin as a plasma extender, a supplement of total parenteral nutrition, and a pharmacologic substance is controversial. Common errors include administering albumin to patients with hypoalbuminemia and never administering albumin to patients regardless of their circulating protein status. Experimental and clinical data addressing the use of albumin were collected, and the therapeutic use of albumin is reviewed.

Findings.—Exogenous albumin in not considered an ideal colloid. The effects of albumin on plasma volume expansion are somewhat unpredictable; this is especially true in pathologic states with leaky capillary membranes. There is no benefit from albumin on many types of tissue edema. Albumin supplementation has no effect on outcome.

Conclusions.—Albumin may have unique properties that make it useful, but more research is needed to confirm this. Because of its high cost and lack of specific benefits, routine use of albumin is currently not supported. Edema physiology and albumin as a volume plasma expander, a supplement of total parenteral nutrition, and a substance with pharmacologic properties are also discussed.

▶ This article is a good review of the therapeutic indications for albumin supplementation. I agree with the author's conclusions that there is no clear-cut benefit of exogenous albumin on tissue edema and that the routine use of albumin as a volume expander is not justified.

W.W. Souba, M.D., Sc.D.

Evaluation of Early Enteral Feeding in Children Less than 3 Years Old With Smaller Burns (8–25 Per Cent TBSA)
Trocki O, Michelini JA, Robbins St, Eichelberger MR (Children's Natl Med Ctr, Washington, DC)
Burns 21:17–23, 1995   8–31

Background.—The nutritional management of children younger than 3 years with burn injury is complicated by many factors, including nutritional demands for rapid growth, the immaturity of the gastrointestinal tract, small gastric volume, and limited body stores of protein and other nutrients. There is very little information available about the nutritional management of these children. Although early enteral feeding has been proved safe and effective in adults, this has not been proved in very young children. The safety and efficacy of early enteral nasogastric feeding of high protein content in very young children with burn injury were evaluated.

Methods.—In 10 children younger than 3 years with burns covering 8% to 25% total body surface area, enteral tube feeding was started when the patient was stabilized. Tube feeding and oral intake were recorded, and resting energy expenditure was measured weekly. Tolerance to nasogastric feeding was monitored.

Results.—The patients tolerated high protein intake without harmful effects on liver and renal function. The incidence of gastrointestinal complications related to feeding was low. The children required 2 weeks of supplemental nasogastric feeding, which provided two thirds of the total energy intake and three fourths of the protein intake. The mean measured resting metabolic expenditure was 1.3 times the predicted resting metabolic expenditure despite the children's smaller burns. A mean energy intake of 92% of recommended daily allowances for energy, or 1.7 times predicted resting metabolic expenditure, maintained body weight. Mean protein intake was 4.3 g/kg/day with a nonprotein-calorie ratio of 114:1. Plasma concentrations of prealbumin, albumin, and transferrin were low the first week after burn injury; the high protein intake raised these visceral proteins to the normal range.

Discussion.—Aggressive, early postburn nasogastric feeding is safe and effective in these patients. Recommended daily allowance requirements for energy are adequate for supporting these children, although 3 times the amount of protein may be necessary to support visceral protein synthesis. This high level of protein had no short-term harmful effects on liver and renal function.

▶ Aggressive early enteral nutrition in the burned patient is now common practice in most burn units. Alexander et al.[1] studied 18 children with large burns who were randomized to a normal diet (controls) or a diet supplemented with milk whey protein. The study group was small and received more nutrients intraluminally and fewer nutrients IV than did the control group, but children receiving the high nitrogen diet displayed improved hepatic synthetic function, fewer bacteremic days, and improved survival. Burn victims require at least twice the amount of protein in the diet to approach nitrogen equilibrium as do normal individuals,[2] and some centers provide their burn patients considerably more.

W.W. Souba, M.D., Sc.D.

References

1. Alexander JW, MacMillan BG, Stinnett JD, et al: Beneficial effects of aggressive protein feeding in severely burned children. *Ann Surg* 192:505–517, 1980.
2. Cunningham JJ, Lydon MK, Russell WE: Calorie and protein provision for recovery from severe burns in infants and young children. *Am J Clin Nutr* 51:553–557, 1990.

Total Energy Expenditure During Total Parenteral Nutrition: Ambulatory Patients at Home Versus Patients With Sepsis in Surgical Intensive Care
Koea JB, Wolfe RR, Shaw JHF (Auckland Hosp, New Zealand; Shriners Burns Inst, Galveston, Tex; Univ of Tex, Galveston)
Surgery 118:54–62, 1995   8–32

Objective.—If patients receiving total parenteral nutrition (TPN) are not to be underfed or overfed, the calories provided should equal the total energy expenditure (TEE) of the patient. In the past, TEE has been estimated because there was no way to measure it. The doubly labeled water method allows the calculation of TEE from the differential elimination rates of isotopic hydrogen and oxygen. Because these elimination rates are proportional to total-body carbon dioxide, TEE can be calculated if the respiratory quotient (RQ) is known. The results of direct measurement of TEE with the doubly labeled water method are presented.

Methods.—Isotopes were administered IV to 4 patients with sepsis aged 27 to 68 who were receiving TPN and to 4 patients with chronic intestinal failure aged 47 to 56 who were receiving home parenteral nutrition (HPN). Total-body water and TEE were calculated and compared with resting energy expenditure (REE).

Results.—Resting energy expenditure calculated by the Harris-Benedict equation (REE HB) in patients with sepsis was significantly lower than either REE calculated by indirect calorimetry (REE CAL) or TEE determined by the doubly labeled water method. In HPN patients there was no significant difference between REE HB and REE CAL, but both were significantly lower than TEE (Fig 2).

ENERGY EXPENDITURE
(K cal / Kg / Day-1)

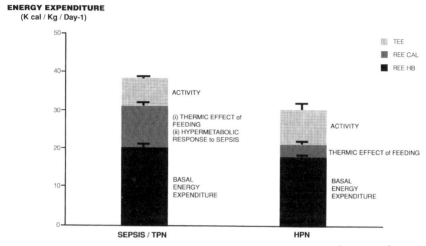

FIGURE 2.—Components of total energy expenditure *(TEE)* in patients with sepsis and patients receiving home parenteral nutrition. *Abbreviations: REE CAL,* resting energy expenditure calculated by indirect calorimetry; *REE HB,* REE calculated by the Harris-Benedict equation. (Courtesy of Koea JB, Wolfe RR, Shaw JHF: Total energy expenditure during total parenteral nutrition: Ambulatory patients at home versus patients with sepsis in surgical intensive care. *Surgery* 118:54–62, 1995.)

Conclusion.—In patients with sepsis, TEE is approximately 1.4 times REE CAL. Sepsis appears to increase REE by 20%, and rehabilitation activity requirements add an additional 30%. In patients with HPN, REE HB and REE CAL are within 10%.

Prognosis of Patients With Nonmalignant Chronic Intestinal Failure Receiving Long-Term Home Parenteral Nutrition

Messing B, Lémann M, Landais P, Gouttelbeel MC, Gérard-Boncompain M, Saudin F, Vangossum A, Beau P, Guédon C, Barnoud D, Beliah M, Joyeux H, Bouletreau P, Robert D, Matuchansky C, Leverve X, Lereebous E, Carpentier Y, Rambaud JC (Hôpital Saint-Lazare, Paris; Hôpital Necker, Paris; Hôpital Paul Lamarque, Montpellier, France; et al)
Gastroenterology 108:1005–1010, 1995   8–33

Introduction.—Previous studies have suggested that long-term survival is good with home parenteral nutrition (HPN) for patients with nonmalignant intestinal failure. However, their ultimate survival and the associated prognostic factors other than primary disease diagnosis are unclear. The survival and prognostic factors of 217 adult patients receiving HPN for chronic intestinal failure were studied.

Methods.—The patients were enrolled in 9 European HPN programs from 1980 through 1989. All had chronic intestinal failure that was not caused by either cancer or AIDS. Their mean age was 47 years, and the overall median duration of HPN was 19 months. Updated data for 1991 were available for all patients. Multivariate analysis was performed to assess prognostic factors for survival.

Results.—There were 73 deaths during the study, 11% of which were related to complications of HPN. The probability of survival was 91% at 1 year, 70% at 3 years, and 62% at 5 years. The independent variables associated with a reduced risk of death were patient age less than 40 years, starting HPN after 1987, and absence of chronic intestinal obstruction. For patients less than 60 years old who were enrolled after 1983—who might be considered candidates for small-bowel transplantation—the 2-year survival rate was 90%.

Conclusions.—When conducted under the control of specialized centers, HPN has good long-term efficacy and safety for patients with non-malignant chronic intestinal failure. The prognosis with HPN compares favorably with recently reported survival results of small-bowel transplantation. At present, it may be best to consider small-bowel transplantation for only those HPN patients at increased risk of mortality caused by HPN complications, such as extensive thrombosis of the superior vena cava, severe metabolic disturbances, or advanced liver disease.

▶ Nitrogen and calorie requirements in patients maintained on TPN are determined primarily by the patients' body surface area and energy expenditure. These determinations are important to avoid the consequences of overfeeding. Unless use of the gut is contraindicated (bowel obstruction, severe diarrhea, high-output enterocutaneous fistula, very low birth weight infant, severe acute pancreatitis, severe enteritis, inadequate luminal surface area, feeding intolerance), enteral nutrition is always the initial route of choice for nutrient administration.[1] Unfortunately, enteral nutrition is not used in all eligible patients with a functional gut.

There is little doubt that parenteral nutrition support is indicated when adequate food intake is not possible for long periods of time. In certain patients with specific intestinal disorders,[2] the long-term provision of parenteral nutrients to prevent death from starvation is lifesaving and is therefore justified. Such therapy is expensive and can be associated with complication such as bone demineralization, electrolyte disturbances, and catheter sepsis.

W.W. Souba, M.D., Sc.D.

References

1. Moore FA, Feliciano DV, Andrassy RJ, et al: Early enteral feeding, compared with parenteral, reduces postoperative septic complications. *Ann Surg* 216:172–183, 1992.
2. Gouttelbeel MC, Saint-Aubert B, Astre C, et al: Total parenteral nutrition needs in different types of short bowel syndrome. *Dig Dis Sci* 31:718–723, 1986.

Insertion of a Transpyloric Feeding Tube During Laparotomy in the Critically Injured: Rationale and Plea for Routine Use
Boulanger BR, Brennemann FD, Rizoli SB, Nayman R (Univ of Toronto)
Injury 26:177–180, 1995   8–34

Background.—Clinical and experimental evidence favors early enteral feeding in critically injured patients. The insertion of a transpyloric feeding tube has several advantages over other techniques of enteral access and nutritional support. Not only is the feeding tube easy to place intraoperatively, it is also safe, reliable, and cost-effective. The technique and its indications and contraindications are described.

> *Technique.*—Insertion of the nasojejunal (NJ) feeding tube is done after a laparotomy for trauma is completed and the abdomen is ready to be closed. The enteral feeding tube used is a single-lumen, radiopaque, polyurethane tube with a tungsten-weighted tip. The wire within the tube is left in place during insertion. After removing the standard nasogastric tube, the anesthesiologist passes the feeding tube through the nose into the stomach. The surgeon then guides the tip through the pylorus into the duodenum. The feeding tube can often be advanced beyond the ligament of Treitz into the proximal portion of the jejunum. With this step accomplished, the surgeon holds the NJ tube in place as the anesthesiologist slowly and carefully removes the guide wire. Once the tube is in position, it is taped securely to the nose, and a standard sump gastric tube is reinserted via the nose or mouth by the anesthesiologist. While the patient is in the critical care unit, the feeding tube should be intermittently flushed with water to preserve patency until continuous enteral feeding is begun. Plain radiographs are not needed to check feeding tube position in the critical care unit. Feeding may be started almost immediately and increased to meet nutritional requirements. Nasojejunal feeding is continued until the patient is able to tolerate oral feeding. Additionally, the NJ tube can be left in place while oral feeding trials are undertaken.

Indications and Contraindications.—Indications for intraoperative insertion of the NJ feeding tube include anticipated extended endotracheal intubation, a need for multiple delayed operations, patients with head injuries precluding safe oral or gastric feeding, and those with premorbid gastric motility disorders. Absolute contraindications include patients with basal skull fractures and hemodynamic or metabolic instability at the conclusion of laparotomy, whereas relative contraindications include patients with facial fractures or abnormal duodenal anatomy. Enteral feeding may also be contraindicated in patients with jejunal or ileal injuries and pancreatic damage.

Conclusions.—Although enteral feeding delivered via a transpyloric tube is well tolerated, even in patients with intra-abdominal and retroperitoneal injuries, this technique is currently underused. Routine use of this simple, safe, and effective procedure should be considered during trauma laparotomies.

Fluoroscopically Guided Nasoenteric Feeding Tube Placement Versus Bedside Placement
Hillard AE, Waddell JJ, Metzler MH, McAlpin D (Univ of Missouri, Columbia)
South Med J 88:425–428, 1995   8–35

Background.—The establishment of adequate nutritional status is an important aspect of therapy in debilitated chronically ill patients. This study compares the benefits, disadvantages, and cost of different methods of enteral feeding tube placement, both fluoroscopic and bedside placement.

Method.—A 4-year retrospective study of 368 nasoenteric feeding tube placements was carried out. Radiology department computer and chart reviews were made to identify patients, to determine the time taken to successfully place the tube, and to assess when adequate nutritional intake was obtained through the enteric feeding tube. Relative costs, time to placement, repeat rate, and complications were evaluated.

Results.—During the 4-year study period, 126 fluoroscopic placements and 242 bedside placements were made. Ninety-one percent of the fluoroscopic procedures were successful, whereas only 17% of the bedside placements were initially successful. The average time between initial placement and the initiation of feeding was 28.1 hours for the bedside method and 7.5 hours for fluoroscopy. Of the patients who had bedside placement, 114 had repeated placement because of patients or staff pulling out feeding tubes, whereas only 40 of the patients who had initially successful fluoroscopic placement required repeat placement. Fluoroscopic placement resulted in fewer complications than did bedside placement and was found to be less expensive by $139.97.

Conclusion.—The results of this study show that in patients who require immediate feeding and who have a high risk of aspiration, fluoroscopically placed feeding tubes are associated with fewer complications, allow earlier feeding, and are more cost-effective than bedside placement feeding tubes.

Gastric Emptying in Critically Ill Patients Is Accelerated by Adding Cisapride to a Standard Enteral Feeding Protocol: Results of a Prospective, Randomized Controlled Trial
Spapen HD, Duinslaeger L, Diltoer M, Gillet R, Bossuyt A, Huyghens LP (Vrije Universiteit Brussel, Brussels, Belgium)
Crit Care Med 23:481–485, 1995   8–36

Introduction.—Critical illness imposes significant metabolic stress resulting in rapid loss of weight and muscle mass and compromising the patient's immunity. Therefore, these patients should receive early nutritional support, preferably enterally. However, providing early nutrition may be complicated by delayed or absent gastric motility in many critically ill patients. A prospective, randomized, controlled trial studied the effect of a new prokinetic agent, cisapride, on gastric emptying.

Methods.—Twenty-one critically ill, sedated, and mechanically ventilated patients were given enough enteral feeding liquid to satisfy individual protein/caloric intake requirements via a nasogastric tube. Ten patients received only the enteral nutrition, and 11 patients also received cisapride. Gastric residues were measured 2 hours after the end of nutritional infusion each day. Bedside scintigraphic gastric emptying studies were performed on the fifth and seventh days after instillation of technetium-99m–labeled nutrition.

Results.—The 2 groups were comparable in age, body weight, antibiotic treatment, and patient acuity. The enteral nutrition group had a significantly higher mean gastric residue measurement than the cisapride group (94.5 vs. 17.7 mL). Scintigraphic studies revealed a significant delay in gastric emptying on days 5 and 7 in the enteral nutrition group as compared with the cisapride group (78 vs. 40 minutes). The 2 groups had a comparable prevalence of loose stools and overt diarrhea. The enteral nutrition group had 6 patients with significant vomiting and 3 with abdominal distension, which did not occur in the cisapride group.

Discussion.—Mean gastric emptying times were significantly faster in the cisapride group than in the enteral nutrition group. However, further comparative and placebo-controlled studies are required to confirm a treatment benefit before advocating generalized use.

▶ Several techniques of enteral nutrition are commonly used in patients in the hospital and in the home setting. Transnasal feeding catheters for intragastric feeding intubation are popular adjuncts for providing nutritional support by the enteral route. Intragastric feedings provide several advantages for the patient. The stomach has the capacity and reservoir for bolus feedings. The major risk of intragastric feeding is the regurgitation of gastric contents resulting in aspiration into the tracheobronchial tree. Placement of the feeding tube through the pylorus into the fourth portion of the duodenum reduces the risk of regurgitation and aspiration of feeding formulas.

A permanent feeding gastrostomy should be considered in patients requiring long-term enteral nutrition (altered sensorium) and in patients with unresectable carcinomas of the head and neck or esophagus. Percutaneous endoscopic gastrostomy to provide access for gastric feeding can be performed without the need for a laparotomy or general anesthesia. Ascites, coagulopathies, and intra-abdominal infections are relative contraindications.

A feeding catheter jejunostomy should be considered following any major upper abdominal procedure if prolonged enteral nutrition support is anticipated. Jejunal feeding catheters can be used immediately for feeding purposes following surgery. Catheter care with routine flushing is essential to ensure adequate patency. The catheter can be removed at the bedside at the desired time by simple traction, and the resulting fistula should close within several days.

W.W. Souba, M.D., Sc.D.

Recovery After Laparoscopic Colonic Surgery With Epidural Analgesia and Early Oral Nutrition and Mobilisation
Bardram L, Funch-Jensen P, Crawford ME, Kehlet H (Hvidovre Univ Hosp, Copenhagen)
Lancet 345:763–764, 1995   8–37

Background.—In patients undergoing conventional open colonic surgery, hospital duration is approximately 8 to 10 days, and postoperative fatigue can lead to several weeks of convalescence and impaired functional activity. Minimally invasive techniques such as laparoscopic surgery combined with epidural analgesia and early oral nutrition and mobilization may result in reduced hospital stay and less postoperative pain. The combined effects of laparoscopic surgery, epidural analgesia, and early oral nutrition and mobilization were thus investigated in a group of elderly patients undergoing elective colon resection surgery.

Patients and Methods.—Nine elderly patients over 70 years of age were included. Before surgery, a thoracic epidural catheter was inserted between T7 and T9. After undergoing laparoscopic colonic resection for neoplastic disease, patients received continuous epidural 0.25% bupivacaine, 4 mL/hr for 48 hours, and oral tenoxicam, 20 mg/day for 6 days. Opioids were avoided because of their effects on gastrointestinal function. Normal oral food intake enriched by an enteral protein solution was permitted in the immediate postoperative period, and early mobilization was enforced according to a fixed schedule.

Results.—Pain during mobilization was minimal during the entire postoperative period. Besides the scheduled administration of 20 mg tenoxicam daily, 3 patients required 1 to 5 tablets of 10 mg morphine, and 3 received occasional paracetamol. Patients were out of bed for a median of 6 hours on day 1 and 8 hours on day 2 after surgery. The median oral intake was 2,500 mL together with 2 to 3 meals from day 1 postoperatively. Vomiting did not occur in any patient, and only 2 patients experienced slight nausea. Bowel function was normal after day 2 in 7 patients; 1 patient had no bowel function on days 3 to 6. Six and 2 patients were discharged on postoperative days 2 and 3, respectively. After discharge, patients regained normal activities quickly and were mobilized for nearly 12 hours beginning on postoperative day 3. At 1 month postoperatively, all patients had returned to normal functional levels. All patients reported satisfaction with their postoperative course and indicated that they would recommend this procedure to others.

Conclusions.—A combined strategy of laparoscopic surgery, continuous epidural blockade, and early oral nutrition and mobilization helps expedite postoperative recovery in elderly patients undergoing elective colon resection surgery.

▶ Kehlet's group has studied the role of epidural anesthesia in the metabolic response to surgery for many years. This study demonstrates that the combination of laparoscopic colectomy, continuous epidural blockade, and early oral nutrition and mobilization improves recovery after major elective surgery. The key may be to avoid postoperative ileus. If this approach proves to be safe and effective in larger trials and results in early discharge with no increased morbidity, it will likely be used in the United States in the not too distant future.

W.W. Souba, M.D., Sc.D.

9 Growth Factors and Wound Healing

Introduction

Poor wound healing prolongs hospital stay and contributes to an increase in morbidity and mortality. Why some wounds heal quickly and normally whereas others heal poorly is not entirely understood. Poor wound healing, whether it be a cutaneous wound, a bowel anastomosis, or an inflammatory focus (pneumonia) in the lung, is more frequently observed in patients undergoing emergency as opposed to elective surgery. Consider some of the differences between elective and emergency surgery that may result in wound complications.

Knowledge of wound healing problems has progressed from recognition of the importance of tissue oxygenation to our current understanding of the role of peptides that modulate the normal healing process. In the past decade over 100 compounds have been identified that modulate the healing of wounds. There has been an explosion of literature on these compounds, and the genes encoding for the biosynthesis of many of these peptides have been cloned. The hope is that these advances in the basic science of growth factors will have clinical applicability that will improve patient care and diminish morbidity and cost.

Differences in Wounding Between Elective Surgery and Accidental Injury

Insult	Elective Surgery	Accidental Injury (Trauma)
Tissue damage	Minimal; tissues are dissected with care and reapproximated	Can be substantial; tissues usually torn or ripped and debridement often necessary
Hypotension	Uncommon; preoperative hydration used and fluid status carefully monitored intraoperatively	Fluid resuscitation often not immediate; blood loss can be substantial and lead to shock, which may impair healing
Local elaboration of growth factors	? Appropriate for normal healing	? Inappropriate
Wound complications	Uncommon; prophylactic antibiotics often administered and patients are generally immune competent	More common as a result of contamination, hypotension, and tissue devitalization; immune dysfunction common
Overall stress response	Controlled and of lesser magnitude; starvation better tolerated	Uncontrolled; proportional to the magnitude of the injury; malnutrition poorly tolerated

From a practical standpoint, in general, clinical wound problems become apparent when there is an abnormality in epithelialization, wound contracture, and/or collagen metabolism. These abnormalities may develop secondary to infection, impaired oxygenation, and genetic defects. Methods used to improve wound healing include the use of growth factors, antibiotics, the systemic administration of anabolic agents, and the provision of nutritional support. Meticulous wound care continues to be paramount to proper wound management.

W.W. Souba, M.D., Sc.D.

The Biology of Normal and Abnormal Wound Healing

Adult Skin Wounds in the Fetal Environment Heal With Scar Formation
Longaker MT, Whitby DJ, Ferguson MWJ, Lorenz HP, Harrison MR, Adzick NS (Univ of California, San Francisco; Univ of Manchester, England)
Ann Surg 219:65–72, 1994   9–1

Objective.—Although the ability of the fetus to heal without scarring is well known, the mechanism of wound healing is poorly understood. In an attempt to learn how adult wound healing may be made more fetal-like, the authors studied wound healing of allogeneic skin grafts in fetal lambs.

Methods.—Maternal skin grafts and 120-day-gestation fetal skin were placed in different 60-day-old fetuses, and 40 days later incisional wounds were made in the graft and surrounding fetal skin. Fetal autografts were used as controls. Wounds were harvested 14 days later and examined by light microscopy and immunohistochemical testing with antibodies to collagen types I, II, and III.

Results.—There was no rejection of skin grafts. The adult skin grafts and 120-day fetal skin contained visible scars. The grafted skin from the 60-day-old fetuses showed no scarring.

Conclusion.—Scar-free fetal healing is not due simply to the warm, sterile environment provided by amniotic fluid but to the difference in composition and architecture of the fetal extracellular matrix and fetal cells that can be modulated to heal without scarring.

An Adult-Fetal Skin Interface Heals Without Scar Formation in Sheep
Sullivan KM, Meuli M, MacGillivray TE, Adzick NS (Fetal Treatment Center, San Francisco; Univ of California, San Francisco)
Surgery 118:82–86, 1995   9–2

Objective.—Because of the disfiguring consequences of scarring, investigators look for models of scarless tissue repair. Fetal skin, which heals by regeneration, is such a model. The results of studies of healing of the interface between the edge of a graft of adult sheepskin and fetal recipient skin are presented.

Methods.—In 16 ewes, a 1 × 2-cm maternal graft was sutured to the back of fetal sheep. Similar maternal grafts were rotated 180 degrees and resutured to the abdomens of the ewes, and similar fetal grafts were rotated 180 degrees and resutured to the backs of fetal sheep as controls. At 1, 3, 7, 14, 21, 28, 54, and 63 days the grafts were excised with a 1-cm margin and examined.

Results.—Twelve fetuses and 13 maternal autografts survived. All adult-fetal grafts and fetal autografts healed without scarring. Adult autografts healed with scar formation.

Conclusion.—Adult-fetal grafts heal without scarring, possibly because the adult graft is exposed to fetal growth factors that block the synthesis, binding, or activation of the cytokine transforming growth factor β which is associated with scarring in adult tissue.

A Model of Scarless Human Fetal Wound Repair Is Deficient in Transforming Growth Factor Beta

Sullivan KM, Lorenz HP, Meuli M, Lin RY, Adzick NS (Univ of California, San Francisco)

J Pediatr Surg 30:198–203, 1995   9–3

Objective.—When the skin of human fetuses is injured, it can heal without scarring. The mechanisms of this scarless regeneration may involve a different cell population, extracellular matrix, or cytokine profile. The cytokine transforming growth factor β (TGF-β) is known to promote fibrosis. The role of TGF-β in scarless human fetal wound repair was assessed in an experimental study.

Methods.—The study used an established model in which 16-week-gestation human fetal skin transplanted into a subcutaneous pocket in adult athymic nude mice heals without scarring. Implanted fetal and adult skin grafts were subjected to incisional wounds 7 days after transplantation. The grafts were harvested 1 to 4 weeks later and subjected to immunochemical studies for isoform-nonspecific TGF-β, TGF-β_1, and TGF-β_2. In a subsequent experiment, a 0.01-, 0.1-, 1.0-, or 10.0-μg TGF-β_1 disk was implanted underneath the fetal skin graft when the incisional wound was made.

Results.—The wounded fetal skin grafts healed without scarring and showed no TGF-β staining. Wounds in adult skin grafts healed with scarring and showed isoform-nonspecific staining for TGF-β from 6 hours to 21 days. Staining for TGF-β_1 was apparent from 6 hours to 21 days and for TGF-β_2 from 12 hours to 7 days.

In the second phase of the study, fetal grafts treated with TGF-β_1 showed marked scarring 14 days after the incisional wounds were made. The size of these scars was proportional to the TGF-β_1 dose.

Conclusions.—A relative lack of the cytokine TGF-β may be an explanation for the scarless regeneration of fetal skin after wounding. The fibrosis noted in wound repair after birth may involve an excess of TGF-β.

Scar formation after skin wounding in both children and adults may be reduced by treatment strategies aimed against TGF-β.

▶ These 3 papers from the laboratory of Scott Adzick, M.D., build on earlier contributions the group has made to our understanding of the unique capability of the fetus to heal skin without scar formation. One of the most striking aspects of fetal wounds is that they heal without an inflammatory response and generate a "scarless" repair hallmarked by an organized structural integrity (regeneration) rather than the disorganized scar matrix seen in adults.

Sullivan, a surgical resident working with Adzick, showed that the relative lack of TGF-β, a growth factor elaborated in adult wounds that is known to promote fibrosis, may be one reason why the fetus heals by regeneration rather than scarring. In more recent work (Longaker et al.), it was demonstrated that the more differentiated cells of adult skin cannot be modulated to heal in a scarless manner simply by exposure to the fetal environment. These observations indicate that the fetal environment alone does not confer scarless repair. Possibly, the structure of adult skin (a denser dermis) prevented it from obtaining key growth factors from the fetal environment that would allow it to "turn back the developmental clock." Alternatively, fetal healing may involve different cellular and matrix components than adult repair, and these processes may be independent of the unique fetal environment.

W.W. Souba, M.D., Sc.D.

Epithelial Antibiotics Induced at Sites of Inflammation
Schonwetter BS, Stolzenberg ED, Zasloff MA (Magainin Pharmaceuticals Inc, Plymouth Meeting, Pa)
Science 267:1645–1648, 1995   9–4

Background.—Several previous studies have identified antimicrobial peptides in barrier epithelial cells of various mammalian species. The role of these peptides in host defense is unclear. Invasive infections of the tongue are rare in normal hosts despite the frequency of abrasions to the surface of the tongue. The bovine tongue was studied to determine whether its epithelium produces antibiotics capable of serving as a broad-spectrum chemical shield.

Findings.—A β-defensin peptide termed lingual antimicrobial peptide (LAP) was isolated, and its corresponding complementary DNA was cloned. This antibiotic, which was expressed by the epithelium of the upper surface of the tongue, showed a broad spectrum of antifungal and antibacterial activity. Its mRNA was markedly abundant in the epithelium surrounding naturally occurring tongue lesions. Along with this increased abundance, the cellular hallmarks of acute and chronic inflammation were observed in the underlying lamina propria.

Conclusions.—The cow tongue expresses a broad-spectrum antimicrobial peptide known as LAP. Expression of this peptide is increased at sites of injury or infection, either because of direct stimulation by bacteria or because of production of cytokines at the injury site. Epithelial antimicrobial peptides may play an integral role in the inflammatory response.

▶ The lingual antimicrobial peptide that the authors cloned and showed to have substantial antibacterial and antifungal properties is likely to play an important role in the host defense system of epithelial surfaces. The factors that "upregulate" the expression of lingual antimicrobial peptide mRNA at the site of injury may include locally produced bacterial toxins and/or cytokines.

W.W. Souba, M.D., Sc.D.

Capillary Morphogenesis During Healing of Full-Thickness Skin Grafts: An Ultrastructural Study
Goretsky MJ, Breeden M, Pisarski G, Harriger MD, Boyce ST, Greenhalgh DG (Univ of Cincinnati, Ohio)
Wound Rep Reg 3:213–220, 1995   9–5

Introduction.—Angiogenesis is crucial to wound and graft healing, and conditions that impair angiogenesis also impair healing. The process of angiogenesis involves the outgrowth of endothelial cells to form capillaries that revascularize injured tissues. To better understand the biological mechanisms of graft revascularization, the pattern of capillary growth in full-thickness skin grafts was examined at serial time points.

Methods.—Experiments were performed in adult male Lewis rats in which full-thickness skin was excised to muscle fascia from the hind limbs. A polypropylene mesh was placed on the wound beneath the graft to identify the graft/wound base boundary. Excised skin was then replaced in its original orientation and the autologous graft secured with silk sutures. Vascular casts of the grafts were prepared after the animals were killed at days 3, 5, 7, and 10. The grafts were excised, the tissues digested, and casts examined with scanning electron microscopy (SEM). Tissues infused with the acrylic polymer used to generate vascular casts, but not digested, were studied with transmission electron microscopy (TEM).

Results.—All animals survived the grafting procedure, but 36% of the grafts failed after being dislodged by the rats. Three days after grafting, SEM showed an immature lobular pattern extending from the wound bed through the polypropylene mesh suggestive of capillary ingrowth. Higher magnification demonstrated these lobules to be contiguous with casts of intact vessels. By TEM, the vessels were clearly seen to be filled with the acrylic polymer in proximity to the polypropylene mesh. No large vessels crossed the mesh, which suggests that no signs of direct capillary connection into the graft had occurred. After 5 days the immature lobules were fewer than at day 3. Capillary formation was suggested by the presence of larger buds extending from existing vessels. Cell junctions seen at TEM attached each endothelial cell together and were in full continuity. The immature lobular pattern was absent by day 7. Capillary sprouts were longer, had more extensions, and had depressions representing endothelial cell nuclei. Vascular continuity appeared to be re-established. The vascular plexi had regained full continuity by day 10, with elongated vessels forming vascular loops.

Conclusion.—The ultrastructural findings of this study are consistent with the clinical behavior of skin grafts. At day 3 after engraftment, an immature lobular pattern indicating capillary outgrowth or extracapillary leakage is seen. There is a decrease in immature lobules and an increase in more discrete capillaries at day 5. Vascular integrity is re-established by day 7, and endothelial cell proliferation appears to have subsided by day 10.

Apoptosis Mediates the Decrease in Cellularity During the Transition Between Granulation Tissue and Scar

Desmoulière A, Redard M, Darby I, Gabbiani G (Univ of Geneva; Pasteur Institut, Lyon, France; Wound Foundation of Victoria, Australia; et al)
Am J Pathol 146:56–66, 1995   9–6

Background.—Wound healing by secondary intention is characterized by the contraction of granulation tissue that develops from connective tissue surrounding a damaged or missing area. Cell numbers, especially those of myofibroblasts, decrease as the scar forms. Previous studies of the expression of α-smooth muscle (SM) actin in myofibroblasts have indicated that in the late phases of wound healing, many of these cells exhibit changes consistent with apoptosis.

Objective and Methods.—Whether apoptosis is responsible for the elimination of myofibroblasts during wound healing was examined by performing morphometric studies at the ultrastructural level in 8-week-old Wistar rats with skin wounds made on their middorsal surfaces. Fragmented DNA was sought in granulation tissue samples by an in situ end-labeling technique.

Findings.—The numbers of both myofibroblasts and vascular cells that underwent apoptosis increased as the wounds closed. Apoptotic staining appeared in myofibroblasts 12 days after wounding, the time of peak expression of α-SM actin. Apoptotic cells—evidenced by marginated and condensed chromatin, enlarged endoplasmic reticulum cisternae, and convoluted cell surfaces—became progressively evident 20 and 25 days after wounding (Fig 4). Tissue cellularity was significantly reduced as healing progressed.

Conclusion.—Apoptotic changes may be an important aspect of scar formation after wounding, and their dysregulation may contribute to pathologic scarring.

▶ These 2 elegant studies provide new information about the biology of wound healing. The paper by Goretsky et al. evaluated the vascularity and

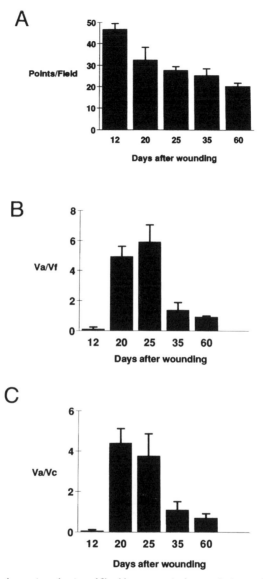

FIGURE 4.—Morphometric evaluation of fibroblast apoptotic changes. **A,** tissue cellularity at different times after wounding. Columns represent the mean ± SE of the number of points per field that fell on cells. **B,** ratio of the relative volume of apoptotic fibroblasts to fibroblasts (*Va/Vf*) at various times after wounding. There is a significant increase in the proportion of apoptotic fibroblasts at 20 and 25 days after wounding. **C,** ratio of the relative volume of apoptotic fibroblasts to all cells (*Va/Vc*) at various times after wounding. An increase in the proportion of apoptotic cells in the wound at 20 and 25 days is evident. (Permission granted: Copyright American Society for Investigative Pathology.)

healing of full-thickness skin grafts. Angiogenesis involves the proliferation and outgrowth of underlying capillaries into the base of the graft to supply oxygen and metabolites for healing. The electron micrographic findings in this study parallel those observed clinically with grafted skin. It takes several days for the grafted skin to "take," and a period of immobilization of the grafted area facilitates new capillary ingrowth into the transplanted skin. By day 7, revascularization is complete, which corresponds with the clinical observation that the graft is now adhered to the site of transfer. This study examined new vessel formation of full-thickness skin grafts and raised the question of whether angiogenesis in partial-thickness grafts is temporally or ultrastructurally different.

Desmoulière and associates studied apoptosis (programmed cell death) during wound healing, specifically its role in decreasing cellularity between the transition from granulation tissue to scar. In particular, endothelial cell fibroblasts decrease in number during the process of scar formation. The authors showed that apoptosis of granulation tissue occurs after wound closure and affects target cells consecutively rather than being a single wave of cellular disappearance. The mechanism of orderly programmed cell death during wound healing may involve the expression of certain genes (c-Myc and/or the mammalian counterpart of ced-3). The study raises the question of impaired apoptosis in patients with keloids or hypertrophic scars.

W.W. Souba, M.D., Sc.D.

Angiogenic Factors Stimulate Mast-Cell Migration
Gruber BL, Marchese MJ, Kew R (State Univ of New York, Stony Brook; Northport Veterans Med Ctr, New York)
Blood 86:2488–2493, 1995   9–7

Introduction.—It appears that early accumulation of mast cells locally at tissue sites potentiates vessel growth, but it is not known why this happens. It has previously been shown that transforming growth factor β is the most potent chemotactic factor yet to be described for mast cells. The ability of platelet-derived growth factor AB, vascular endothelial cell growth factor, basic fibroblast growth factor, and platelet-derived endothelial cell growth factor (PD-ECGF) angiogenic factors (at picomolar or less concentrations) to induce mast cell chemotaxis was observed.

Methods.—Chemotaxis assay was performed by quantifying mast cell migration in vitro. An enzyme immunoassay was done to determine whether the angiogenic factors induced mast cell degranulation. Each experiment was performed twice on duplicate samples.

Results.—Each of the factors tested induced directed migration in vitro with a typical bell-shaped dose-response curve (Fig 1). However, the mast cells were essentially unresponsive to epidermal growth factor. Checkerboard analysis indicated that PD-ECGF was more chemokinetic than chemotactic in its activity. The only angiogenic factor that stimulated histamine release, as well as chemotaxis, was PD-ECGF. Chemotactic

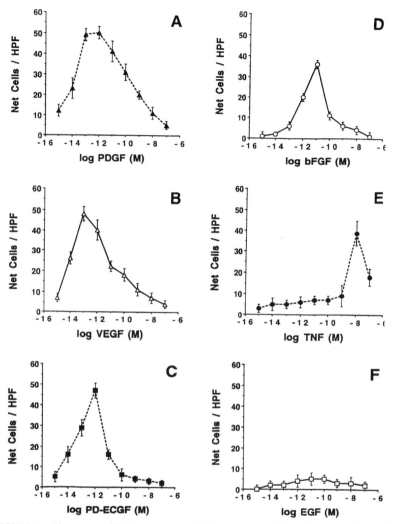

FIGURE 1.—Chemotaxis of C57 mouse mast cell line to angiogenic/growth factors. Mast cells (4 million/mL) in the assay buffer (Opti-MEM plus 1% bovine serum albumin) were allowed to migrate toward the indicated concentration of platelet-derived growth factor AB (*PDGF;* **A**), vascular endothelial cell growth factor (*VEGF;* **B**), platelet-derived endothelial cell growth factor (*PD-ECGF;* **C**), basic fibroblast growth factor (*bFGF;* **D**), tumor necrosis factor α (*TNF;* **E**), or epidermal growth factor (*EGF;* **F**) for 3 hours at 37°C plus 5% CO_2. Numbers represent means ± SEM (n = 3–5) of total cells per high-power field (*HPF*) (×400). (Courtesy of Gruber BL, Marchese MJ, Kew R: Angiogenic factors stimulate mast-cell migration. *Blood* 86:2488–2493, 1995.)

responses were effectively dampened by the tyrosine kinase inhibitor genistein. However, inhibition of G-protein–coupled receptors by pertussis toxin had no effect.

Conclusion.—This is the first known report to indicate that a broad family of angiogenic factors may influence mast cells to facilitate new vessel formation. Further investigation is needed to determine their biological effects on mast cell physiology.

The Role of Transforming Growth Factor-β in the Conversion From "Scarless" Healing to Healing With Scar Formation

Houghton PE, Keefer KA, Krummel TM (Pennsylvania State Univ, Hershey)
Wound Rep Reg 3:229–236, 1995   9–8

Background.—Wound healing in the fetus lacks the inflammation, fibroplasia, and deposition of collagen characteristic of adult healing. This "scarless" fetal repair may be explained by the decreased availability or inactivity of transforming growth factor β (TGF-β) during fetal life. A previous study had shown that isolated fetal mouse limbs wounded at day 14 of gestation (term, 20 days) heal without evidence of a scar whereas wounded day 18 fetal mouse limbs produce abundant disorganized collagen deposition in the dermis, called scar formation. Using this model, a study was conducted to examine the mediators responsible for the conversion of "scarless" wound healing to healing with scar formation.

Methods.—Wounded day 14 and day 18 fetal forelimbs were grown in a serum-free organ culture system. Day 14 limbs received either phosphate-buffered saline (PBS) solution or human recombinant TGF-β_1 (1

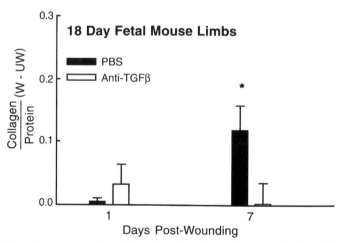

FIGURE 3.—Change over baseline of the collagen/protein ratio in wounded regions of day 18 limbs where baseline was considered to be the ratio determined in the unwounded region of the same limb. Wounded limbs were treated daily with topical administration of phosphate-buffered saline (*PBS, filled bars*) or anti–transforming growth factor β (*Anti-TGFβ, open bars*). The *asterisk* denotes that the collagen/protein ratio was significantly greater in wounded than in unwounded regions of day 18 limbs treated for 7 days with only PBS ($P < 0.005$, paired Student's t test). Values represent means ± SEM.

$$\frac{\text{Collagen (W} - \text{U)}}{\text{Protein}} = \frac{\text{Collagen (wounded)}}{\text{Protein}} = \frac{\text{Collagen (unwounded)}}{\text{Protein}}$$

(Courtesy of Houghton PE, Keefer KA, Krummel TM: The role of transforming growth factor-β in the conversion from "scarless" healing to healing with scar formation. *Wound Rep Reg* 3:229–236, 1995.)

µg/mL) daily. Day 18 limbs received either PBS solution or neutralizing antibody to TGF-β (1 µg/mL) daily. The amount of scar formation in cross sections of limbs was studied qualitatively with Masson's trichrome stain for collagen fibers and quantitatively by spectrophotometric analysis of Sirius red and fast green dyes, which bind to collagen and noncollagen protein, respectively.

Results.—Both qualitative and quantitative analyses showed abundant collagen deposition in day 18 as compared with day 14 limbs 7 days after wounding. This scar formation on day 18 limbs was attenuated by the administration of anti–TGF-β (Fig 3). The wound matrix of anti–TGF-β–treated day 18 limbs mimicked the normal architecture of the un-wounded dermis. Furthermore, TGF-β$_1$ administration to day 14 wounded limbs induced the formation of a wound matrix that was composed of relatively high collagen levels. The scar in TGF-β$_1$–treated day 14 limbs was in marked contrast to the PBS-treated day 14 wounded limbs, which underwent a regenerative type of repair.

Conclusion.—In this in vitro model, TGF-β in the local wound environment is responsible, at least in part, for the conversion of "scarless" fetal repair to adult-like healing with scar formation.

Differential TNF Secretion by Wound Fibroblasts Compared to Normal Fibroblasts in Response to LPS

Fahey TJ III, Turbeville T, McIntyre K (Univ of Texas Southwestern, Dallas)
J Surg Res 58:759–764, 1995   9–9

Objective.—The role of fibroblasts in wound healing is to promote wound contraction and collagen synthesis. In addition, studies have shown that fibroblasts can release cytokines and growth factors. The authors hypothesize that fibroblasts may also be capable of secreting cytokines in response to stimulation by endotoxin. The results of a study investigating the tumor necrosis factor (TNF) secreting capability of wound fibroblasts are presented.

Methods.—Wound fibroblasts were obtained from wound granuloma sponges that had been embedded into the flanks of 7- to 8-week-old female BALB/c mice. Normal fibroblasts were also obtained from untreated mice. Cells were stimulated with lipopolysaccharide (LPS). L929 fibroblast cytotoxicity assays and messenger RNA analyses were performed.

Results.—Wound fibroblasts secreted significant levels of TNF in response to LPS stimulation whereas dermal fibroblasts did not. A TNF response could be seen as soon as 4 hours after LPS stimulation and coincided with the induction of TNF mRNA. When dermal fibroblasts and wound fibroblasts were each incubated in wound fluid, again only the wound fibroblasts retained the ability to secrete TNF (Fig 5).

Conclusion.—Wound fibroblasts have an altered phenotype as compared with normal dermal fibroblasts. The fact that wound fibroblasts secrete TNF established that they initiate or sustain the inflammatory

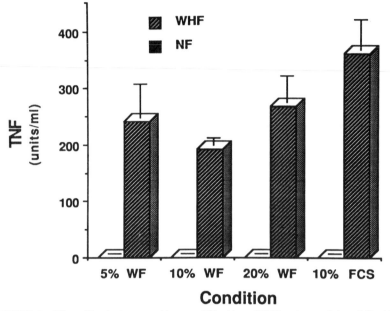

FIGURE 5.—Effect of incubating wound-harvested fibroblasts (*WHF*) and normal dermal fibroblasts (*NF*) with wound fluid (*WF*) before stimulation with lipopolysaccharide (LPS). Wound fluid was harvested and cells were incubated with the indicated concentration of wound fluid or fetal calf serum (*FCS*) for 48–72 hours before stimulation with 1 µg/mL LPS under serum-free conditions. Despite preincubation with wound fluid, NF still did not secrete any detectable levels of TNF into the supernatant fluid. The data represent mean (± SEM) TNF in units per milliliter of supernatant after LPS stimulation (performed in triplicate) of the indicated groups. (Courtesy of Fahey TJ III, Turbeville T, McIntyre K: Differential TNF secretion by wound fibroblasts compared to normal fibroblasts in response to LPS. *J Surg Res* 58:759–764, 1995.)

process and possibly fibrosis and scarring. Additional research is planned to study cell surface markers and the mechanism of response to LPS.

Wound Healing in the Transforming Growth Factor-β_1–Deficient Mouse

Brown RL, Ormsby I, Doetschman TC, Greenhalgh DG (Shriners Burns Inst, Cincinnati, Ohio; Univ of Cincinnati, Ohio)
Wound Rep Reg 3:25–36, 1995   9–10

Objective.—Transforming growth factor β_1 (TGF-β_1) is involved in wound repair by modulating cellular responses. It stimulates fibroblast proliferation and inhibits matrix degradation. To examine the role of TGF-β_1 in tissue repair, wound healing studies were conducted in TGF-β_1–deficient mice.

Methods.—Severe wasting syndrome developed in these mice at approximately 3 weeks of age. At 10 days of age, the deficient animals and control animals were wounded by excising a 0.5 × 0.5-cm section of skin from the back. The percentage of wound closure over a period of 10 days was determined. Reverse transcriptase–polymerase chain reaction was performed to determine messenger RNA transcripts for TGFs, interleukins, and tumor necrosis factor in wounded and unwounded skin and in liver.

Results.—There were no differences in wound closure between control and mutant mice until day 10. Whereas control animals gained weight, the mutant mice began to lose weight beginning at day 6. A defect in tissue repair was observed in the mutant mice, which were observed to have a thinner, less vascularized, but extensively inflamed tissue base. Transforming growth factor β_2 was expressed in control mice but not in mutant mice.

Conclusion.—Without TGF-β_1 regulation, there is an overwhelming inflammatory response accompanied by wasting that contributes to impaired wound healing.

▶ These papers collectively address the role of several growth factors/ cytokines in regulating the wound healing response. Gruber and colleagues (Abstract 140-96-9–7) showed that several angiogenic factors (platelet-derived growth factor, fibroblast growth factor, vascular endothelial cell growth factor) in vivo promote vascular growth by stimulating the recruitment of mast cells that sustain the angiogenic process. Transforming growth factor β, another potent mast cell recruiter, was studied by Houghton and colleagues (Abstract 140-96-9–8), who noted that the presence of this growth factor in the local wound environment is partially responsible for the conversion of scarless healing to scar formation. Similarly, Brown and colleagues (Abstract 140-96-9–10) noted impaired wound healing in TGF-β_1 knockout mice, an observation that was not apparent until after day 10. The authors noted marked inflammation of the wounds accompanied by a severe wasting syndrome and induction of interleukin-1 (IL-1) and IL-6. That cytokines can modulate wound healing was shown by Fahey et al. (Abstract 140-96-9–9), who demonstrated that wound fibroblasts are capable of secreting tumor necrosis factor, which initiates a profound inflammatory response that may lead to scarring. It is very likely that all of these growth factors work coordinately in a complex fashion to modulate wound healing.

Although the biology of wound healing is complicated and incompletely understood, advances in our knowledge of the molecular biology of growth factors has enhanced our understanding of the regulation of normal and abnormal wound healing immensely. The hope is that these advances in the basic science of growth factors will lead to translational studies that will improve wound healing in the clinical setting.

W.W. Souba, M.D., Sc.D.

Effect of Ischemia on Growth Factor Enhancement of Incisional Wound Healing
Wu L, Mustoe TA (Northwestern Univ, Chicago)
Surgery 117:570–576, 1995   9–11

Introduction.—Several growth factors, including transforming growth factor β (TGF-β), platelet-derived growth factor BB (PDGF-BB), and basic

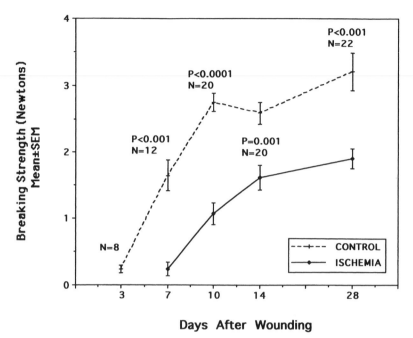

Days After Wounding

FIGURE 2.—Breaking strengths of incisions were measured at days 3, 7, 10, 14, and 28 after wounding. Healing was significantly impaired through day 28 after wounding by tissue ischemia, and the lag phase was delayed from day 3 under normal conditions to about day 7 under ischemic conditions. Paired Student's t test was used for statistical analysis. (Courtesy of Wu L, Mustoe TA: Effect of ischemia on growth factor enhancement of incisional wound healing. *Surgery* 117:570–576, 1995.)

fibroblast growth factor (bFGF), have been shown to be present at wound sites and also to play a role in wound healing. Enhancement in incisional wound healing by these growth factors has been shown, however, under varying conditions. These conditions make comparisons of the effect of different growth factors difficult. A reproducible incisional wound model was developed and used to evaluate the effects of growth factors on wound healing under ischemic conditions.

Methods.—An ischemic wound healing model was developed in rabbit ears by the placement of incisions with interruption of dermal circulation. The contralateral ear was used as a nonischemic control during development of the model. After development of the model, the incision was treated topically with growth factor, either recombinant human TGF-β, recombinant human PDGF-BB, recombinant bFGF, or recombinant Kaposi's fibroblast growth factor (K-FGF), under ischemic and nonischemic conditions. The contralateral ear served as a control and was treated with vehicle only. Breaking strength measurements, histologic studies, and venous blood gas measurements were performed on harvested tissue at 3, 7, 10, 14, and 28 days after wounding during development of the model and on days 10 and 14 during wound healing.

Results.—During development of the model, return to normal color occurred after 15 days of wounding in the ischemic ear, with indirect hypoxia maintained for 14 days. Wound healing was found to be impaired for at least 28 days after wounding in the model, with a significant reduction in breaking strength in the ischemic model when compared with nonischemic controls (Fig 2). Impairment in wound healing was also shown by histologic studies. At day 10 after wounding, TGF-β, PDGF-BB, and K-FGF resulted in an increase in breaking strength in nonischemic tissue. At day 10 and day 14, PDGF-BB was found to be ineffective under ischemic conditions. Basic FGF was found to be ineffective under both ischemic and nonischemic conditions 10 days after wounding; however, K-FGF was effective under both conditions. The greatest percent increase in breaking strength under both ischemic and nonischemic conditions was shown by TGF-β when compared with matched controls.

Conclusion.—The model developed by using an ischemic and a non-ischemic incisional wound in the rabbit ear was found to be an effective reproducible model for evaluating the effects of growth factors on wound healing. Two growth factors, K-FGF and TGF-β, were found to have beneficial effects under ischemic conditions; however, 2 other growth factors showed no benefit under ischemic conditions. Ischemia appears to be an important factor that affects the action of growth factors in wound healing.

▶ The authors used a rabbit ear incisional model to study the effects of ischemia on growth factor effects. They demonstrated that certain growth factors are ineffective under conditions of ischemia. This is an important observation that suggests that the topical application of growth factors to nonhealing wounds to accelerate healing may require adequate oxygenation of the tissues. The dual use of hyperbaric oxygen and growth factors may be a useful combination in some situations.

W.W. Souba, M.D., Sc.D.

Basic Research with Clinical Applicability

Dose-Response Study of the Effect of Growth Hormone on Mechanical Properties of Skin Graft Wounds

Jørgensen PH, Bang C, Andreassen TT, Flyvbjerg A, Ørskov H (Univ of Aarhus, Denmark)
J Surg Res 58:295–301, 1995   9–12

Background.—A recent study showed that mechanical strength development of a full-thickness skin graft was decreased by 40% to 60%, as compared with ordinary incisional wounds. Prompted by a previous report that treatment with biosynthetic human growth hormone (b-hGH) increased the mechanical strength of skin incisional wounds in normal rats after 4 days of healing, the present study examined the effect of b-hGH on

TABLE 2.—Dimensions of the Grafts After Treatment With Saline (NaCl) and
Biosynthetic Human Growth Hormone

Experimental group	n	Length (mm)	Width (mm)	Adherence to the wound bed	
				Number of grafts fully adherent	Number of grafts not fully adherent
Saline	9	3.38 (0.06)	1.82 (0.04)	3	6
2.0 mg b-hGH	9	3.43 (0.06)	1.85 (0.05)	8*	1
4.0 mg b-hGH	9	3.44 (0.05)	1.93 (0.03)*	8*	1
8.0 mg b-hGH	11	3.49 (0.01)	1.95 (0.03)*	8	3
16.0 mg b-hGH	10	3.48 (0.01)	1.93 (0.04)*	7	3

Note: Treatment started 7 days before graft induction and continued until testing after 7 days of healing. Values are means (SEM).
* $P < 0.05$ vs. the saline group.
Abbreviation: b-hGH, biosynthetic human growth hormone.
(Courtesy of Jørgensen PH, Bang C, Andreassen TT, et al: Dose-response study of the effect of growth hormone on mechanical properties of skin graft wounds. J Surg Res 58:295–301, 1995.)

compromised wound healing in a model without exogenously applied metabolic disturbances, i.e., diabetes mellitus.

Methods.—Female Wistar rats were randomly assigned to treatment with saline or b-hGH at 2.0, 4.0, 8.0, and 16.0 mg/kg/day starting 7 days before surgery and continuing to 7 days after surgery. On the left side of the dorsal skin, a 35 × 20-mm full-thickness skin graft was raised and replaced in situ. After 7 days of healing, the skin was tested mechanically.

Results.—When compared with the saline group, the maximum load and maximum stiffness correlated positively with the dose of b-hGH, being increased by 40% and 47%, respectively, in the 8.0-mg group and by 34% and 48%, respectively, in the 16.0-mg group. All grafts adhered to the wound bed, and the number of grafts with full adherence was significantly increased in the b-hGH–treated animals, particularly in the 2.0- and 4.0-mg groups (Table 2). Preoperatively, b-hGH at doses of 2.0 and 4.0 mg counteracted the decline in serum insulin-like growth factor type 1 (IGF-1) seen in the saline group, and serum IGF-1 levels even increased in the 8.0- and 16.0-mg groups. There were no significant changes in serum IGF-1 in any groups after the operation when compared with preoperative values. Blood glucose was not affected by b-hGH. Treatment with b-hGH counteracted the weight loss seen postoperatively; the saline group showed an 8% weight loss and the 2.0-mg b-hGH group a 3% weight loss, whereas no significant changes were seen in the other b-hGH groups.

Conclusion.—Treatment with b-hGH can improve the compromised healing seen in skin grafts in terms of increased mechanical strength in the graft wounds after 7 days of healing.

Increased Wound-Breaking Strength Induced by Insulin-Like Growth Factor I in Combination With Insulin-Like Growth Factor Binding Protein-1
Jyung RW, Mustoe TA, Busby WH, Clemmons DR (Washington Univ, St Louis, Mo; Northwestern Univ, Chicago; Univ of North Carolina, Chapel Hill)
Surgery 115:233–239, 1994   9–13

Objective.—Growth factors are thought to play a key role in inflammation and wound healing. Previous studies have found that polypeptide growth factors can accelerate wound repair in rodent models. The ability of insulin-like growth factor binding protein type 1 (IGFBP-1) to modify the wound healing response to insulin-like growth factor type I (IGF-I) was assessed, as was the influence of the phosphorylation state of IGFBP-1.

Methods.—Linear incisions were made in the dorsal skin of Sprague-Dawley rats, in which model transforming growth factor β and platelet-derived growth factor accelerate wound healing. The incisions were treated directly with IGF-I alone or with a combination of IGF-I and IGFBP-1. The effects were assessed by histologic analysis of breaking strength and hydroxyproline quantification.

Results.—Whereas IGF-I alone did not affect wound breaking strength, the combination of IGF-I and IGFBP-1 increased it by 33%. On its own, IGFBP-1 had no effect. Dephosphorylated IGFBP-1 showed full biological activity, whereas phosphorylated IGFBP-1 was ineffective. Wound hydroxyproline content increased by 67% in wounds treated with IGF-I plus dephosphorylated IGFBP-1, whereas those treated with IGF-I plus phosphorylated IGFBP-1 showed no effect.

Conclusions.—In a rat model, IGF-I is found to be a potent stimulator of incisional wound healing. However, its effects are demonstrable only when given in combination with one of its specific binding proteins. Although binding proteins can modulate the bioactivity of IGF, they do not define the extent to which it is needed for normal wound repair.

Perioperative Growth Hormone Improves Wound Healing and Immunologic Function in Rats Receiving Adriamycin
Harrison LE, Port JL, Hochwald S, Blumberg D, Burt M (Mem Sloan Kettering Cancer Ctr, New York)
J Surg Res 58:646–650, 1995   9–14

Objective.—Chemotherapy affects the host immunologic condition and wound healing ability and may lead to additional morbidity and mortality. Because reports indicate that growth hormone (GH) promotes wound healing and improves immunologic performance, this study was conducted to examine the effect of perioperative GH administration on wounds and immunologic function in rats receiving Adriamycin.

Methods.—A total of 47 animals received a standard 1-cm gastrotomy and were implanted with a wound sponge. Twenty rats received chemo-

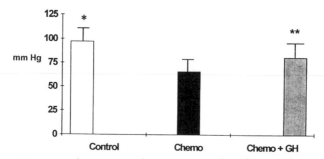

FIGURE 1.—Laparotomy bursting strength. *P < 0.05 vs. chemotherapy (*Chemo*) alone, chemotherapy plus growth hormone (*GH*); **P < 0.05 vs. chemotherapy alone. (Courtesy of Harrison LE, Port JL, Hochwald S, et al: Perioperative growth hormone improves wound healing and immunologic function in rats receiving Adriamycin. *J Surg Res* 58:646–650, 1995.)

therapy, 15 received chemotherapy and GH, and 12 animals were used as controls. Wound sponge hydroxyproline content was determined. Delayed-type hypersensitivity was determined by using the footpad response to dinitrochlorobenzene. Natural killer cell activity was determined from splenocytes.

Results.—There were 7 deaths in the chemotherapy group and 3 in the chemotherapy + GH group. Both groups lost significantly more weight and had significantly lower gastrotomy bursting strengths, lower hydroxyproline levels in wound sponges, and lower splenic weights than did the control group (Fig 1). Gastrotomy bursting strength, hydroxyproline levels, and splenic weights were significantly lower in the chemotherapy group than in the chemotherapy + GH group (Fig 4). Delayed-type hypersensitivity was significantly depressed in the chemotherapy group as compared with the chemotherapy + GH and control groups. Natural killer cell activity was significantly higher in the chemotherapy + GH group than in the chemotherapy group.

Conclusion.—Growth hormone administered concurrently with chemotherapy improves healing and immunologic function.

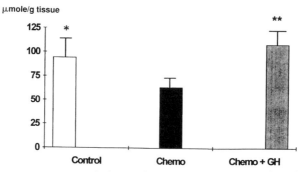

FIGURE 4.—Gastric anastomotic hydroxyproline content. *P < 0.05 vs. chemotherapy (*Chemo*) alone; **P < 0.05 vs. chemotherapy alone. *Abbreviation: GH,* growth hormone. (Courtesy of Harrison LE, Port JL, Hochwald S, et al: Perioperative growth hormone improves wound healing and immunologic function in rats receiving Adriamycin. *J Surg Res* 58:646–650, 1995.)

▶ Growth hormone has potent growth-promoting properties and exerts these effects via stimulation of IGF-1. Several human studies support the contention that growth hormone may be beneficial in some clinical settings. In burned children, growth hormone has been shown to accelerate healing of the donor site.[1] Byrne et al.[2] demonstrated the ability of exogenous growth hormone to enhance the accrual of lean body mass in patients requiring nutritional rehabilitation. The anabolic properties of growth hormone in conjunction with its minimal side effects and the ability to synthesize recombinant growth hormone make the utility of growth hormone and/or IGF-1 in certain clinical settings quite promising.

W.W. Souba, M.D., Sc.D.

References

1. Herndon DN, Barrow RE, Kunkel KR, et al: Effects of recombinant growth hormone on donor-site healing in severely burned children. *Ann Surg* 212:424–431, 1990.
2. Byrne T, Morrisey TB, Gatzen C, et al: Anabolic therapy with growth hormone accelerates protein gain in surgical patients requiring nutritional rehabilitation. *Ann Surg* 218:400–409, 1993.

In Vivo Characterization of Interleukin-4 as a Potential Wound Healing Agent
Kucukcelebi A, Harries RH, Hennessey PJ, Phillips LG, Broemeling LD, Listengarten D, Ko F, Narula S, Robson MC (Univ of Texas Med Branch/ Shriners Burns Inst, Galveston; Research Inst, Kenilworth, NJ)
Wound Rep Reg 3:49–58, 1995   9–15

Introduction.—In human and rat fibroblasts, the synthesis of collagen types I and III and fibronectin is increased by interleukin-4 (IL-4). The cells needed for normal wound healing produce and use IL-4, and fibroblasts are the final common effector cells in most phases of tissue repair. The effectiveness of IL-4 treatment was assessed in various in vivo models of impaired soft tissue repair.

Methods.—Three wound models in Sprague-Dawley rats were studied: acute excisional wounds and chronic granulating wounds inoculated with *Escherichia coli* and incisional wounds in animals with streptozocin-induced diabetes. The open wounds were treated with topical recombinant murine or human IL-4, 0.1, 1.0, or 10.0 μg/cm^2 per wound for 5 or 10 days. The incisional wounds were treated with the same doses at the time of the incision. The various groups were compared with untreated controls in terms of time to wound closure or wound breaking strengths.

Results.—The presence of *E. coli* impaired the process of wound contraction. This effect was reversed by recombinant murine IL-4 in all doses tested. In noncontaminated wounds, treatment with recombinant murine IL-4 did not enhance the closure of noncontaminated wounds. Mouse IL-4 decreased wound breaking strength in acute excisional wounds, except in contaminated wounds treated with 1.0 pg/cm² of IL-4. For both diabetic and normal incisional wounds, 1.0 µg of recombinant IL-5 improved wound breaking strength.

Conclusions.—Interleukin-4 may aid in accelerating wound closure, especially wounds in which healing is impaired. Interleukin-4 seems to have a pleiotropic effect on wound breaking strength under various conditions. This effect may involve not only fibroblast activity but also the ratio of cross-linked to total collagen content in the wound. The authors plan further studies of the mechanisms of IL-4 in wounds for the purpose of starting clinical trials in humans.

▶ Interleukin-4 is secreted by several cell types, including mast cells, and plays a central role in wound healing by stimulating angiogenesis. Interleukin-4 also stimulates the synthesis and secretion of extracellular matrix proteins by fibroblasts. It has been detected in healing wounds and therefore it almost certainly participates with numerous other growth factors in regulating wound healing. The clinical applicability of this cytokine in wound repair has yet to be tested.

W.W. Souba, M.D., Sc.D.

Exogenous Transforming Growth Factor-Beta Amplifies Its Own Expression and Induces Scar Formation in a Model of Human Fetal Skin Repair
Lin RY, Sullivan KM, Argenta PA, Meuli M, Lorenz HP, Adzick NS (Univ of California, San Francisco)
Ann Surg 222:146–154, 1995   9–16

Background.—Wounded fetal skin can heal without scarring, although the mechanisms of scarless healing are unknown. Human fetal skin that is subcutaneously transplanted to an adult athymic mouse and then wounded heals without scarring, but similarly transplanted adult skin heals with scarring. Transforming growth factor β_1 (TGF-β_1) may have a key role in scar formation. To determine this role, the expression of human TGF-β_1 mRNA was analyzed.

Methods.—Human transforming growth factor β_1 mRNA expression was examined by in situ hybridization in fetal wounds, fetal wounds treated with exogenous TGF-β_1, and adult wounds. Species-specific cell types in the wound were determined by immunohistochemistry.

Results.—Expression of TGF-β_1 mRNA resulted from wounding adult skin. No expression was observed in wounded fetal skin. When exogenous TGF-β_1 was added to fetal skin, TGF-β_1 mRNA expression in fetal fibroblasts began; an inflammatory response as seen in adults was noted, and the skin healed with scarring.

Conclusions.—Transforming growth factor β_1 has an important role in scar formation. Research in wound healing will help deepen the understanding of the biology of scar and scarless healing. Anti-TGF-β strategies may contribute to eventual scarless healing in adults.

Safety and Effect of Transforming Growth Factor-β₂ for Treatment of Venous Stasis Ulcers

Robson MC, Phillip LG, Cooper DM, Lyle WG, Robson LE, Odom L, Hill DP, Hanham AF, Ksander GA (Univ of Texas, Galveston; Celtrix Pharmaceuticals Inc, Santa Clara, Calif)
Wound Rep Reg 3:157–167, 1995   9–17

Background.—Transforming growth factor β₂ (TGF-β₂) promotes healing in animals and induces a local accumulation of connective tissue formation when injected intradermally in humans. Two clinical trials were conducted to assess the safety and effect of topical application of TGF-β₂ purified from bovine bone (bTGF-β₂) in chronic leg ulcers associated with venous stasis.

Study Design.—Noninfected chronic venous ulcers with a surface area between 1 and 25 cm² were treated 3 times per week for up to 6 weeks. The first study was a 2-arm, open-label, placebo-controlled trial in which 15 patients received topical intraulcer application of either bTGF-β₂, 0.5 mg/cm² in a lyophilized collagen matrix, or placebo consisting of lyophilized collagen vehicle without active drug. After no safety issues arose in that trial, a 3-arm, randomized, observer-blinded protocol was conducted in 36 patients who received topical intraulcer application of bTGF-β₂ at a dose of 2.5 µg/cm², vehicle placebo alone, or standard dressing of Xeroform gauze. Standardized elastic compression was applied to all test extremities. The rate of reduction of the ulcer area was measured by planimetry.

Outcome.—There were no serious safety-related events in either trial. Ulcers treated with bTGF-β₂ demonstrated an improvement in the quality and quantity of granulation tissue before epithelialization that was not seen in placebo-treated ulcers. In both trials, the mean area of ulcers treated with bTGF-β₂ continuously decreased during treatment, whereas control ulcers exhibited impaired healing. In the open-label trial, the mean rate of closure of ulcers treated with bTGF-β₂ was significantly greater than that of ulcers treated with placebo (Fig 3). Likewise, in the second trial, ulcers treated with bTGF-β₂ demonstrated an enhanced reduction in ulcer area. However, because of a higher variability in patient response and a greater placebo effect, the differences between treatment groups were not significant. The rate of closure in the placebo group was not different from that in the standard dressing group, thus indicating that the vehicle was not injurious to healing. Global assessment in the 2 trials favored treatment of ulcers with bTGF-β₂, although the differences were not statistically significant.

Conclusions.—At doses of 0.5 to 2.6 mg/cm², bTGF-β₂ is safe as a topically applied agent in a collagen matrix vehicle and demonstrates a

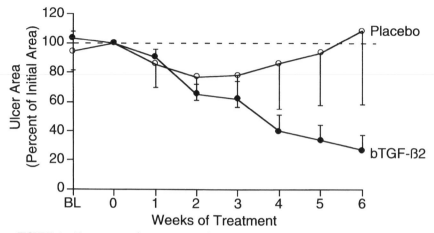

FIGURE 3.—Time course of venous stasis ulcer closure in an open-label study. Ulcer area was measured by planimetry and is expressed as a percentage of the area at the time of the first treatment (*dashed line*). *Abbreviations: bTGF-β₂*, bovine bone transforming growth factor β; BL, area at the time of baseline measurement. Variation is shown as SEM (Courtesy of Robson MC, Phillip LG, Cooper DM, et al: Safety and effect of transforming growth factor-β₂ for treatment of venous statis ulcers. *Wound Rep Reg* 3:157–167, 1995.)

positive effect on closure of venous stasis ulcers. Based on the mean rate of ulcer closure and initial ulcer area, it is projected that continued treatment with bTGF-β₂ could reduce the time for complete healing by a factor of 2- to 7-fold as compared with placebo or standard dressing. Further large multicenter trials are needed to define the potential utility of TGF-β₂ in accelerating closure of chronic dermal ulcers.

► These 2 articles have focused on the role of TGF-β in wound healing. The approach, however, was different—Lin and colleagues point out that expression of TGF-β mRNA is apparent after wounding of adult skin whereas TGF-β mRNA upregulation was not detectable in fetal skin after wounding. They suggest that TGF-β is responsible in part for scar formation in adults. Robson and associates, on the other hand, suggest that exogenous TGF-β may promote connective tissue formation in wounds and propose that large-scale clinical trials be initiated to determine the potential use of topical TGF-β on the healing of chronic dermal ulcers.

W.W. Souba, M.D., Sc.D.

Wound Healing in Clinical Practice

Factors Influencing Wound Dehiscence After Midline Laparotomy

Mäkelä JT, Kiviniemi H, Juvonen T, Laitinen S (Oulu Univ Hosp, Finland)
Am J Surg 170:387–390, 1995   9–18

Background.—Wound dehiscence after abdominal surgery can prolong hospital treatment and is associated with higher mortality rates. Retention sutures can prevent wound disruption. Patients who are at high risk of

TABLE 2.—Distribution of Preoperative Risk Factors in the Wound Dehiscence and Control Groups

Risk Factor	Dehiscence Group	Control Group
Hypoalbuminemia	31	10*
Obesity	20	16
Chronic heart disease	18	12
Anemia	18	5†
Chronic lung disease	12	4‡
Malnutrition	10	2§
Intestinal obstruction	7	2
Jaundice	4	3
Chronic alcoholism	2	0
Use of steroids	2	0
Diabetes	0	2
Mean preoperative hospital stay	4	2
Range	0–13	0–8

* The 95% confidence interval (CI) for the difference is 26.8–62.4.
† The 95% CI for the difference is 16.9–57.5.
‡ The 95% CI for the difference is 2.1–31.2.
§ The 95% CI for the difference is 3.9–29.5.
(Reprinted by permission of the publisher from Mäkelä JT, Kiviniemi H, Juvonen T, et al: Factors influencing wound dehiscence after midline laparotomy, *Am J Surg* 170:387–390, Copyright 1995 by Excerpta Medica Inc.)

wound dehiscence and who might benefit from the use of retention sutures were identified in a retrospective study.

Methods.—Data from 48 patients in whom wound dehiscence developed after midline laparotomy during a 5-year period were compared with data from 48 control patients matched for operative indication, age, and sex.

Results.—Patients in whom wound dehiscence developed had significantly prolonged hospital stays. Of 41 patients with preoperative hypoalbuminemia, wound dehiscence developed in 31 (Table 2). Hypoalbuminemia, anemia, malnutrition, chronic lung disease, and emergency procedures were significantly associated with wound dehiscence. Postoperative factors significantly associated with wound dehiscence were intestinal paralysis, increased coughing, vomiting, and repeated urinary catheterization (Table 4). Nonsignificant variables were obesity, chronic heart disease,

TABLE 4.—Postoperative Risk Factors in Relation to Wound Dehiscence and *P* Values by Fisher's Exact Test

Risk Factor	Dehiscence Group	Control Group	*P* Value
Intestinal paralysis	27	4	0.0004
Coughing	21	5	0.0037
Vomiting	17	3	0.0008
Repeated urinary catheterization	13	4	0.0303

(Reprinted by permission of the publisher from Mäkelä JT, Kiviniemi H, Juvonen T, et al: Factors influencing wound dehiscence after midline laparotomy, *Am J Surg* 170:387–390, Copyright 1995 by Excerpta Medica Inc.)

diabetes, alcoholism, preoperative intestinal obstruction, jaundice, systemic and local infection, use of steroids, type of incision, operating time, and type of wound closure. The risk of wound dehiscence developing increased as the number of risk factors increased.

Conclusions.—Internal retention sutures are recommended for patients with 3 or more risk factors for wound dehiscence. Closure of abdominal wounds is also discussed in detail.

▶ The authors have identified nontechnical factors that predispose to post-operative midline abdominal wound dehiscence. Unlike the findings of some previous studies, obesity, wound infection, and the use of steroids were not significant risk factors for the development of wound dehiscence in this study. The authors suggest the prophylactic use of retention sutures in patients with more than 3 risk factors since more than half of these patients developed a postoperative fascial disruption. This recommendation seems justified since wound dehiscence is associated with a marked prolongation of hospital stay, a huge increase in costs, and a higher incidence of future incisional hernias.

W.W. Souba, M.D., Sc.D.

Slowing of Wound Healing by Psychological Stress

Kiecolt-Glaser JK, Marucha PT, Malarkey WB, Mercado AM, Glaser R (Ohio State Univ, Columbus)
Lancet 346:1194–1196, 1995   9–19

Background.—Previous studies have shown stress-related changes in cellular immune function, including cytokine production, which is important in tissue repair. The effects of stress on wound healing were studied in those caring for a relative with Alzheimer's disease.

Methods.—Thirteen women who were caregivers for a spouse or parent with Alzheimer's disease and 13 healthy control women matched for age and income were given uniform wounds with a 3.5-mm punch biopsy on the nondominant forearm. Wound healing was monitored with photographs and the response to hydrogen peroxide, both repeated every 2–8 days. Complete healing was determined when peroxide no longer induced foaming. The proinflammatory cytokine response was evaluated in both groups by measuring the interleukin-1β response in heparinized blood to sterile saline, *Salmonella typhimurium* lipopolysaccharide, recombinant tumor necrosis factor α (TNF-α), and granulocyte-macrophage colony-stimulating factor (GM-CSF). Stress was measured in the 2 groups with a 10-item scale.

Results.—Complete wound healing took 24% longer in caregivers than in controls (48.7 vs. 39.3 days) (Fig 1). Caregivers also produced significantly less interleukin-1β than did controls in response to lipopolysaccharide, but not to TNF-α or GM-CSF. The caregivers also had significantly higher stress scores than did controls.

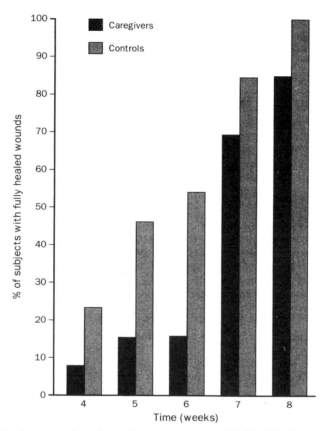

FIGURE 1.—Percentage of caregivers and controls whose wounds had healed with time (range, 24–68 days). (Courtesy of Kiecolt-Glaser JK, Marucha PT, Malarkey WB, et al: Slowing of wound healing by psychological stress, 346(5):1194–1996, copyright by *The Lancet* Ltd. 1995.)

Conclusions.—Stress is associated with significant delays in wound healing, which may be related to reduced production of interleukin-1β. Stress-related changes in immune function and wound healing could have clinical importance in expectations for surgical recovery.

▶ This study evaluated a small number of subjects, but the results are quite interesting as they suggest that emotional stress can impair wound healing. Previous studies have documented the relationship between stress and vulnerability to infectious disease.[1]

W.W. Souba, M.D., Sc.D.

Reference

1. Ader R, Cohen N, Felten R: Psychoneuroimmunology: Interactions between the nervous system and the immune system. *Lancet* 345:99–103, 1995.

Management of Traumatic Cutaneous Defects by Using a Skin-Stretching Device

Boden BP, Buinewicz BR (Temple Univ, Abington, Pa; Abington Mem Hosp, Pa)
Am J Orthop 24:27–30, 1995   9–20

Purpose.—Large skin defects frequently require skin grafts, regional flaps, or microsurgical reconstruction, all of which may cause significant morbidity and prolonged hospitalization. Use of a skin-stretching device as an alternative method of closing traumatic soft tissue defects in orthopedic patients is reported.

Technique and Results.—Nine patients underwent the skin-stretching procedure for treatment of 10 acute soft tissue defects. The skin-stretching device applied cyclic tension to the wound edges until the desired amount of stretching was obtained, at which point the skin was closed with a standard suturing technique. Nine of 10 wounds had healed without complication by an average of 9 weeks after the procedure. Dehiscence of 1 wound occurred, although the defect eventually healed by secondary intention. If skin stretching had not been used, 5 wounds would have required flap reconstruction and 5 would have required skin grafts. With skin stretching, cosmetic appearance was maintained and patient hospital stay was shorter.

Discussion.—The skin-stretching technique uses intermittent periods of stretching and relaxation to encourage skin to stretch beyond its inherent extensibility. The skin edges do not require undermining, which reduces the risk of vascular insufficiency. Oxygen saturation at the wound margins is a concern; if the blood supply is tenuous, the skin should be closely observed for blanching and pulse oximetry should be performed at the wound margins. The skin-stretching technique may have future additional applications, including alleviating the need for small open wounds to heal by secondary intention, reducing the risk of dehiscence in wounds closed under tension, allowing primary closure of ulcers, and lengthening the level of an amputation stump with a skin deficit. If the procedure is performed in the operating room, most patients can be discharged on the first postoperative day. Furthermore, skin stretching bears the potential to be conducted under local anesthesia. Skin grafting and free tissue reconstruction require considerably longer hospital stays and do not provide the ideal match in skin color and hair-bearing properties possible with skin stretching.

▶ This technique may obviate the need for a skin graft or a free tissue flap in selected patients. It is associated with a considerably shorter hospital stay. In defects with a tenuous blood supply, this technique may be contraindicated.

W.W. Souba, M.D., Sc.D.

10 Gastrointestinal

Esophagus and Stomach
INTRODUCTION

The modern era of surgical therapy for esophageal and gastric diseases began in the mid-1940s with the treatment of pyloroduodenal disease by Lester R. Dragstedt of the University of Chicago. His pioneering contributions to gastric and duodenal physiology allowed these principles to be applied to surgical practice. Many of his surgical pupils, including the late Edward R. Woodward, were instrumental in refining technical approaches and therapies directed at the management of benign (ulcers, fistulas, obstruction, hemorrhage, and achalasia) and malignant diseases of these organs. The first treatment of achalasia is credited to Thomas Willis in 1674 when he used ordinary esophageal bougienage to treat this physiologic obstruction. In 1939, Browne and McHardy advised forceful dilatation to treat achalasia by disruption of the lower esophageal sphincter with pneumatic dilators. Subsequently, the use of hydrostatic dilators was reported in 1951 by Olsen and Harrington. Credit must be given to Heller, who in 1913 formulated the physiologic operation of esophagomyotomy for the treatment of achalasia, despite a number of failed operations on the distal end of the organ for this disorder. Zaaijer modified the operation in 1923 to a single esophageal incision; Ellis and colleagues are credited with the development of transthoracic esophagomyotomy for treatment of the disease.

Despite the extraordinary advances in the treatment of various benign and malignant diseases of the esophagus and stomach, it was not until the post–World War II era that esophageal and gastric surgeons separated and appreciated the complex variability in physiologic function of the 2 organs. Thereafter, these investigators further described the variabilities of intrinsic diseases specific to these organs, thus allowing the evolution of modern scientific therapeutic approaches. The contributions of Ingelfinger and associates and Code and colleagues in the 1950s advanced the knowledge base to enable understanding of the importance of physiology to therapeutic decisions. Implicit in management was the physiologic separation of duodenal and gastric ulceration. Thereafter, surgeons involved in the care of esophageal and gastric diseases could more properly document the natural history of these diseases, which supported the fundamental physiologic basis for selection of patients for operative approaches. This pioneering era for management of diseases of the esophagus, stomach, and duodenum encouraged the surgeon to emphasize anatomical and physiologic principles to define technical approaches to these organs for enhancement of postoperative outcome.

Barrett's esophagus, a condition in which normal squamous epithelium of the distal portion of the esophagus is replaced with metaplastic columnar epithelium continuous with the gastric mucosa, was described independently in 1957 by Barrett and Lortat-Jacob. Previously, the association between adenocarcinoma and ectopic gastric mucosa was recognized in 1952. Hameeteman and associates estimate an incidence of adenocarcinoma in Barrett's esophagus to be 1 in 52 patient-years—a 125-fold increase in risk of carcinoma when compared with the general population. Abstract 10–1 describes the importance of the emerging molecular biology technology in providing an intermediate biomarker for Barrett's esophagus. The putative tumor suppressor gene p53 has been the most commonly implicated (60%) immunoreactive oncogene in mammalian neoplasms. This study by Jones and associates noted an increase in p53 immunoreactivity as the histologic classification progressed toward adenocarcinoma that was highly specific. Progression to high-grade dysplasia may be predictable based upon the p53 immunoreactivity for this molecular marker. The long-established preneoplastic injury of caustic ingestion leading to esophageal carcinoma creates both functional and long-term disability. A report (Abstract 10–2) from Izmir, Turkey, relates the extraordinary experience with esophageal strictures in children following caustic esophageal burns. This study suggests that for the pediatric population, retrosternal colon interposition provides excellent results with little overall morbidity and mortality. Preoperative staging of esophageal cancer with endoscopic ultrasound is reported by investigators at Georgetown University (Abstract 10–3). This technique appears safe and allows complete ultrasonographic examination of the esophagus, mediastinum, and celiac nodes and adds prognostically important data to patient management. Abstract 10–4 (Fig) identifies the incidence and overall results of the management of tracheoesophageal fistula and/or esophageal atresia (TEF-EA) at Indiana University. The authors note that the high rate of gastroesophageal reflux in the pediatric population following the surgical therapy is related to anastomotic shortening of the esophagus or to intrinsic esophageal dysmotility. The authors report that these improved surgical approaches with state-of-the-art anesthesia and intensive care management are contributory to the improved survival in these difficult lesions. The report by Robertson et al. from McGill University (Abstract 10–5) further verifies that abnormal lung function, especially of the restrictive type, is frequent in infants who survive TEF-EA repair in the neonatal period. Of interest, the authors note that the causes of the pulmonary function abnormalities seen in these patients still remain unexplained and do not correlate with pulmonary function.

Prior to the 19th century, attempts at hiatal hernia surgery emphasized anatomical correction rather than physiologic restoration of function.

Harrington (1928) emphasized correction of the anatomical defect and closure of the diaphragmatic hiatus. This approach influenced surgical therapy for hiatal hernia for more than 2 decades. Allison (1951) is credited with describing gastroesophageal reflux as etiologic for many of the symptoms experienced by patients with hiatal hernia; moreover, Allison was among the first to use the term "reflux esophagitis." The report by Watson and associates (Abstract 10–6) provides convincing evidence that reflux can be controlled by a 120-degree anterolateral fundoplication, even when performed laparoscopically. This variation in technical approach, when compared with the 360-degree Nissen fundoplication or the 240- to 270-degree Toupet technique, suggests that the method is much simpler and safer than the traditional Nissen fundoplication. However, long-term follow-up and outcome results are essential before recommending this technical improvement as the "standard" open/laparoscopic approach for gastroesophageal reflux disease.

Abstract 10–7 suggests that there is greater augmentation of lower esophageal sphincter (LES) pressure by the laparoscopic approach and that this technique improves complete LES relaxation. The technical variations of these approaches and the advantages of advanced laparoscopic surgical skills are detailed in Abstract 10–8. Surgeons performing antireflux procedures, whether open or laparoscopic, should have expertise and experience in posterior fundoplasty approaches for patients with poor esophageal contractility. These variants and corrective surgical approaches are emphasized in this report.

Fonkalsrud and associates at UCLA (Abstract 10–9) emphasize the importance of gastroesophageal fundoplication for symptomatic children who have both gastroesophageal reflux and delayed gastric emptying. These investigators document the importance of consideration of these procedures in the majority of neurologically impaired children who require a feeding gastrostomy.

Following the introduction of vagotomy as definitive therapy for duodenal ulcer disease by Dragstedt in 1945, antrectomy with truncal or selective vagotomy emerged as the superior procedure because of its low recurrence rate (2%–5%). Alternatives to gastric resection include more conservative approaches with retention of the stomach and duodenum to ensure diminution in postgastrectomy symptoms. Although parietal cell vagotomy (PCV) and proximal gastric vagotomy (PGV) have been observed to have the lowest operative mortality and morbidity and the fewest postoperative sequelae, these procedures remains demanding, technically exacting, and time-consuming and are considered to be associated with a high risk of ulcer recurrence (15%–25%). Abstract 10–10 describes an innovative, novel technical approach to therapy for peptic ulcer disease. This technique has important implications for laparoscopic management of peptic ulcer disease. Given the significant contributions of North American and European surgeons to the management of duodenal ulcer disease, Abstract 10–10 further suggests that surgeons take a new role in prospective analysis for the management of peptic ulcer disease. These authors provide supportive retrospective data that are encouraging and give excellent postoperative results for the management of symptoms when posterior truncal vagotomy and anterior gastric wall stapling are combined. Long-term recommendations of these techniques can only be proposed following the completion of prospective trials. In contradistinction, the long-term retrospective study by Jordan and Thornby of the Baylor College of Medicine in Houston, Texas (Abstract 10–11), confirms that the combination of PCV and omental patch closure of perforated pyloroduodenal ulcers remains an excellent choice of therapy for patients who by virtue of their age and fitness and the status of their peritoneal cavity are candidates for definitive surgery. These techniques provide definitive therapy for the large number of patients who might subsequently have required a second operation if only simple closure were performed.

The surgical literature continues to embrace the increasing application of indications and cost comparisons associated with therapy for morbid obesity. Martin and associates (Abstract 10–12) provide an important study to document, in a well-designed manner, the cost-effectiveness of these weight reduction procedures. Fundamental to this concept is the improvement in quality of life, employee performance, and job stability. The import of this study is its bearing on the managed care environment and its continual effort to control costs at the expense of patient satisfaction, access to patient care, morbidity-mortality, and employment satisfaction. The pressure of managed care and HMO corporations to justify cost enhancement must be balanced with important outcome data studies, as that provided by Martin et al.

Abstracts 10–13 and 10–14 describe the safety and excellent technical results with laparoscopic repair of hypertrophic pyloric stenosis. The results of these prospective randomized studies have to be compared with the results of the open time-honored operation described by Fredet and Ramstedt. The laparoscopic approach to esophageal achalasia is the subject of Abstracts 10–15 and 10–16. These investigators approach the repair with balloon dilatation of the esophagus. The report by Ancona et al. (Abstract 10–15) is the first large comparison trial of achalasia repair with laparoscopic vs. the conventional open Heller-Dor technique. The short-term results of the closed approach appear comparable to those of the well-established open technique. Cost-effective outcome data and long-term results are essential to confirm the validity of these reports.

Kirby I. Bland, M.D.

Potential Application of p53 as an Intermediate Biomarker in Barrett's Esophagus

Jones DR, Davidson AG, Summers CL, Murray GF, Quinlan DC (West Virginia Univ, Morgantown)
Ann Thorac Surg 57:598–603, 1994   10–1

Background.—Patients with Barrett's esophagus and dysplasia are at increased risk of esophageal adenocarcinoma. However, it has been difficult to predict whether adenocarcinoma will develop in a patient without dysplasia or with only low-grade dysplasia. Mutations of the p53 tumor suppression gene have been identified in several carcinomas and have been detected in patients with esophageal lesions, including Barrett's esophagus and adenocarcinoma. p53 protein accumulation may serve as an intermediate biomarker in esophageal carcinogenesis.

Methods.—Immunohistochemical analysis with an anti-p53 monoclonal antibody was performed with 100 esophageal specimens from patients with Barrett's esophagus (73 without dysplasia, 20 with low-grade dysplasia, and 7 with high-grade dysplasia), 10 specimens from patients with adenocarcinoma, and 35 specimens from patients with chronic esophagitis. The antibody reacted with both the wild-type and mutant forms of p53. The p53 immunoreactivity in each group of patients was compared.

Results.—No tissue from patients with chronic esophagitis exhibited p53 immunoreactivity. There was p53 immunoreactivity in 10% of the specimens from patients with Barrett's esophagus and no dysplasia, in 60% of the patients with low-grade dysplasia, in all of the patients with high-grade dysplasia, and in 70% of the patients with adenocarcinoma.

Discussion.—Ten percent of the patients with Barrett's esophagus and mild dysplasia had immunoreactivity to p53, which suggests that the p53 mutation occurs early in the neoplastic progression. The percentage of patients with p53 immunoreactivity increased with increasing dysplasia, which suggests that measuring p53 immunoreactivity is a reliable marker of the carcinogenic process. Therefore, p53 immunoreactivity can be used to predict which patients with Barrett's esophagus will have malignant progression. Further studies should assess the possible role of p53 as a target for chemotherapy.

▶ This paper addresses the issue of genetic mutations in more extensively studied tumor suppressor genes such as p53. It may become a useful adjunct in the decision-making tree of the timing for surgical intervention in Barrett's esophagus. The appeal of this paper resides in the fact that increased p53 immunoreactivity would be a more objective method than the degree of dysplasia. Although controversy exists as to whether or not p53 mutations affect prognosis in adenocarcinoma, the late occurrence in carcinogenesis of p53 mutations would imply that surgical resection might be warranted in selected cases with low-grade dysplasia and p53 overexpression.

V.E. Pricolo, M.D.

Oesophagoplasty in the Treatment of Caustic Oesophageal Strictures in Children

Mutaf O, Özok G, Avanoglu A (Ege Univ, Izir, Turkey)
Br J Surg 82:644–646, 1995   10–2

Introduction.—Esophageal burns from caustic ingestion are common among children in western and southern Turkey. Although the majority of these patients can be adequately managed with early esophageal dilatation, some patients require extensive reconstructive surgery. The surgical techniques performed in a large series of patients are reported.

Methods.—A total of 932 children aged 1–10 years were admitted between 1975 and 1992 with a diagnosis of esophageal burn. Patients with acute burns were managed with starvation, antibiotic coverage, and IV fluids for the initial 24–48 hours, with oral fluids begun when the patient began swallowing saliva. Esophageal dilatation was first attempted 21 days after the burn. Patients who required dilatation more frequently than every 3 weeks were considered nonresponders. Of the 932 children, 111 did not respond to dilatation and were treated surgically. Of these patients, 80 underwent retrosternal colon interposition, 10 underwent right thoracic retrohilar colon interposition, 18 underwent segmental resection and end-to-end esophagoesophagostomy, and 3 underwent jejunal interposition to the esophagus (Table 1). Of the 80 patients treated with retrosternal colon interposition, 19 received right colon transplants and 61 received left colon transplants; the procedure was done in a single stage in 12 patients and in 2 stages in 68 patients.

Results.—Among the patients who underwent retrosternal colon interposition, cervical anastomotic stenosis occurred in 50% of the patients with the single-stage procedure and in 10% of the patients with the 2-stage

TABLE 1.—Management of 111 Children With Caustic
Esophageal Strictures

Type of Procedure	*n*
Retrosternal colon interposition	80
Right colon	19
Left colon	61
Single-stage procedure	12
Two-stage procedure	68
Right thoracic retrohilar colon interposition	10
Segmental resection and end-to-end esophago-esophagostomy	18
Jejunal interposition to esophagus	3

(Courtesy of Mutaf O, Özok G, Avanoglu A: Esophagoplasty in the treatment of caustic esophageal strictures in children. *Br J Surg* 82:644–646, 1995, Blackwell Science Ltd.)

procedure, and cervical anastomotic leakage occurred in 8% of the patients with the single-stage procedure and in 1% of the patients with the 2-stage procedure. Anastomotic revision was required most frequently with the single-stage retrosternal colon interposition procedure. Three of the 80 patients who underwent retrosternal colon interposition and 1 of the 18 patients who underwent segmental resection and end-to-end esophagoesophagostomy died during follow-up of sepsis associated with procedure complications. Long-term morbidity occurred in 26 patients and included the inability to swallow, a cervical lump and minor respiratory distress during swallowing, acquired pectus carinatum, nocturnal emesis, prone position sleeping preference, and occasional melena.

Discussion.—Retrosternal colon transposition with a staged esophagocolostomy at the cervical end is the procedure of choice among patients who do not respond adequately to dilatation therapy. Staging substantially reduces the risk of cervical anastomotic stenosis.

▶ Caustic burns of the esophagus have now all but disappeared in Western Europe and North America with the widespread use of child-proof bottles of household products. In view of this, the present series from Izmir, Turkey, is both impressive and frightening: 932 children in 7 years (about 3 cases a week), all 10 years old or younger, 93 of whom (more than 1 a month) eventually required esophageal replacement. Their procedure of choice is retrosternal colon interposition (left or right colon), and their results certainly justify this choice: only 1 cervical leak and 10% cervical stenosis when they used a staged approach. The long-term results in 26 of these patients are not excellent, but certainly in keeping with other reports.

F.I. Luks, M.D.

Endoscopic Ultrasound for Staging Esophageal Cancer, With or Without Dilation, Is Clinically Important and Safe

Kallimanis GE, Gupta PK, Al-Kawas FH, Tio LT, Benjamin SB, Bertagnolli ME, Nguyen CC, Gomes MN, Fleischer DE (Georgetown Univ, Washington, DC)
Gastrointest Endosc 41:540–546, 1995   10–3

Objective.—Although endoscopic ultrasonography (EUS) has made it easier to stage esophageal cancer, its diagnostic capabilities are limited in patients with esophageal stenosis. In 1 study, dilation followed by endosonography has been associated with a perforation rate of 24%. The authors present a review of their experience using EUS and dilation to stage esophageal cancer.

Methods.—Preoperative staging of esophageal cancer with EUS was performed on 63 patients (16 women) aged 22 to 82 by using 7.5- to 12-MHz, 13-mm-diameter echoendoscopes. The staging results of EUS were compared with the results of CT, surgery, and bronchoscopy. The esophagus was easily passable in 39 patients (group I). Of 10 patients with impassable stenoses (group II), 3 underwent dilation. All 14 patients in group III with impassable strictures underwent dilation. A pediatric scope passed through the stenosis was dilated sequentially to maximum resistance with 27 F or 30 F Bard polyvinyl dilators. Complications were recorded.

Results.—Squamous cell carcinoma was diagnosed in 32 patients, adenocarcinoma in 29, leiomyosarcoma in 1, and lymphoma in 1. Malignancies were located in the upper third in 8 patients, midesophagus in 32, and distal third in 23. Thirty-one of 39 group I patients were correctly classified by EUS for an overall accuracy of 79%. Endoscopic ultrasonography could not pass beyond the strictures in the 3 patients in group II who underwent dilation. The remaining 7 did not undergo dilation. Staging accuracy of EUS in this group was 50%. Endoscopic ultrasonography was performed in all group III patients and had a staging accuracy of 86% and a celiac lymph node staging accuracy of 79%. Endoscopic examinations were accurate in 33% of the patients before dilation. After dilation, staging accuracy increased by 53%. There were no severe complications, but 3 patients had transient hypertension, 4 had hypotension, 10 had tachycardia, 6 had brachycardia, and 2 had desaturation.

Conclusion.—Preoperative staging of esophageal cancer by EUS is a useful adjunct to traditional staging methodologies. Dilation increases the diagnostic capability of EUS in patients with esophageal stenoses and is a safe procedure.

▶ This interesting review addresses the challenging topic of nonoperative staging of esophageal cancer. In recent years, EUS has become an important and fairly reliable tool in the preoperative evaluation of gastrointestinal malignancies, as well as some nonmalignant conditions (e.g., fistulas). The major point emphasized by this paper is the safety of endoscopic dilatation followed by EUS staging in patients with esophageal stenosis.

The importance of passing the ultrasound probe across the stricture is seen in the increase in diagnostic accuracy from approximately 33% to 86% in a group of patients with passable stenosis after dilatation. Of note, neither dilatation nor EUS increased morbidity or mortality in this patient series. The major limitation of this study is that the excellent results, unfortunately, have not been reproduced by other endoscopists, who have reported a much higher perforation rate (approximately 25%) and lower overall diagnostic accuracy (approximately 60% to 70%). With more widespread availability of this technology and increasing diagnostic experience, it is anticipated that EUS will become a standard step in the staging of most gastrointestinal malignancies.

V.E. Pricolo, M.D.

Analysis of Morbidity and Mortality in 227 Cases of Esophageal Atresia and/or Tracheoesophageal Fistula Over Two Decades

Engum SA, Grosfeld JL, West KW, Rescorla FJ, Scherer LRT III (Indiana Univ, Indianapolis)
Arch Surg 130:502–508, 1995   10–4

Introduction.—Two hundred twenty-seven infants with esophageal atresia and/or tracheoesophageal fistula (TEF) were studied retrospectively from 1971 to 1993. The average gestation was 38 weeks, with an average birth weight of 2,581 g. The most common variant seen was type C found in 78% of the patients, followed by type A in 13% and type E in 6% (Fig). A majority of the infants had associated anomalies, the most common of which were cardiac anomalies in 38%, musculoskeletal anomalies in 19%, and renal and CNS anomalies in 15%.

Operative Repair.—The vast majority of patients with type C anomalies, 160, underwent TEF division with primary esophageal repair. Fourteen type A patients underwent initial cervical esophagostomy and gastrostomy tube placement with subsequent colon interposition, and 9 patients received daily esophageal dilatation and delayed end-to-end esophageal anastomosis. Type D and E anomalies were all repaired primarily. Of the 2 patients with type B defects, 1 required cervical esophagostomy only and the other was treated by primary end-to-end repair. Eighty-one percent of primary repairs of type A, B, C, or D anomalies were done with a single-

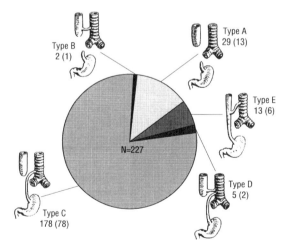

FIGURE.—Incidence of esophageal atresia (EA) and/or tracheoesophageal fistula (TEF) by anatomic type. Type C was the most common anomaly observed. Values are numbers (%) of patients. Type A, pure EA; type B, EA with proximal TEF; type C, EA with distal TEF; type D, EA and both proximal and distal TEF; type E, H-type TEF without EA. (Courtesy of *Archives of Surgery,* May 1995, 130:502–508, Copyright 1995, American Medical Association.)

TABLE 3.—Birth Weight and Survival

Birth Weight, g	No. of Patients	Survival, No. (%)
≤1000	0	0
1001–1500	16	15 (94)
1501–2000	39	36 (92)
2001–2500	44	39 (89)
>2500	100	98 (98)

Note: Weight data were complete on 199 patients. Birth weight was not a prognostic indicator of survival.
(Courtesy of *Archives of Surgery*, May 1995, 130:502–508 Copyright 1995, American Medical Association.)

layer end-to-end anastomotic technique. The 17% of repairs done with a Haight 2-layer telescopic technique occurred earlier in the series. Esophageal contrast studies were obtained 6 to 8 days postoperatively.

Results.—Thirty five patients suffered anastomotic leaks, although only 2 required operative intervention. Patients suffering leaks were more prone to stricture development, and the baseline rate of stricture formation for all procedures remained high at 35%. Gastroesophageal reflux occurred in 58% of the patients, with most treated medically although a significant portion required an additional procedure. Tracheomalacia occurred in 15% of the patients, postoperative bradycardia or apnea in 10%, and wound infection in 7%. The overall rate of survival was 95%, with the incidence of mortality apparently unrelated to birth weight (Table 3). When stratified into Waterston risk group categories, the study population demonstrated better than expected survival.

Discussion.—The high rate of gastroesophageal reflux may relate to anastomatic shortening of the esophagus or to intrinsic esophageal dysmotility. Severe tracheomalacia requiring tracheostomy or aortopexy is believed to be associated with type B, C, or D anomalies; however, the overall incidence of tracheomalacia in this series was approximately equal for type A, C, and E patients. Improved survival rates over those predicted by Waterston suggest that these criteria have been rendered out of date by technological advances in neonatal care.

▶ This impressive series summarizes several decades of tracheoesophageal fistula repair at a single institution and echoes the worldwide experience with this anomaly. None of the findings and statements in this study are really new, but the sheer number of patients gives it the authority of a work of reference.

F.I. Luks, M.D.

Late Pulmonary Function Following Repair of Tracheoesophageal Fistula or Esophageal Atresia

Robertson DF, Mobaireek K, Davis GM, Coates AL (McGill Univ, Montreal)
Pediatr Pulmonol 20:21–26, 1995   10–5

Background.—Past experience shows that in infants who successfully undergo repair of tracheoesophageal fistula with esophageal atresia (TEF-EA), restrictive and obstructive pulmonary changes frequently develop, and these patients are also at risk of hyperreactive airway disease.

Objective and Methods.—The risk of respiratory dysfunction was examined in 25 unselected patients who in the years 1962–1985 survived TEF-EA repair. The age range at the time of review was 7–28 years. In 10 instances a sibling was available for assessment. The participants were interviewed about bronchial symptoms and underwent standard pulmonary function studies. Bronchial challenge testing was done with methacholine.

Findings.—Growth was significantly impaired in the TEF-EA group. Respiratory symptoms were present in 72% of the study group and 50% of the control subjects. Although average lung function parameters were all within the normal range, function was significantly less than in the sibling controls (Fig 1). Half the study patients had abnormal pulmonary function; 3 had obstructive and 9 had restrictive changes. Airway hyperreactivity was not significantly more prevalent in the TEF-EA group. Abnormal lung function could not be related to the presence of esophageal stricture, a history of gastroesophageal reflux, or the occurrence of tracheomalacia or recurrent pneumonia. It was also unrelated to the type of surgery performed and the duration of mechanical ventilation in the postoperative period.

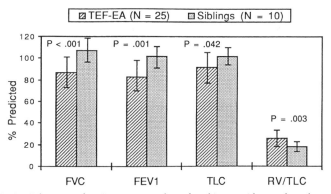

FIGURE 1.—Pulmonary function test results of subjects with esophageal atresia (*EA*)/ tracheoesophageal fistula (*TEF*) and control siblings. *Abbreviations: FVC*, forced vital capacity; *FEV1*, forced vital capacity in 1 second; *TLC*, total lung capacity; *RV*, residual volume; *FRC*, functional residual capacity. (Courtesy of Robertson DF, Mobaireek K, Davis GM, et al: Late pulmonary function following repair of tracheoesophageal fistula or esophageal atresia. *Pediatr Pulmonol* 20:21–26, copyright 1995. Reprinted by permission of John Wiley & Sons, Inc.)

Conclusion.—Abnormal lung function, especially restrictive change, is frequent in those who survive repair of TEF-EA in the neonatal period. The abnormalities tend to be mild, however, and are not related to increased respiratory symptoms.

▶ This interesting study supports the conventional wisdom about patients with esophageal atresia: these are problem children, even when the repair is easy. The authors propose a primary bronchopulmonary etiology for the respiratory handicap in these patients. The fact that 100% of patients with TEF have abnormal acid clearance (leading to gastroesophageal reflux, or at least to microaspiration) and the mechanical restrictions of a thoracotomy (up to a 30% incidence of scoliosis in some long-term series) may further explain their results.

F.I. Luks, M.D.

Laparoscopic 'Physiological' Antireflux Procedure: Preliminary Results of a Prospective Symptomatic Objective Study
Watson A, Spychal RT, Brown MG, Peck N, Callander N (Royal North Shore Hosp, Sydney, New South Wales, Australia)
Br J Surg 82:651–656, 1995   10–6

Introduction.—The laparoscopic approach has been applied to antireflux surgery. Although the floppy modification of the Nissen fundoplication is effective in correcting resistant gastroesophageal reflux, it is associated with a significant risk of complications, particularly gas bloating, an inability to belch or vomit, and dysphagia. The physiologic antireflux procedure with a laparoscopic approach was developed to reduce the complication rate while maintaining efficacy. The feasibility of this procedure was evaluated prospectively in 26 patients.

Surgical Procedure.—The procedure includes the same steps as in the open operation: transhiatal dissection to produce a long intra-abdominal segment, a posterior crural repair with the long intra-abdominal segment fixed to the crural repair, accentuation of the angle of His, and a 120-degree anterolateral fundoplication. Five cannulas were placed, with 1 located 4 cm above the umbilicus for the telescope, 1 located 4 cm below the left costal margin in the anterior axillary line for retraction of the stomach and the sling around the esophagus, 1 located just below the right costal margin in the anterior axillary line for the retroesophageal dissection and liver retraction, 1 located high in the epigastrium right of the midline for the initial liver retraction and for the receiving needle holder, and 1 located high in the epigastrium left of the midline and functioning as the main operating port.

Methods.—The laparoscopic physical antireflux procedure was attempted in 26 patients with resistant gastroesophageal reflux disease. All patients underwent esophageal manometry and 24-hour ambulatory esophageal and gastric pH monitoring, as well as symptom evaluation, before and after surgery.

Results.—Of the 26 patients, the procedure was completed successfully in 23. The procedure required a mean operating time of 2.3 hours and a mean postoperative hospital stay of 3.8 days. Return to work occurred in a mean of 1.8 weeks. Complications included pneumothorax in 3 patients, esophageal perforation in 1, and solid food bolus obstruction in 2. The mean symptom score was improved from 6.2 to 0.6. In no patient did gas bloating or an inability to belch or vomit develop. Lower esophageal sphincter pressure increased from 8.4 to 11.5 mm Hg. The number of patients with the lower esophageal sphincter within the abdomen increased from 54% to 92%. Of the 14 patients with pH monitoring data, all had physiologic esophageal acid exposure postoperatively. The postoperative manometric and pH values were similar to those measured in 30 asymptomatic controls.

Conclusions.—The laparoscopic physiologic antireflux procedure is feasible in the majority of patients, but not all. Although the incidence of perioperative complications is higher than that occurring after the open operation, it is lower than that achieved with Nissen fundoplication. The early results are comparable to those of the open operation. More study is required to determine the long-term results.

▶ Surgical repair of reflux disease is based on 3 surgical principles: (1) posterior closure of the hiatus, (2) lengthening of the intra-abdominal esophagus, and (3) creation of a complete or incomplete ring around the intra-abdominal esophagus. The size of the fundal ring, initially 360 degrees as described in the Nissen fundoplication, was reduced to 240–270 degrees by Toupet and others. By using an incomplete ring, the incidence of gas bloating and postoperative dysphagia was reduced while maintaining satisfactory elimination of reflux. Now Watson and coworkers have provided convincing evidence based on preoperative and postoperative manometric and pH studies that reflux can be controlled by a 120-degree anterolateral fundoplication, even when performed laparoscopically.

Unfortunately, this study contains few patients and does not compare the 120-degree fundoplication with the gold standard floppy Nissen fundoplication in a randomized trial. Should such data become available and confirm the results of this study, the 120-degree wrap would be a much simpler and safer alternative to the Nissen fundoplication since mobilization of the greater curvature of the stomach by division of the short gastric vessels would be unnecessary.

J.F. Amaral, M.D.

Clinical and Physiologic Comparison of Laparoscopic and Open Nissen Fundoplication

Peters JH, Heimbucher J, Kauer WKH, Incarbone R, Bremner CG, De-Meester TR (Univ of Southern California, Los Angeles)
J Am Coll Surg 180:385–393, 1995   10–7

Purpose.—Laparoscopic Nissen fundoplication has been demonstrated to be a safe and effective procedure for gastroesophageal reflux disease. However, no studies have compared the clinical and physiologic outcomes of laparoscopic and open Nissen fundoplication. Such a comparison was performed in 81 patients.

Methods.—The study included 47 patients who underwent laparoscopic Nissen fundoplication from 1991 to 1994 and 34 patients who had the open procedure from 1986 to 1994. A standardized questionnaire and a modified Visick Index were used to assess symptoms. Some patients in each group underwent postoperative pH monitoring and manometry to assess physiologic outcome.

Results.—Heartburn was the primary symptom in 55% of the patients, dysphagia in 11%, and regurgitation in 9%; 25% of the patients had atypical symptoms. Operative time was 218 minutes in the laparoscopic group and 168 minutes in the open group. The mean duration of hospitalization was 4.7 and 9.2 days, respectively. The symptomatic outcomes of surgery were graded as excellent to good in 84% of both groups, with nearly all patients having relief of their primary symptom. Five operations in each group were considered failures. On physiologic assessment, postoperative lower esophageal sphincter (LES) pressure was 21 mm Hg in the laparoscopic group and 12 mm Hg in the open group. There was no significant difference in augmentation of sphincter length. Seventy-one percent of the patients in the laparoscopic group could not completely relax their LES after fundoplication as compared with 32% of the open group.

Conclusions.—Laparoscopic and open fundoplication yield similar symptomatic outcomes. The laparoscopic operation is associated with greater augmentation of LES pressure and a low prevalence of sphincter relaxation. As the trend toward minimally invasive surgery continues, physiologic assessment before antireflux surgery becomes more and more important.

▶ This important study by Peters and colleagues confirms the efficacy of laparoscopic Nissen fundoplication in the treatment of gastroesophageal reflux disease, not only by documenting the safety and efficacy of the procedure but also by comparing the outcomes with those observed after open procedures. While the data for this study are retrospective and non-randomized, there should be little doubt that the laparoscopic approach to treating gastroesophageal reflux disease has become the standard.

Two findings of this study are particularly interesting: the greater augmentation of LES pressure by the laparoscopic approach and the marked reduction in complete LES relaxation in the laparoscopic group. As pointed out by the authors, it is likely that these 2 findings, at least in part, account for the greater postoperative dysphagia observed in the laparoscopic group. Among possible reasons for these findings cited by the authors, incomplete mobilization of the short gastric vessels and improper wrapping of the body rather than the fundus seem most likely to account for the findings.

J.F. Amaral, M.D.

A 270 Degree Laparoscopic Posterior Fundoplasty in the Treatment of Gastroesophageal Reflux
Mosnier H, Leport J, Aubert A, Kianmanesh R, Idrissi MSS, Guivarc'h M (Hôpital Foch, Suresnes, France; Hôpital Louis Mourier, Colombes, France)
J Am Coll Surg 181:220–224, 1995   10–8

Objective.—Although the Nissen fundoplication procedure for the treatment of gastroesophageal reflux is more effective than medical treatment for up to 2 years in improving symptoms, there is a 10% incidence of side effects, including postoperative dysphagia and gas bloating. Results of a study evaluating the performance and outcome of a laparoscopic 270-degree posterior fundoplasty combined with closure of the crura are discussed.

Methods.—The procedure was performed on 51 patients (21 women) aged 19 to 76 with resistant gastroesophageal reflux, paraesophageal hernia, or both.

> *Technique.*—The esophagus is exposed and the crura secured behind the esophagus by 2 or 3 standard polyglactin resorbable sutures. The posterior gastric valve is secured on the left and right side of the esophagus by 1 and 2 rows of sutures, respectively. Patients were examined at 2 weeks, 4 months, 1 year, and 2 years. At 4 months, incompetence of the esophageal sphincter was monitored by fibroscopy, pH metric reflux, and manometry.

Results.—Forty-two patients had an incompetent sphincter. One patient required conversion to an open laparotomy, and 1 patient had intraoperative pulmonary aspiration of gastric juice. No patient died perioperatively. All but 1 patient were evaluated between 4 and 6 months after surgery. A Nissen or Nissen-Rossetti fundoplasty is the preferred technique because it requires fewer knots, although the posterior fundoplasty simplifies the gastric valve tightening process. The floppy Nissen procedure results in no major dysphagia but requires sectioning of all short vessels and can lead to hemostasis in obese patients. Operating time decreases with experience.

Conclusion.—The 270-degree posterior fundoplasty leads to no mortality or major morbidity. It is less complex than the floppy Nissen procedure. Dysphagia and gas bloating syndrome are rarer with the floppy Nissen procedure. Return of function in patients with a 270-degree procedure is rapid, and there is no long-term deterioration.

▶ Mosnier et al. provides us with a small but well-studied group of patients who underwent a posterior fundoplication for reflux esophagitis. Two important points can be made from this study. First, patients with gastroesophageal reflux disease who are well studied and well selected will in general have excellent results no matter what technique is used to create the gastroesophageal valve. Second, all surgeons doing antireflux surgery either by open means or laparoscopically should have a posterior fundoplication of some sort in their armamentarium. The reason for this is the logical application of the posterior fundoplication to patients with poor esophageal contractility.

The authors provide an excellent comparison of the Nissen fundoplication to the posterior fundoplication with respect to technical difficulties. These are summarized as a need for many more sutures with the posterior fundoplication and added time and risk for division of the short gastric blood vessels for Nissen fundoplication. The latter appears improved by the use of ultrasonically activated coagulating shears, which reduce the time needed for short gastric vessel division by reducing instrument changes.

The technique as described by the authors seems simple and straightforward given advanced laparoscopic surgical skills. In addition, one is tempted to propose that it be used more often than it has been given the absence of dysphagia and gas bloating. However, a question is certainly raised by the authors' use of absorbable sutures in creating the fundoplication. Given the need for lifelong survival of the fundoplication, nonabsorbable sutures would seem to be a better choice.

J.F. Amaral, M.D.

A Combined Hospital Experience With Fundoplication and Gastric Emptying Procedure for Gastroesophageal Reflux in Children
Fonkalsrud EW, Ellis DG, Shaw A, Mann CM, Black TL, Miller JP, Snyder CL (Univ of Calif, Los Angeles; Fort Worth Children's Med Ctr, Tex)
J Am Coll Surg 180:449–455, 1995   10–9

Objective.—Children with gastroesophageal reflux (GER) frequently require surgery. Delayed gastric emptying (DGE) often accompanies GER, particularly in children with neurologic impairment. About half these children benefit from a gastric emptying procedure (GEP) with or without fundoplication. The results of a retrospective review of the surgical treatment of children with both GER and DGE are presented.

Methods.—In 2 pediatric surgery centers, 1,200 patients 18 and younger underwent surgery for GER. Gastroesophageal fundoplication (GEF) was performed in 871 and GEF plus GEP in 286. A repeat GEF with GEP was performed in 30 patients. A total of 78% of the patients had major medical problems, including CNS damage, cerebral palsy, microencephaly, congenital heart disease, pharyngeal swallowing problems, esophageal atresia, and Down syndrome. The most accurate method for quantitating the severity of GER was the 24-hour esophageal pH monitoring test, which was performed on 1,162 patients. On esophagoscopy and biopsy, 102 of 156 patients were shown to have esophagitis, and 53 of 87 patients undergoing manometric studies had low esophageal sphincter pressure. A total of 241 of 451 patients undergoing gastric emptying tests showed delayed emptying with retention of more than 50% of the isotope meal at 90 minutes.

Results.—All operated patients had relief of emesis, and failure-to-thrive infants gained a significant amount of weight. Approximately 90% of the patients with pulmonary symptoms experienced improvement or cure, and 92% of those with asthma improved. Only 51 patients experienced recurrent GER as a result of fundoplication breakdown, 14 of these occurring in neurologically impaired children and 4 in patients who had received GEP as well as GEF. Recurrent symptoms or alkaline reflux has not been seen in patients followed as long as 14 years.

Conclusion.—Combined GEP and GEF in children with GER and DGE gave excellent results even in neurologically impaired children. Reconstruction of malfunctioning fundoplications puts children at high risk for vagal nerve paresis. Concomitant GEP should possibly be performed in the case of secondary fundoplication.

▶ This very large series comes from one of the most fervent advocates of gastric emptying procedures (pyloroplasty and, more recently, pyloromyotomy) to help in the treatment of gastroesophageal reflux. Although their results in neurologically impaired children are excellent by anybody's standards, it is not clear whether the added gastric emptying procedure can be credited for this. The authors did not explicitly describe when a gastric emptying procedure was performed, based on objective results from gastric emptying studies. Considering the large number of procedures these authors perform yearly, the absence of randomization or a control group is unfortunate.

F.I. Luks, M.D.

Anterior Gastric Wall Stapling Combined With Posterior Truncal Vagotomy in the Treatment of Duodenal Ulcer
van Hee R, Mistiaen W, Hendrickx L, Blockx P (Univ of Antwerp, Belgium; Stuivenberg Gen Hosp, Antwerp, Belgium; Univ Hosp of Antwerp, Belgium)
Br J Surg 82:934–937, 1995   10–10

Background.—Although highly selective vagotomy (HSV) is a safe and effective surgical treatment of duodenal ulcers with few side effects, it is a time-consuming procedure requiring great technical expertise. A simplified technique combining posterior truncal vagotomy with anterior gastric stapling has been developed. The technique can be performed more quickly, yet offers protection of the anterior nerve of Latarget and more complete parietal cell denervation than HSV. The effect of this technique on gastric secretion and emptying, recurrence, and clinical parameters was studied in patients with peptic ulcer.

Methods.—Anterior gastric stapling with posterior truncal vagotomy was performed on 32 patients with duodenal ulcers refractory to medical treatment. Acid secretion in the gastric aspirate was measured before and after surgery under basal conditions and after pentagastrin stimulation. Gastric emptying rates for liquids and solids were determined. Clinical results were assessed with the modified classification of Visick.

> *Surgical Procedure.*—The posterior vagal trunk is severed. Then 3 sutures are placed just below and transverse to the cardia. With gentle traction, the sutures form a full-thickness fold of the gastric wall, which is stapled tangentially. A 1-cm full-thickness section of the stomach is excised outside the device. The procedure is performed again on the lesser curve along a longitudinal line.

Results.—Of the 25 patients with clinically classified results, 21 were graded good or excellent. Gastric acid production was reduced to less than 20% of preoperative values under basal conditions and to 36% of preoperative values at peak output. Gastric half-emptying times more than doubled for solids, and retention increased by more than 40% after 30 minutes, although liquid gastric emptying did not change.

Conclusions.—Posterior truncal vagotomy with anterior gastric stapling reduces basal and peak acid output even more than HSV, probably because of the complete denervation of the posterior wall, and results in clinical and motility effects that are comparable to the results of HSV. It has the additional benefit of being a simpler, quicker operation requiring less technical expertise.

▶ This study by van Hee and colleagues has important implications for the laparoscopic management of peptic ulcer disease. The results of this open surgical study document a significant reduction in basal and maximum acid output and excellent postoperative results by Visick grading when posterior truncal vagotomy and anterior gastric wall stapling are combined in the management of peptic ulcer disease.

Laparoscopic posterior truncal vagotomy and anterior gastric wall stapling have been proposed over the more tedious alternatives available: posterior truncal vagotomy and seromyotomy, which risks gastric mucosal perforation; posterior truncal vagotomy and anterior highly selective vagotomy, which risks bleeding; and highly selective vagotomy, which is time-consuming. Given the encouraging results provided by van Hee and colleagues, a prospective trial of a laparoscopic approach appears warranted in the near future.

J.F. Amaral, M.D.

Perforated Pyloroduodenal Ulcers: Long-Term Results With Omental Patch Closure and Parietal Cell Vagotomy

Jordan PH Jr, Thornby J (Baylor College of Medicine, Houston)
Ann Surg 221:479–488, 1995   10–11

Introduction.—The use of definitive surgery for the treatment of duodenal ulcers at the time of perforation is controversial. Most definitive treatment involves removal of the pyloroantral pump that regulates gastric emptying, which puts the patient at risk for adverse postoperative sequelae. However, parietal cell vagotomy (PCV) preserves the pyloroantral pump and is rarely associated with untoward symptoms. Long-term results are reported in 107 patients with perforated pyloroduodenal ulcers who underwent omental patch closure and PCV.

Methods.—The mean patient age of 103 male and 4 female patients was 48.5 years. The mean duration of ulcer symptoms before perforation was 3.5 years. Patients underwent annual follow-up for up to 21 years after omental patch closure and PCV. Gastric analysis was performed during each visit after patient consent. Endoscopy was performed on patients suspected of having a recurrent ulcer.

Results.—There was 1 operative death (0.9%) in a 61-year-old patient with ulcer symptoms for 6 years before perforation. Ninety-three patients were available for follow-up for 2–21 years. The probability rate for ulcer recurrence was 7.4%. There was a 1.9% reoperative rate. The postoperative gastric sequelae were minor. At the time of their last evaluation, all but 4 patients were graded Visick I or II.

Conclusion.—Long-term follow-up of this series of patients indicates that the combination of omental patch closure and PCV is an excellent choice for treatment in patients with perforated pyloroduodenal ulcers. Parietal cell vagotomy to treat perforated ulcers has no significant postoperative sequelae and a mortality rate similar to that of a simple closure. The choice of this surgery at the time of perforation should depend on the presence or absence of risk factors and not on whether the ulcer is acute or chronic.

▶ This excellent series reports outstanding functional results and very low morbidity, reoperative rate, and ulcer recurrence. In an era where intractable ulcers are rarely seen since the advent of protein pump inhibitors (omeprazole) and *Helicobacter pylori* therapy, it is likely that perforated ulcers may become the most common indication for surgical intervention. It is essential that this operation be taught in its fine technical aspects to surgical residents across the country.

V.E. Pricolo, M.D.

Comparison of the Costs Associated With Medical and Surgical Treatment of Obesity

Martin LF, Tan T-L, Horn JR, Bixler EO, Kauffman GL, Becker DA, Hunter SM
(Pennsylvania State Univ, Hershey; Louisiana State Univ, New Orleans)
Surgery 118:599–607, 1995   10–12

Introduction.—The need to reduce health care costs has led to many studies evaluating the cost-effectiveness of various therapies over a long-term period. The long-term effectiveness and cost-effectiveness of the medical and surgical management of obesity were compared, with at least a 2-year follow-up of patients.

Methods.—Between 1984 and 1991, 464 obese patients were evaluated and given a choice of surgical or medical management. The medical management program included weekly behavioral modification therapy plus a 12-week supplemented fast, then a 10-week transitional phase of gradual reintroduction of food and a 52-week maintenance phase with a very low-calorie diet. The surgical management program consisted of a Roux-en-Y gastric bypass procedure, with patients consuming the same very low-calorie diet before and after the surgery for at least 1 week. Of the 464 patients, 362 completed the program and were monitored for at least 2 years. The costs were calculated retrospectively and were established at approximately $3,000 annually for the medical program and $24,000 for the surgical program. The cost of achieving successful weight loss, defined as the loss of at least 33% of the excess weight, was then calculated.

Results.—The patients in the 2 management programs had different biopsychosocial profiles, which was only partly related to different patterns of insurance reimbursement. Weight loss curves were initially steep in both groups but stopped abruptly for the patients in the medical group and slowed for the patients in the surgical group when they stopped using the very low-calorie diet. Five years after beginning treatment, 89% of the surgical group and 21% of the medical group had maintained successful weight loss. By the sixth year, the cost of medical treatment was greater than that of surgical treatment.

Conclusions.—Surgical management is more efficacious and cost-effective than medical management for the achievement and long-term maintenance of weight loss in obese patients.

▶ This extremely important study by Martin and co-workers begins to document in a well-designed study what all surgeons doing bariatric surgery suspect: surgical therapy is more cost-effective for weight loss than medical therapy when the patient is morbidly obese. This finding is particularly important as we enter the era of managed care. Currently, insurers are usually not supportive of paying for obesity therapy, whether it be medical or surgical. This nearsighted approach fails to acknowledge the marked improvements in obesity-related illness such as diabetes, hypertension, arthritis, and heart disease such that medical therapy is not needed and health dollars for these illnesses are saved. The authors note that a true accounting of the cost of a particular form of therapy vs. no therapy is extremely complex and expensive. Nonetheless, it is imperative that these studies be performed as we enter a managed care era to avoid further discrimination in health care benefits provided the morbidly obese.

J.F. Amaral, M.D.

A New Technique for Laparoscopic Repair of Hypertrophic Pyloric Stenosis
Castañón J, Portílla E, Rodriguez E, González V, Silva H, Ramos A (Instituto Mexicano del Seguro Social, Guadalajara, Mexico)
J Pediatr Surg 30:1294–1296, 1995
10–13

Introduction.—Pyloric traumamyoplasty is a relatively new technique that has been used to treat hypertrophic pyloric stenosis since 1987 with satisfactory results. When prehensile force is applied with Babcock clamps on the hypertrophied pylorus, the force tears the hypertrophic fibers, creates grooves on either side of the pyloric olive, and opens the outflow channel to the duodenum. Perforation of the mucosa does not occur, which is the most frequent complication of Fredet-Ramstedt pyloromyotomy.

Technique.—A modified 10-mm laparoscopic Babcock clamp was inserted through a midline epigastric incision. The left hepatic lobe was raised with the clamp and the pylorus grasped from its avascular antimesenteric portion. Firm, continuous force was applied to the clamp until rupture of the hypertrophic muscle was seen and felt. This procedure was repeated on the sides of the first lesion to form 2 grooves in the anterior and posterior portions of the pylorus. An intact mucosa was observed when the opening of both grooves was viewed. Pylorus spreaders were not used and intraperitoneal sutures were not needed.

Results.—This technique was performed in 17 patients with hypertrophic pyloric stenosis. Twelve patients were younger than 30 days and 7 patients weighed less than 3.5 kg. The mean weight of the patients was 3.75 kg. Four months postoperatively, the mean weight of 12 patients was 7.162 kg and all patients showed adequate development and weight. No gastric or duodenal perforation or pyloric hemorrhage occurred. There were 2 wound infections, 1 suture dehiscence, and 1 peritoneal fluid leak. There were no deaths. Surgical time averaged 30 minutes.

Discussion.—Gastric emptying is important for obtaining easy access to the pyloric olive. Only 2 incisions were used in each patient and laparotomy was not needed to corroborate pyloric repair. Laboratory training is important for this technique. This procedure is easy and quick and does not use cutting instruments. It is an attractive alternative for treating hypertrophic pyloric stenosis.

▶ Yet another new technique—instead of incising and splitting the pyloric muscle, it is now crushed. Although it is an interesting alternative, this and other laparoscopic reports do not ask what was wrong with the "old" pyloromyotomy.

F.I. Luks, M.D.

Early Experience With Laparoscopic Pyloromyotomy for Infantile Hypertrophic Pyloric Stenosis

Najmaldin A, Tan HL (Royal Children's Hosp, Melbourne, Australia)
J Pediatr Surg 30:37–38, 1995   10–14

Introduction.—The proven safety and effectiveness of the open Ramstedt pyloromyotomy in the treatment of infantile hypertrophic pyloric stenosis (IHPS) has been largely unchallenged in spite of the known complications of open surgery. Advances in laparoscopy have opened this technique to the treatment of IHPS. The results of the use of laparoscopic pyloromyotomy for 37 infants with IHPS are reported.

Methods.—The instruments used were designed by H.L. Tan and Karl Storz. After induction of general anesthesia, carbon dioxide is insufflated through a 4-mm port inserted in a periumbilical incision. Two accessory 4-mm ports were used for manipulation and pyloromyotomy. The duodenum is stabilized and a seromuscular incision is made at the duodenal end and extended proximally.

Results.—The babies averaged 6 weeks of age and weighed 4.5 kg. The technique was successful in all 37 babies. No technical failures, bleeding, or perforations occurred. The operation averaged 29 minutes and the infants were first fed 5.2 hours after the operation. The hospital stay averaged 28 hours. All infants were asymptomatic at the 1- and 6-week follow-up.

Conclusion.—Initially the length of the procedure was 1 hour but has been reduced to as little as 15 minutes with experience. The incisional scar is minimal. There is a need for a comparative study between this and the open procedures. The laparoscopic procedure is safe and can be performed successfully in infants with IHPS. The surgeon must pay particular attention to detail and use the proper instruments.

▶ Since its first description 5 years ago, laparoscopic pyloromyotomy has been defended only by H.L. Tan and colleagues and by J.-L. Alain's group from Limoges, France. This approach rivals but does not surpass open pyloromyotomy in operative time, postoperative return to oral feeding, and hospital stay, and one cannot help seeing in this "new" technique an attempt to find the pediatric equivalent of laparoscopic cholecystectomy: a single surgical indication prevalent enough to provide sufficient laparoscopic experience to the pediatric surgeon. Whether or not laparoscopic pyloromyotomy will ever replace the time-honored operation described by Fredet and Ramstedt—and one doubts that it will—these authors and their French colleagues have demonstrated that laparoscopic surgery can be safely performed in infants and neonates.

F.I. Luks, M.D.

Esophageal Achalasia: Laparoscopic Versus Conventional Open Heller-Dor Operation
Ancona E, Anselmino M, Zaninotto G, Costantini M, Rossi M, Bonavina L, Boccu C, Buin F, Peracchia A (Univ of Padua, Italy; Univ of Milan, Italy)
Am J Surg 170:265–270, 1995 10–15

Objective.—Laparoscopic surgery for the treatment of esophageal achalasia appears to have significant advantages in reducing surgical trauma and postoperative discomfort and improving appearance. However, there have been no direct comparisons of the laparoscopic and conventional open approaches. A retrospective comparison of the laparoscopic and open Heller-Dor operations for primary esophageal achalasia was performed.

Methods.—The analysis included 17 patients who underwent the laparoscopic Heller-Dor procedure and a matched group of 17 patients who had the open Heller-Dor procedure. The 2 procedures were compared for duration, morbidity, postoperative course, and hospital costs. The 6-month results of clinical follow-up and manometric and pH monitoring were compared as well.

Results.—Mean operative time was 178 minutes for the laparoscopic procedure and 125 minutes for the open procedure. Neither operation was associated with any mortality or major morbidity. Patients in the laparoscopic group had less postoperative pain and a shorter duration of ileus. The median postoperative hospital stay was 4 days in the laparoscopic group and 10 days in the open group. The median time for return to normal activity was 14 and 30 days, respectively. One patient in the laparoscopic group had recurrent dysphagia during follow-up, and 1 patient in the open group had gastroesophageal reflux. Both procedures significantly decreased lower esophageal sphincter pressure. The average total cost was about $2,700 for the laparoscopic approach and $3,100 for the open approach.

Conclusions.—For patients with primary laparoscopic achalasia, the laparoscopic Heller-Dor procedure offers short-term results similar to those of the conventional open technique. However, the laparoscopic approach can significantly reduce surgical trauma and hospital costs. Long-term follow-up studies are needed, as are cost-benefit analyses.

▶ These 2 articles by investigators in Milan and Padua, Italy, provide a significant contribution to the surgical management of achalasia via an abdominal approach. Rosati et al. emphasize a key step in preventing mucosal perforation by dilating the esophagus with a balloon. One should also consider the use of a bougie or a flexible endoscope. It is also remarkable that the overall incidence of mucosal perforation in this series was 25%. Fortunately, most can be repaired laparoscopically.

Ancona and colleagues provide us with the first large comparative study of open and laparoscopic Heller myotomy with a Dor fundoplication. In addition to documenting the efficacy of laparoscopy in the treatment of achalasia, this study adds to the growing literature that supports an abdominal rather than thoracic approach to the treatment of achalasia.

J.F. Amaral, M.D.

Laparoscopic Approach to Esophageal Achalasia
Rosati R, Fumagalli U, Bonavina L, Segalin A, Montorsi M, Bona S, Peracchia A (Univ of Milan, Italy)
Am J Surg 169:424–427, 1995   10–16

Introduction.—The Dor antireflux procedure with a Heller myotomy is considered the surgical treatment of choice for esophageal achalasia. Although this operation has been done as open surgery, a laparoscopic approach has also been successful. Several technical details considered important in open surgery must also be accomplished for a successful laparoscopic approach. The important technical maneuvers used in the performance of a successful laparoscopic Heller-Dor procedure are described.

Methods.—After trocar placement, a flexible esophagoscope is introduced. Mild distension of the lower portion of the esophagus and cardia is then accomplished with the use of a low-compliance balloon dilator. After myotomy of the esophageal wall, the right edge of the myotomy is lifted to allow for dissection of the muscular layer from the submucosa and a 5- to 6-cm extension of the myotomy cranially. A 1.5- to 2-cm extension of the myotomy caudally below the cardia is then performed to identify the transectable proximal oblique cardia muscle fibers. Construction of the anterior fundoplication is accomplished with suturing of the anterior fundic wall to the left muscular edges of the myotomy and then to the right muscular edges. This laparoscopic Heller-Dor procedure has been performed on 25 patients with grade I, II, or III achalasia. Laparotomy was required in 3 patients because of a mucosal tear in 2 and difficulty in exposing the hiatal region in 1. At the 1-month follow-up, postoperative dysphagia scores revealed 20 patients with no symptoms (grade 0), 4 patients with mild symptoms (grade 1), and 1 patient with moderate symptoms (grade 2). Preoperatively, 24 patients had moderate or severe symptoms of dysphagia.

Discussion.—The laparoscopic approach to performing the Heller-Dor procedure provides satisfactory clinical and functional results. A reduction in postoperative pain and earlier recovery are advantages of the laparoscopic approach over open surgery. However, because of the lack of tactile perception with the laparoscopic technique, performance of myotomy may be more difficult and have an increased risk of mucosal tear or incomplete myotomy. In these cases, an open surgical procedure may be required.

Hepatobiliary, Pancreas and Spleen

INTRODUCTION

The advent, introduction, and implementation of laparoscopic procedures in general surgery has established its primacy in the management of acute and chronic cholecystitis over the past 8 years. Moreover, a fundamental alteration in the management of gallstones and cholecystitis has occurred in the past decade. Presently, the majority of surgeons and internists concur that cholecystectomy is the therapy of choice for cholelithiasis and is preferable to gallstone chemical dissolution and extracorporeal shock wave lithotripsy (ESWL), which represent inferior methodologies for satisfactory long-term outcome. In 1991, the favorable reports of minicholecystectomy suggested the procedure to be superior to the open technique. Synchronously in the United States and the United Kingdom, laparoscopic cholecystectomy was being introduced and became the new benchmark standard by which other technologies would be compared. Abstracts 10–17 to 10–20 review various applications of laparoscopic cholecystectomy and the techniques used by various surgeons in clinics throughout western Europe and North America for clearance of stones from the hepatobiliary tree and management of acute/chronic cholecystitis.

The randomized trial by McGinn and associates of Southampton University Hospital (United Kingdom) (Abstract 10–17) provides evidence in a prospective analysis that patients undergoing the laparoscopic procedure have faster recovery and less need for analgesic medication. Predictably, the laparoscopic approach had higher complication and conversion rates when compared with the open minicholecystectomy procedure. The consistent feature is that return to work and normal activities is accelerated by the laparoscopic approach when compared with minicholecystectomy (e.g., open incision less than 8 cm). This result continues to be an important feature of laparoscopic approaches, with advantages being a reduction in analgesia administration and convalescent time and rapid return to the work environment. Peters and associates of UCLA (Abstract 10–18) retrospectively analyzed 746 laparoscopic cholecystectomies and noted that inflammation and adhesions and/or the need for clearance of the common bile duct (CBD) are the most common reasons for conversion to the open technique. Abstracts 10–21 and 10–22 describe the increasing necessity for recognition of CBD stones prior to laparoscopic cholecystectomy intervention. The management of impacted cystic or CBD stones with transcystic duct exploration or laparoscopic CBD exploration is evolving; these advanced laparoscopic principles will be increasingly applied by the majority of laparoscopic surgeons. These abstracts emphasize the increasing complexities of stone retrieval and the necessity for surgeons to familiarize themselves with the applications of selective endoscopic retrograde cholangiopancreatography (ERCP) for individuals undergoing laparoscopic cholecystectomy. The important message provided by the authors of several of these abstracts is that preoperative ERCP is *not* necessary in the majority of patients, even if there is suspicion of CBD stones, as intraoperative cholangiography, together with a variety of alternatives for retrieval of these stones, allows successful management in all but a very few cases. For these failures, the excellent imaging provided by postoperative ERCP remains a viable option for patients with retained stones. In most institutions, if ERCP cannot be performed within 24 hours, patients without cholangitis or obstructive symptoms may be discharged for outpatient ERCP following the laparoscopic procedure. The high success rate of ERCP for clearance of the CBD is being increasingly realized in the majority of clinics in western Europe and North America.

The sobering consequences of bile duct injury following laparoscopic cholecystectomy is emphasized in Abstracts 10–21 to 10–22. Abstract 10–23 by Schol et al. notes a 25% incidence of early stricture (mean of 134 days after repair) and a 6% early mortality following bile duct injury. Recognition of CBD injury demands definition of the hepatobiliary anatomy by radiographic and/or ERCP approaches. Repair should be reconstructed as a biliary-enteric anastomosis unless the injury is partial or complete without loss of duct tissue or length and repaired at the time of injury. This situation may lend itself to primary ductal repair. Recognition of the necessity for ductal repair at laparoscopic cholecystectomy is fait accompli evidence of need for an open approach and immediate primary repair over T-tube decompression. Patients at prolonged intervals after common duct injury with evidence of a significant inflammatory response should have treatment by drainage and resolution of the infectious process *prior to* intervention and repair. These authors also identify that the majority of postoperative biliary leaks result from cystic duct necrosis rather than isolated clip dislodgement. Early identification of a biliary leak following laparoscopic surgery is managed most efficaciously by identification of the leak with a diisopropyliminodiacetic acid (DISIDA) scan. Identification of a leak within an intact biliary system may be managed by relaparoscopy, at which time the leak, if identified, may be repaired and drained. The presence of biliary discontinuity on a DISIDA scan requires ERCP to further determine the location and extent of the injury. Thereafter, stenting of the distal duct prior to open surgical repair is advisable.

Abstract 10–25 reports the satisfaction index of patients with laparoscopic cholecystectomy. A choice between the laparoscopic approach and ESWL or open cholecystectomy, when properly presented, will favor the laparoscopic approach. Further, the report by McMahon and associates from Scotland (Abstract 10–25) suggests that laparoscopic and minilaparotomy cholecystectomy both result in patient satisfaction and symptomatic benefit in at least 90% of patients with symptomatic cholelithiasis. Patients who reported poor outcomes were more likely to have suffered postoperative complications; these individuals also had lower quality-of-life scores with concomitant high anxiety and depression scores. In this cost-effective managed care environment era, financial consideration and patient satisfaction outcome should be evaluated for these 2 approaches with comparison in a randomized prospective trial.

As for adults, therapy for hemorrhagic portal hypertension in the pediatric population has undergone evolution over the past decade. Evans and associates (Abstract 10–27) at Emory University suggest that selective distal splenorenal shunts for intractable variceal bleeding in pediatric patients plays a major role in the management of portal hypertension. This approach is well tolerated and advised and provided high survival rates among these children with variceal hemorrhage unresponsive to medical management. Additional evidence of the advantage of the ileocolic conduit in managing ascending cholangitis and improving patient survival and quality of life is evident in the report of infants with biliary atresia from Keio University in Tokyo (Abstract 10–28). The Kasai hepatoportoenterostomy remains an important first-line therapy for infants with biliary atresia despite improved patient survival following hepatic transplantation.

The increasing recognition of molecular biology to enhance diagnostic and therapeutic approaches to the hepatobiliary tree has been further emphasized with the report by Berthélemy and associates of France (Abstract 10–29). The putative K-*ras* oncogene mutation in samples of pancreatic juice were useful in differentiating between pancreatic cancer and noncancerous pancreatic diseases. Mutations were evident in the majority (77%) of patients with pancreatic tumors. The increasing application of molecular biology to other hepatobiliary and gastric sites will almost surely follow inasmuch as mutations of oncogenes and a loss of the tumor suppressor gene p53 may precede clinical, biochemical, and radiologic evidence of an established neoplasm. In all organ systems, however, the clinical implications of these molecular biological results require comprehensive review and confirmation prior to global therapeutic recommendations.

Abstract 10–30 emphasizes the emerging improvement in mortality figures for the Whipple pancreaticoduodenectomy and notes that reduction in surgical complications and improved patient survival with excellent quality of life are attainable. The ultrastructural, biochemical, and functional correlates of histologic changes that initiate pancreatitis following hypercalcemia were reviewed by Frick and associates (Abstract 10–31). These authors observed that hypercalcemia induces pancreatic injury via a secretory block; the resultant physiologic consequences include an accumulation of secretory proteins and possible evidence of activation of proteases that initiate pancreatitis. These histologic and ultrastructural evaluations will enhance the physiologic explanations of pancreatitis and its prevention. The timing of laparoscopic cholecystectomy in patients recovering from gallstone pancreatitis is the subject of Abstract 10–32. These authors determined that early surgery is safe in patients with mild pancreatitis. However, when 3 or more of Ranson's criteria are evident, surgery within the first week following admission is ill advised and associated with an enhanced operative complication frequency and increased probability of conversion to an open procedure with prolongation of hospital stay. The tenets of this important paper should be considered in the practice of the majority of surgeons and residents in general surgery. There is increasing evidence to suggest that these patients often benefit from early ERCP and papillotomy within the first 24–48 hours of diagnosis.

Recognition of pancreatic injury in children by CT evaluation is the subject of Abstract 10–33. Ultrasonography also represents a noninvasive, sensitive, and reliable test to detect splenic cysts in children. Partial splenectomy and splenorrhaphy are excellent options for patients to allow splenic preservation for epidermoid cysts of the spleen. Increasing application of laparoscopic splenectomy will almost surely follow in the pediatric population (Abstracts 10–34 to 10–36). Laparoscopic splenectomy in this younger patient population represents a safe alternative to open splenectomy, has few complications, and is being shown in a number of studies to be cost-effective and well accepted.

Randomized Trial of Laparoscopic Cholecystectomy and Mini-Cholecystectomy

McGinn FP, Miles AJG, Uglow M, Ozmen M, Terzi C, Humby M
(Southampton Univ Hosps Trust, England)
Br J Surg 82:1374–1377, 1995   10–17

Introduction.—Both laparoscopic cholecystectomy and minicholecystectomy have had favorable results. The relative safety and treatment benefits of the 2 procedures were studied prospectively.

Methods.—All patients scheduled to undergo elective cholecystectomy after June 1991 were eligible. Those who participated were randomly assigned to either laparoscopic cholecystectomy or minicholecystectomy. The amount of analgesia, time required for return to normal activities and to work, and rates of complications and conversion to open cholecystectomy were compared in the 2 groups.

Results.—A total of 310 patients participated; 155 patients were allocated to each of the treatment groups. The 2 groups had no significant differences in age, sex, and body mass index. Conversion to open cholecystectomy was required for 13% of the laparoscopic group and 4% of the minicholecystectomy group. The laparoscopic procedure required a median of 24 minutes longer to perform than did minicholecystectomy. Patients in the laparoscopic group required significantly less postoperative opiate treatment but a comparable amount of nonsteroidal anti-inflammatory medication as the minicholecystectomy group. Among the patients with successful procedures, the length of inpatient stay was significantly reduced in the laparoscopic cholecystectomy group (median, 2 vs. 3 days). However, when patients requiring conversion to open cholecystectomy were included in the analysis, there was no significant difference between groups in hospital stay. The laparoscopic group had a significantly faster return to activities and to work. The complication rate was 9% in the laparoscopic group and 3% in the minicholecystectomy group.

Conclusions.—When compared with patients undergoing minicholecystectomy, patients undergoing laparoscopic cholecystectomy had a faster recovery and needed less analgesic medication but had a higher complication and conversion rate. Therefore, neither procedure is clearly superior to the other.

▶ This large analysis of patients (n = 310) having elective cholecystectomy had a higher conversion rate to open cholecystectomy with the laparoscopic technique (13% vs. 4%); complications were also more frequent with the laparoscopic approach (9% vs. 3%). The majority of studies conclude, as did these authors, that hospital stay will be reduced for either the laparoscopic cholecystectomy or the minicholecystectomy when compared with the traditional open methodology. In this U.K. study at Southampton University Hospital, no significant cost difference was evident between the 2 techniques. Table 4 of this study confirms that analgesia administration and time back to work from convalescence were reduced with the laparoscopic cholecystectomy. The faster return to work with resumption of normal activities has an enormous social and financial impact on society and has to be one of the major considerations in outcome data as to the advisability and selection of the laparoscopic approach over minicholecystectomy.

K.I. Bland, M.D.

Reasons for Conversion From Laparoscopic to Open Cholecystectomy in an Urban Teaching Hospital
Peters JH, Kraidadsiri W, Incarbone R, Beremn CG, Froes E, Ireland AP, Crookes P, Ortega AE, Anthone GA, Stain SA (Univ of Southern California, Los Angeles)
Am J Surg 168:555–559, 1994   10–18

Introduction.—A standard procedure in the general practice of surgery is laparoscopic cholecystectomy. Most of the time the procedure is successful; however, a number of patients must be converted to the open technique. This increases time, cost, and the number of complications. Improvement in technique has reduced the complications associated with early attempts at the laparoscopic procedure as well as improved decisions to convert to the open procedure. This retrospective study was designed to determine the factors for conversion to an open cholecystectomy.

Methods.—Over a 2.5-year period, 746 patients underwent laparoscopic cholecystectomy and 101 patients were converted to an open cholecystectomy. From a review of the charts of the patients, symptoms, blood profiles, mode of admission, intraoperative notes, and complications were all recorded.

Results.—The reasons for converting to an open cholecystectomy were age greater than 60 (odds ratio, 2.2), elevated total bilirubin (odds ratio,

TABLE 4.—Multivariate Analysis of Risk Factors for Conversion From Laparoscopic to Open Cholecystectomy

Characteristic	Odds Ratio	95% Confidence Interval
Acute cholecystitis	14.4	8–26.8
Suspected common duct stone	11.3	4.1–30.2
Total bilirubin	2.6	1.3–4.9
Age >60	2.3	1.1–5.1

(Reprinted by permission of the publisher from Peters JH, Kraidadsiri W, Incarbone R, et al: Reasons for conversion from laparoscopic to open cholecystectomy in an urban teaching hospital. *Am J Surg* 168:555–559, Copyright 1994 by Excerpta Medica Inc.)

2.6), suspected common bile duct stones (odds ratio, 11.3) and acute cholecystitis (odds ratio, 14.4) (Table 4). The typical patient was male, admitted through the emergency room, and over 60 years of age with preoperative diagnoses of acute cholecystitis and common bile duct stones. Laboratory findings included elevated levels of alkaline phosphatase, total bilirubin, and alanine aminotransferase, and aspartate aminotransferase and a thickened gallbladder wall on ultrasound examination.

Conclusion.—The most common reasons for converting to the open procedure were related to inflammation and adhesions that were secondary to severe disease, as well as the need for clearing the common bile duct. The person likely to need conversion was a patient who was admitted to the emergency department, had been managed nonoperatively, and had a diagnosis of acute cholecystitis.

▶ These authors have demonstrated in an analysis of over 746 laparoscopic cholecystectomies performed from January 1991 to May 1993 that the most common reason for conversion to open cholecystectomy was inflammation and adhesions secondary to severe acute and chronic disease. In addition, patients who are admitted to the emergency department, particularly if they had been managed nonoperatively for a period of time and had a preoperative diagnosis of acute cholecystitis, are more likely to require conversion to open cholecystectomy. Multivariate analysis demonstrated that acute cholecystitis and suspected common bile duct stones are the most common reasons for conversion from laparoscopic to open cholecystectomy. Overall, a difficult dissection was contributory in about 55% of the conversions from laparoscopic to open cholecystectomy. In my experience, acute cholecystitis is the most common reason for conversion to an open cholecystectomy. After decompression of the gallbladder, if adequate traction cannot be made on the cystic duct, to demonstrate the cystic duct–gallbladder junction I feel that it is important that these procedures be converted to an open procedure to avoid potential damage to the common bile duct. An overall conversion rate of approximately 50% has been my experience in patients who have acute cholecystitis.

H.H. Simms, M.D.

Selective Use of ERCP in Patients Undergoing Laparoscopic Cholecystectomy

Rieger R, Sulzbacher H, Woisetschläger R, Schrenk P, Wayand W (Ludwig Boltzmann Inst, Linz, Austria)
World J Surg 18:900–905, 1994   10–19

Introduction.—Controversy has continued over whether stone-related disease in the gallbladder and common bile duct (CBD) is best managed by surgery alone or by preoperative biliary endoscopy. A number of approaches to CBD stones have been proposed since the advent of laparoscopic cholecystectomy (LCH).

Series.—The role of preoperative endoscopic retrograde cholangiopancreatography (ERCP) was examined in 1,140 consecutive patients having LCH. Endoscopic retrograde cholangiopancreatography was attempted in 128 patients, 11% of those operated on, and was successful in 121 cases.

Results.—Endoscopic retrograde cholangiopancreatography was performed before laparoscopy in 106 patients (9.3%). It identified CBD stones in 56 patients and benign papillary stenosis in 5. All but 3 of these 61 patients underwent endoscopic sphincterotomy and stone extraction, followed (after 1½ days on average) by LCH. The remaining 3 patients required open exploration of the CBD. Two of the patients without duct stones were unexpectedly found to have ampullary or pancreatic cancer. Endoscopic retrograde cholangiopancreatography was done at varying times after LCH in 22 patients, 8 of whom were found to have retained stones in the CBD. None of the patients having perioperative ERCP died, but pancreatitis developed in 2 after endoscopic sphincterotomy.

Conclusion.—Until laparoscopic clearance of the CBD becomes a reality, LCH in conjunction with ERCP and sphincterotomy if indicated is a useful approach to patients with CBD stones.

▶ Despite the performance of laparoscopic cholangioscopy and stone extraction, this technique has not gained widespread acceptance. Furthermore, it is not always technically possible or successful. Therefore, a role still exists for selective use of ERCP in patients with a high risk of choledocholithiasis in the preoperative phase. A multitude of papers have addressed the risk of a "positive cholangiogram" at the time of laparoscopic cholecystectomy. It is certainly preferable to perform ERCP and papillotomy before laparoscopic cholecystectomy; however, its performance in the postoperative phase may still be successful in over 90% of patients, especially those with small stones.

V.E. Pricolo, M.D.

Bile Duct Stones in the Laparoscopic Era: Is Preoperative Sphincterotomy Necessary?

Phillips EH, Liberman M, Carroll BJ, Fallas MJ, Rosenthal RJ, Hiatt JR (Univ of California, Los Angeles)
Arch Surg 130:880–886, 1995   10–20

Introduction.—Several approaches to managing patients with suspected common bile duct stones (CBDSs) undergoing laparoscopic cholecystectomy (LC) have been developed. The various management approaches were assessed retrospectively, particularly as they related to preoperative evaluation, intraoperative management, and secondary treatment strategies.

Methods.—The records of 1,231 patients who underwent LC between 1989 and 1995 were reviewed. They included 1214 patients who underwent intraoperative fluorocholangiography (IOC). Of the 1231 patients, 320 (26%) had preoperative serum chemistry or ultrasonography indicators suspicious for CBDS. Of these, CBDS were confirmed in 99 (31%). Of the 911 patients with no preoperative indicators of CBDS, IOC detected CBDS in 46 (5%).

Results.—Of the 320 patients with suspected CBDS, 9 underwent preoperative endoscopic retrograde cholangiography and attempted endoscopic sphincterotomy; these were successful in 5 patients and detected CBDS in 4. The most common technique for removing CBDS was laparoscopic transcystic duct exploration, which was successful in 91% of the patients and was associated with the shortest postoperative hospital stay, the least morbidity, and the lowest incidence of retained stones. Endoscopic sphincterotomy was most useful as a secondary treatment strategy. It was successful in 91% of the postoperative attempts, compared with 56% of the preoperative attempts and 50% of the intraoperative attempts to remove CBDS.

Discussion.—Endoscopic duct radiography can be performed successfully in 88% to 100% of the patients undergoing laparoscopic cholecystectomy, but CBDS are detected in only 33% to 50% of these patients. Laparoscopic transcystic duct exploration may be appropriate in more than 85% of patients with suspected CBDS, resulting in complications in only 2% of this series, no mortality in patients younger than 65 years, and a 1.7% mortality rate in patients older than 65 years. However, it is contraindicated in patients with small or friable cystic ducts, stones larger than 9 mm in diameter, or stones proximal to the cystic duct entry into the common bile duct. These patients may be more effectively managed with laparoscopic choledochotomy, open common bile duct exploration, drainage procedures, or postoperative endoscopic sphincterotomy. Because the most common reason for unsuccessful endoscopic sphincterotomy is the inability to cannulate the sphincter, the placement of a cystic duct tube allowing the use of a guide wire can ensure the postoperative removal of CBDS.

▶ The use of laparoscopic cholecystectomy has provided us with many alternatives for the management of common bile duct stones. This article by Phillips and colleagues details their management of common bile duct stones determined for the most part at the time of laparoscopic cholecystectomy. The important message provided by the authors is that preoperative ERCP is not needed in most patients, even if there is a suspicion of common duct stones, since intraoperative cholangiography together with a variety of alternatives to common duct stone management will successfully treat the problem in all but a few cases. For the failures, postoperative ERCP remains a viable option. In addition, the authors provide a strong and possibly biased case in support of intraoperative transcystic duct common bile duct exploration. Unfortunately, they do not provide any cost data with respect to transcystic exploration versus postop ERCP. Furthermore, the data provide only short-term follow-ups. It is also unclear from the manuscript why a patient who undergoes a laparoscopic cholecystectomy and postoperative ERCP should have a mean length of hospital stay of 10.5 days. In our institution, if ERCP cannot be performed within the next 24 hours, the patient is usually discharged for outpatient ERCP. The rather low success ratio for ERCP when intraoperative (50%) or preoperative (56%) leaves one wondering why, since accepted success rates in the literature are in the 88 to 100% range.

J.F. Amaral, M.D.

Management of Common Bile Duct Stones in the Era of Laparoscopic Cholecystectomy
Miller RE, Kimmelstiel FM, Winkler WP (St Luke's-Roosevelt Hosp Ctr, New York)
Am J Surg 169:273–276, 1995   10–21

Introduction.—Among patients undergoing cholecystectomy, 10% to 20% have common bile duct stones. Such patients have traditionally been treated with open cholecystectomy and common bile duct exploration. However, these patients have been increasingly managed with a laparoscopic approach. Patients undergoing laparoscopic cholecystectomy (LC) were studied retrospectively to determine the prevalence and indications for common bile duct stones and to review the treatment of calculous biliary tract disease.

Methods.—The records of 217 patients who underwent LC over an 18-month period were reviewed. Of these 217 patients, 37 (17%) patients underwent preoperative endoscopic retrograde cholangiopancreatography (ERCP) with or without endoscopic sphincterotomy. Endoscopic retrograde cholangiopancreatography was performed in patients with the following indications: clinical jaundice, gallstone pancreatitis, abnormal liver function tests suggestive of biliary tract obstruction, and ultrasound evidence of biliary ductal dilatation. The relative risk of common duct stones was calculated in relation to each of these indications.

Results.—Nineteen patients (8.6%) had confirmed stones in the bile ducts. Stones were found in 1.1% of the patients with none of the identified risk factors, 55% of those with clinical jaundice, 9% of those with gallstone pancreatitis, 18% of those with abnormal liver function tests and normal ultrasound findings, 82% of those with abnormal liver function tests and ultrasound evidence of dilated ducts, and 100% of those with ultrasound visualization of stones. Therefore, 51% of the patients with risk factors suggestive of common duct stones had confirmed stones. Only 2 patients without preoperative risk factors were found postoperatively to have stones in the bile duct. There was only 1 complication (complication rate, 2.7%) of ERCP, and ERCP was unsuccessful in clearing the stones from the common bile duct in only 1 patient (2.7%).

Conclusions.—Bile duct stones were found in 51% of the patients with known risk factors for choledocholithiasis and only 1.1% of the patients without these risk factors. Endoscopic retrograde cholangiopancreatography had a 97% success rate for cannulation and stone clearance and a 2.7% complication rate. Preoperative ERCP can reduce the risk of subjecting the patient to 2 general anesthetics to remove common bile duct stones postoperatively.

▶ The authors provide us with this preoperative evaluation of 37 patients with findings suggestive of common duct stones who underwent preoperative ERCP prior to laparoscopic cholecystectomy. The authors use their high success rate and low complication rate to support their conclusion that preoperative ERCP is a safe and effective method of clearing the bile duct prior to laparoscopic cholecystectomy and imply that it should be done under these circumstances. Furthermore, the authors add the small risk of a second anesthesia if postoperative ERCP fails to clear the bile duct.

Unfortunately, the criteria they used disclosed common duct stones in only 22 of 37 patients treated (59%). In addition, their criteria resulted in 16.6% of the patients who required preoperative ERCP undergoing laparoscopic cholecystectomy. These same data can be used to argue against preoperative ERCP—a high number of patients subjected to a costly procedure who do not need it. The real issue raised by this study, but not addressed by it, is given the increasing number of surgeons who have the advanced laparoscopic skills to perform transcystic duct exploration and the availability of ERCP at or near most hospitals, when will it be unacceptable to only be able to do a laparoscopic cholecystectomy? If one never tries to apply these more advanced techniques, they will never be accepted and learned. It seems the time has come to establish complete intraoperative and postoperative endoscopic management of common duct stones as the standard.

J.F. Amaral, M.D.

Outcome of 49 Repairs of Bile Duct Injuries After Laparoscopic Chole-cystectomy

Schol FPG, Go PMNYH, Gouma DJ (Univ Hosp Maastricht, The Netherlands; Academic Med Ctr, Amsterdam)
World J Surg 19:753–757, 1995   10–22

Objective.—Bile duct injury during laparoscopic cholecystectomy can lead to complications such as bile leakage, cholangitis, biliary cirrhosis, and recurrent, possibly disabling strictures. Bile duct injuries and their repair procedures and outcomes are evaluated in this study.

Methods.—One survey of 6,076 laparoscopic cholecystectomies identified 49 bile duct injuries and classified them as class I (tangential lesion), class II (clip injury), and class IIIa (bile duct transection without tissue loss), class IIIb (bile duct transection with tissue loss), and class IV (injury of 1 of the hepatic ducts). Detection of the injury during the primary operation or later during a second procedure was noted. Repairs were categorized as end-to-end anastomosis of the bile duct with or without T-tube drainage and biliodigestive anastomosis. Early complications included bile leakage at the anastomotic site, hemorrhage, wound infection, intra-abdominal infection, and death. Late complications consisted of repair site strictures.

Results.—The survey showed an incidence of 0.81% for bile duct injuries after introduction of laparoscopic cholecystectomy in the Netherlands. This study found a 25% stricture rate within a year after various repairs. Most patients received emergency care in a nonspecialized center and may experience more strictures in the future. The literature reports a higher rate of biliodigestive anastomoses because it includes secondary procedures. In this study the complication rate was similar for the 2 types of repair. Both types of repair had the same complication rates, probably because of the limited number of patients involved. Bile duct injuries can be confirmed at laparotomy and must be repaired immediately with a simple suture repair or end-to-end anastomosis (class I, II, IIIa) unless impairment of bile duct vasculature increases the anastomotic stricture. A (double) biliodigestive anastomosis is often necessary after class IIIb or IV injuries and frequently leads to stricture formation. Sometimes a biliodigestive anastomosis is the only recourse. If inflammation is present, and end-to-end repair may provide temporary drainage because of the high likelihood of anastomotic stricture development. At a later stage, biliodigestive anastomosis is frequently necessary. Percutaneous drainage is recommended for severe class IIIb and IV injuries, followed by an elective biliodigestive anastomosis when the inflammation has resolved. This study found that immediate treatment with biliodigestive anastomosis leads to a high incidence of complications.

Conclusion.—Because treatment of bile duct injuries leads to a high incidence of stricture at the site of the anastomosis, analysis indicates that the most successful treatment involves end-to-end anastomosis for less severe injuries or temporary internal drainage for more severe injuries followed by a biliodigestive anastomosis once the inflammation has resolved.

▶ Schol and colleagues provide us with the sobering consequences of bile duct injury following laparoscopic cholecystectomy—a 25% incidence of early stricture at a mean of 134 days after repair and a 6% early mortality. They also provide us with 3 important tenets of biliary reconstruction for bile duct injury. Repair should be a biliodigestive anastomosis unless the injury is partial or complete with no tissue loss and repaired at the time of the injury. These situations can be managed by primary repair. Second, patients who have a significant inflammatory process from the common duct injury should first be cooled down by drainage rather than undergo immediate repair.

Numerous studies have documented the strong correlation between experience as judged by the number of cases performed and the incidence of bile duct injury. Since laparoscopic cholecystectomy has become the gold standard and has been widely performed for the past 5 years, it is likely that the significant incidence of 0.81% in their study will be markedly reduced. Important steps in achieving this goal are carefully identifying the cystic duct–gallbladder junction, no energized dissection in the hepatoduodenal ligaments, cholangiography as indicated, and overall meticulous dissection close to the gallbladder wall.

J.F. Amaral, M.D.

The Ability of Laparoscopic Clips to Withstand High Intraluminal Pressure

Deans GT, Wilson MS, Brough WA (Stepping Hill Hosp, Stockport, England)
Arch Surg 103:439–441, 1995   10–23

Objective.—Displacement or migration of laparoscopic clips may possibly be responsible for 2% of postoperative bile leaks and some cases of postoperative obstructive jaundice, although there is no direct evidence for such slippage. The possibility that complications might be the result of slippage of metal or absorbable clips was studied under high transluminal pressures in both a porcine and human model.

Methods.—In anesthetized pigs, segments of artery and vein from splenic, renal, and mesenteric vessels were occluded by titanium or polydioxanone clips and connected to a system capable of delivering a pressure of 300 mm Hg. Pressure was increased until the clip released, the vessel burst, or a pressure of 300 mm Hg was attained. The experiment was repeated in in situ porcine gallbladders and in freshly removed human gallbladders.

Results.—A force of 2 and 4 newtons is required to displace clips in the transverse and axial directions from Silastic tubing. None of the clips subjected to intraluminal pressures of 300 mm Hg was displaced during the study. Other investigators have found that 11% to 34% of laparoscopy clips could be displaced by a transverse pulling force, but this does not represent the clinical situation. One report showed that major vessels occluded for 1 day with an absorbable clip could withstand pressures of 171 mm Hg but that arteries ligated with a suture required 4 days to achieve independent security and could withstand a pressure of only 88 mm Hg before leaking. In addition to pressure consideration, absorbable clips produce less of an inflammatory reaction than do titanium clips, although both single titanium and absorbable clips properly applied appear to prevent leakage. After 24 hours, even if displacement does occur, the vessel is not likely to leak. Bile leakage after traditional cholecystectomy is thought to result from ischemic necrosis of the cystic duct remnant; this also explains why clips do not migrate from the cystic artery.

Conclusion.—Bile leakage after laparoscopic cholecystectomy is most likely the result of necrosis of the cystic bile duct rather than displacement or removal of the clip.

▶ Deans et al. provide us with a simple study that gives us very important information, namely, clips do not face off vessels or tubular structures when correctly placed, even at very high and unphysiologic pressures. Despite this proof, we do see during surgery the occasional dislodgment of a clip spontaneously and the frequent presence of free clips. Therefore, it is reasonable to wonder why this occurs.

The answer most likely resides in the "correct placement of clips." Structures that are to be clipped should be completely dissected prior to clipping so that the clip completely encircles the structure and metal touches metal on the open side of the clip after closure. Placement of clips on structures that are wider than the clip, or thicker than the open radius of the clip, are likely to slip off. The latter situations should be handled with staples or ties.

Another possible answer that likely accounts for the finding of free clips during surgery relates to the manipulation of clips during retraction, dissection and aspiration. The force required to dislodge clips in a transverse manner is not great, as is known by the simple maneuver of removing an improperly placed clip. Therefore, the prudent surgeon should exercise extreme care when manipulating tissue that has been previously clipped.

The most disturbing part of their finding is the conclusion that most postoperative bile leaks result from cystic duct necrosis rather than clip dislodgment since it is difficult to envision how to prevent it. A catch-22 situation exists in which we must skeletonize the duct wall in order to ensure secure clip closure and at the same time not devascularize it. In addition, we could clip the duct above the usual feeding branch to the cystic duct from the cystic artery, but that might result in the cystic duct stump syndrome. Possibly the answer is to make every effort to clip the cystic duct near the common duct so that there is little cystic duct to necrose.

J.F. Amaral, M.D.

Management of Bile Leaks After Laparoscopic Cholecystectomy

Barton JR, Russell RCG, Hatfield ARW (Middlesex Hosp, London)
Br J Surg 82:980–984, 1995   10–24

Introduction.—The rise of laparoscopic cholecystectomy has focused new attention on the problem of bile duct injuries. It has been suggested that the new operation increases the risk of bile duct damage, although the evidence for this claim is debatable. Many cholecystectomy-related bile duct injuries can be managed endoscopically. A review of bile duct injuries occurring after laparoscopic cholecystectomy and their management is reported.

Methods.—From 1991 to 1993, the authors' unit performed a total of 4,039 endoscopic retrograde cholangiopancreatography procedures, 2,838 of which were therapeutic. The study period covered a time during which most surgeons in the area were learning laparoscopic cholecystectomy. All procedures were entered prospectively into a computerized database, which was reviewed to identify patients with a biliary problem after laparoscopic cholecystectomy. Records of these cases were reviewed to identify their history, diagnosis, treatment, and outcomes.

Patients.—Twenty-four patients with bile leaks after laparoscopic cholecystectomy were identified. The initial operations were considered to be complicated in 16 cases. Eleven patients had injuries to the cystic duct alone, 5 had complete hepatic duct obstruction, and 8 had high bile duct leaks. Endoscopic management consisting of stenting in 7 cases and sphincterotomy in 4 was successful in all patients with cystic duct leaks. For the patients with complete obstruction, endoscopic or percutaneous techniques were used to manage postoperative problems in 2 cases and to prepare for surgery in 3 cases. All 8 patients with high bile duct leaks were managed endoscopically, 7 by stenting and 1 by sphincterotomy. Healing appeared to be better with stenting than with sphincterotomy alone. None of the patients died. At 3 months' to 3 years' follow-up, all patients but 1 had normal biliary function.

Conclusions.—Bile duct injuries are relatively uncommon in patients undergoing laparoscopic cholecystectomy. When such injuries are suspected, they should be managed by a combination of interventional radiology and endoscopic intervention techniques. Only patients with complete obstruction of the biliary tree are likely to need surgery. When stenting is performed for bile duct leaks, it seems best to leave the stent in place for 2 months before removing it.

▶ This study by Barton and colleagues is one of a growing list of retrospective or prospective nonrandomized studies that provide data to support the contention that all bile leaks after laparoscopic cholecystectomy require management by a combination of interventional radiology and endoscopy. As is the case in all previous studies, there are no data to show the failure of other methods, most notably relaparoscopic intervention, no comparison of length of hospital stays among various potential modalities, and most importantly, a bias that interventional radiologic and endoscopic techniques are *interventions* that the authors do not consider *surgery.*

Our personal experience is that most bile leaks following laparoscopic surgery are most efficaciously treated by an initial diisopropyliminodiacetic acid (DISIDA) scan. If the scan shows an intact biliary system with a leak, the patient is relaparoscoped, at which time the site of the leak is found, repaired, and drained. Patients treated in such a manner are discharged 1 to 2 days following the laparoscopy. The presence of biliary discontinuity on DISIDA scan requires endoscopic retrograde cholangiopancreatography (ERCP) to determine the location of the injury and stenting of the distal duct for intraoperative recognition. Therefore, although the approach the authors recommend will work, the reader should consider other alternatives that will reduce pain, suffering, and hospitalization for the patient. Furthermore, let's stop kidding ourselves that ERCP is less of an intervention than a laparoscopy.

J.F. Amaral, M.D.

Symptomatic Outcome 1 Year After Laparoscopic and Minilaparotomy Cholecystectomy: A Randomized Trial
McMahon AJ, Ross S, Baxter JN, Russell IT, Anderson JR, Morran CG, Sunderland GT, Galloway DJ, O'Dwyer PJ (Univ of Aberdeen, Scotland; Southern Gen Hosp, Glasgow, Scotland; Gartnavel Gen Hosp, Glasgow, Scotland; et al)
Br J Surg 82:1378–1382, 1995   10–25

Background.—Symptomatic improvement occurs in 90% of the patients undergoing cholecystectomy, but approximately 33% have continued symptoms. Although laparoscopic cholecystectomy has become the technique of choice for the treatment of symptomatic cholelithiasis, the long-term outcomes of laparoscopic and open cholecystectomy have not been compared. The symptomatic outcome 1 year after surgery was assessed in patients undergoing laparoscopic and minilaparotomy cholecystectomy.

Methods.—All patients undergoing elective cholecystectomy for symptomatic cholelithiasis at 5 hospitals were eligible for random assignment to treatment with either laparoscopic or minilaparotomy cholecystectomy. One year after surgery, questionnaires assessing symptomatic outcome were sent to participating patients. The questionnaires addressed quality of life, general health, anxiety, and depression.

Results.—A total of 299 patients were randomized to minilaparotomy (148 patients) or laparoscopy (151 patients). The 2 groups had similar indications for surgery and duration of symptoms. Conversion to open cholecystectomy was required in 10% of the laparoscopy group and 9% of the minilaparotomy group. Complication rates were similar in the 2 groups. At least 90% of both groups reported symptomatic benefit. Nevertheless, more than half of the patients reported abdominal pain, about a quarter reported flatulence, and about a quarter reported dyspepsia. The laparoscopic cholecystectomy group reported nonsignificantly more epigastric pain and significantly more heartburn, and the laparotomy group reported nonsignificantly more right upper quadrant pain. Complete symptomatic relief was reported by 64% of the patients with severe preoperative pain but only 41% of those with mild preoperative pain. Of the 20 patients with a poor outcome, only 1 had rated the outcome as poor at 3 months after surgery. These patients had a high rate of complications, lower general health perception, greater postoperative limitations, poorer social functioning, and higher anxiety and depression scores than those with a good outcome.

Conclusions.—Although there are clear short-term advantages associated with laparoscopic cholecystectomy, when compared with minilaparotomy cholecystectomy, long-term symptomatic improvement is not superior with laparoscopy. Cholecystectomy may bring less symptomatic improvement in patients with mild symptoms than in patients with severe symptoms preoperatively.

▶ This randomized controlled analysis of 299 patients for laparoscopic cholecystectomy vs. minilaparotomy for cholecystectomy evaluated symptoms via a questionnaire in a high proportion of contactable patients. Expectantly, patients who acknowledged a "poor outcome" were found more commonly to have suffered postoperative complications; therefore, these patients had lower quality-of-life scores. Of interest, the patients with poor outcome reports also had a higher depression score and a higher anxiety index. The significant short-term advantages of laparoscopic cholecystectomy over minilaparotomy cholecystectomy will no doubt be differentiated in the next decade of prospective analyses. The study further confirms that patients exhibiting mild symptoms are less likely to benefit from cholecystectomy (with either technique) than are those who have severe symptoms, which is of no surprise to the readership. Patient-directed options and cost-effective implications will almost surely determine the technical approaches available to surgeons treating individuals with symptomatic cholelithiasis.

K.I. Bland, M.D.

Involvement of Platelet Activation Factor in Microcirculatory Disturbances After Global Hepatic Ischemia
Minor T, Isselhard W, Yamaguchi T (Univ of Cologne, Germany)
J Surg Res 58:536–540, 1995   10–26

Introduction.—Recent evidence suggests that early microcirculatory failure upon postischemic reperfusion may play a pivotal role in liver transplantation. It is likely that platelet activating factor (PAF) is involved in the pathophysiologic processes during ischemia/reperfusion of the liver because of its proinflammatory effects and contraction of the isolated

Moving?

I'd like to receive my *Year Book of Surgery* without interruption.
Please note the following change of address, effective:

Name: _____

New Address: _____

_____

City: _____ State: _____ Zip: _____

Old Address: _____

_____

City: _____ State: _____ Zip: _____

Reservation Card

Yes, I would like my own copy of *Year Book of Surgery*. Please begin my subscription with the current edition according to the terms described below.* I understand that I will have 30 days to examine each annual edition. If satisfied, I will pay just $70.95 plus sales tax, postage and handling (price subject to change without notice).

Name: _____

Address: _____

City: _____ State: _____ Zip: _____

Method of Payment
○ Visa   ○ Mastercard   ○ AmEx   ○ Bill me   ○ Check (in US dollars, payable to Mosby, Inc.)

Card number: _____ Exp date: _____

Signature: _____

LS-0908

*Your *Year Book* Service Guarantee:

When you subscribe to the *Year Book*, we'll send you an advance notice of future volumes about two months before they publish. This automatic notice system is designed to take up as little of your time as possible. If you do not want the *Year Book*, the advance notice makes it quick and easy for you to let us know your decision, and you will always have at least 20 days to decide. If we don't hear from you, we'll send you the new volume as soon as it's available. And, of course, the *Year Book* is yours to examine free of charge for 30 days (postage, handling and applicable sales tax are added to each shipment.).

BUSINESS REPLY MAIL
FIRST CLASS MAIL   PERMIT No. 762   CHICAGO, IL

POSTAGE WILL BE PAID BY ADDRESSEE

Chris Hughes
Mosby-Year Book, Inc.
200 N. LaSalle Street
Suite 2600
Chicago, IL 60601-9981

NO POSTAGE
NECESSARY
IF MAILED
IN THE
UNITED STATES

portal vein. The effects of antagonism of PAF were observed in male Wistar rats to determine whether they modified the postischemic micro-circulation of the liver and how much vascular endothelial and parenchymal hepatocellular integrity could be improved.

Methods.—Rats were anesthetized and the common bile duct cannulated with polyethylene tubing and divided distally. Blood flow to the left and median liver lobes was interrupted for 60 minutes by cross-clamping the corresponding vessels with a vascular clamp. An IV injection of 5 mg/kg of body mass of the PAF-antagonist BN52021 was given in saline solution to the treatment group before induction of liver ischemia. Reperfusion was started by removal of the clamp and lasted 30 minutes. Animals were sacrificed at the following intervals: before induction of ischemia, at the end of 60 minutes of regional hepatic ischemia in situ, or after 30 minutes of postischemic reperfusion in vivo. At each interval, the left liver lobe was freeze-clamped to acquire blood samples for biochemical assay.

Results.—Serum activities of alanine aminotransferase and purine nucleoside phosphorylase were low during the ischemic period and rose sharply upon reperfusion, with massive leakage upon restoration of blood flow (Table 1). Tissue perfusion was noted in the early reperfusion period after 60 minutes of warm ischemia in untreated livers. However, after 10 minutes of application of BN52021, significant amelioration of erythrocyte flux occurred, nearly to control values. High amounts of peroxidase activity, indicating notable neutrophil infiltration into the liver tissue, was observed in untreated livers. This was significantly reduced but not eliminated by antagonization of PAF. During ischemia, tissue adenosine triphosphate (ATP) fell to very low levels in the treated and untreated groups. However, ATP tissue concentrations at the end of reperfusion were 50% higher in the treated than the untreated group. Although the levels did not reach significance, the sum of adenine nucleotides was also higher in the treated than the untreated group after reperfusion. A significant increase in

TABLE 1.—Liver Tissue Levels of Adenosine Triphosphate and the Sum of Adenine Nucleotides In Situ, at the End of 60 Minutes of Normothermic Ischemia, and at the End of a Consecutive 30-Minute Reperfusion Period

	In Situ ($n \geq 6$)	Ischemia ($n = 3$)	Reperfusion ($n \geq 6$)
ATP (μmol/g dry mass)			
Untreated		0.58 ± 0.11	4.03 ± 1.37
	10.30 ± 0.78		
BN52021		0.67 ± 0.34	$6.12 \pm 1.73^*$
SAN (μmol/g/dry mass)			
Untreated		8.75 ± 0.61	9.42 ± 1.29
	15.44 ± 0.88		
BN52021		8.53 ± 1.81	10.9 ± 1.10

* $P < 0.05$ vs. untreated.
Abbreviations: ATP, adenosine triphosphate; *SAN*, sum of adenine nucleotides.
(Courtesy of Minor T, Isselhard W, Yamaguchi T: Involvement of platelet activation factor in microcirculatory disturbances after global hepatic ischemia. *J Surg Res* 58:536–540, 1995.)

hepatic bile production after reperfusion was observed in the treated group as compared with the untreated group.

Conclusion.—Upon reperfusion, a significant improvement in hepatic global recovery was observed in rat livers treated with the PAF antagonist BN52021. The use of PAF-antagonizing approaches should be considered for clinical use in liver surgery.

▶ This study is one of the first to analyze the involvement of platelet activating factor in ischemia/reperfusion injury of the liver. In a rat model a specific platelet activating factor antagonist, BN52021, resulted in a significant reduction in postischemic enzyme loss into the serum from the vascular endothelium and the hepatic parenchyma. The authors also demonstrated a significant increase in hepatic bile production and tissue levels of ATP. Laser Doppler flowmetry revealed a significant improvement in erythrocyte flux. This study is one of the first to provide evidence implicating platelet activating factor in ischemia/reperfusion damage to the vascular endothelium, and the results are presumably due to altered microvascular reperfusion. This study fits nicely with the concept that platelet activating factor also plays a significant role in nonocclusive mesenteric ischemia and suggests that future therapies with platelet activating factor antagonists should be employed; however, to the best of my knowledge to date, no prospective randomized clinical trials have been performed in man in the area of ischemia/reperfusion in utilizing platelet activating factor inhibitors.

H.H. Simms, M.D.

Selective Distal Splenorenal Shunts for Intractable Variceal Bleeding in Pediatric Portal Hypertension
Evans S, Stovroff M, Heiss K, Ricketts R (Emory Univ, Atlanta, Ga)
J Pediatr Surg 30:1115–1118, 1995   10–27

Introduction.—During the past decade, endoscopic sclerotherapy has emerged as the treatment of choice for children with hemorrhagic portal hypertension. Because of the efficacy of sclerotherapy, only children with refractory hemorrhage are managed with surgical shunting. A 10-year experience with surgical shunting used for the emergent care of such children is reported.

Methods.—The medical records of all children who underwent porto-systemic shunting for intractable hemorrhagic portal hypertension despite extensive medical treatment between 1983 and 1994 were reviewed. Medical therapy had included restoration of blood volume, correction of the coagulopathy, splanchnic vasoconstriction, and sclerotherapy. Either a distal splenorenal shunt (DSRS) or a mesocaval shunt was used.

Results.—Ten shunts were placed in 9 patients, including 8 selective DSRS and 2 nonselective mesocaval shunts; all successfully relieved the acute hemorrhage. Six of the patients had intrahepatic disease, 2 had portal vein thrombosis, and 1 had splenic vein thrombosis. No intraoperative deaths occurred, but 2 patients with advanced disease died subsequently. Of the 9 patients, 3 underwent subsequent orthotopic liver transplantation (OLT), after which 1 died. In 1 child with a mesocaval shunt, fulminant hepatic failure and profound encephalopathy developed several weeks after the procedure. In no patients with selective shunting did encephalopathy develop.

Discussion.—Distal splenorenal shunt have a role in the management of children with emergent hemorrhagic portal hypertension. Benefits include a low rate of hepatic encephalopathy and rebleeding and preservation of liver function. A DSRS can often be life-sustaining in patients awaiting OLT because it avoids the porta hepatis, unlike nonselective shunts.

▶ The division of pediatric surgery at Emory reminds us that portosystemic shunts still have a place in the treatment of children with portal hypertension. Not surprisingly, they favor the Warren shunt; others have advocated mesocaval interposition grafts, particularly in small children. While this series tries to revive shunt operations, it is also a testimony to their demise: less than 1 procedure a year. Now that both less (sclerotherapy) and more aggressive (liver transplantation) options exist, few centers can report a very large experience (the recently published papers by Drs. Orloff notwithstanding). In their conclusion, the authors point out a new role for portosystemic shunts: as a bridge to transplantation.

F.I. Luks, M.D.

Outcomes of Ileocolic Conduit for Biliary Drainage in Infants With Biliary Atresia: Comparison With Roux-en-Y Type Reconstruction

Endo M, Watanabe K, Hirabayashi T, Ikawa H, Yokoyama J, Kitajima M (Keio Univ, Tokyo)
J Pediatr Surg 30:700–704, 1995   10–28

Introduction.—This study compares the complication rate and long-term outcome in infants treated for biliary atresia with an ileocolic conduit as opposed to Roux-en-Y reconstruction. An ileocolic conduit was created in 24 infants (IC group), with the proximal end of a 30-cm portion of ileum anastomosed to the porta hepatis and the distal 10 cm of the ascending colon vented to the abdominal wall. The other 16 infants received a 40- to 60-cm Roux-en-Y hepatoportoenterostomy (RY group), 5 of which featured a double Roux-en-Y and a Suruga II diverting stoma. At 1 year, if the patients had no further episodes of cholangitis, both complete and partial diverting conduits were internalized. In the IC group, an end-to-side anastomosis of the colonic end of the ileocolic conduit with the second segment of duodenum was performed. In the RY group, the stomal limb of the double Roux-en-Y was resected and closed and the Suruga II diverting stoma was attached to the distal limb. The biliary atresia prognostic index (BAPI) was used to score the condition of the

TABLE 2.—Postoperative Outcomes

	Ileocolic Conduit (n = 23)	Roux-en-Y (n = 16)
Bile excretion obtained	23 (100%)	16 (100%)
Jaundice disappeared	20 (87.0%)	10 (62.5%)
Current survival	15 (65.2%)	7 (43.8%)

(Courtesy of Endo M, Watanabe K, Kirabayashi T, et al: Outcomes of ileocolic conduit for biliary drainage in infants with biliary atresia: Comparison with Roux-en-Y type reconstruction. *J Pediatr Surg* 30:700–704, 1995.)

patients on 4- to 15-year follow-up, as well a Z score that factored in height and weight. Postoperative cholangitis was defined as high fever without an obvious source, with or without decreased hepatic function.

Results.—Bile excretion was obtained in 100% of the infants studied (Table 2). However, only 87.0% in the IC group and 62.5% in the RY group became anicteric. On follow-up, the survival rate was 65.2% in the IC group and 43.8% in the RY group. The incidence of cholangitis after stomal closure was 53.3% in the IC group vs. 83.3% in RY patients who had a partial or complete diverting stoma and 70% in RY patients without a stoma. The incidence of cholangitis thereafter tended to diminish with time in both groups. In 53.3% of the 4-year survivors in the IC group there was a BAPI of less than 25, as opposed to 28.6% in a similar segment of the RY group. As regards physical development, both groups showed a pattern of decreased height relative to weight, with both parameters far below normal.

Discussion.—The persistence of episodic cholangitis in both study groups, even during periods of complete diversion, suggests that the mechanism of this infection may be more complicated than simple ascension of intestinal loop bacteria into the biliary system. Antireflux procedures appear to alleviate the morbidity of these infections rather than eradicate them. Regarding long-term outcome, the ileocolic conduit offered improved survival and lower biliary atresia prognostic indices than did the Roux-en-Y procedures.

▶ Cholangitis with biliary atresia is probably as much a factor of poor bile flow as enteric reflux into the bile ducts. Certainly, complete diversion of bile flow did not eradicate cholangitis in the present series (if anything, it made it worse: 87% vs. 70%). In spite of this, many surgeons still interpose 1 or more anticholangitis barriers (diverting stoma, intussuscepted valve, or as shown here, the ileocecal valve). The results reported herein are excellent (62% to 87% long-term resolution of jaundice) but cannot convincingly be attributed solely to this ileocecal conduit.

F.I. Luks, M.D.

Identification of K-*ras* Mutations in Pancreatic Juice in the Early Diagnosis of Pancreatic Cancer

Berthélemy P, Bouisson M, Escourrou J, Vaysse N, Rumeau JL, Pradayrol L
(Institut Natl de la Santé et de la Recherche Médicale, Toulouse, France)
Ann Intern Med 123:188–191, 1995   10–29

Introduction.—Pancreatic malignancy is usually diagnosed in the advanced stage. The development of new early diagnostic assays for this fifth leading cause of death from cancer would be welcome. A high incidence of activating point mutations of the K-*ras* 12th codon has been observed in large groups of pancreatic tumors. Pure pancreatic juice collected during endoscopic retrograde cholangiopancreatography was collected to evaluate the diagnostic value of identification of K-*ras* mutations in differentiating benign from malignant pancreatic disease.

Methods.—Endoscopic ductal aspiration of cells or brush cytology was done on the following patients undergoing endoscopic retrograde cholangiopancreatography for diagnostic or therapeutic reasons: group 1, 24 patients with no pancreatic disease; group 2, 29 patients with nontumoral pancreatic disease; and group 3, 22 patients with pancreatic tumor. K-*ras* genes were analyzed by polymerase chain reaction (PCR)-mediated restriction fragment length polymorphism and direct sequencing.

Results.—All group 1 and group 2 patients had a normal sequence for the K-*ras* 12th codon. Seventeen of 22 patients in group 3 had mutations. Two of these 17 patients with a mutation of the K-*ras* 12th codon had no evidence of pancreatic cancer at the first examination. However, pancreatic tumors developed in both 18 and 40 months, respectively, after PCR analysis.

Conclusion.—This investigation gives the first direct evidence that K-*ras* mutation occurs early in the development of pancreatic cancer. Further analysis is needed, but identification of K-*ras* mutations in samples of pancreatic juice may prove useful in differentiating between pancreatic cancer and noncancerous pancreatic diseases.

▶ This interesting paper proposes yet another clinical application of genetic mutational analysis in the diagnosis and treatment of cancer patients. Our laboratory has demonstrated the correlation between K-*ras* mutations and prognosis in pancreatic cancer. K-*ras* mutations have been identified in fecal samples and might be of use in early detection of colorectal cancer. One limiting factor is the relatively low occurrence of such mutations, which would lead to high specificity but potentially low sensitivity in the early diagnosis of pancreatic cancer.

V.E. Pricolo, M.D.

Quality of Life, Nutritional Status, and Gastrointestinal Hormone Profile Following the Whipple Procedure

McLeod RS, Taylor BR, O'Connor BI, Greenberg GR, Jeejeebhoy KN, Royall D, Langer B (Univ of Toronto)
Am J Surg 169:179–185, 1995   10–30

Introduction.—There is a perception that the Whipple procedure is associated with a high mortality and morbidity rate despite a mortality rate of 0% to 5%. An investigation was done to evaluate the quality of life, nutritional status, and gastrointestinal hormone profile of 25 patients who underwent the Whipple procedure.

Methods.—The control group consisted of patients who underwent a cholecystectomy. Instruments for measuring quality of life were the Time Trade-Off Technique (to estimate the utility of a given health state as perceived by the general public), Direct Questioning of Objectives, Gastrointestinal Quality of Life Index, Sickness Impact Profile, Physician Global Assessment, and the Visick Scale. Nutritional assessment was determined by the Subjective Global Assessment, skinfold anthropometry, and height and weight. Blood glucose and gastrointestinal hormones were measured.

Results.—No patients in the control group required a reoperation, but 2 patients in the Whipple group required surgery for wound dehiscence and biliary fistula, respectively. Slightly more patients in the Whipple group than the control group experienced heartburn and greasy bowel movements and were restricted in the quantity of food they could ingest. One patient in each group complained of mild early or late dumping. Scores from both groups, not significantly different, indicated near normal well-being. Fasting, peak postprandial, and integrated release of plasma gastrin was significantly lower in patients undergoing the standard Whipple procedure than in those in the pylorus-sparing Whipple and control groups. Patients in both Whipple groups had significantly lower fasting concentrations of serum pancreatic polypeptide than did controls.

Conclusion.—Long-term studies of patients with a Whipple procedure have focused on survival, not quality of life. Patients in this series had nearly normal well-being and good nutritional status. Most gastrointestinal symptoms are mild and infrequent.

▶ Is the cure worse than the disease? This is the question asked by these authors in regard to pancreaticoduodenectomy. The importance of the assessment of the quality of life following surgical procedures is now well recognized. This article demonstrates that not only can Whipple procedures be performed with relatively low mortality, but one can also expect excellent quality of life and nutritional status following this procedure. The authors are to be commended for undertaking this study and for their excellent results.

W.G. Cioffi, M.D.

Hypercalcemia Causes Acute Pancreatitis by Pancreatic Secretory Block, Intracellular Zymogen Accumulation, and Acinar Cell Injury

Frick TW, Mithöfer K, Castillo CF, Rattner DW, Warshaw AL (Univ of Zurich Hosp, Switzerland; Massachusetts Gen Hosp, Boston)
Am J Surg 169:167–172, 1995   10–31

Background.—Acute pancreatitis can be caused by hypercalcemia. To investigate the pathophysiology and pathomorphology of pancreatitis, hypercalcemia was induced in rats, followed by examination of the histochemical changes that occurred in that state.

Methods.—Eight Wistar rats were administered an infusion of 0.6 mmol/kg/hr of $CaCl_2$ or physiologic saline over a 12-hour period. After infusion, some pancreatic tissue was removed, stained, and examined under a JEOL 100-CX electron microscope; the remaining pancreatic tissue was homogenated and examined for DNA, lactate dehydrogenase (LDH), protein, amylase, and calcium content. Pancreatic juice was har-

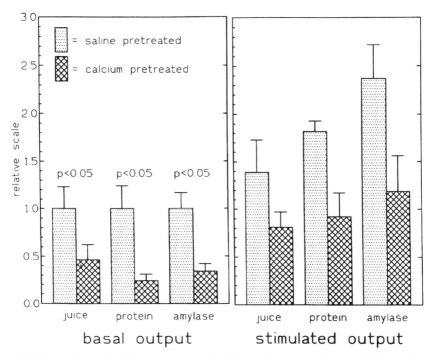

FIGURE 3.—Pancreatic juice volume, pancreatic juice protein output, and pancreatic juice amylase output of rats after 12 hours of calcium infusion (n = 4, *hatched bars*) and controls (n = 4, *dotted bars*). **Left,** basal secretion for 1 hour. **Right,** stimulated secretion (cerulein, 0.25 µg/kg) for 1 hour. Results are expressed as relative changes as compared with control values of basal secretion (control values = 1, mean ± SEM). Differences in the hourly volume, protein output, and amylase output during basal secretion are statistically significant. (Reprinted by permission of the publisher from Frick TW, Mithöfer K, Castillo CF, et al: Hypercalcemia causes acute pancreatitis by pancreatic secretory block, intracellular zymogen accumulation, and acinar cell injury. *Am J Surg* 169:167–172, Copyright 1995 by Excerpta Medica Inc.)

vested for biochemical determinations of volume, protein, amylase output, and protein composition by gel electrophoresis. Data were interpreted with the two-tailed Student's t test.

Results.—When compared with saline-treated rats, pancreatic tissue harvested from calcium-treated rats exhibited structural changes. The acinar cells were filled with zymogen granules from the apical region to the basolateral space. Also evident were cell alterations such as chromatin clumping and cytosolic vacuole formation. In some cases, the cell structure was so disrupted that it was not visible. Although there is no significant difference in the DNA and LDH contents and ratios that occurred between groups, the protein/DNA and amylase/DNA ratios were higher in calcium-treated rats. Animals receiving calcium had lower basal secretion of pancreatic juice (Fig 3). Total calcium was not affected by pretreatment.

Discussion.—Pancreatic secretion is inhibited by a long (12-hour) infusion of calcium, similar to the hyperstimulation of the pancreas that occurs with cerulein administration. This finding suggests that hyperstimulation of the pancreas by hypercalcemia may be the pathogenetic mechanism of acute pancreatitis.

▶ These authors investigated the role of hypercalcemia in contributing to the pathomorphology and pathophysiologic changes associated with acute pancreatitis. In a rat animal model, animals were randomized to receive either calcium chloride or saline with subsequent examinations of pancreatic tissue and pancreatic exocrine output. The authors demonstrated that the tissue calcium content and ratio of lactate dehydrogenase to DNA was unchanged after calcium infusion but that the ratios of total protein to DNA and amylase to DNA were significantly larger. Of importance, ultrastructural examination demonstrated an accumulation of zymogen granules in the acinar cells, large autophagic granules containing remnants of condensing vacuoles. Their findings support the hypothesis that hypercalcemia induces pancreatic injury via a secretory block, accumulation of secretory proteins, and possibly activation of proteases. In my opinion, this study further supports the concept that patients with asymptomatic hypercalcemia secondary to hyperparathyroidism should clearly have a parathyroidectomy to lower their calcium levels as acute hypercalcemia appears to contribute to the pathophysiologic changes associated with acute pancreatitis.

H.H. Simms, M.D.

Timing of Laparoscopic Surgery in Gallstone Pancreatitis
Tang E, Stain SC, Tang G, Froes E, Berne TV (Univ of Southern California, Los Angeles)
Arch Surg 130:496–500, 1995   10–32

Patients.—The results of laparoscopic cholecystectomy were reviewed in 126 women and 16 men with gallstone pancreatitis who underwent the procedure in 1991–1993. Serum amylase averaged 1,616 U/L at the time of admission. The patients, whose average age was 39.5 years, all had surgery more than 48 hours after admission when the pancreatitis had resolved. Twenty-five patients had endoscopic retrograde cholangiopancreatography preoperatively, and common duct stones were removed in 10 cases.

Results.—Of 20 patients who had severe pancreatitis on the basis of 3 or more of Ranson's criteria, 9 had laparoscopic cholecystectomy attempted within a week after being admitted. Conversion to open surgery was necessary in 6 of these 9 patients. The 11 other patients with severe disease were operated on more than a week after admission, and only 2 of them required open cholecystectomy. The postoperative stay was significantly shorter when surgery was delayed (2.3 vs. 5.4 days). The timing of surgery did not influence the postoperative stay in patients with less severe pancreatitis. Management of 8 of these patients (6.6%) was converted to open surgery.

Conclusion.—Laparoscopic cholecystectomy may be safely performed after acute gallstone pancreatitis has resolved. If severe pancreatitis is present, the procedure should be delayed for at least 1 week.

▶ As one would expect, the advent of laparoscopic surgery has not changed the natural history of biliary gallstone disease and its complications. However, the availability of the laparoscopic technique has certainly increased the frequency of laparoscopic cholecystectomies performed around the world. As one might expect, patients with more severe pancreatitis did not do well if operated on within the first week after intervention. There is ample evidence that suggests that these patients might benefit from early ERCP and papillotomy within the first 24–48 hours of hospitalization.

V.E. Pricolo, M.D.

CT Diagnosis of Pancreatic Injury in Children: Significance of Fluid Separating the Splenic Vein and the Pancreas

Sivit CJ, Eichelberger MR (Children's Natl Med Ctr, Washington, DC; Case Western Reserve Univ, Cleveland, Ohio)
AJR Am J Roentgenol 165:921–924, 1995   10–33

Background.—It has been proposed that the presence of fluid between the pancreas and the splenic vein on CT scanning is a sensitive measure of pancreatic injury. Nevertheless, a number of children without such injury have had fluid in the anterior pararenal space.

Objective.—Contrast CT findings were reviewed in 25 children with confirmed injuries of the pancreas, often the result of a motor vehicle accident. Twenty-nine other children who were evaluated after blunt trauma had fluid in the anterior pararenal space but no evidence of pancreatic injury.

Findings.—Fifteen of the 25 children with pancreatic injury (60%) had fluid separating the splenic vein and pancreas. All of them had further

CT-detected changes associated with injury, which in all cases but 1 included fluid in the anterior pararenal space. Twelve of the 15 children had laceration or transection of the pancreatic parenchyma, and 8 had fluid in the lesser sac. All but 3 of the 10 children without fluid separating the splenic vein and pancreas also had CT evidence of pancreatic injury. Fourteen of the children without pancreatic injury (48%) had fluid separating the splenic vein and pancreas in addition to fluid in the anterior pararenal space. All of them also had other CT abnormalities, and 6 had injury to the spleen, liver, and/or kidney.

Discussion.—When fluid is present for any reason in the anterior pararenal space surrounding the pancreas, it may dissect between the pancreas and the splenic vein. Pancreatic injury is one cause of fluid at this site, but not the only one. Hypovolemic shock and injury to a solid intraperitoneal viscus are other possibilities. This finding by itself is not a reliable indicator of pancreatic injury.

▶ Computed tomography may be the best there is, but it is less than perfect for the diagnosis of retroperitoneal injuries—and this coming from one of the leading institutions in pediatric trauma imaging!

F.I. Luks, M.D.

Splenic Preservation in the Management of Splenic Epidermoid Cysts in Children
Tsakayannis DE, Mitchell K, Kozakewich HPW, Shamberger RC (Harvard Med School, Boston)
J Pediatr Surg 30:1468–1470, 1995   10–34

Background.—Splenic cysts in general are relatively rare. In areas where hydatid disease is endemic, most true cysts are parasitic in origin. One fourth of nonparasitic cysts are congenital epidermoid lesions; they are seen mainly in children. Conventionally these cysts are managed by splenectomy, but conservation of the spleen has increasingly been adopted as complications of splenectomy in children are recognized.

Series.—Nineteen children with congenital splenic cysts were encountered in the years 1914–1993. The 10 girls and 9 boys had a median age of 12 years.

Clinical Aspects.—Five of the cysts were incidental findings; 2 patients had a history of trauma. Eleven children had abdominal pain and 9 had a mass. All symptomatic children had a cyst exceeding 8 cm in size. None of the children had cyst-related complications. Nine children in whom splenic cysts were diagnosed before 1973 underwent total splenectomy. Two of those seen since 1983 had hemisplenectomy and in 3 others the cyst was excised. In 2 cases the splenic artery was clamped during surgery. Abdominal pain consistently resolved postoperatively, and there were no complications. All 3 conservatively treated children who were reassessed 3–6 months postoperatively had continued splenic function and normal platelet counts.

Discussion.—Ultrasonography is a noninvasive, sensitive, and relatively inexpensive means of diagnosing splenic cysts in children. The best time to remove an asymptomatic epidermoid cyst remains uncertain.

▶ This (small) series of splenic preservation for epidermoid cysts confirms the feasibility of partial splenectomy and splenorrhaphy. There were no hilar cysts in this group of patients; unroofing of the cyst and marsupialization work well in these circumstances.

F.I. Luks, M.D.

Operative Strategy in Laparoscopic Splenectomy
Cadiere GB, Verroken R, Himpens J, Bruyns J, Elfira M, De Wit S (Saint-Pierre Hosp, Free Univ of Brussels, Belgium)
J Am Coll Surg 179:668–672, 1994   10–35

Introduction.—The location of the spleen in the deep recesses of the abdominal cavity make exposure difficult during laparotomy. Although the spleen can be exposed by a left thoracotomy, postoperative pain and accessory spleens are difficult to locate. The use of laparoscopy would seem to be an alternative surgical procedure.

Methods.—Over a 2-year period, 17 patients aged 11–80 years underwent laparoscopic splenectomy. The reasons for splenectomy were idiopathic thrombocytopenic purpura, HIV related, spherocytosis, necrosis of a wandering spleen, splenic polycystosis and sickle cell trait. The patients with thrombocytopenia were given high-dose immunoglobulins IV to increase their platelet count. The volume of the spleens ranged from 90 to 1,200 mL.

Technique.—General anesthesia is required. The patient is positioned supine with the legs fully abducted and the knees bent on a table with a 20-degree reversed Trendelenburg tilt and a 45-degree tilt to the right. The surgeon stands between the legs of the patient with assistants on either side of the patient. Five trocars are used (Fig 2): a 10-mm trocar above the umbilicus, a 5-mm trocar in the right subcostal region, a 5-mm trocar in the left subcostal region, a 10-mm trocar between the first and third trocars, and a 10-mm trocar under the xiphoid. Also needed are an optical system, probes to retract the liver and stomach, grasping forceps, and a coagulation hook. The second assistant (on the left) retracts the stomach. Ligaments are dissected and then the short gastric vessels are clipped. The hilar vessels are isolated and ligated separately. The spleen is placed into a plastic bag and removed through the lower left trocar site.

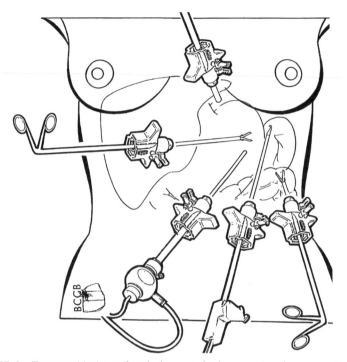

FIGURE 2.—Trocar positioning and tool placement for laparoscopic splenectomy. (Courtesy of Cadiere GB, Verroken R, Himpens J, et al: Operative strategy in laparoscopic splenectomy. *J Am Coll Surg* 179:688–672, 1994. By permission of the *Journal of the American College of Surgeons.*)

Results.—The operations lasted from 90 minutes to 6 hours, averaging 3 hours. The laparoscopic procedure had to be converted to laparotomy in 2 patients because of parenchymal bleeding. In 3 patients, injured blood vessels could be controlled laparoscopically. Only 2 patients had accessory spleens. The postoperative course was uneventful in 11 of the 15 successful procedures. There were 2 operative complications. One was an evisceration of an omental fringe and 1 was a left pneumothorax. The 2 medical complications were bronchitis and confusion with agitation. All patients had bowel sounds the first postoperative day. The hospital stay averaged 3 days, ranging from 2 to 16 days.

Comment.—Based on this series of 15 successful surgeries, there was one important technical aspect. The spleen must be fully mobilized before dissection of the hilum.

▶ These authors report a critical analysis of the operative strategy in laparoscopic splenectomy. After 15 successful laparoscopic splenectomies, the most important technical aspect seems to be full mobilization of the spleen before the hilum is dissected. The authors have provided a very nice technical approach to laparoscopic splenectomy. However, they have not addressed the important issue of splenosis. I think that the indication for a splenectomy is critically important in deciding whether or not a laparoscopic splenectomy should be performed. If one is performing a laparoscopic splenectomy for idiopathic thrombocytopenic purpura (ITP), then shedding of splenic cells is a potential complication in the peritoneal cavity with resultant splenosis and possible recurrent ITP. In contrast, if one is performing a laparoscopic splenectomy for sickle cell disease with autoinfarctions of the spleen, then shedding of splenic cells may be less important. This important issue of the shedding of splenic cells with possible resultant splenosis at long-term follow-up has not really been addressed in the laparoscopic literature and remains a potential complication of laparoscopic splenectomy.

H.H. Simms, M.D.

Pediatric Laparoscopic Splenectomy
Moores DC, McKee MA, Wang H, Fischer JD, Smith JW, Andrews HG (Loma Linda Univ, Calif; Kaiser Permanente Med Ctr, Fontana, Calif)
J Pediatr Surg 30:1201–1205, 1995
10–36

Background.—Increasing evidence shows that laparoscopic techniques can be successfully applied to children. Laparoscopic methods are associated with less postoperative pain, reduced ileus, fewer pulmonary complications, and shorter hospital stays. Such techniques also appear to be useful for elective splenectomy in patients with hematologic disease or for staging in those with Hodgkin's lymphoma. A series of laparoscopic splenectomies is described.

Methods and Findings.—Twelve children treated consecutively since 1993 were reviewed retrospectively. The patients ranged in age from 3 to 16 years. Diagnoses were hereditary spherocytosis in 5 patients, idiopathic thrombocytopenia purpura in 4, and autoimmune thrombocytopenia, β-thalassemia, and sickle cell anemia in 1 each. The outcomes of this group were compared with those of 20 children undergoing open splenectomy for a similar spectrum of diseases. Total operative time and estimated blood loss were greater in the patients undergoing laparoscopic splenectomy, although the amount of IV analgesia needed in the first 48 hours was comparable. Patients undergoing open splenectomy had significantly longer times to oral intake followed by regular diet and longer overall hospital stays. There were no long-term complications in either group.

Conclusions.—Laparoscopic splenectomy can be performed effectively, efficiently, and at a reasonable cost in the hands of experienced laparoscopic surgeons. When compared with open splenectomy, laparoscopic splenectomy has a more benign postoperative course and the potential for fewer long-term complications in children requiring splenectomy.

▶ The authors demonstrate that laparoscopic splenectomy is possible even in very young children. This is not truly a comparative study, of course, since the open splenectomy group is historical and some of the criteria (analgesia requirements, hospital stay) are subjective. When the recovery time (shorter in younger patients regardless of the approach), length of scar, blood loss, cost of the operation, technical difficulty, and learning curve are weighed against each other, one gets the sense that laparoscopic vs. open splenectomy is really the dealer's choice. There is no doubt, however, that laparoscopic splenectomy is feasible, safe, and here to stay.

F.I. Luks, M.D.

Abdomen and Small Bowel

INTRODUCTION

Increasing utilization of state-of-the-art imaging technology has enhanced diagnostic accuracy in preoperative, intraoperative, and postoperative states. The surgeon of the 1990s must have an in-depth knowledge base regarding the appropriate applications of directed imaging procedures, together with knowledge of their sensitivities and specificities for diagnostic procedures. Abstract 10–37 from the Kyorin University School of Medicine in Tokyo reports the first prospective study to evaluate sensitivity of the "streaky density" within the mesentery on abdominal CT as a diagnostic finding of ruptured small bowel following blunt abdominal trauma. This important analysis has special significance for traumatologists and general surgeons as a method for identification of occult small intestinal rupture resulting from the most common variant of trauma (blunt) in North America.

Abstracts 10–39 through 10–42 evaluate hernial and/or abdominal wall defects and their management in the adult and pediatric populations. Abstract 10–39 provides the readership with a large prospective multicenter trial of laparoscopic inguinal herniorrhaphy. The authors confirm that laparoscopic hernia repair via the transabdominal or total extraperitoneal approach effectively corrects the hernia with an acceptable complication rate. The unique presentations by Lawrence et al. and Barkun and colleagues (Abstracts 10–40 and 10–41) evaluate 2 randomized, prospective trials of the utility of laparoscopic vs. open inguinal herniorrhaphy. Unequivocally, the laparoscopic procedure is more costly in both studies; this added expense appears to have provided only a small improvement in postoperative pain with a reduction in analgesic usage. As with any "steep" learning curve, a high rate of misadventure and subsequent complications is to be expected. Deans and co-workers (Abstract 10–42) provide a review of recurrent laparoscopic hernias that confirms the previous findings of Phillips and colleagues in the larger, multicenter trial sponsored by Society of American Gastrointestinal Endoscopic Surgeons (SAGES). This abstract details the mechanisms of failure of laparoscopic herniorrhaphy, which are often similar to those identified in open hernia repairs. This important analysis reinforces the concept that the direct space must be reinforced for indirect hernia repair in all subjects, with the exception of young patients. Analysis of abdominal wall defects in infants by Tunell et al. of the University of Oklahoma (Abstract 10–43) suggests that survival rates in patients with abdominal wall defects is favorable; deaths occur mainly in patients with coexisting lethal or multiple congenital anomalies. These authors recount the important observation that re-operative surgery is necessary principally for individuals who have post-closure abdominal wall hernias and for those with bowel atresia at birth. Quality of life in survivors of major abdominal wall defects is patient perceived and entirely satisfactory in the majority. The authors emphasize that reoperations are usually unnecessary after school age.

Abstracts 10–45 through 10–48 are replete with common surgical disorders experienced in the pediatric population. The report by Misra et al. of Ireland (Abstract 10–45) suggests that transperitoneal closure of the internal ring is a reliable and safe operative approach in infants for whom the alternative inguinal approach is difficult. The authors noted that these situations include hernias that are irreducible or hernias in which dissection of the cord would risk damage to the vas deferens or the testicular vessels.

Abstract 10–46 evaluates malrotation in older children to determine proper management and outcome. Of significance, 41% of the patients were observed to have either a volvulus or internal hernia at exploration that was not clearly demonstrable by the diagnostic tests selected. Surgery was highly effective in alleviating chronic symptoms in these children, and the authors confirm that surgical therapy is clearly indicated in older children with proven malrotation. Prompt intervention eliminates the possibility for loss of bowel from volvulus or internal hernia, both of which may not be evident on diagnostic radiographic studies.

Additional management problems with small-bowel disease are reviewed in Abstracts 10–47 and 10–48. Enterostomy may be a lifesaving procedure in newborns with acute bowel perforation, obstruction, and necrosis that arise from a variety of acquired or congenital disorders. Further, a stoma may be required at any level of the gastrointestinal tract. Weber and associates of St. Louis University School of Medicine (Abstract 10–47) confirm that enterostomy is a potentially morbid condition in the newborn and is prone to complications. The authors recommend closure of the enterostomy only when the child is in satisfactory nutritional condition. In this study, 2 relatively simple measures of nutrition (percent weight gain over 30 days and serum albumin level) predicted risk for postoperative complications following stoma closure. Necrotizing enterocolitis (NEC) is currently the most common etiology of perforation of the gastrointestinal tract in the neonate. Harms et al. of the University of Göttingen, Germany (Abstract 10–48), analyze the clinical findings and course of 5 patients with idiopathic spontaneous perforation of the small bowel and compare these findings with the course seen in NEC. The excellent results of this study, given the inherent risk of operating on small premature infants, are noteworthy; this approach confirms the advisability of early diagnosis and prompt surgical intervention for salvage of these critically ill infants.

In view of the frequency of the diagnosis of acute appendicitis in both adults and infants of both genders, the increasing application of laparoscopic appendectomy requires in-depth scrutiny and is the subject of Abstracts 10–49 to 10–51. The retrospective review of nonrandomized patients by Apelgren and associates of Michigan State University (Abstract

10–49) noted increased operating time and cost for the laparoscopic group. However, hospital stay and wound infection rates were not significantly different in either group. The authors conclude in this retrospective analysis that laparoscopic appendectomy is *not* superior to the open approach. Abstracts 10–50 and 10–51 are among the first prospective randomized studies to evaluate open vs. laparoscopic appendectomy. Martin and associates of the University of Miami School of Medicine (Abstract 10–50) conclude that laparoscopic appendectomy is comparable to the open technique with regard to complications, hospital stay, cost, and return to activity and the work environment. This prospective analysis also concludes that laparoscopic appendectomy does *not* offer significant benefit over the open approach for the routine patient with suspected appendicitis. The tenet of this argument is further emphasized by Ortega et al. (Abstract 10–51) in their randomized prospective comparison. This study is somewhat biased in that the technique is performed by highly skilled laparoscopic surgeons who do not represent the expertise or experience of the *average* general surgeon in North America. The value and place of laparoscopic appendectomy will continue to be debated until there is an integration of cost-effective data, hospital length of stay, and disability outcomes to recommend its usage in treatment of the average patient with suspected appendicitis. Future prospective randomized trials conducted by multicenter study groups on a larger scale are encouraged to resolve this important issue.

Kirby I. Bland, M.D.

Early Diagnosis of Small Intestine Rupture From Blunt Abdominal Trauma Using Computed Tomography: Significance of the Streaky Density Within the Mesentery
Hagiwara A, Yukioka T, Satou M, Yoshii H, Yamamoto S, Matsuda H, Shimzazki S (Kyorin Univ, Tokyo; Japan; Saiseikai Kanagawaken Hosp, Yokohama, Japan)
J Trauma 38:630–633, 1995   10–37

Background.—Diagnoses of intestinal ruptures are often difficult in patients with a consciousness or sensory disturbance and may be delayed in patients with multiple injures. Detection of a streaky density within the mesentery on abdominal CT was prospectively evaluated for its ability to improve diagnoses of ruptured small intestines in patients experiencing blunt abdominal trauma.

Patients and Methods.—Four hundred thirty patients underwent enhanced CT within 3 hours after blunt abdominal injuries. Scanning was done in 1-cm-thick sections from the diaphragmatic dome to the pelvis. In patients with a streaky density within the mesentery, the outline of the alimentary tract was traced from the third portion of the duodenum to the end of the ileum. The position of the ruptured small intestine observed on the CT slice was compared with that noted during surgery. The CT scans were also evaluated for free air in the abdominal cavity. Clinical decisions were not based on the presence of the mesenteric sign. Rather, clinical findings and the presence of free air in the diagnostic images were used to determine whether patients should undergo surgery.

Results.—Ruptures of the small intestine were noted in 13 patients, 9 of whom had a streaky density within the mesentery. Abdominal free air was detected by CT in only 6 of the 13 patients. The sensitivity of the mesenteric sign was thus 69% as compared with 46% for free air alone. None of the patients without small intestinal rupture had a streaky density within the mesentery, yielding a specificity of 100% for this sign. The diagnostic sensitivity of small intestinal rupture by the presence of the mesenteric sign, free air, or both was 85%—significantly higher than that of free air only. In 8 of the 13 patients, ruptures were detected at a mesenteric site at surgery. In all 8 patients, the streaky density within the mesentery was noted on CT. Bleeding and cellular infiltration along the mesenteric vasculature were observed on histopathologic examination of the area with the mesenteric sign. This appearance may be associated with direct injury and chemical irritation of the mesentery resulting from intestinal rupture.

Conclusions.—The streaky density within the mesentery, which can be detected early after blunt abdominal trauma, has a high sensitivity for intestinal rupture of a mesenteric site and may be particularly useful for diagnosis in patients whose physical signs are difficult to assess.

▶ A common complaint against the routine use of CT in the evaluation of blunt abdominal trauma is its lack of sensitivity in detecting hollow viscous injury. In this small series, the sensitivity of a streaky density within the mesentery for small intestinal rupture was 69% with a 100% specificity. When this finding was used in conjunction with free air, the sensitivity increased to 85%. Although the numbers are small, such studies are important to define nuances in the use of CT in the evaluation of blunt trauma patients.

W.G. Cioffi, M.D.

Prophylactic Mesalamine Treatment Decreases Postoperative Recurrence of Crohn's Disease
McLeod RS, Wolff BG, Steinhart AH, Carryer PW, O'Rourke K, Andrews DF, Blair JE, Cangemi JR, Cohen Z, Cullen JB, Chaytor RG, Greenberg GR, Jaffer NM, Jeejeebhoy KN, MacCarty RL, Ready RL, Weiland LH (Univ of Toronto; Toronto Hosp; Mayo Clinic, Rochester, Minn; et al)
Gastroenterology 109:404–413, 1995   10–38

Background.—About 80% of patients with Crohn's disease eventually need surgery. Unfortunately, the disease often recurs after such treatment.

The value of mesalamine in reducing the risk of recurrent Crohn's disease after surgical resection was investigated.

Methods.—One hundred sixty-three patients with no evidence of residual disease after surgical resection were enrolled in the study. By random assignment, patients received 1.5 g mesalamine twice a day or placebo within 8 weeks of surgery. Maximum follow-up was 72 months.

Findings.—Symptomatic recurrence was documented in 31% of the patients in the active treatment group as compared with 41% of those in the control group. The relative risk of recurrence in the treatment group was 0.63 by an intention-to-treat analysis and 0.53 by an efficacy analysis. In addition, the endoscopic and radiologic rate of recurrence was significantly reduced, with relative risks of 0.65 and 0.64 in the 2 respective analyses. One serious side effect—pancreatitis—was documented in the mesalamine group.

Conclusions.—Mesalamine effectively reduces the symptomatic, endoscopic, and radiologic rate of recurrence after surgery for Crohn's disease. Additional research is needed to determine the best pharmacologic agents and dosage for prophylaxis and whether prophylaxis is of value in patients with residual disease after surgery.

▶ Maintenance therapy after surgical intervention for Crohn's disease has become an issue of importance. Since the aim of surgical therapy cannot be to eradicate the disease but simply to palliate its symptoms, it only follows that the disease left behind should continue to be treated. Ideally, one would want to choose a medical therapeutic regimen with minimal side effects and adequate tolerance for long-term maintenance.

V.E. Pricolo, M.D.

Laparoscopic Inguinal Herniorrhaphy: Results of a Multicenter Trial
Fitzgibbons RJ Jr, Camps J, Cornet DA, Nguyen NX, Litke BS, Annibali R, Salerno GM (Creighton Univ, Omaha, Neb)
Ann Surg 221:3–13, 1995   10–39

Introduction.—Several laparoscopic procedures have been developed in the wake of the successful introduction of laparoscopic cholecystectomy. However, there is considerable controversy regarding the benefits of laparoscopic inguinal herniorrhaphy. The feasibility of this procedure was investigated in a phase II trial in order to assess the need for a prospective randomized controlled trial comparing it with conventional hernia repair.

Methods.—A total of 686 patients with 869 hernias underwent hernia repair at 19 institutions and were followed for more than 1 year. The 21 investigators chose 1 of 3 standardized laparoscopic techniques: transabdominal preperitoneal laparoscopic inguinal herniorrhaphy, intraperitoneal onlay mesh laparoscopic herniorrhaphy, or totally extraperitoneal laparoscopic herniorrhaphy.

Results.—Only 1 laparoscopic procedure required a change to open repair because of an intraoperative complication. The mean operating times were 70 minutes for unilateral repair and 90.6 minutes for bilateral repairs. There was no significant difference in length of stay among the 3 procedures, with most patients (93%) discharged within 24 hours after surgery. There were complications related to laparoscopy in 5.4% of the patients, including episodes of bleeding in 24, abdominal wall hematomas in 8, bowel perforation in 1, and bladder laceration requiring open repair in 1 patient. There were patient complications in 6.7%; most of them were urinary difficulties (5.8%), including dysfunction, retention, or infection. Herniorrhaphy complications occurred in 17.1% and included groin, testicular, or leg pain, seroma with or without aspiration, groin hematoma, hydrocele, wound infection, prosthesis infection, and transection of the vas deferens. The incidence of leg pain was related to the surgeon's laparoscopic experience. There was a recurrence rate of 4.5%.

Conclusions.—Laparoscopic inguinal herniorrhaphy is effective and safe and has a low early failure rate. However, a small number of patients may require a second abdominal procedure to treat complications. A randomized prospective controlled trial comparing the results of laparoscopic and conventional repair of inguinal hernias is warranted.

▶ Fitzgibbons and colleagues provide us with the second large prospective multicenter trial of laparoscopic inguinal herniorrhaphy. The conclusions are similar to those of the Society of American Gastrointestinal Endoscopic Surgeons (SAGES) study in that laparoscopic hernia repair via the transabdominal or totally extraperitoneal approach effectively corrects the hernia with an acceptable complication rate. The unmentioned caveat to these conclusions is that this is true when performed by highly skilled laparoscopic surgeons with a large experience, which is the case in this and the SAGES study. The study also raises 2 very important and disturbing findings. First and foremost is the need for laparotomy in fewer than 1% of the patients and, second, the high incidence of nerve injury during the laparoscopic approach. The former problem may be resolved in the future by use of the totally extraperitoneal approach, which does not enter the abdomen, and the latter may be eliminated by the surgeon gaining more experience with the anatomy of the area.

Although the authors call for a controlled randomized trial comparing the laparoscopic approach with the open method, such a study is fraught with difficulties such as establishing the open hernia repair to be used as a standard, what the surgeon's experience level should be, how to truly blind the study so that biases can be eliminated, and making the study of large enough size and duration to quiet critics.

J.F. Amaral, M.D.

Randomised Controlled Trial of Laparoscopic Versus Open Repair of Inguinal Hernia: Early Results

Lawrence K, McWhinnie D, Goodwin A, Doll H, Gordon A, Gray A, Britton J, Collin J (Univ of Oxford, England)
BMJ 311:981–985, 1995

10–40

Introduction.—Because open herniorrhaphy can be performed on an outpatient basis and rarely causes severe pain or morbidity, the benefits of laparoscopic herniorrhaphy are unclear and controversial. The safety, short-term outcome, and cost of laparoscopic and conventional repair of inguinal hernia were compared.

Methods.—A total of 124 patients with a primary, unilateral inguinal hernia were randomly assigned to treatment with either laparoscopic transabdominal preperitoneal prosthetic mesh repair or the 2-layer modified Maloney darn. The rate of short-term complications was the primary measure of safety. In addition, pain scores and the use of analgesics were recorded for the first 7 postoperative days, and quality of life was assessed at 10 days and 6 weeks after surgery. The costs of the 2 procedures were compared.

Results.—Postoperative complications occurred in 7 patients (12%) in the laparoscopic group and in 1 patient (2%) in the open repair group. The laparoscopic repair group had significantly lower pain scores during movement and coughing, but not at rest. Findings at 10 days and 6 weeks indicated that pain diminished most rapidly in the laparoscopic group. There was no statistically significant difference in the median time to return to work or normal activity. The mean operating time was substantially longer for laparoscopic than for open repair (72 vs. 32 minutes). The total surgical costs were significantly greater for laparoscopic than for open repair, largely because of differences in operating time and the use of consumable materials.

Discussion.—When compared with open repair, laparoscopic repair of inguinal hernia is associated with reduced postoperative muscular pain and improved quality of life. However, the risk of short-term complications was greater with the laparoscopic procedure, which also had higher costs. Before laparoscopic hernia repair is adopted widely, further studies should evaluate long-term recurrence.

Laparoscopic Versus Open Inguinal Herniorrhaphy: Preliminary Results of a Randomized Controlled Trial

Barkun JS, Wexler MJ, Hinchey EJ, Thibeault D, Meakins JL (McGill Univ, Montreal)
Surgery 118:703–710, 1995

10–41

Introduction.—Although preliminary reports support the feasibility of laparoscopic repairs of inguinal hernias, the benefits of this approach have not been proved. Therefore, the short-term efficacy and effectiveness of open (OH) and laparoscopic (LH) herniorrhaphy approaches were compared in a prospective randomized controlled trial.

Methods.—A total of 92 patients with a unilateral, nonrecurrent inguinal hernia were stratified by age (younger or older than 50 years) and randomly assigned to treatment with either OH or LH. Preoperative and postoperative data were collected prospectively by direct patient interviews conducted by third-party observers. Operative data were obtained from the surgeon immediately after the procedure and confirmed with data from the operative records. Outcome evaluations included the duration of convalescence, measures of postoperative pain, duration of hospital stay, quality of life, and morbidity. The cost-effectiveness of the 2 treatment approaches was compared.

Results.—There were 49 patients treated with OH and 43 treated with LH. No significant differences were found between the 2 groups in any of the baseline variables except that the LH group anticipated a shorter convalescence. The duration of the procedure was comparable in the 2 groups, and the surgeons reported similar satisfaction. There were no statistical differences in the duration of hospitalization (1 day in both groups) or convalescence (9.6 days in the LH group and 10.9 days in the OH group). Patients in the LH group required less postoperative narcotic administration than did patients in the OH group. The LH group reported significantly greater improvement in the quality of life as measured by 1 of 2 instruments. There were complications in 22.5% of the LH patients and 11.9% of the OH patients during a median follow-up of 14 months. The total direct costs were approximately $500 greater for LH than for OH.

Conclusions.—The feasibility of the laparoscopic approach to inguinal hernia repair was confirmed. When compared with the OH approach, the LH approach resulted in less postoperative pain and a possibly greater improvement in quality of life, but no benefit in convalescence. Because of the greater costs of the laparoscopic approach, it should be used selectively.

▶ Lawrence et al. and Barkun et al. provide us with 2 randomized trials of laparoscopic vs. open hernia repair that have essentially the same conclusions despite taking place on 2 different continents. The procedure costs significantly more in the laparoscopic group in both studies. This added expense resulted in only a small improvement in postoperative pain and analgesic use in both of these studies. Most importantly, neither study documented earlier return to work for the laparoscopic group despite less pain. Given these findings, why do laparoscopic hernia repairs?

J.F. Amaral, M.D.

Recurrent Inguinal Hernia After Laparoscopic Repair: Possible Cause and Prevention

Deans GT, Wilson MS, Royston CMS, Brough WA (Stepping Hill Hosp, Stockport, England)
Br J Surg 82:539–541, 1995   10–42

Background.—As many as 20% of patients in the United Kingdom who undergo inguinal hernia repair suffer recurrences over the long term. Once a hernia has recurred, the risk of later failure may be as great as 35%, with considerable morbidity and economic loss resulting. Reportedly there are few recurrences when inguinal hernia is repaired with prosthetic mesh. Mesh may be inserted laparoscopically to promote rapid rehabilitation.

Series.—Recurrence developed in 10 of 800 patients whose inguinal hernias were repaired laparoscopically by a transperitoneal approach and who were followed for 2 years. An 11th patient had recurrent hernia after laparoscopic repair elsewhere. The patients had a median age of 57 years when seen with recurrent hernia; the median interval after initial repair was 13 months. Eight patients had a primary indirect inguinal hernia. One had bilateral hernias repaired with mesh, and 2 patients had mesh repair of a recurrent hernia after initial open repair.

Operative Findings.—In all cases a single staple had been used to fix a 6 × 11-cm piece of mesh to the pubic ramus. Dissection proceeded only to the pubic tubercle. All patients had a medial recurrence, with the mesh rolled up away from the inside of the ramus toward the inferior epigastric artery, and exposing Hesselbach's triangle. It appeared that the staple had been dislodged.

Management.—A second piece of polypropylene mesh measuring 9 × 13 cm was placed in the preperitoneal space and extended medially well past the midline of the pubic symphysis. Its inferior border was tucked beneath the ramus and the lateral border double-breasted over the original mesh. The new mesh was secured to the inferior pubic ramus with 3 staples. The median operating time was 45 minutes.

Outcome.—There were no complications, and all patients were discharged the day after surgery. No patient has had a further recurrence during follow-up for 3–16 months.

Recommendations.—When laparoscopic hernia repair is performed with prosthetic mesh, the mesh should be placed up to or across the midline and fixed to the inferior pubic ramus with at least 3 staples. Mesh measuring at least 9 × 13 cm should be used. Bilateral hernias are repaired with a segment of mesh measuring at least 9 × 28 cm.

► Deans and co-workers provide us with a small group of recurrent laparoscopic hernias that confirm the reason for recurrence found by Phillips and colleagues in a much larger multicenter trial sponsored by Society of American Gastrointestinal Endoscopic Surgeons (SAGES). These reasons are that the mesh was too small, there were too few staples, and the staples pulled out. The patients in the study of Deans et al. are also interesting in that all recurrences noted were medial direct hernias in patients who had undergone indirect hernia repairs. This finding is the same as that observed after conventional, open hernia repairs and reinforces the concept that the direct space must be reinforced in an indirect hernia repair in all but the young to prevent future recurrence.

The data in this study are also encouraging in that the early recurrence rate for laparoscopic hernia repair was 1.2% at a mean of 13 months of follow-up. This recurrence rate is in agreement not only with 2 large published multicenter trials by Fitzgibbons and SAGES but also with most series of open hernia repair performed in nonspecialized centers. The data also support the beliefs of Stoppa for bilateral preperitoneal mesh repair in that 1 large piece of mesh is recommended rather than 2 separate pieces. As more information is gained with respect to laparoscopic hernia repair, the more these approaches seem the same as open anterior repairs.

J.F. Amaral, M.D.

Abdominal Wall Defects in Infants: Survival and Implications for Adult Life
Tunnell WP, Puffinbarger NK, Tuggle DW, Taylor DV, Mantor PC (Univ of Oklahoma, Oklahoma City; Children's Hospital of Oklahoma, Oklahoma City)
Ann Surg 221:525–530, 1995   10–43

Objective.—There are few long-term studies of the surgical outcome for newborns with abdominal wall defects. The results of a review of survival, morbidity, and quality of life in newborns surgically treated for omphalocele gastroschisis are presented.

Methods.—Between January 1975 and December 1984, 66 infants were treated for gastroschisis and 28 for omphalocele.

Results.—One patient with omphalocele did not have surgery and died. Of the remaining 93, 11 died in the hospital, 20 were lost to follow-up, and the remainder were followed for 10–20 years. Complete initial closure was achieved in 21 of 28 gastroschisis patients and in 47 of 66 omphalocele patients, with staged closure used rarely. Seven omphalocele patients died, 5 because of lethal anomalies, 1 because of injury to the hepatic vein during surgery, and 1 because of bronchopulmonary dysplasia. Four gastroschisis patients died, 2 because of "too tight" closure resulting in pulmonary failure, 1 of midgut volvulus at 1 month, and 1 of sudden infant death syndrome at 2½ months. There were 31 reoperations in 19 children—13 in omphalocele patients and 18 in gastroschisis patients—2 of which were performed for nonabdominal problems. The use of mechanical ventilation and total parenteral nutrition decreased the incidence of pulmonary death. Coexisting lethal conditions and reoperation were the main causes of morbidity and mortality. All 19 patients with bowel atresia or abdominal wall hernias required a reoperation by the age of 6. The incidence of reoperation declines with age. At follow-up, the health of these patients is good, although 40% reported shortness of stature and inadequacy in sports or social activities. The gastrointestinal problems reported by 50% of the gastroschisis patients were self-limiting and tended to decrease with age.

Conclusion.—The survival rate in these patients is favorable. Reoperation before the age of 6 is common in patients with bowel atresia or abdominal wall hernias. Quality of life is good and tends to improve with age.

▶ The results of this long follow-up confirm what most pediatric surgeons have always believed (or at least hoped): most problems associated with abdominal wall defects will manifest themselves within the first years of life. Both omphalocele and gastroschisis have a similarly excellent long-term outcome; the patients with omphalocele who died did so early from associated anomalies. Of interest is 1 patient with gastroschisis in whom midgut volvulus developed. Although all children with abdominal wall defects have some form of intestinal malrotation, it is often suggested that this does not have to be corrected because children with gastroschisis "never" volvulize: this is apparently not true anymore.

F.I. Luks, M.D.

Nonfluoroscopic Reduction of Intussusception by Air Enema
Wang G, Liu XG, Zitsman JL (Jilin Province Hosp, China; Beijing Inst, China; Beijing Med Univ, China; et al)
World J Surg 19:435–438, 1995   10–44

Introduction.—The standard nonsurgical treatment of intussusception is a barium enema. In recent years, pneumatic reduction with air and fluoroscopic guidance has been used increasingly, and diagnosis has been aided by ultrasonography. The possibility of performing air reduction of intussusception without fluoroscopy was explored.

Methods.—Over a 4-year period, 224 children between the ages of 6 weeks and 4 years were diagnosed and treated for intussusception. It was diagnosed by history and physical examination and confirmed in 40 patients with ultrasonography. A balloon catheter connected to a self-controlled intussusception reduction instrument was used to deliver pressure at 50 mm Hg with air, held for several minutes, and released. The pressure was increased by increments of 10 mm Hg when necessary. Three patients required pressures of 110 mm Hg to reduce the intussusceptions. Successful reduction was determined by disappearance of the mass or of abdominal distension, passage of nonbloody stool, sound of gas entering the reduced bowel, excretion of ingested charcoal, and/or ultrasonographic confirmation.

Results.—Nonoperative pneumatic reduction without fluoroscopy was successful in 217 of the 224 patients. Seven patients required surgical reduction for a 96.9% success rate without surgery. There were no complications or deaths. Discharge occurred after 2–4 hours of observation in 192 patients and after 9–12 hours in 25 patients.

Conclusions.—Intussusception could be diagnosed clinically in 82.1% and was confirmed with ultrasonography in 17.9%. The intussuscepted bowel was reduced in 96.9% of the children by using carefully monitored pneumatic reduction without exposing the patients to ionizing radiation.

▶ After having introduced air enema reduction to the Western world, Chinese pediatric surgeons now go one step further: pneumatic reduction without the need for radiation exposure and postreduction observation as an outpatient. This very cost-efficient approach seems to work very well, indeed; they achieved an impressive 97% reduction rate. Although not as huge as the 6,000-patient series from Shanghai, this study comprises a large enough number of cases to be convincing.

F.I. Luks, M.D.

Transperitoneal Closure of the Internal Ring in Incarcerated Infantile Inguinal Hernias

Misra D, Hewitt G, Potts SR, Brown S, Boston VE (Royal Belfast Hosp for Sick Children, Ireland)
J Pediatr Surg 30:95–96, 1995   10–45

Introduction.—Between 14% and 24% of pediatric inguinal hernia (IH) cases in infants result in incarceration. The difficult dissection of the spermatic cord may cause damage to the vas or vessels. Problems associated with the preperitoneal approach can be avoided with the transperitoneal closure of the internal ring (TPIR). This paper reports on 14 consecutive babies with difficult incarcerated IH.

Methods.—A transverse incision was made 2 cm superior to the deep ring and the peritoneum opened. The internal ring and inguinal canal were recognized. The bowel was gently returned to the peritoneal cavity. From within, a pursestring suture was placed around the internal ring to avoid the vas and testicular vessels. Abdominal closure was performed in a typical manner.

Results.—In the 6-year period 1987–1992, IH was diagnosed in 251 patients under 6 months of age, with 59 (24%) having incarceration. Transperitoneal closure of the internal ring was performed in 14 infants. One infant had an elective herniotomy with a recurrence the next day that required TPIR. The other 13 had 15 IHs, 14 of which were incarcerated. Three of the IHs were reduced with induction of general anesthesia. The remaining 11 were reduced after laparotomy. No resections were required. The vas and vessels were avoided. The average operating time was 20 minutes. There were no infections or complications. Follow-up ranged from 6 weeks to 3 years, averaging 9 months.

Conclusion.—In babies for whom the alternative approaches to IH would be difficult, TPIR is a safe and reliable operation. In babies when the anticipated dissection would be difficult because of edema or hemorrhage or when intestinal resection may be needed, TPIR should be considered.

▶ Closing the internal inguinal ring from within elegantly avoids tearing the "wet tissue paper" of a hernia sac and injuring the already edematous cord structures. The transperitoneal approach allows resection of ischemic bowel loops, but as shown by the authors, this is rarely necessary. In the end, a laparotomy (instead of an extraperitoneal inguinal approach) may be a small price to pay if recurrence and testicular damage can thus be prevented. The only objection to this series is its prohibitive rate of irreducibility: 14 out of 59, or 24%, whereas more than 90% of incarcerated inguinal hernias in children should be reducible. In fact, the only hernias that cannot be reduced preoperatively are those requiring bowel resection intraoperatively.

F.I. Luks, M.D.

Malrotation in the Older Child: Surgical Management, Treatment, and Outcome
Maxson RT, Franklin PA, Wagner CW (Univ of Arkansas, Little Rock)
Am Surg 61:135–138, 1995   10–46

Background.—In newborns with intestinal malrotation, there are clear indications for surgery. However, there is debate over the management of older children with malrotation. Some authors maintain that incidentally detected malrotation is harmless, whereas others recommend prompt surgery for all patients with abnormalities of rotation and fixation, even asymptomatic cases. Twenty-two cases of intestinal malrotation in older children are reviewed.

Patients.—The patients were seen over a 15-year period at 1 children's hospital. They represented nearly one fourth of the patients who underwent surgery for intestinal malrotation during this time. The age range was 3 to 23 years, with an average age of 9 years. The initial symptoms included vomiting in 68% of the patients, colicky abdominal pain in 55%, and diarrhea in 9%. Hematemesis and constipation each occurred in only 5% of the patients. The symptoms had been present for an average of 28 months.

Findings.—Except for 1 case recognized at exploratory laparotomy for intestinal duplication, all cases of intestinal malrotation were diagnosed at upper gastrointestinal radiography. All patients underwent a Ladd's procedure with appendectomy. Forty-one percent of the patients were found at surgery to have a volvulus or internal hernia that was not detected preoperatively, and 2 patients had ischemic bowel necessitating intestinal resection. There was no perioperative mortality, and wound infection in 1 patient was the only postoperative complication. Sixty-four percent of the patients obtained complete relief from their symptoms, and all had at least partial relief of chronic symptoms. Symptoms resolved in all patients with volvulus or internal hernia.

Conclusions.—Older children with proven intestinal malrotation should receive surgical treatment. Surgery avoids the chance of bowel loss from volvulus or internal hernia, which are common surgical findings that are not always detected on preoperative radiographs. Surgery is very effective in relieving the chronic symptoms of malrotation as well.

▶ The most important message of this paper is that 4 of the 22 "older" patients with malrotation had midgut volvulus, 2 of them with ischemic bowel. While an upper gastrointestinal contrast study was diagnostic of malrotation in all, it failed to demonstrate the—potentially catastrophic—volvulus. This was recently demonstrated by Touloukian as well. Therefore, surgical intervention for malrotation appears wise at any age.

F.I. Luks, M.D.

Enterostomy and Its Closure in Newborns
Weber TR, Tracy TF Jr, Silen ML, Powell A (St Louis Univ, Mo)
Arch Surg 130:534–537, 1995   10–47

Introduction.—Although enterostomy is commonly performed in newborns with acute bowel perforation, necrosis, or obstruction, its complications and outcome have been examined only minimally. Therefore, enterostomy and its closure in newborns were reviewed over a 6-year period.

Methods.—Of the 109 newborns who underwent enterostomy between 1988 and 1993, 41% were younger than 32 weeks' gestation and 18% were younger than 28 weeks' gestation. The procedures performed were jejunostomy in 31 (28%), ileostomy in 62 (57%), and colostomy in 16 (15%) for the treatment of necrotizing enterocolitis, intestinal atresia, idiopathic perforation, intestinal volvulus, or meconium ileus. Most (81%) of the enterostomies were exteriorized, and a distal mucous fistula was used in 90%. Complications, function, and need for revision of the enterostomies were monitored until closure of the ostomy or patient death. Weight gain during the 30 days before closure and the serum albumin level 7–10 days before closure were evaluated in each child.

Results.—Within 48 days of the surgery, 16% of the patients died, all of causes unrelated to the enterostomy or its closure. In the remaining patients, complications requiring revision developed in 34% of those who underwent jejunostomy, in 26% of those who underwent ileostomy, and in 23% of those who underwent colostomy. The enterostomy was closed 14–65 days after the procedure in 92 patients, with death occurring in 4 of these patients 14–145 days after closure from chronic respiratory failure or liver failure (probably related to prolonged total parenteral nutrition). There were closure complications, including anastomotic dehiscence, anastomotic stricture, and/or wound infection, in 44% of the remaining patients with jejunostomies, 43% of the patients with ileostomies, and 25% of the patients with colostomies. There were significant differences in both weight gain and serum albumin levels before closure in the patients with necrotizing enterocolitis who had anastomotic dehiscence as compared with those without dehiscence.

Discussion.—Enterostomy complications and anastomotic breakdown were most common in patients who had the diagnosis of necrotizing enterocolitis, which is indicative of its severity and long-term effects. There was a 23% to 34% stoma complication rate, with a higher risk of closure complications in patients with a low serum albumin level and/or poor weight gain. Therefore it is suggested that closure of an enterostomy occur only when the patient's nutritional condition is satisfactory.

▶ The substantial complication rate of temporary ostomies is being recognized more and more frequently and has led many surgeons to favor primary anastomosis in such varied conditions as penetrating colonic trauma, endorectal pull-through and pouch procedures, and even necrotizing enterocolitis of the newborn. Ostomies are therefore used in the sickest patients, which may contribute to this 23% to 34% complication rate. Not surprisingly, jejunostomies fared worse. While the authors emphasize the importance of adequate nutritional status before ostomy closure, they fail to mention one of the difficult problems associated with proximal enterostomies: high output resulting in brittle water and electrolyte homeostasis and an inability to achieve optimal nutrition, which often leads to a catch-22 situation regarding the ideal timing of closure.

F.I. Luks, M.D.

Idiopathic Intestinal Perforations in Premature Infants Without Evidence of Necrotizing Enterocolitis
Harms K, Lüdtke F-E, Lepsien G, Speer CP (Univ of Göttingen, Germany)
Eur J Pediatr Surg 5:30–33, 1995   10–48

Introduction.—The most common cause of neonatal gastrointestinal perforation is necrotizing enterocolitis (NEC). Five patients with idiopathic, spontaneous intestinal perforation are described. The course of these patients is compared with the typical course of NEC.

Methods.—Of 260 premature, very low birth weight infants, severe NEC developed in 7 (2.6%), only 1 of whom had intestinal perforation and 5 (1.9%) required laparotomy for spontaneous intestinal perforation. All the patients were very premature (25–28 weeks' gestation). All were fed parenterally. Four of the 5 patients with spontaneous intestinal perforation were treated with IV indomethacin, 3 before and 1 after intestinal perforation. The course of these 5 patients was followed.

Results.—None of the 5 patients had signs of peritonitis or abdominal distension. Four of the 5 patients had gray-green skin in the inguinal region and flanks as their initial symptom. Ultrasonography revealed ascites in 3 infants. Radiologic studies showed pneumoperitoneum in all 5 patients but no signs of NEC (pneumatosis intestinalis or portal gas bubbles). At surgery, 4 patients had only 1 perforation in the medial or distal portion of the ileum with no macroscopic abnormalities in the rest of the intestine. The remaining patient had 2 perforations separated by 3 cm. Postoperative septicemia with disseminated intravascular coagulopathy developed in 1 patient who died on the second day after surgery.

Discussion.—Laparotomy in premature infants was most frequently indicated for the management of a spontaneous, idiopathic intestinal perforation. The patients did not exhibit any of the typical initial symptoms of NEC, including guarding, bloody stools, abdominal distension, and microcirculatory problems. Nor did they have typical radiographic or laboratory findings, including decreased leukocyte and neutrophil counts. However, the patients did have similar risk factors to patients with NEC, including extreme prematurity and severe respiratory distress. The pathogenesis of both NEC and spontaneous perforation may involve mesenteric hypoperfusion. It has been suggested that these 2 disorders may be different manifestations of the same disease process. Patients with spontaneous gastrointestinal perforations have a good prognosis with early diagnosis.

▶ In necrotizing enterocolitis, the best surgical candidates are those infants with a single, isolated perforation. Whether the present series represents a different entity or a *forme très fruste* of necrotizing enterocolitis is debatable; the distinction is also not very important since both conditions are still "idiopathic." The authors' results are excellent given the inherent risks of operating on very small premature infants. However, their definition of a very low birth weight infant is a little too generous and in 1995 should probably not include babies over 1,000 g. Finally, peritoneal drainage as a safer alternative to laparotomy in the tiniest of infants would have been worth mentioning.

F.I. Luks, M.D.

Laparoscopic Is Not Better Than Open Appendectomy
Apelgren KN, Molnar RG, Kisala JM (Michigan State Univ, East Lansing)
Am Surg 61:240–243, 1995   10–49

Background.—As experience with laparoscopic appendectomy continues to grow, more and more general surgeons are using this procedure. The benefits of this approach over open appendectomy are not, however, as apparent as those associated with laparoscopic vs. open cholecystectomy. The role and advantages of laparoscopic vs. open appendectomy in the management of appendicitis and right lower quadrant pain were retrospectively reviewed.

Patients and Methods.—Nonrandomized patients undergoing open or laparoscopic appendectomy for simple acute appendicitis were included. Pregnant patients, those under 16 years of age, and those with a ruptured appendix were excluded. All procedures were performed by 2 attending surgeons between April 1991 and February 1993. Patient age, gender, operating room time, hospital costs and stay, negative appendectomy rate, wound infection rates, and time to return to normal activities were reviewed and compared between surgical groups.

Results.—Patient age was similar between groups. There were significantly more females in the laparoscopic group: 68% vs. 39% in the open appendectomy group. Mean operating room time and hospital costs were significantly higher for the laparoscopic group: 84.5 minutes and $6,838 vs. 56.5 minutes and $5,430 for the open appendectomy group, respectively. Average hospital stay was 2.5 days for the laparoscopic patients and 3 days for the open appendectomy group, and average time to return to normal activities was 16.6 days and 17.6 days, respectively. None of the patients in the laparoscopic group experienced wound infection, as opposed to 2% in the open group. These differences were not significant. Patients in the laparoscopic group had a negative appendectomy rate of 37% vs. 12% for the open group.

Conclusions.—Laparoscopic appendectomy is more costly than open appendectomy and offers no evident clinical benefits over the latter approach. Further experience with laparoscopic appendectomy will help clarify its role in the management of patients with appendicitis and right lower quadrant pain.

▶ As more experience is gained in advanced laparoscopic surgery, laparoscopic appendectomy is being employed on a more frequent basis. Unfortunately, the advantages of laparoscopic appendectomy are not as clear-cut as those for laparoscopic cholecystectomy. This nonrandomized study compared open and closed appendectomy and found no advantage to the closed technique in conjunction with increased cost. Clearly, the ability to perform a procedure does not justify its use, and in this case it appears that increased cost without shorter postoperative stays or a quicker return to normal activity does not justify performing this procedure at present, especially in the era of managed care.

W.G. Cioffi, M.D.

Open Versus Laparoscopic Appendectomy: A Prospective Randomized Comparison
Martin LC, Puente I, Sosa JL, Bassin A, Breslaw R, McKenney MG, Ginzburg E, Sleeman D (Univ of Miami, Fla)
Ann Surg 222:256–262, 1995   10–50

Background.—Although the laparoscopic approach is well accepted for the treatment of cholelithiasis, the efficacy and indications for laparoscopic appendectomy are still at issue. Previous studies have suggested that laparoscopic appendectomy can significantly shorten hospital stay when compared with the conventional open operation. Open was compared with laparoscopic appendectomy in a prospective, randomized study.

Methods.—The study included 169 patients aged 15 years or older in whom acute appendicitis was diagnosed over a 9-month period. The patients were randomized to a laparoscopic or open surgical approach: 81 and 88 patients, respectively. Both groups received preoperative antibiotics. Operative time—defined as the time from incision to full wound closure—was compared for the 2 groups, as were hospital stay and the time for return to normal activity. Patients requiring conversion from laparoscopic to open appendectomy were considered separately.

Results.—The demographic characteristics of the 2 groups were similar. Sixteen percent of the laparoscopic group required conversion to open surgery. Acute appendicitis was present in 80% of the open group and 77% of the laparoscopic group; perforative appendicitis were present in 24% and 12%, respectively. Operative time was 82 minutes in the open group vs. 102 minutes in the laparoscopic group. Hospital stay was significantly longer in the open group, 4.3 vs. 2.2 days. Although hospital stay was not significantly different for patients who had acute appendicitis vs. those who had a normal appendix but with pelvic inflammatory disease, there was a significant difference for patients with perforative appendicitis: 9.5 days in the open group vs. 1.5 days in the laparoscopic group. The mean hospital cost was $7,227 for open vs. $6,077 for laparoscopic appendectomy. The laparoscopic group had no increase in their complication rate. There were no differences in return to normal activity.

Conclusions.—Laparoscopic and open appendectomy are similar in terms of hospital complications, hospital stay, cost, return to activity, and return to work. Operative time is significantly longer with the laparoscopic approach. Diagnostic laparoscopy may be useful for selected patients with vague clinical findings, such as women of childbearing age or obese patients, but laparoscopic appendectomy does not offer any significant benefit over open appendectomy for the routine appendicitis patient.

▶ The study by Martin et al. is very interesting in that even though it shows open appendectomy to be better than laparoscopic appendectomy in 1 measured parameter and laparoscopic appendectomy better in only 1 (length of hospital stay), they conclude that there is no reason in the study to advocate laparoscopic appendectomy. Clearly, there is also no reason to advocate open appendectomy, and in fact, the hospital stay with perforated appendicitis treated by open surgery is much longer and suggests that the laparoscopic route may be better.

The problems with this study are multiple but, most importantly, center on uncontrolled bias. It is impossible to blind patients as to the procedure they had since this information is known to the patients when they look at their bandages. This clearly introduces bias from the patients, nurses, families, and doctors taking care of them. In the future, randomized studies of laparoscopic procedures should be blinded by putting the same bandage on all.

Although many of the parameters are marginally longer than that of other studies, this is explained by the fact that residents performed the procedures. Furthermore, it is noted that the attending staff was the same for both. Unfortunately, we do not know what the experience of the attending staff was in laparoscopic surgery in general and, in particular, laparoscopic appendectomy. Perhaps this is reflected in the high conversion rate to open appendectomy of 16%. Of further note, converted cases took only 17 minutes more than open cases. Since open cases took 81.7 minutes, the small increase in operative time with conversion over laparoscopy suggest that little time was spent on the laparoscopic portion. Finally, what percentage of open cases were converted? Who needed a larger or different incision and what impact did that have?

The bottom line of this study is that, in general, patients went home sooner after a laparoscopic appendectomy and, in particular, after perforated appendicitis. This occurred without an increase in cost. Therefore, why not do laparoscopic appendectomies?

J.F. Amaral, M.D.

A Prospective, Randomized Comparison of Laparoscopic Appendectomy With Open Appendectomy
Ortega AE, Hunter JG, Peters JH, Swanstrom LL, Schirmer B, and the Laparoscopic Appendectomy Study Group (Univ of Southern California, Los Angeles; Emory Univ, Atlanta, Ga; Oregon Health Sciences Univ, Portland; et al)
Am J Surg 169:208–213, 1995   10–51

Introduction.—Laparoscopic appendectomy (LA) techniques have been developed, but their advantages are not established, largely because traditional open appendectomy (OA) itself requires only a small incision. Therefore, the advantages and disadvantages of LA were compared with those of OA in patients with presumed appendicitis. In addition, the effectiveness of the 2 most popular LA techniques, i.e., using either ligatures or linear stapling, was compared.

Methods.—A total of 253 patients with a clinical diagnosis of appendicitis or right lower quadrant pain of uncertain etiology were randomly assigned to treatment with either LA with stapling (LAS), LA with catgut ligatures (LAL), or OA. Data on pain, complications, and outcome were collected prospectively.

Results.—The operative findings confirmed acute appendicitis in 65.6%, perforated appendicitis in 17.4%, and normal appendices in 67.9%, with no significant differences in the proportion of each diagnosis in the 3 treatment groups. The mean operative time was significantly longer with the 2 laparoscopic procedures than with the open procedure. In the 2 laparoscopic groups, 6.6% of the patients required conversion to OA, with equal occurrence in the LAL and LAS groups. The group treated with LAL had a greater rate of intraoperative fecal soilage and postoperative emesis than did the groups treated with LAS or OA, whereas the group treated with OA had a greater rate of wound infection. Intra-abdominal abscesses occurred in 2 patients in the LAS group, 4 patients in the LAL group, and none in the OA group. The mean length of stay was comparable in the 3 groups, but patients in the OA group required an average of 5 additional days to return to full activity. The patients required pain medication for a similar number of days in the 3 treatment groups, but the 2 laparoscopic groups reported significantly lower pain scores than the OA group, on visual analogue pain scales.

Conclusions.—Laparoscopic appendectomy has significant benefits over OA, especially when performed with a linear stapler. The benefits include less pain and shorter convalescence. Its disadvantages are longer operative time and greater surgical costs. More research is needed to determine the long-term cost-effectiveness of LA.

▶ The laparoscopic appendectomy study group provides us with the largest series of patients to date randomized to open or laparoscopic appendectomy. The data provided document slightly longer operative times for laparoscopic procedures, but less pain, earlier discharges, less wound infection, and earlier return to normal activities. Despite these findings, the data are difficult to interpret in light of 3 shortcomings of the study. First, there are no cost data provided for the 3 groups. Although the authors argue that this was not possible because of the multicenter nature of the trial, some idea of cost could have been provided by making a relative comparison at each site. This cost information is crucial since the significant reductions in length of hospital stay and convalescence were less than 1 day and 5 days, respectively. What should that be worth given a potential increased cost of the laparoscopic approach documented in other studies? Second, to what extent are the advantages in pain, discharge, and convalescence the result of uncontrollable biases present in a study such as this, which is randomized but not biased? Third, these results are from highly skilled laparoscopic surgeons. What would the results be for the average general surgeon who at present has few advanced laparoscopic skills? Until these questions are answered, the value and place of laparoscopic appendectomy will continue to be debated.

J.F. Amaral, M.D.

The Role of Cefoxitin Prophylaxis in Chronic Pilonidal Sinus Treated With Excision and Primary Suture
Søndenaa K, Nesvik I, Gullaksen FP, Furnes A, Harbo SO, Weyessa S, Søreide JA (Rogaland Central Hosp, Stavanger, Norway; Deaconess Hosp, Bergen, Norway; County Hosp, Molde, Norway)
J Am Coll Surg 180:157–160, 1995   10–52

Background.—Postoperative wound complications often follow excision of chronic pilonidal sinuses. In this study, patients were treated with prophylactic cefoxitin before excision and suture of the pilonidal sinuses to determine the drug's effect on postoperative infection.

Methods.—Cefoxitin-treated patients (n = 78) in this multicenter study were randomly selected to receive IV cefoxitin prophylaxis. No prophylaxis was given to patients in the control group (N = 75). Two grams of the drug was given within one-half hour of the operation. Preoperative cultures were completed in 86 patients at 1 hospital. Seven days after surgery, the sutures were removed by a nurse and the wound was inspected. Complications, wound infection, and healing time were noted. Healing was defined as a dry wound with complete approximation of the edges within 2 weeks; a wound that took from 2 to 4 weeks to heal was recorded as a minor complication. Data were evaluated by using chi-square tests with the Yates' correction.

Results.—Aerobic organisms were cultured from 28% of the patients in whom cultures had been performed; anaerobes were cultured from 43% of the patients. Within 4 weeks, 69% of the cefoxitin-treated patients had healed as compared with 64% of the controls. Two patients in each group had a recurrence. Eighty-seven patients without complications healed within 2 weeks. Sixty-one patients with complications healed in a median of 6.6 weeks. The most frequent complication was partial and slight separation of the wound and drainage. More complications occurred in patients who did not have a straight midline incision, particularly those who required more than 1 incision.

Discussion.—These findings indicate that 2 g of preoperative cefoxitin does not influence the short-term course of patients undergoing this procedure. This group of patients had a high rate of complications, which suggests that primary closure of the wound is not indicated for chronic pilonidal sinus tracts.

▶ The purpose of this article was to determine the role of perioperative antibiotic prophylaxis in improving results after treatment for chronic pilonidal sinuses. One hundred fifty-three patients with chronic pilonidal sinuses were operated on with radical excision and primary suture and randomized to receive a single dose of antibiotic prophylaxis of 2 g of cefoxitin IV or no prophylaxis. Results of this study demonstrated an equal number of complications in both groups of patients. Forty-four percent of the patients with cefoxitin had complications as compared with 43% without cefoxitin, and the most common complication was partial and slight separation of the wound and unusual discharge. Sixty-nine percent of the patients with prophylaxis healed within 4 weeks, whereas 64% healed without antibiotics, and in a follow-up period of 6–30 months, 2 patients in each group did not heal their wounds. Two patients (3%) in the group with cefoxitin had recurrences, as opposed to 5 patients (7%) in the group without prophylaxis. The immediate and short-term results after excision and primary suture for chronic pilonidal sinus are not influenced significantly by a single dose prophylaxis of 2 g of cefoxitin. In addition, the large number of complications in these patients would suggest that primary closure is not indicated for chronic pilonidal sinuses and that healing by secondary intention may ultimately result in a lower incidence of complications.

H.H. Simms, M.D.

Colorectum and Anus

INTRODUCTION

The importance of a proper colonic bowel preparation is the subject of Abstract 10–53. This blinded, prospective, randomized analysis from the Division of Colon and Rectal Surgery at Grant Medical Center in Columbus, Ohio, finds equivalent efficacy in bowel preparation with a variety of cathartics: (1) peroral, orthograde polyethylene glycol–electrolyte lavage solution; (2) a similar solution with oral metoclopramide; and (3) oral sodium phosphate. The authors note that abdominal symptoms and bowel preparation were not influenced by the addition of metoclopramide. This important analysis confirmed that the oral sodium phosphate preparation is less expensive, better tolerated and more likely to be completed than either of the other preparations. Further, the importance of early feeding and its safety following elective colorectal surgery was subjected to a randomized prospective trial by Reissman et al. of the Cleveland Clinic (Florida) Colorectal Department (Abstract 10–54). This important study indicates that early oral feeding following elective colorectal surgery is safe and well tolerated by the majority of patients. These data suggest that the cost-effectiveness of the technique is a benefit to patients in routine care and should be considered an important feature of postoperative management in otherwise uncomplicated patients. Cost-effectiveness of surgical procedures is further exemplified in Abstract 10–55, which suggests that the use of patient-controlled analgesia (PCA) following uncomplicated colectomy objectively increases the risk of prolonged postoperative ileus. The implications of prolongation of the ileus with its attendant demands and the necessity of in-hospital stay for provision of IV fluid resuscitation are evident. The consideration for use of PCA must be re-evaluated as the return of normal bowel function was delayed a mean of 0.9 days.

Senagore et al. (Abstract 10–56) provide a prospective evaluation of the experience of a single team of surgeons in 60 consecutive laparoscopic-assisted colectomies. Learning curves increase stepwise as surgeons progress to more complex (extended) resections. With mastery of this technical approach, it appears that operation expenses, conversion to the open method, and length of stay decreased. Of interest, the time of first oral intake decreased from 3.9 ± 2.4 days to 1.6 ± 0.9 days ($P < 0.05$) and contributed to this improvement in cost-effectiveness and reduced length of stay. Therapy for inflammatory bowel disease and preneoplastic colonic polyposis with technically successful approaches to complete total abdominal proctocolectomy and reconstruction with an ileal pouch–anal anastomosis is undergoing increasing scrutiny due to the increasing number of reports of pouchitis. The report by Sandborn et al. (Abstract 10–58) observed that fecal concentrations of bacteria, bile acids, and short-chain fatty acids were similar in patients with and without pouchitis, thus suggesting that these factors are not the sole etiology of this problem. Of interest, patients with the ileoanal anastomosis had higher ratios of anaerobes/aerobes and higher concentrations of anaerobic gram-negative rods than did patients who were reconstructed with an ileostomy. The review by Fazio and colleagues (Abstract 10–59) from the Cleveland Clinic Foundation in Ohio reports a large experience with the ileal pouch–anal anastomosis and associated complications and physiologic function. This approach to inflammatory bowel disease and familial adenomatous polyposis resulted in good to excellent functional results and quality of life in the majority of these patients. The low mortality rate of 1% and the overall morbidity rate (63%) suggest that this technique is a state-of-the-art approach to these formidable inflammatory and preneoplastic disease processes.

The analysis by Miller and associates of the General Infirmary at Leeds, England (Abstract 10–61), evaluates anorectal function following rectal excision and stapled coloanal anastomosis for rectal carcinoma. This study identified important features that may predict a poor outcome. While the majority of patients with rectal adenocarcinoma desire and can be treated with sphincter preservation surgery, the distal or midrectal anastomosis may result in fecal leakage and urgency of defecation in up to 50% of patients. To determine the etiology and correlates of poor outcome, these investigators evaluated the functional results following low anterior resection with coloanal anastomosis; these studies assessed anorectal physiologic function in terms of sensory, motor, and reflex activity. Poor function was significantly more common in women than in men; these results suggest that occult damage to the sphincter may have occurred *prior to* the low anterior resection, especially in multigravid patients. The import of this study is that both genders, especially women, should have an investigation *prior to* the operation by means of manometry and endoanal ultrasonography, both of which are sensitive and reliable methods for determining the anatomy and physiologic competency of the anal sphincter. A profound reduction in the resting anorectal pressure gradient preoperatively suggests that these abnormal values will only be exaggerated with distal low anterior resection. Thus these preoperative measurements may allow the surgeon the opportunity to predict functional outcome with great reliability following coloanal anastomosis and, perhaps, determine whether construction of a colonic J-pouch reservoir is advisable.

Kirby I. Bland, M.D.

Colonoscopic Bowel Preparations: Which One? A Blinded, Prospective, Randomized Trial
Golub RW, Kerner BA, Wise WE Jr, Meesig DM, Hartmann RF, Khanduja KS, Aguilar PS (Grant Med Ctr, Columbus, Ohio)
Dis Colon Rectum 38:594–599, 1995   10–53

Introduction.—When compared with traditional 2-day preparations of clear liquids, laxatives, and enemas, the preoral, orthograde, polyethylene glycol–electrolyte lavage solutions (PEG-ELSs) have become the preferred bowel-cleansing agents before endoscopic and surgical procedures on the colon and rectum. However, patients tend to have difficulty with drinking the large PEG solution volumes, and many experience nausea, vomiting, abdominal fullness, cramps, anal irritation, and sleep loss. Patients were randomized to 1 of 3 bowel preparation regimens to determine which would provide greater patient acceptance while maintaining similar or improved effectiveness and safety in 329 patients undergoing elective ambulatory colonoscopy.

Methods.—Patients were prospectively randomized to group 1, 4 L of PEG-ELS; group 2, PEG-ELS and oral metoclopramide; or group 3, oral sodium phosphate. Groups were age and sex matched.

Results.—The preparations were completed by 91% of all patients. Significant sleep loss was experienced by 16% of all patients. There were no significant between-group differences in complaints of nausea, vomiting, abdominal cramps, anal irritation, or quality of the preparation. Oral sodium phosphate was tolerated better than the other preparations. Significantly more patients were able to complete the preparation, and fewer group 3 patients complained of abdominal fullness. Sodium phosphate was 4 times less expensive than either PEG-ELS preparation.

Conclusion.—The 3 regimens were equally effective, reliable, and well tolerated. However, oral sodium phosphate was less expensive, better tolerated, more likely to be completed, and considerably cheaper than either PEG-ELS preparation.

▶ Finally, a blinded prospective randomized trial on such a common clinical question. As one would expect, all regimens were found to be equally effective. The extreme variation in patients' ability to tolerate 1 regimen or another certainly warrants discussion with individual patients. Interestingly, the oral sodium phosphate preparation was not only less expensive and better tolerated but also more likely to be completed than either of the other preparations, most likely a result of the total volume to be ingested. Its potential side effects, especially in terms of electrolyte imbalances, must warn against its routine use.

V.E. Pricolo, M.D.

Is Early Oral Feeding Safe After Elective Colorectal Surgery? A Prospective Randomized Trial
Reissman P, Teoh T-A, Cohen SM, Weiss EG, Nogueras JJ, Wexner SD
(Cleveland Clinic Florida, Fort Lauderdale)
Ann Surg 222:73–77, 1995   10–54

Introduction.—Early feedings have been shown to be safe and well tolerated after laparoscopic colectomy. The safety, tolerability, and outcome of early oral feedings after elective colorectal procedures were prospectively assessed.

Methods.—All patients undergoing elective laparotomy with either colon or small bowel resection over a 16-month period were randomized to 1 of 2 groups: in group 1, early oral feeding, all patients were given a clear liquid diet on the first postoperative day and advanced to a regular diet as tolerated; in group 2, regular feeding, nothing was taken by mouth until resolution of ileus, then a clear liquid diet followed by a regular diet as tolerated. The nasogastric tube was removed immediately after surgery from all patients in both groups. Vomiting, bowel movements, nasogastric tube reinsertion, time of regular diet consumption, complications, and length of hospitalization were recorded. If patients had 2 episodes of vomiting of more than 100 mL over a 24-hour period in the absence of bowel movements, the nasogastric tube was reinstated. Postoperative ileus was considered resolved after a bowel movement in the absence of abdominal distension or vomiting.

Results.—There were 80 patients in group 1 and 81 patients in group 2. Early feedings were well tolerated in 63 group 1 patients. These patients were advanced to a regular diet within the next 24 to 48 hours. There were no significant differences between group 1 and group 2 patients in the rate of vomiting, 21% vs. 14%; rate of nasogastric tube reinsertion, 11% vs. 10%; length of ileus, 3.8 vs 4.1 days; length of hospitalization, 6.2 vs. 6.8

TABLE 4.—Mean Length of Hospitalization After Laparoscopic Colectomy

Author	No. of Patients	Mean Hospitalization (Days)
Lointier	6	10
Milsom	9	7
Tate	11	12.3
Van Ye	14	9.1
Corbitt	17	4.0
Vara-Thorbeck	18	7.6
Larach	18	8.4
Franklin	19	7.4
Quattlebaum	20	4.4
Scoggin	20	5
Peters	24	4.8
Musser	24	8.5
Etienne	35	9
Senagore	38	7
Monson	40	8
Phillips	51	4.6
Zucker	65	4.4
Wexner	74	7
Total	506	6.8
Present study (open colorectal procedures)		
Regular feeding	81	6.8
Early feeding	80	6.2

(Courtesy of Reissman P, Teoh T-A, Cohen SM, et al: Is early oral feeding safe after elective colorectal surgery? A prospective randomized trial. *Ann Surg* 222:73–77, 1995.)

days; or overall complication rate, 7.5% vs. 6.1%. Patients in group 1 tolerated a regular diet significantly earlier than did group 2 patients—2.6 vs. 5.0 days.

Conclusion.—Early oral intake after elective abdominal colorectal surgery was safe and well tolerated by the majority of the patients. In a collective series from the literature, 506 patients who underwent laparoscopic colectomy had a mean hospital stay of 5.8 days (Table 4). This finding is similar to that of group 2 patients and 0.6 days longer than that of group 1 patients in the present series.

▶ This provocative study addresses the issue of whether the length of hospital stay after elective colorectal surgery is influenced by the duration of postoperative ileus or, rather, by surgeons' habits. Clinical series of laparoscopic colon resections boasted a shorter hospital length of stay based on feeding patients earlier. However, the flaw of those studies was their comparison with historical controls. Greater emphasis has been placed on early postoperative discharge by pressure exerted on physicians by third-party payers. This paper elegantly demonstrates that early postoperative feeding is just as safe after "open" as it is after laparoscopic colorectal surgery and that surgical technique alone is not likely to have a significant influence on the duration of postoperative ileus.

V.E. Pricolo, M.D.

Patient-Controlled Analgesia and Prolonged Ileus After Uncomplicated Colectomy

Petros JG, Realica R, Ahmad S, Rimm EB, Robillard RJ (St Elizabeth's Med Ctr, Boston; Harvard School of Public Health, Boston)
Am J Surg 170:371–374, 1995   10–55

Purpose.—During a 4-year period, the mean duration of postoperative ileus after uncomplicated colon surgery had increased at this hospital, even though there had been no important changes in patient population or surgical technique during that period. The purpose of this study was to identify risk factors for prolonged postoperative ileus after uncomplicated colectomy.

Patients.—The study population consisted of 182 men and 176 women with a mean age of 62 years who had undergone uncomplicated colon resection. Of these 358 patients, 186 received postoperative IV patient-controlled analgesia (PCA) with morphine or meperidine, and 172 were given postoperative IM morphine or meperidine every 3 hours as needed. Prolonged ileus was defined as ileus lasting 7 days or more. Postoperative ileus was considered resolved at the first postoperative passage of flatus or stool or after tolerance of a clear liquid diet.

Results.—There was no significant relationship between prolonged postoperative ileus and age, gender, operating time, or the type or amount of analgesic agent used for analgesia. After controlling for confounding factors, however, patients who used postoperative PCA had significantly higher rates of ileus at 7, 6, and 5 days after surgery than those who received IM analgesia. The mean duration of ileus was 5.5 days in the PCA group and 4.6 days in the IM group. Thus the use of PCA was associated with a mean delay in the resolution of postoperative ileus of 0.9 days. Performance of a right colectomy decreased the time to postoperative ileus resolution by an average of 0.4 days as compared with other types of colon resection.

Conclusions.—The use of postoperative PCA after uncomplicated colon resection increases the risk of prolonged postoperative ileus.

▶ The introduction of PCA in the past decade has significantly simplified postoperative pain management after major abdominal surgery. Patients derive a significant psychological benefit from controlling their own analgesics, and the nursing time consumption, as well as local complications (e.g., nerve injury, hematomas) of IM injections, is avoided altogether. This provocative study suggests that PCA significantly prolongs postoperative ileus and therefore recovery and hospitalization after uncomplicated colon surgery.

Patients reviewed during this study certainly represent an adequate sample; however, the retrospective nature of the work questions the possible influence of other factors not entered into account. A prospective randomized study on this topic published by Rogers in 1990 failed to demonstrate a similar adverse effect of PCA on the return of gastrointestinal motility. Clearly, in this era of cost containment, any factor that may adversely affect the length of hospital stay should be further evaluated, and a large, prospective, randomized study comparing IM and PCA postoperative analgesia is warranted.

V.E. Pricolo, M.D.

What is the Learning Curve for Laparoscopic Colectomy?
Senagore AJ, Luchtefeld MA, Mackeigan JM (Michigan State Univ, East Lansing)
Am Surg 61:681–685, 1995   10–56

Objective.—There is a learning curve associated with laparoscopic colectomy, but little information is available about the variables that affect the learning experience. This prospective study reviews the experience of 1 surgical team with the first 60 consecutive laparoscopic-assisted colectomies.

Methods.—The 60 patients were divided into 3 groups of 20 patients each. Data on age, sex, indication for the procedure, prior major abdominal surgery, type of resection, operative time, operating room cost, time to first passage of flatus, time to first bowel movement, time to first oral intake, length of hospital stay, complications, conversion rate, and hospital costs were collected.

Results.—Male/female ratios and ages were similar among the groups. There was a higher incidence of abdominal surgeries in groups 2 and 3 than in group 1. The 5 intraoperative complications occurred in group 2, and the conversion rate was highest in this group. Mean operating time decreased by 25 minutes with group 3. The postoperative complication rate was highest in group 1 and included atelectasis, pneumonia, and prolonged ileus. Pulmonary complications decreased from 30% in group 1 to 5% in groups 2 and 3. When compared with groups 1 and 2, group 3 had a significantly shorter time to flatus, and the first bowel movement. Time to first oral intake decreased significantly from 3.9 days in group 1 to 3.3 in group 2 and 1.7 in group 3. Similarly, the length of hospital stay decreased from 6.8 to 6.6 to 4.2 days. Operating room charges decreased from group 1 ($3,003) to group 2 ($2,988) but increased to the highest level with group 3 ($4,215). Overall hospital charges decreased from $13,965 to $14,063 to $11,860.

Conclusion.—The learning curve increases stepwise as surgeons begin with good-risk patients and progress to patients with more complex resections. Learning requires mastery of technical skills, proper surgical instruments, and individualized postoperative care.

▶ The authors set out to show and conclude in this article that there is a learning curve for laparoscopic colectomy and that the curve occurs incrementally by surgeons doing laparoscopic colectomy. Unfortunately, they fail to address the more important question of what this curve is. For example, how many cases should one do, what role does previous laparoscopic surgery experience have, and what exactly is mastery of laparoscopic colectomy.

By far, colectomy is currently the most technically demanding procedure performed with any frequency by laparoscopy. It is hard to imagine that any learning curve for laparoscopic colectomy would be more than hundreds of cases given the complexity and numerous resective options available.

The authors also raise a second and very provocative issue, that of the postoperative learning curve. Their perception that we must not only change the way we do the operation but also the way we take care of these patients is undoubtedly correct. What is intriguing is to consider the changes in the management of open colectomy patients. Our present paradigm for the management of open colectomy patients is clear liquids only after flatus and discharge after bowel movement. It would not be surprising to see a shift in the future to the current laparoscopic paradigm of early feeding and early discharge. After all, what does a patient do following open colectomy in the hospital after the first 36 to 48 hours, and more importantly, what do we do for the patient?

J.F. Amaral, M.D.

Posterior Plication of the Rectum for Rectal Prolapse in Children

Tsugawa C, Matsumoto Y, Nishijima E, Muraji T, Higashimoto Y (Kobe Children's Hosp, Japan)
J Pediatr Surg 30:692–693, 1995   10–57

Introduction.—Fourteen children aged 1 to 12 years underwent posterior rectal plication for persistent rectal prolapse on defecation that required manual reduction. All patients had failed a regimen of conservative management.

Technique.—The natal cleft was incised with the patient in a jackknife position. Parasagittal and levator muscle fibers were divided in the midline by electrocautery, with the center of the external sphincter left untouched. Two thirds of the rectal circumference was dissected free and 10 to 15 cm was dissected vertically. The distal rectal wall was also dissected, as low beneath the external sphincter as possible. Three or four longitudinal U-shaped mattress sutures using 3-0 or 4-0 double-armed Prolene were placed in the freed two thirds of the rectal wall. As these sutures were pulled up for tying, the rectum was folded in on itself in an accordion fashion and the sutures were approximated to the surface of the sacrum. Muscle fibers and the wound were closed without drainage.

Results.—There was only 1 recurrence of prolapse during the follow-up period of 3 months to 12 years, this occurring transiently in a patient with myelomeningocele 2 weeks postoperatively. One patient had a wound infection requiring subcutaneous drainage, but otherwise no complications were reported.

Discussion.—Posterior rectal plication appears to be a simple and effective technique for treating rectal prolapse. The reefing of the rectum prevents prolapse while allowing the atonic, stretched muscle fibers to recover their tone and function.

▶ This elegant procedure is a spin-off of the posterior sagittal anorectoplasty, and the authors stress Dr. Pena's credo to "always stay in the midline" to avoid neuromuscular damage. While their operation makes sense, so do most of the other 100 procedures for rectal prolapse they refer to. It is to be seen, therefore, whether the posterior rectal reefing technique will stand the test of longer follow-up, particularly in older, neurologically impaired children.

F.I. Luks, M.D.

Fecal Bile Acids, Short-Chain Fatty Acids, and Bacteria After Ileal Pouch–Anal Anastomosis Do Not Differ in Patients With Pouchitis

Sandborn WJ, Tremaine WJ, Batts KP, Pemberton JH, Rossi SS, Hofmann AF, Gores GJ, Phillips SF (Mayo Clinic, Rochester, Minn; Univ of California, San Diego)
Dig Dis Sci 40:1474–1483, 1995   10–58

Objective.—Because an ileal reservoir alters the fecal bacterial flora as well as the fecal content of bile acids and short-chain fatty acids (SCFAs), an attempt was made to relate the pouch content of fecal bacteria, bile acids, and SCFAs to pouch inflammation in 25 patients.

Patients.—Pouchitis developed in 10 patients with ulcerative colitis who underwent an ileal pouch–anal anastomosis (IPAA). Five others had IPAA without pouchitis. Five patients had IPAA for familial adenomatous polyposis; they also were free of pouchitis. Finally, 5 patients having a Brooke ileostomy for ulcerative colitis served as a control group.

Methods.—Pouchitis was considered to be present when a patient scored 7 or higher on an 19-point scale of disease activity. Aerobic and anaerobic organisms were cultured quantitatively. Total aqueous-phase bile acids were estimated by thin-layer chromatography and an enzymatic 3α-OH hydroxysteroid dehydrogenase method. The fecal content of SCFAs was estimated by gas-liquid chromatography.

Results.—All patients undergoing IPAA had greater ratios of anaerobic organisms to aerobes and higher concentrations of gram-negative anaerobic rods than the ileostomy patients. There were no other group differences in bacteria, aqueous-phase bile acids, or fecal SCFAs. Patients with pouchitis and those who were unaffected had comparable fecal contents of bacteria, bile acids, and SCFAs.

Conclusion.—Pouchitis in patients undergoing IPAA is not chiefly a result of fecal stasis and consequent changes in luminal contents. Instead, pouchitis may represent recurrent ulcerative colitis.

▶ This interesting paper addresses the unresolved issue of pouchitis after restorative proctocolectomy. The etiology and pathogenesis of this condition continue to elude us. This study confirms the previously known fact that patients with an IPAA had higher ratios of aerobes over anaerobes and a higher concentration of anaerobic gram-negative rods. The fact that fecal bile acids, short-chain fatty acids, and total bacteria did not differ does not exclude the fact that mediators of anaerobic bacteria metabolism may be involved in the pathogenesis of this condition which warrants further investigation.

V.E. Pricolo, M.D.

Ileal Pouch-Anal Anastomoses Complications and Function in 1005 Patients
Fazio VW, Ziv Y, Church JM, Oakley JR, Lavery IC, Milsom JW, Schroeder TK
(Cleveland Clinic Found, Ohio)
Ann Surg 222:120–127, 1995   10–59

Introduction.—Since its introduction in 1978, restorative proctocolectomy with ileal pouch–anal anastomosis (IPAA) has become an established operation for patients with chronic ulcerative colitis and familial adenomatous polyposis. The results of a large series of patients over an 11-year period are reported.

Methods.—Charts of 1,005 patients who underwent IPAA from 1983 to 1993 were reviewed. Histopathologic preoperative diagnoses were ulcerative colitis in 858, familial adenomatous polyposis in 62, indeterminate colitis in 75, and miscellaneous in 10. Data collected included demographics, type and duration of disease, previous surgeries, indications for and type of surgery, postoperative pathologic diagnosis, and early and late complications. Annual follow-up included functional and quality-of-life questionnaires, physical examination, and biopsies of the pouch and transitional zone.

Results.—Histopathologic postoperative diagnoses were ulcerative colitis in 812, familial adenomatous polyposis in 62, indeterminate colitis in 54, Crohn's disease in 67, and miscellaneous in 10. The histopathologic diagnoses were changed for 25 patients during a mean follow-up of 35 months. The overall mortality rate was 1%. Of those who died, there were 4 early and 6 late deaths. One death (0.1%) was related to pouch necrosis and sepsis. The overall morbidity rate was 62.7%. Six-hundred thirty patients experienced 1,218 complications. Of these, 27.5% were early complications and 50.5% were late complications. Twenty-four percent of the patients experienced a reoperation, and 6.8% had septic complications. The ileal pouch was removed in 34 patients (3.4%). It was nonfunctional in 11 patients (1%). Most patients (93%) indicated that functional results and quality of life were good to excellent. Questionnaire results were similar in patients with ulcerative colitis, familial adenomatous polyposis, indeterminate colitis, and Crohn's disease. Patients whose surgeries were done between 1983 and 1988 had functional results and quality of life similar to those whose surgeries occurred after 1988.

Conclusion.—Patients in this series who underwent restorative proctocolectomy with an IPAA had low mortality rates and major morbidity rates. Patient satisfaction was high and functional results were generally good.

▶ This large retrospective review, second in size only to that of the Mayo Clinic, presents an overview of restorative proctocolectomy and ileal pouch–anal anastomosis. The authors state that since 1988 they have used the double-staple technique with preservation of 1–2 cm of the columnar epithelium above the dentate line in the vast majority of their patients.

Interestingly, although they state that this stapled technique is associated with fewer complications and better postoperative sphincter pressure when compared with the hand-sewn technique, there is no functional difference in quality of life between patients operated on between 1983 and 1988 and those operated on after 1988. It is unfortunate that such an institution with such a large volume did not undertake any prospective randomized comparison study.

V.E. Pricolo, M.D.

Unexpected Death From Enterocolitis After Surgery for Hirschsprung's Disease
Marty TL, Matlak ME, Hendrickson M, Black RE, Johnson DG (Univ of Utah, Salt Lake City; Sunrise Hosp, Las Vegas, Nev)
Pediatrics 96:118–121, 1995   10–60

Introduction.—Enterocolitis is the leading cause of death in patients with Hirschsprung's disease, even with the recent advances in early diagnosis and surgical treatment. Preoperative enterocolitis can occur in 15% to 50% of patients and is associated with a 20% to 50% mortality rate. Postoperative enterocolitis is reported in 2% to 33% of patients and is associated with a mortality rate of up to 30%. Five cases of postoperative enterocolitis with deceptively mild symptoms but resulting in unexpected death are reported.

Case Reports.—Postoperative enterocolitis occurred in 37 of 135 infants and children treated for Hirschsprung's disease over a 12-year period (incidence, 27.4%) and resulted in death in 5 (13.5%). These patients included 4 males and 1 female. The diagnosis of Hirschsprung's disease was established in all 5 within the first 6 months of life. None had any comorbidities and none had long-segment Hirschsprung's disease. They underwent routine surgical reconstruction and had no postoperative complications. One patient had a history of preoperative enterocolitis. Low-grade fever, diarrhea, and vomiting developed in the infants between 3 weeks and 20 months after surgery. Within 2–4 days of the onset of symptoms, they had seizures or cardiac arrest and died.

Discussion.—The outcomes of these children may have been improved if they had been admitted to the pediatric ICU earlier. Although primary care physicians are aware of the risk of enterocolitis in association with Hirschsprung's disease, they may be less likely to recognize it postoperatively. However, enterocolitis can develop even several years after surgical reconstruction. The surgical protocol has been revised to include better parental and referring physician education. Parents are instructed to perform prophylactic saline rectal irrigations twice daily for 3 months and once daily for another 3 months, which is the period with the highest incidence of postoperative enterocolitis.

▶ As stated by the authors, enterocolitis (the most feared complication of Hirschsprung disease) can occur before diverting colostomy, as well as after the definitive pull-through procedure. Aggressive treatment of this complication has dramatically decreased fatal outcomes, the rate of which was once believed to be 50%. However, the mortality rate is not yet 0%; it is still in the double digits, particularly if long-term vigilance is allowed to weaken.

F.I. Luks, M.D.

Factors That Influence Functional Outcome After Coloanal Anastomosis for Carcinoma of the Rectum
Miller AS, Lewis WG, Williamson MER, Holdsworth PJ, Johnston D, Finan PJ (Gen Infirmary, Leeds, England)
Br J Surg 82:1327–1330, 1995   10–61

Introduction.—Although most patients with rectal carcinoma can be treated with sphincter-saving surgery, up to half may experience fecal leakage and urgency of defecation after low anterior resection. Patients who underwent low anterior resection with coloanal anastomosis were studied to determine the relationship between postoperative functional outcome and anorectal motor, sensory, and reflex function.

Methods.—Thirty patients who were treated for rectal carcinoma with anterior resection over a 10-year period were studied. Anal sphincter function was evaluated at a median of 11 months after surgery. The station pull-through technique was used to measure anal pressure. Neorectal capacity was measured by inflating a balloon, placed with its lower edge 5 cm from the anal verge, with air until discomfort or a strong desire to defecate occurred. The response of the entire length of the anal sphincter was measured to assess the rectoanal inhibitory reflex. Sensation in the upper, middle, and lower portions of the anal canal was measured with manometry. The patients were questioned about bowel frequency, defecation urgency, anal soreness, and fecal leakage. Their functional result was categorized as either perfect continence (11 patients) or fecal leakage with or without urgency of defecation (19 patients).

Results.—The anal canal had a median maximum resting pressure of 80 cm H_2O in patients with good function and 51 cm H_2O in patients with poor function and a median maximum squeeze pressure of 160 cm H_2O in patients with good function and 102 cm H_2O in patients with poor function. The pressure required for maximal inhibition of the anal sphincter was significantly lower than the pressure within the lower part of the sphincter during reflex inhibition in patients with good function and was significantly higher than the pressure throughout the length of the anal sphincter in patients with poor function. The maximum tolerated air volume was 98 mL in patients with good function and 65 mL in patients with poor function. Patients with poor function had significantly less sensation in the upper portion of the anal canal. The patients with poor outcome were predominantly women.

Discussion.—A disproportionate number of women undergoing low anterior resection had a poor functional outcome. The significant sensory neuropathy in these patients suggests that preoperative occult sphincter injury, possibly related to childbirth, may compromise the outcome of sphincter-saving surgery in patients with rectal carcinoma. Preoperative manometric and endoanal ultrasonographic evaluation of the anatomy of the anal sphincter and assessment of the rectoanal inhibitory reflex may be useful for predicting functional outcome after coloanal anastomosis and in surgical planning.

▶ The authors correctly emphasize that a high proportion of women have poor functional results following low anterior resection with coloanal anastomosis. We would agree that antecedent occult sphincter injury, perhaps by the trauma of obstetrics, will strongly influence the outcome of the coloanal anastomosis of sphincter preservation surgery for cancer. This study gives strong credence to the findings that preoperative assessment of anal-sphincter function prior to low anterior resection is essential when sphincter preservation is desired or anticipated. The study further concludes that preoperative evaluation with manometry and endoanal ultrasonography provides objective parameters to the clinician for preoperative selection of appropriate candidates for the coloanal reconstruction. Only with consistent and aggressive surveillance of eligible candidates will superior outcome results be achieved with the technique.

K.I. Bland, M.D.

11 Oncology

Introduction

This has been a very productive year in the surgical and basic science literature. While not every selection for this portion of the YEAR BOOK is a landmark paper, I have tried to select manuscripts that will have an impact on the everyday practice of a busy surgeon treating various malignancies. Some selections are contributions made through large clinical trials, some introduce innovative technical contributions, and still others make significant basic science observations. While these may not be definitive studies, they will clearly have a major impact on the practice of surgery now and in the future.

In the breast section, several large trials verify breast conservation as being equivalent treatment to mastectomy for early-stage breast cancer. Several manuscripts comment about the importance of obtaining negative surgical margins and the impact that positive margins may have on outcome. Patients requiring mastectomy can be treated with breast reconstruction by having immediate transverse rectus abdominis musculocutaneous flap reconstruction. This provides superb results and does not hinder the detection of recurrence or delay adjuvant therapies. p53 antibody detection may have predictive value in selecting patients with higher risk of recurrence. Thoracic epidural anesthesia appears to be a safe alternative to general anesthesia for breast surgery and breast reconstructive procedures.

With respect to colorectal tumors, radioimmunoguided surgery cannot only be an aid to detection of recurrence but can also serve as an adjunct to accurate surgical staging. We have revisited the question of stapled vs. hand-sewn anastomosis and have shown that intraoperative ultrasound is currently among the most accurate means of detection of colorectal metastasis in the liver. With respect to rectal cancer, several trials utilizing various aspects of preoperative radiation therapy in high or low dose, with or without chemotherapy, can clearly downstage tumors, will most likely diminish local recurrence, and may have a positive impact on survival. Identification for timing and selection of patients is presented. This therapy is associated with a higher incidence of toxicity and morbidity. Quite a number of very elegant manuscripts describe the results of coloanal reconstruction following resection for very low rectal tumors. Alternatives such as full-thickness local excision and J-pouch reconstruction are discussed. Adaptation of these techniques into the treatment of patients with invasive rectal cancers will provide excellent treatment, but not at the expense of sphincter ablation.

Once again, significant advances have been made in the genetic changes of colorectal tumors by using hereditary nonpolyposis colon cancer syndrome as a model. Similarly, changes in the cell surface glycoprotein (CD44) may play an important role in the transformation of normal mucosa to carcinoma. Treatment of gastric cancers remains a very difficult clinical problem. The importance of adequate and accurate staging, as well as the important pathologic features of lymphatic vessel invasion, margin involvement, and lymph node metastases, is emphasized. In addition, however, other newer diagnostic markers, such as epidermal growth factor and transforming growth factor α may help in the selection of patients who may benefit from adjuvant therapies. Identification of the molecular events that occur in the transformation of normal gastric mucosa to gastric carcinoma are also discussed.

Several very large, very well done trials documenting survival in pancreatic carcinoma are presented. These trials are significant as they identify factors that may play an important role in improving survival. Once again, by utilizing molecular techniques, somatic genetic mutations are being associated with the development of pancreatic carcinoma. Further work will establish a genetic model and provide the possibility to intervene in this disease with genetic therapies.

Technical aspects of liver resection as well as clinical trials in hepatocellular carcinoma are presented. New techniques such as sentinel lymph node biopsy and lymphoscintigraphy in melanoma patients are discussed. Clinical and pathologic parameters associated with survival characteristics in truncal and retroperitoneal soft tissue sarcoma are presented. Once again, by using the polymerase chain reaction technique, new molecular markers are being identified that will aid in the accurate diagnosis and staging of patients with sarcoma.

In summary, this year has witnessed many significant clinical and technical contributions in the surgical management of various solid malignancies. In addition, however, significant advances are being utilized in the identification of genetic and molecular markers in breast, gastric, and pancreatic carcinoma and in soft tissue sarcoma. Familiarity with these genetic changes and molecular markers will not only provide a basis for alternative treatments for patients with solid tumors but more immediately will also aid in the accurate staging and selection of patients for more intensive treatments.

Timothy J. Eberlein, M.D.

Carcinoma of the Breast

Manuscripts selected in this section vary widely, with their subject matter indicative of the diversity of diagnosis and treatment of carcinoma of the breast. The selected manuscripts will touch on multiple topics that will have practical implications in the current management of carcinoma of the breast.

T.J. Eberlein, M.D.

Breast-Conserving Surgery for Breast Cancer: Patterns of Care in a Geographic Region and Estimation of Potential Applicability
Foster RS Jr, Farwell ME, Costanza MC (Univ of Vermont, Burlington; Vermont Cancer Ctr, Burlington)
Ann Surg Oncol 2:275–280, 1995   11–1

Background.—Research had amply established by 1989 that survival is similar in patients with local disease treated with either breast conservation surgery (with or without radiation therapy) or mastectomy. It has been hypothesized that breast cancer screening would result in the detection of more early-stage breast cancers that could be managed with breast-conserving therapy. Data from a state database were analyzed to determine the proportion of patients eligible for breast-conserving surgery before and after the widespread availability of screening mammography.

Methods.—Data were collected on the method of cancer detection, age, clinical staging, tumor size, and node status for patients with pathologically diagnosed breast cancer treated in 1975–1984 and 1989–1990 at university and community hospitals and were related to patterns of breast-conserving surgery.

Results.—Detection by mammography increased from 2% in 1975–1984 to 36% in 1989–1990. Noninvasive disease was found in 2.3% of the patients in 1975–1984 and 8.4% in 1989–1990. In addition, patients in whom cancer was diagnosed in 1989–1990 tended to have smaller tumors and earlier clinical and pathologic stages than patients in whom cancer was diagnosed in 1975–1984. Management with breast-conserving surgery increased overall from 8.6% in 1975–1984 to 42% in 1989–1990. In 1989–1990, staging and patient age distributions were similar in the university and community hospital settings (Table 2). However, the use of breast-conserving surgery varied in association with both staging and hospital type. At university hospitals in 1989–1990, breast-conserving surgery was performed on 68% of the patients who were at least 70 years old and 75% of the younger patients. Age was a significantly more limiting factor in the use of breast-conserving surgery in community than in university hospitals. Applying the age and stage selection criteria for breast-conserving surgery at university hospitals in 1989–1990 to the patients treated in 1975–1984 resulted in an estimate of 67% of the earlier patients who could have been treated with breast-conserving surgery.

Discussion.—Most patients could be appropriately treated with breast-conserving surgery regardless of whether their breast cancer is detected with screening mammography. However, universal screening mammography would increase the number of patients eligible for breast conservation.

TABLE 2.—Breast-Conserving Surgery in Vermont Breast Cancer Patients 1989–1990

Patient Category	University Hospital Stage %	n	BCS %	Community Hospitals Stage %	n	BCS %
Clinical TNM stage						
0 (TIS)	10*	26	85	6	23	48
I	56	154	86	54	205	27
II	26	70	60	30	112	13
III	4	12	33	5	17	12
IV	4	11	0	5	19	5
All patients staged and unstaged		283			400	
All invasive cancers		247†	73		359	22
Invasive breast cancer pathologic diameter (cm)						
<2		111†	87		162	32
2–5		102	72		145	15
>5		10	20		12	0
Axillary nodes histologically negative		120†	82		156	17
Axillary nodes histologically positive		68†	56		111	14
No resection of axillary nodes (invasive cancers): age (yrs)						
<50		6	50		6	50
50–69		16	69		14	50
>69		31	84		36	61

Note: Variation in totals is due to missing data.
* Chi-square analysis of stage distribution for university hospital vs. community hospitals shows no significant difference.
† Indicates $P < 0.001$ by chi-square analysis.
Abbreviations: BCS, breast-conserving surgery; *TIS,* tumor in situ.
(Courtesy of Foster RS Jr, Farwell ME, Costanza MC: Breast-conserving surgery for breast cancer: Patterns of care in a geographic region and estimation of potential applicability. *Ann Surg Oncol* 2:275–280, 1995.)

Regional variations in the use of breast-conserving surgery are related more to local community factors and individual physician attitudes than to regional variations in patient characteristics.

▶ It is now widely accepted that for stage I/II carcinoma of the breast, breast-conserving surgery renders similar survival results as does mastectomy. However, there is considerable variability with regard to the rate of breast-conserving surgery among individual surgeons and geographically. This has been documented by the American College of Surgeons, as well as in this study from diagnosed breast cancers from all general hospitals in the state of Vermont. This study showed that age and stage of disease had less influence on the rate of breast-conserving surgery than did local community factors and physician attitudes. Two thirds of the women in the state were actually eligible for breast-conserving surgery. As higher utilization of mammographic screening becomes prevalent nationwide and there is further downstaging of disease at the time of presentation, these physican attitudes will become even more important in determining the rate of breast-conserving surgery.

T.J. Eberlein, M.D.

The Importance of the Lumpectomy Surgical Margin Status in Long Term Results of Breast Conservation

Smitt MC, Nowels KW, Zdeblick MJ, Jeffrey S, Carlson RW, Stockdale FE, Goffinet DR (Stanford Univ, Calif; Redwood Microsystems, Menlo Park, Calif)

Cancer 76:259–267, 1995   11–2

Background.—In appropriately selected patients with early-stage breast cancer, freedom from relapse and overall survival are comparable in patients treated with lumpectomy and radiation therapy or with mastectomy. However, long-term local failure rates have varied considerably after lumpectomy and radiation therapy. The influence of the microscopic resection margin on long-term local control was examined retrospectively.

Methods.—The records of 289 women with 303 stage I and II invasive carcinomas of the breast who were treated with lumpectomy and radiation therapy between 1972 and 1992 were examined. The surgical margins on the initial biopsy and any re-excision specimens were classified as either positive, close (within 2 mm of the margin), negative, or indeterminate. The actual probabilities of local and metastatic disease-free and overall survival were calculated. The risk of local relapse was calculated for each

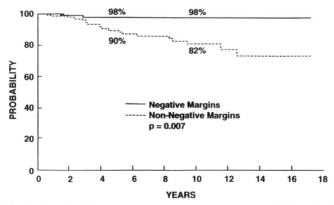

FIGURE 2.—Freedom from local recurrence by margin status: negative, *solid line*; all others, *dashed line*. (Courtesy of *Cancer*, from Smitt MC, Nowels KW, Zdeblick MJ, et al., copyright © 1995. Reprinted by permission of Wiley-Liss, Inc., a division of John Wiley & Sons, Inc.)

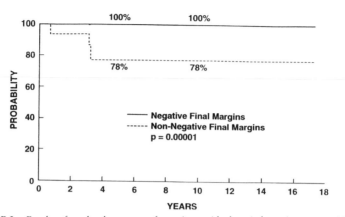

FIGURE 3.—Freedom from local recurrence for patients with close, indeterminate, or positive initial margins who underwent re-excision with negative final margins (*solid line*) or nonnegative final margins (*dashed line*). (Courtesy of *Cancer*, from Smitt MC, Nowels KW, Zdeblick MJ, et al., copyright © 1995. Reprinted by permission of Wiley-Liss, Inc., a division of John Wiley & Sons, Inc.)

margin status classification and for re-excision. The importance of other potential prognostic factors for local recurrence was analyzed overall and for patients with negative and nonnegative surgical margins.

Results.—The actuarial freedom from local recurrence was 94% at 5 years and 87% at 10 years. Rates of freedom from distant recurrence and overall survival were 83% at 10 years. The probability of local control in the groups defined by final margin status were as follows: 98% for negative margins, 84% for close margins, 100% for focally positive margins, 91% for indeterminate margins, and 91% for diffuse or unknown positive margins. At 10 years, the probability of local control was 98% in patients with negative margins and 82% in patients with all other margin classifications (Fig 2). Overall, the local control probability at 10 years for patients undergoing re-excision was 97% as compared with 84% for patients not undergoing re-excision. Among patients with nonnegative

TABLE 2.—Relationship of Extensive Intraductal Component and Margin Status to Re-excision Findings

	% Residual Carcinoma
Whole group	42
EIC present	82
EIC absent	31
Initial margin	
Negative	25
Close	7
Focal positive	28
Other positive	46
Indeterminate	45

Abbreviation: EIC, extensive intraductal component.
(Courtesy of *Cancer*, from Smitt MC, Nowels KW, Zdeblick MJ, et al., copyright © 1995. Reprinted by permission of Wiley-Liss, Inc., a division of John Wiley & Sons, Inc.)

margins initially who underwent re-excision, the 10-year probability of local control was 100% for those with a negative final margin status and 78% for those with a nonnegative final margin status (Fig 3). Univariate analysis for the entire study group identified final margin status, N stage, histologic type, and adjuvant therapy with tamoxifen or chemotherapy as potentially prognostic. Final margin status and the use of chemotherapy were significant prognostic factors in multivariate analysis (Table 2).

Conclusions.—Achieving negative surgical margins, either initially or with re-excision, is the most important predictor of local control in patients undergoing lumpectomy and radiation for early-stage breast cancer.

▶ This is a retrospective study showing the long-term importance of attaining negative margins. This has practical importance, especially with the increase in core needle biopsies and/or fine-needle aspiration (FNA) as a means of diagnosing cancers. This study shows that local control at 10 years was 98% for patients with negative surgical margins. It did not appear to matter whether the negative margins were attained at the time of the first operation or at the time of re-excision. This emphasizes the point that whichever strategy one uses to treat breast cancer patients, be it incisional biopsy, core biopsy, or FNA, the importance of attaining negative margins is paramount for long-term local control. Obviously, the extent of surgical excision of a known malignancy is best guided by gross intraoperative pathologic evaluation. Our own policy at the Joint Center is to offer re-excision to patients who have positive margins prior to administering radiation therapy.

T.J. Eberlein, M.D.

Ten-Year Results of a Comparison of Conservation With Mastectomy in the Treatment of Stage I and II Breast Cancer
Jacobson JA, Danforth DN, Cowan KH, D'Angelo T, Steinberg SM, Pierce L, Lippman ME, Lichter AS, Glatstein E, Okunieff P (Natl Cancer Inst, Bethesda, Md; Univ of Michigan, Ann Arbor; Georgetown Univ Hosp, Washington, DC; et al)
N Engl J Med 332:907–911, 1995   11–3

Objective.—Because it remains uncertain whether breast conservation treatment is as effective as mastectomy in women with early-stage breast cancer, the National Cancer Institute conducted a randomized trial in the years 1979–1987 to compare these 2 approaches in 247 women with clinical stage I and II breast cancers.

Study Plan.—A total of 237 patients were randomized and have been followed for a median of just over 10 years. Conservation treatment included lumpectomy, axillary dissection, and irradiation. Women randomized to mastectomy also underwent axillary dissection. Radiotherapy consisted of 4,500–5,040 cGy to the whole breast delivered in 180-cGy fractions 5 days a week. Patients with node involvement received cyclophosphamide and doxorubicin.

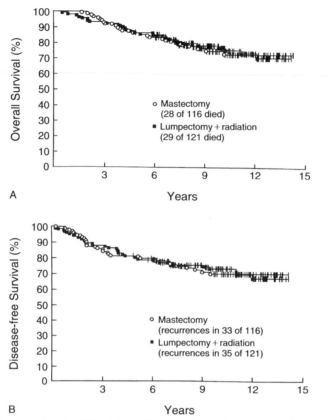

FIGURE 1.—Overall survival (**A**) and disease-free survival (**B**) in the 2 groups. *Tick marks* indicate the lengths of follow-up for patients who had not died (**A**) or had a recurrence of disease (**B**). Wider bars indicate overlapping tick marks. (Reprinted by permission of *The New England Journal of Medicine*, from Jacobsen JA, Danforth DN, Cowan KH, et al: Ten-year results of a comparison of conservation with mastectomy in the treatment of stage I and II breast cancer. *N Engl J Med* 332:907–911, Copyright 1995, Massachusetts Medical Society.)

Results.—Disease-free survival and overall survival were comparable in the 2 treatment groups (Fig 1). The disease-free survival rate at 10 years was 69% in the mastectomy group and 72% for those assigned to conservation treatment. Locoregional recurrence as an isolated first event developed in 4% of the patients in each group but was more frequent in the mastectomy group when patients with concomitant distant disease were included (Fig 2). The risk of recurrence limited to the ipsilateral breast after lumpectomy was 18% at 10 years. The only factors significantly predicting disease-free survival were tumor stage and axillary node involvement.

Conclusions.—These results affirm those obtained in 5 similar randomized trials. Lumpectomy combined with axillary node dissection and radiotherapy eliminates stage I/II breast cancer as effectively as mastectomy does.

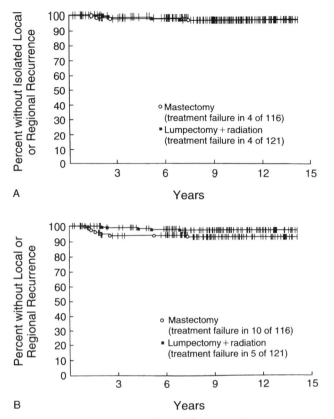

FIGURE 2.—Local or regional recurrences as isolated first events (**A**) or as any component of a first event (**B**) in the 2 treatment groups. Data were censored on patients with recurrences confined to the ipsilateral breast and successfully treated. *Tick marks* indicate follow-up times for patients who had not had recurrences. (Reprinted by permission of *The New England Journal of Medicine*, from Jacobsen JA, Danforth DN, Cowan KH, et al: Ten-year results of a comparison of conservation with mastectomy in the treatment of stage I and II breast cancer. *N Engl J Med* 332:907–911, Copyright 1995, Massachusetts Medical Society.)

▶ This series is an update of a previously published series from the National Cancer Institute. It affirms what the National Surgical Adjuvant Breast Project, Milan, Italy, as well as multiple other series have stated—that breast conservation is as effective in the treatment of stage I and II breast cancer as mastectomy. It is noteworthy that at 10 years, the actuarial rate of recurrence of cancer confined to the ipsilateral breast was 18%. In this series, salvage mastectomy was extremely effective in eliminating disease. It is also noteworthy that all 10 patients in the mastectomy group who had local or regional failure also had systemic disease, yet only 8 of the 20 patients with recurrence of cancer within the breast after breast-conserving therapy had distant metastasis—an interesting finding that raises some questions regarding the biology of the disease as well as selection of patients. Thus whether the patient receives breast conservation therapy or mastectomy, the patient can expect similar survival benefit as long as the treatment is adequate.

T.J. Eberlein, M.D.

Ten-Year Results in 1070 Patients With Stages I and II Breast Cancer Treated by Conservative Surgery and Radiation Therapy
Mansfield CM, Komarnicky LT, Schwartz GF, Rosenberg AL, Krishnan L, Jewell WR, Rosato FE, Moses ML, Haghbin M, Taylor J (Thomas Jefferson Univ, Philadelphia, Pa; Univ of Kansas, Kansas City)
Cancer 75:2328–2336, 1995   11–4

Background.—Although the value of radiation therapy in the conservative treatment of early-stage breast cancer is well documented, many surgeons continue to perform mastectomy because they believe that it provides better local control. Local control in a large series of patients with early-stage breast cancer treated conservatively by surgery and irradiation was reported.

Methods.—The 1,070 patients were treated between 1982 and 1994. Median follow-up was 40 months. All underwent wide local excision and lower lymph node dissection followed by radiation therapy. An external beam dose of 4,500 cGy was delivered to the whole breast at 180 cGy/5 days/wk. Another boost dose of 2,000 cGy was delivered to the tumor bed at the time of lumpectomy by an ^{192}Ir implant or electron beam therapy after external beam therapy.

Findings.—Disease-specific survival rates were 97% at 5 years and 90% at 10 years among women with stage I disease and 87% and 69%, respectively, for women with stage II disease. Local control rates at 5 and 10 years were 93% and 85%, respectively, for patients with stage I cancer and 92% and 87% for those with stage II cancer. Premenopausal status and estrogen receptor–negative status were risk factors for local failure in

---

TABLE 8.—Factors That Influence Local Control

Risk Factor	P Value	RR
Menopause (*pre/post & peri)	0.001	2.36
Estrogen receptor (*neg/pos)	0.01	2.26
Margins (*pos/neg)	0.06	2.09
Age (*<55/>55)	0.11	0.64
Stage (*I/II)	0.19	1.40
Breast technique (*electron/implant)	0.21	0.72
Intraductal (*neg/pos)	0.30	1.31
Progesterone receptor (*pos/neg)	0.36	1.38
Nodes (*pos/neg)	0.47	1.24
Chemotherapy (*no/yes)	0.92	0.97

* Worse risk.
Abbreviation: RR, relative risk.
(Courtesy of *Cancer*, from Mansfield CM, Komarnicky LT, Schwartz GF, et al., copyright © 1995. Reprinted by permission of Wiley-Liss, Inc., a division of John Wiley & Sons, Inc.)

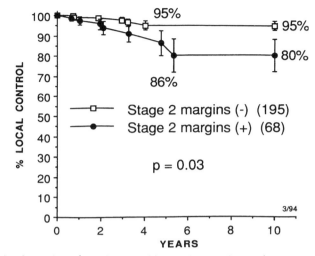

FIGURE 3.—Comparison of negative vs. positive margins in patients with stage II carcinoma of the breast. (Courtesy of *Cancer*, from Mansfield CM, Komarnicky LT, Schwartz GF, et al., copyright © 1995. Reprinted by permission of Wiley-Liss, Inc., a division of John Wiley & Sons, Inc.)

univariate analysis (Table 8). Premenopausal status and margin status were significant in multivariate analysis (Fig 3).

Conclusions.—These 10-year outcomes in patients with early-stage breast cancer treated conservatively with surgery and radiation therapy are at least as good as those associated with mastectomy. More surgeons should offer conservative treatment as an alternative to women with stages I and II breast cancer.

▶ This is a very large series from Thomas Jefferson University Hospital of patients treated with breast conservation and radiation therapy. While disease-specific survival and local control rates diminish as stage increases, premenopausal status and margin involvement were significant with respect to local failure. An additional finding from this study was that a boost dose of radiation, which is now fairly standard in most institutions, may decrease the risk of local recurrence without increasing morbidity or decreasing cosmesis.

T.J. Eberlein, M.D.

Randomized Trial of Chemoendocrine Therapy Started Before or After Surgery for Treatment of Primary Breast Cancer

Powles TJ, Hickish TF, Makris A, Ashley SE, O'Brien MER, Tidy VA, Casey S, Nash AG, Sacks N, Cosgrove D, MacVicar D, Fernando I, Ford HT (Royal Marsden Hosp, Sutton, Surrey, England)

J Clin Oncol 13:547–552, 1995

11–5

Introduction.—Several studies have established the value of adjuvant cytotoxic chemotherapy or tamoxifen in reducing the risk of relapse and mortality in patients with primary breast cancer. The results also suggest that combination therapy with both tamoxifen and chemotherapy may further improve outcome. It has been suggested that neoadjuvant treatment with systemic endocrine therapy and chemotherapy before surgical treatment may improve outcome and may reduce the extent of surgical treatment required. The effects of neoadjuvant therapy were compared with those of adjuvant therapy in women with operable primary breast cancer.

Methods.—Patients under 70 years of age with palpable primary operable breast cancer confirmed by fine-needle aspiration cytology were randomly assigned to be treated with either primary surgery followed by adjuvant chemoendocrine therapy within 3–6 weeks or primary chemoendocrine therapy for 3 months before and 3 months after primary surgery. Both groups were also treated with radiotherapy if required. The size of the primary tumor was monitored clinically during presurgical treatment in the patients receiving neoadjuvant systemic therapy.

Results.—Of the 212 randomized patients, 200 were assessable. Among the patients in the neoadjuvant group, 85% had an objective response, with a complete or nearly complete response in most of them and no differences between the 2 chemotherapy regimens in results. These patients also experienced significant reductions in tumor size, tumor stage, and clinical axillary node status when compared with patients in the adjuvant group (Table 3). The patients in the neoadjuvant group demonstrated objective reductions in tumor size in 81% of the measurable tumors with mammography and in 88% of the measurable tumors with ultrasound. Measurements of the excised tumors revealed tumors smaller than 2 cm in 86% of the neoadjuvant patients vs. 43% of the adjuvant patients. There was a complete pathologic response in 10% of the neoadjuvant patients. This downstaging resulted in reduced requirements for mastectomy. The median follow-up of 28 months was too short to adequately assess the effect on relapse and mortality.

Discussion.—Neoadjuvant therapy produced a high objective response rate and a significant reduction in surgical requirements, including the need for mastectomy. More study of the relapse rate, disease-free survival rate, and overall survival rate is needed before neoadjuvant therapy can be advised.

TABLE 3.—Clinical Downstaging and Surgical Requirements According to
Clinical Stage and Tumor Size

Tumor Characteristic	No. of Adjuvant Patients (n = 99)	No. of Neoadjuvant Patients	
		Prechemotherapy (n = 101)	Postchemotherapy (n = 101)
Clinical size (cm)			
0.1–1.0	2 ⎫ 10%	2 ⎫ 9%	62 ⎫ 81%
1.1–2.0	8 ⎭	7 ⎭	20 ⎭
2.1–3.0	42	43	11
3.1–4.0	32	25	3
4.1–5.0	7	21	4
>5.0	8	3	1
Tumor stage			
T0–T1	10	9	82*
T2	81	89	18
T3	8	3	1
Node stage			
N0	85	79	98†
N1a	8	14	0
N1b	6	8	3

* $P < 0.001$.
† $P < 0.001$.
(Courtesy of Powles TJ, Hickish TF, Makris A, et al: Randomized trial of chemoendocrine therapy started before or after surgery for treatment of primary breast cancer. *J Clin Oncol* 13:547–552, 1995.)

▶ This is a randomized prospective trial looking at the response to neoadjuvant therapy. It is the first to include small primary cancers as well. This study and others have shown that neoadjuvant chemotherapy can reduce the requirement for mastectomy; however, it will take a very large trial, such as the National Surgical Adjuvant Breast Project B-18 trial, to study disease-free and overall survival implications. In a biological sense, this type of therapy may be an ideal opportunity to study various biological markers of breast cancer and their response to chemotherapies and perhaps develop newer strategies for prediction of treatment and survival. Simply treating all patients with neoadjuvant chemotherapy, while expedient, may negate the opportunity to biologically study these patients and identify the most appropriate population to utilize this type of therapy.

T.J. Eberlein, M.D.

Intraductal Carcinoma (Ductal Carcinoma In Situ) of the Breast: A Comparison of Pure Noninvasive Tumors With Those Including Different Proportions of Infiltrating Carcinoma
Moriya T, Silverberg SG (Kawasaki Med School, Kurashiki, Japan; George Washington Univ, Washington, DC)
Cancer 74:2972–2978, 1994   11–6

Introduction.—Although ductal carcinoma in situ (DCIS) is a noninvasive carcinoma arising in the duct structures, it may be found in combination with infiltrating ductal components (IDCs) that invade the surrounding stroma. It has been suggested that the relative proportion of DCIS to IDCs may predict prognosis, with a lower proportion of IDCs associated with a better prognosis. Studies have also suggested that the comedo-type DCIS has a greater potential of progressing to infiltrating carcinoma. To investigate these associations, the histologic type was identified in pure DCIS samples and in the DCIS components of mixed DCIS/IDC cases.

Methods.—Records and glass slides were reviewed from 85 pure DCIS lesions and 64 mixed DCIS/IDC lesions. Histopathologic analysis determined the proportion of IDCs, subtype, nuclear grade, mitoses, the presence of lobular cancerization, and the presence or type of stromal reaction.

Results.—With pure DCIS, the histopathologic subtype was more frequently micropapillary with and without necrosis or cribriform with and without necrosis. With mixed DCIS/IDC, the histopathologic subtype of the DCIS component was more frequently solid with necrosis, solid, and comedo. The solid subtype was more frequently found in the mixed lesions when the proportion of DCIS was lower than 50%, whereas comedocarcinoma was found more frequently in lesions with a greater than 50% proportion of DCIS than among either pure DCIS lesions or lesions with a greater invasive component. Pure DCIS lesions were more likely to have well-differentiated nuclei and no mitotic figures than were mixed lesions. Both periductal stromal inflammation and multifocality were more common with mixed DCIS/IDC lesions than with pure DCIS lesions. Of the tumors identified as comedocarcinomas, a solid growth pattern occurred in 68% of the mixed lesions and 32% of the pure DCIS lesions, with a low nuclear grade in 37% of the pure DCIS lesions and 20% of the mixed lesions and central necrosis in 32% of the pure DCIS lesions and 36% of the mixed lesions.

Discussion.—Solid tumors with poorly differentiated nuclei and mitotic activity were associated with increased infiltrating carcinomas and more aggressive progression. These factors appear to be more important than central necrosis in predicting prognosis in patients with DCIS.

▶ I have included this manuscript simply because it raises a controversial issue. Does DCIS progress to infiltrating ductal carcinoma? Here, a solid growth pattern and high nuclear grade seem to predict progression to infiltrating ductal carcinoma. This study suggests that central necrosis, used most frequently in the past to define comedocarcinoma, is the least important factor in distinguishing between carcinomas that are purely intraductal when first diagnosed and those that progress to stromal invasion. Obviously, some cases of DCIS such as the cribriform or micropapillary type may never develop into invasive carcinoma, and likewise, some invasive carcinomas may never progress through an intraductal stage. In a practical sense, these high-grade features underscore the need for thorough mammographic evaluation and attainment of negative margins. They may also imply the need for evaluation of the axilla, especially if the extent of the high-grade DCIS is over 2 cm.

T.J. Eberlein, M.D.

Lobular Carcinoma of the Breast Can be Managed by Breast-Conserving Therapy
Holland PA, Shah A, Howell A, Baildam AD, Bundred NJ (Univ Hosp, South Manchester, England)
Br J Surg 82:1364–1366, 1995   11–7

Introduction.—Breast-conserving surgery is now considered as safe and effective as mastectomy in the management of invasive ductal carcinoma. However, many surgeons are reluctant to treat invasive lobular carcinoma (ILC) with breast conservation because of the difficulties in detecting recurrent disease mammographically and determining the extent of the disease. The incidence of local relapse in patients with ILC was compared retrospectively in a large series of patients treated with either breast conservation or mastectomy.

Methods.—The medical records and pathology reports of all patients with pure ILC treated between 1973 and 1991 were reviewed. Only patients with tumors of 4 cm or smaller were included. Relapse rates were compared in patients who underwent breast conservation by wide local excision and those who underwent mastectomy.

Results.—Of the 226 patients with ILC masses 4 cm or smaller, 52 underwent breast conservation and 174 underwent mastectomy. The 2 groups had a similar median age, tumor size, and proportion of patients given systemic adjuvant therapy. The mastectomy group had significantly more multifocal tumors. Axillary dissection was performed more frequently in the mastectomy group (74%) than in the breast conservation group (48%). However the incidence of involved axillary nodes and axillary recurrence was similar in the 2 groups. Local relapse occurred in 8% of the breast conservation group and 12% of the mastectomy group. The mortality rate was significantly higher in the mastectomy group (22% vs. 10%).

Conclusions.—Breast-conserving surgery was not associated with increased recurrence rates or mortality in patients with ILC and should be considered an appropriate treatment option for selected patients.

▶ This is a retrospective review, and I have selected it simply to emphasize the fact that patients with pure lobular carcinoma of the breast can be adequately and safely managed by breast-conserving therapy. This is not a randomized trial; however, it is a selected series. While infiltrating lobular carcinoma is associated with an increased risk of multifocality, breast conservation is still possible. Careful mammographic evaluation after biopsy as well as careful pathologic evaluation will minimize the risk of breast recurrence following breast-conserving surgery.

T.J. Eberlein, M.D.

Immediate Transverse Rectus Abdominis Musculocutaneous Flap Reconstruction After Mastectomy

Wilkins EG, August DA, Kuzon WM Jr, Chang AE, Smith DJ (Univ of Michigan, Ann Arbor)
J Am Coll Surg 180:177–183, 1995   11–8

Introduction.—Immediate breast reconstruction after mastectomy offers the advantage of lower postoperative psychological morbidity and avoids the necessity of additional anesthesia and hospitalization. A retrospective review was done to examine the early and long-term outcomes of immediate unilateral and bilateral transverse rectus abdominis musculocutaneous (TRAM) breast reconstruction.

Methods.—Preoperative planning for the combined ablative and reconstructive procedures required a collaborative effort between the surgical oncologist and plastic surgeon. When possible, mastectomy incisions were designed to maximally conserve skin and underlying soft tissue. When feasible (and without compromise of carcinoma resection), every effort was made to preserve the inframammary fold and the underlying pectoralis major for reconstruction. Both pedicle and free TRAM breast reconstructions were reviewed.

Results.—The median patient age was 46 years, with a range of 25–64 years. Fifty-three patients underwent 73 immediate TRAM flap reconstructions. The procedure was bilateral in 20 patients. Fifty simple mastectomies and 23 modified radical mastectomies were performed in 53 patients. Twenty-three patients underwent free TRAM flap procedures and 31 patients received 46 pedicle TRAM flaps. There were no total flap losses or major cardiopulmonary complications. The overall complication rate was 26% (29% for pedicle TRAM flaps and 22% for free TRAM flaps) (Table 2). Median follow-up was 22.6 months. All patients employed preoperatively resumed their occupations postoperatively.

Conclusion.—Pedicle TRAM flap and free TRAM flap procedures immediately after mastectomy are safe and viable surgical interventions for patients desiring reconstruction at the time of mastectomy. The free

TABLE 2.—Complications

Complication	Pedicle TRAM, $n=31$	Free TRAM, $n=22$
Mastectomy flap necrosis	2	3
Partial TRAM flap necrosis	2	0
Marginal necrosis donor site	1	1
Flap cellulitis	1	0
Donor site hernia	2	1
Fat necrosis	1	0
Total	9 (29)	5 (22)

Note: Numbers in parentheses are percentages.
Abbreviation: TRAM, transverse rectus abdominis musculocutaneous flap.
(By permission of the *Journal of the American College of Surgeons.*)

TRAM flap has considerable promise and needs further study of its advantages over pedicle TRAM flaps.

▶ There are many advantages to immediate breast reconstruction. While it may be inconvenient to schedule, the fact that the patient is never without a breast and the overall preservation of self-image have led to the development of many new techniques. Use of the TRAM flap reconstruction (pedicle or free) has an additional advantage as the size of the reconstructed breast can be tailored very specifically to the opposite breast. Yet a potential complication of this type of reconstruction is necrosis of the native breast skin, which underscores the importance of coordination of technical effort between the surgeon performing the mastectomy and the surgeon performing the reconstruction. Newer utilization of a skin-sparing mastectomy coupled with this type of reconstruction can provide superb results. While not commented upon in this manuscript, other series show that there is no delay in beginning adjuvant therapies, nor is there an increased risk of recurrence or a delay in diagnosis of recurrence because of the reconstruction.

T.J. Eberlein, M.D.

Tamoxifen Use in Breast Cancer Patients Who Subsequently Develop Corpus Cancer Is Not Associated With a Higher Incidence of Adverse Histologic Features
Barakat RR, Wong G, Curtin JP, Vlamis V, Hoskins WJ (Mem Sloan-Kettering Cancer Ctr, New York; Cornell Univ, Ithaca, NY)
Gynecol Oncol 55:164–168, 1994   11–9

Introduction.—Patients with breast cancer are typically treated with tamoxifen, a nonsteroidal antiestrogen. However, tamoxifen, which can act as an estrogen agonist, has been implicated in the development of endometrial carcinoma with high-grade lesions or high-risk histologic

TABLE 2.—Histologic Distribution of Corpus Cancer According to
Tamoxifen Use

Histology	Tamoxifen	No Tamoxifen
Endometrioid	16 (70%)	34 (68%)
Adenosquamous	1 (4%)	3 (6%)
Clear cell	0 (0%)	2 (4%)
Papillary serous	1 (4%)	3 (6%)
Mesodermal mixed	5 (22%)	6 (12%)
Leiomyosarcoma	0 (0%)	2 (4%)
Total	23 (100%)	50 (100%)

(Courtesy of Barakat RR, Wong G, Curtin JP, et al: Tamoxifen use in breast cancer patients who subsequently develop corpus cancer is not associated with a higher incidence of adverse histologic features. *Gynecol Oncol* 55:164–168, 1995.)

TABLE 3.—Distribution by Histologic Grade of Endometrial Carcinoma*

Histologic Grade	Tamoxifen	No Tamoxifen
1	11 (65%)	19 (51%)
2	2 (12%)	11 (30%)
3	4 (23%)	7 (19%)
Total	17 (100%)	37 (100%)

* Includes endometrioid and adenosquamous cancers.
(Courtesy of Barakat RR, Wong G, Curtin JP, et al: Tamoxifen use in breast cancer patients who subsequently develop corpus cancer is not associated with a higher incidence of adverse histologic features. *Gynecol Oncol* 55:164–168, 1995.)

findings. A retrospective study evaluated the possible association between tamoxifen treatment and a more aggressive endometrial carcinoma.

Methods.—The medical records of 77 patients with invasive breast cancer and subsequent endometrial cancer treated between 1980 and 1992 were reviewed. They were divided into 2 groups: 27 had received tamoxifen (23 for at least 1 year) and 50 had not been treated with tamoxifen. Data regarding the grade, stage, and histology of uterine tumors were gathered and compared. The groups were also compared for the interval between the diagnosis of breast cancer and that of endometrial cancer and for survival.

Results.—The 2 groups did not differ significantly in median survival after hysterectomy or in mortality from corpus cancer (22% in the tamoxifen group vs. 26% in the no-tamoxifen group). The median interval between the breast and corpus cancer diagnoses was 4.6 years for the tamoxifen group and 6.7 years for the no-tamoxifen group, but the difference was not statistically significant. In the tamoxifen group, 65% of the patients had stage I endometrial carcinoma, 9% were at stage II, 22% were at stage III, and 4% were at stage IV. In the no-tamoxifen group, 74% of the patients had stage I endometrial carcinoma, 2% were at stage II, 16% were at stage III, 6% were at stage IV, and 2% were unstaged. The distribution of histologic types was very similar in the 2 groups, with most patients having endometrial adenocarcinomas (Table 2). There were no significant grading differences in the endometrial adenocarcinomas in the

TABLE 4.—Relationship Between Grade of Endometrial Adenocarcinoma and Depth of Myometrial Invasion in Tamoxifen-Treated Patents*

Myometrial Invasion	Grade 1	Grade 2	Grade 3	Total	
Inner 1/3	16	5	0	21	(46%)
Middle 1/3	3	3	2	8	(17%)
Outer 1/3	0	2	3	5	(11%)
Unknown	3	3	6	12	(26%)
Total	22 (48%)	13 (28%)	11 (24%)	46	(100%)

* Includes 9 series plus the present one.
(Courtesy of Barakat RR, Wong G, Curtin JP, et al: Tamoxifen use in breast cancer patients who subsequently develop corpus cancer is not associated with a higher incidence of adverse histologic features. *Gynecol Oncol* 55:164–168, 1995.)

2 groups; only 23% of the tamoxifen group and 19% of the no-tamoxifen group had grade 3 lesions (Table 3). The relationship between endometrial adenocarcinoma grade and depth of myometrial invasion is presented in Table 4.

Conclusion.—These data indicate that women treated with tamoxifen do not have a more advanced stage or grade or more aggressive histologic type of corpus cancer than women with a history of primary breast cancer who were not treated with tamoxifen. Prognosis was not altered by tamoxifen treatment.

▶ This article was selected because of the controversy surrounding the utilization of tamoxifen. The risk of the development of uterine carcinoma associated with tamoxifen is small. This large series from Memorial Sloan-Kettering Cancer Center confirms that the majority of patients with uterine carcinoma associated with tamoxifen use have early-stage cancers. While this was a retrospective series, there was no difference in stage of presentation in patients utilizing tamoxifen or those patients without utilization of tamoxifen. Close surveillance of patients on tamoxifen is key to diagnosing this associated malignancy early.

T.J. Eberlein, M.D.

Prognostic Significance of Circulating P53 Antibodies in Patients Undergoing Surgery for Locoregional Breast Cancer

Peyrat J-P, Bonneterre J, Lubin R, Vanlemmens L, Fournier J, Soussi T (Centre Oscar Lambret, Paris)
Lancet 345:621–622, 1995   11–10

Introduction.—Patients with breast carcinoma often have alterations in the tumor suppressor gene p53. Alterations in p53 have been associated

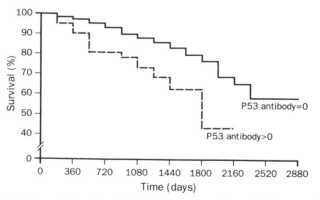

FIGURE.—Overall survival by p53 antibody status. (Courtesy of Peyrat J-P, Bonnterre J, Lubin R, et al: Prognostic significance of circulating p53 antibodies in patients undergoing surgery for locoregional breast cancer, 345(3):621–622, copyright by *The Lancet* Ltd., 1995.)

with reduced survival. Altered p53 in tumor cells can induce the production of serum p53 antibodies. The association between serum p53 antibodies and histopathologic or clinical factors and the prognostic significance of serum p53 antibodies were investigated in patients with breast carcinoma.

Methods.—Plasma was collected from 353 women undergoing surgery for locoregional breast cancer, including axillary dissection. All patients also received radiation therapy; node-positive patients received adjuvant chemotherapy and/or tamoxifen. Serum p53 antigen was identified with enzyme-linked immunosorbent assay with and without p53 antigen. Estrogen and progesterone receptors were also assayed. The patients were followed for a mean of 5.3 years. Actuarial overall survival and relapse-free survival were calculated.

Results.—Of the 353 patients, 42 (12%) had serum p53 antibody. The presence of p53 antibody was significantly negatively correlated with estrogen and progesterone receptors. Patients with p53 antibody in serum had significantly decreased overall survival (Fig). Multivariate analysis revealed that p53 antibody in serum was a significant independent prognostic factor for overall survival, but not for relapse-free survival.

Discussion.—Serologic analysis of p53 antibodies produced results similar to those found with immunohistochemical analysis of p53 alterations. The findings confirmed the incidence, negative association with estrogen and progesterone receptors, and diminished survival seen in breast cancer patients with p53 alterations in other immunohistochemical studies.

▶ p53 is a tumor suppressor gene associated with a number of malignancies, but it has been shown to correlate with tumor aggressiveness and other markers of aggressive biological behavior. This study from France looks at p53 antibody status and by multivariate analysis shows that it is an independent prognostic variable. This series was unselected, but perhaps in a series of node-negative patients, p53 antibody may be important in selecting patients for more aggressive and/or adjuvant therapies. Although p53 antibody was an independent prognostic factor in this study, larger studies may require that this prognostic indicator be combined with other indicators such as angiogenesis, HER2/neu expression, etc.

T.J. Eberlein, M.D.

Thoracic Epidural Anesthesia Improves Outcome After Breast Surgery
Lynch EP, Welch KJ, Carabuena JM, Eberlein TJ (Harvard Med School, Boston)
Ann Surg 222:663–669, 1995   11–11

Background.—Although general anesthesia is typically given to patients undergoing oncologic breast surgeries, thoracic epidural anesthesia appears to be associated with fewer postoperative complications, earlier hospital discharge, and less change in mental status after surgery. The

% of Patients

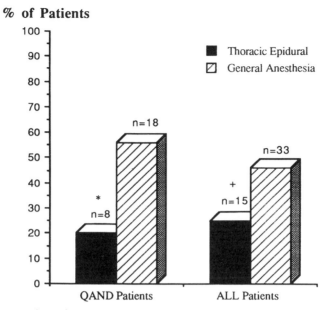

FIGURE 1.—Incidence of postoperative nausea and/or vomiting among patients undergoing quadrantectomy/axillary node dissection and patients undergoing all procedures. The columns represent the percentage of patients in each anesthetic group, and the number of patients is given above each column. *$P < 0.01$ vs. the general anesthesia group. $+P = 0.01$ vs. the general anesthesia group. (Courtesy of Lynch EP, Welch KJ, Carabuena JM, et al: Thoracic epidural anesthesia improves outcome after breast surgery. *Ann Surg* 222:663–669, 1995.)

authors of the present report have used the latter technique since March 1993 and have noted a high level of patient and surgeon satisfaction. Outcomes of patients undergoing thoracic epidural anesthesia were compared with those receiving general anesthesia during breast surgeries in this retrospective review.

Patients and Methods.—One hundred thirty-six consecutive patients undergoing various oncologic breast procedures over a 12-month period were identified and reviewed. All procedures were performed by a single surgeon, with 60 patients (mean age, 53.6 years) receiving thoracic epidural anesthesia and 72 (mean age, 55 years) undergoing general anesthesia. The remaining 4 patients (mean age, 54.1 years) had received both thoracic epidural and general anesthesia. The incidence of nausea and vomiting and time to discharge were compared between groups.

Results.—For all surgical procedures, 25% of the patients receiving thoracic epidural anesthesia experienced nausea and/or vomiting as compared with 46% of those in the general anesthesia group. Among patients undergoing quandrantectomy/axillary node dissection (QAND), 20% of those in the thoracic epidural group had nausea and/or vomiting vs. 56% of those receiving general anesthesia (Fig 1). Thoracic epidural anesthesia was also associated with a statistically significant earlier hospital discharge. Among patients undergoing QAND, 51% of those in the thoracic

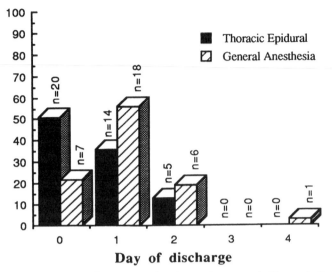

FIGURE 2.—Day of discharge for patients undergoing quadrantectomy/axillary node dissection. The columns represent the percentage of patients in each anesthetic group, and the number of patients is given above each column. (Courtesy of Lynch EP, Welch KJ, Carabuena JM, et al: Thoracic epidural anesthesia improves outcome after breast surgery. *Ann Surg* 222:663–669, 1995.)

epidural group were discharged on the operative day as compared with 22% of those given general anesthesia (Fig 2).

Conclusions.—Thoracic epidural anesthesia is a safe alternative to general anesthesia for patients undergoing oncologic breast procedures. This technique is not associated with neurologic or respiratory complications and may help facilitate postsurgical recovery and decrease procedure-related expenses.

▶ This is one of the first large series of breast cancer patients treated with thoracic epidural anesthesia instead of general anesthesia. With this technique, breast cancer patients as well as patients with more minor plastic reconstruction procedures can be treated as outpatients. There is clearly a learning curve among anesthesiologists. However, once the anesthesiologist is familiar with high thoracic epidural anesthesia and comfortable with dosing the catheter as well as sedative techniques, this can be an extremely safe and cost-effective adjunct to breast cancer surgery. Patients are overwhelmingly enthusiastic for this technique.

T.J. Eberlein, M.D.

MR-Guided Localization of Suspected Breast Lesions Detected Exclusively by Postcontrast MRI

Fischer U, Vosshenrich R, Bruhn H, Keating D, Raab BW, Oestmann JW
(Univ of Göttingen, Germany)
J Comput Assist Tomogr 19:63–66, 1995   11–12

Objective.—Contrast-enhanced MRI is able to visualize lesions in very dense breasts that are not detectable by ultrasound or mammography. A simple MR technique for localizing lesions for preoperative planning purposes is described.

Methods.—Contrast-enhanced MRI was performed on 658 patients to distinguish between malignancies and scars, to exclude malignancies, and to differentiate irregularly shaped densities. Fifteen lesions were found in 14 patients, and these patients underwent preoperative localization with a technique that used nickel sulfate–filled plastic tube skin markers. Four skin markers were placed in the suspected lesion quadrant with the patient bending over, an IV injection of 0.1 mmol/kg of gadopentetate dimeglumine was given, and contrast-enhanced MRI (dynamic 2-dimensional fast low-angle shot) was performed. The procedure was repeated with the patient in a prone position and a nonmagnetic wire of nickel-titanium alloy inserted into the breast as suggested by the skin markers and data from the previous MRI.

Results.—There were no complications. The procedure lasted about an hour and was successful in all patients. Surgical excision yielded 5 invasive carcinomas, 4 fibroadenomas, 2 papillomas, and 4 cases of hyperplasia. Follow-up MRI 3 to 6 months later showed that all lesions had been completely excised.

Conclusion.—Postcontrast MR-guided localization of breast lesions is a useful technique for establishing the coordinates of the lesion for surgical removal and verifying complete excision of the lesion.

▶ Magnetic resonance imaging appears to be a more sensitive, albeit expensive technique for identifying abnormalities of the breast. This manuscript simply shows the utility of being able to do MR-guided localization, similar to the technique used in mammography. Because of the expense, we have tended to utilize MRI, and specifically this technique, when equivocal mammographic findings are present and a definitive approach to the patient cannot be obtained with more conventional techniques. Breast MRI will also be facilitated by the design of more flexible coils to more easily accommodate the breast.

T.J. Eberlein, M.D.

Colorectal Cancer

The following section deals with both colon cancer and rectal cancer. There are lots of diverse articles that deal with new techniques, evaluation of old techniques, trials of preoperative radiation, as well as new molecular markers. Once again, I have tried to select manuscripts that review the literature and, in particular, may have an impact on the everyday surgical management of this common malignancy.

T.J. Eberlein, M.D.

Radioimmunoguided Surgery in Primary Colorectal Carcinoma: An Intraoperative Prognostic Tool and Adjuvant to Traditional Staging
Arnold MW, Young DC, Hitchcock CL, Schneebaum S, Martin EW Jr (Comprehensive Cancer Ctr, Columbus, Ohio; Ohio State Univ, Columbus) *Am J Surg* 170:315–318, 1995   11–13

Rationale.—The Duke classification system has been used to predict survival in colorectal cancer for longer than 6 decades but despite advances in surgical technique and adjuvant chemotherapy, overall survival has not improved very much. Accurate staging by the conventional method requires adequate resection and lymph node sampling. In addition, traditional systems fail to take micrometastatic disease into account. Predictions of survival in individual cases remain very uncertain.

A New Approach.—Radioimmunoguided surgery (RIGS) was undertaken in 31 patients requiring primary resection of a colorectal tumor. The patients were injected with radioiododine-labeled CC49, a monoclonal antibody directed against the tumor-associated mucin glycoprotein TAG-072, about 3 weeks before resection. A RIGS examination was performed with a handheld gamma detector, and the primary tumor was then resected

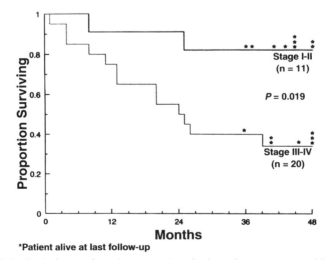

FIGURE 3.—Survival rates after primary resection of colorectal cancer as assessed by traditional staging. (Reprinted by permission of the publisher from Arnold MW, Young DC, Hitchcock CL, et al: Radioimmunoguided surgery in primary colorectal carcinoma: An intraoperative prognostic tool and adjuvant to traditional staging. *Am J Surg* 170:315–318, Copyright 1995 by Excerpta Medica Inc.)

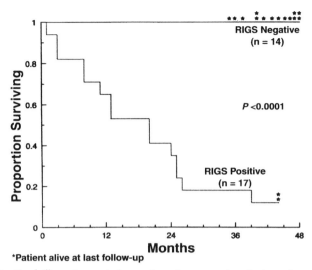

FIGURE 4.—Graph illustrating survival rates after primary resection of colorectal cancer as assessed by the presence (radioimmunoguided surgery [*RIGS*]-positive) or absence (RIGS-negative) of residual RIGS tissue. (Reprinted by permission of the publisher from Arnold MW, Young DC, Hitchcock CL, et al: Radioimmunoguided surgery in primary colorectal carcinoma: An intraoperative prognostic tool and adjuvant to traditional staging. *Am J Surg* 170:315–318, Copyright 1995 by Excerpta Medica Inc.)

along with any other RIGS-positive tissue identified with the probe. Patients were also staged according to the TNM system.

Results.—The patients were followed for 30–54 months after the resection of colon or rectal cancer. All patients had RIGS-positive tissue, including 2 who had no primary tumor left at the time of surgery. All but 4 of the 29 primary tumors were localized by the RIGS procedure. One hundred nine extraregional RIGS-positive sites were identified, with an average of 3.5 sites per patient. Only 41% of these sites were identified by CT scanning. Seventeen of the 31 patients remained RIGS-positive at the end of surgery. These patients tended to have advanced-stage disease; no RIGS-negative patient had stage IV disease (Fig 3). All 14 RIGS-negative patients remained alive 2–4 years postoperatively. In contrast, 15 of the 17 RIGS-positive patients died of disease (Fig 4).

Conclusion.—The RIGS system is a useful supplement to conventional pathologic staging of colorectal cancer, and it provides immediate prognostic information.

▶ The group at Ohio State have popularized RIGS. This technique has been utilized to detect recurrent disease. In the current manuscript, this technique is used as an adjunct to the traditional staging system. All RIGS-negative patients remained alive at the latest follow-up, while RIGS-positive patients died of the disease. This paper offers a more sophisticated technique to detect the presence of micrometastatic tumor, the underlying philosophy-being that complete tumor excision offers the best opportunity for cure. This, however, is true only in patients in whom "all" tumor is excised.

Selection of a monoclonal antibody directed against the colon tumor and the ability to utilize this technique on more than 1 occasion are areas of future development. Obviously, the potential prognostic significance of this technique is balanced by the additional length of surgery as well as additional morbidity resulting from a more extensive resection.

T.J. Eberlein, M.D.

Supraperitoneal Colorectal Anastomosis: Hand-Sewn Versus Circular Staples—A Controlled Clinical Trial

Fingerhut A, Hay J-M, Elhadad A, Lacaine F, Flamant Y (Universitaire de Recherche en Chirurgie, Bois-Colombes, France)
Surgery 118:479–485, 1995   11–14

Introduction.—Circular stapling devices are commonly used for intestinal and colonic anastomoses, although their superiority has not been proved. The morbidity and mortality associated with supraperitoneal col-

TABLE 3.—Early Postoperative Complications

| | Type of Anastomosis | | Total |
	Hand-sewn (74)	Stapled (85)	(159)
Anastomotic leakage			
Roentgenologic alone	4	6	10
Clinical and roentgenologic	0	0	0
Wound abscess	4	2	6
Deep abscess	0	3	3
Generalized peritonitis	0	0	0
Postoperative hemorrhage per anus*	0	5	5
Reoperations	0	4	4
Patients with one or more intraabdominal infective complication(s)	4	5	9
Extraabdominal complications			
Infective†	14	13	27
Noninfective‡	8	12	20
Deaths			
Total	1	1	2
With intraabdominal infective complications	0	0	0

* Two patients required blood transfusion.
† Pulmonary, urinary tract, septicemia, catheter-related infection.
‡ Pulmonary, urinary tract, cardiac, hepatic, and cerebral.
(Courtesy of Fingerhut A, Hay J-M, Elhadad A, et al: Supraperitoneal colorectal anastomosis: Hand-sewn versus circular staples—a controlled clinical trial. *Surgery* 118:479–485, 1995.)

TABLE 4.—Factors Influencing the Safety of Anastomosis

	Type of anastomosis		Total
	Hand-sewn	*Stapled*	
	(74)	*(85)*	*(159)*
Tested for airtightness	16	47	63
Leak detected and	1	4	5
Extra sutures added	1	4	5
Doughnuts verified	0	83	83
Defect detected	0	4	4
Sutures added	0	3	3
Reanastomosis	0	3*	3
Doughnuts not verified	NK	2	2
Protection†			
Diverting colostomy	5	4	9
Omental wrap	16	14	28
Mishaps	0	10	10

* In 2 patients, sutures were added first and then judged to be insufficient.
† Some patients had both.
Abbreviation: NK, not known.
(Courtesy of Fingerhut A, Hay J-M, Elhadad A, et al: Supraperitoneal colorectal anastomosis: Hand-sewn versus circular staples—a controlled clinical trial. *Surgery* 118:479–485, 1995.)

orectal anastomosis with either hand-sewn or circular stapled anastomoses and the efficacy of each technique for leakage protection were compared in a prospective, multicenter study.

Methods.—A total of 149 consecutive patients undergoing immediate supraperitoneal anastomosis after elective left colectomy were randomly assigned to have either hand-sewn (74 patients) or circular stapled (85 patients) anastomoses. Anastomotic leakage, as detected by fecal matter in drainage discharge, sinograms, reoperation, postmortem examination, or a sodium benzoate enema performed on day 7, was compared in the 2 treatment groups. Intraoperative and postoperative morbidity and mortality were also compared.

Results.—One patient in each group died of causes unrelated to intraabdominal complications, for an overall mortality rate of 1.3%. Anastomotic leakage was detected in 4 patients (5%) in the hand-sewn group and 6 patients (7%) in the stapled group. Postoperative hemorrhage, reoperation, and noninfective extra-abdominal complications were nonsignificantly less frequent in the hand-sewn group than in the stapled group (8% vs. 13%). Most other postoperative complications occurred relatively equally in both groups (Table 3). Stapling device mishaps requiring mechanical repair occurred in 10 patients. (Table 4). Anastomotic strictures occurred in 3% of the hand-sewn group and 5% of the stapled group.

Conclusions.—Because stapled anastomoses do not result in reduced clinical anastomotic leakage and are associated with increased intraoperative and postoperative complications, the routine use of circular stapling devices in performing supraperitoneal colorectal anastomoses is not justified.

▶ This is a randomized multicenter trial looking at anastomosis following left colectomy. In general, stapled and hand-sewn anastomoses in this location had similar results except that there were 10 intraoperative mishaps secondary to the mechanical nature of this stapling device and 5 episodes of hemorrhage associated with this stapled group. In spite of this, the anastomosis time was shorter in the stapled group. When carefully performed, as in this trial, there appears to be no advantage to utilizing one technique over the other. Stapled anastomoses are most efficacious in the rectum, where limitations of hand-sewn anastomoses are often critical.

T.J. Eberlein, M.D.

Intraoperative Ultrasonography in Detection of Hepatic Metastases From Colorectal Cancer

Rafaelsen SR, Kronborg O, Larsen C, Fenger C (Odense Univ Hosp, Denmark)
Dis Colon Rectum 38:355–360, 1995   11–15

Background.—Recent studies have reported that 25% of patients with limited liver metastases from colorectal carcinoma and no evidence of spread elsewhere can be cured. The accuracy of intraoperative ultrasonography (IOUS) in the diagnosis and location of liver metastases was compared with measurements of liver enzymes, preoperative ultrasonography (PUS), and surgical exploration.

Methods.—A total of 295 consecutive patients (148 males, 147 females) admitted to the hospital for elective surgery for colorectal carcinoma were studied by IOUS, as well as PUS and measurement of liver enzymes. At surgery, the liver was inspected and palpated by the surgeon, and findings regarding metastases were recorded before the results of PUS were known and before IOUS. The size and location of liver metastases detected by IOUS were recorded. Biopsy was performed on all doubtful lesions before resection. Patients were examined 3 months postoperatively with conventional ultrasonography. If the examination was negative, the patient was considered cured. If the ultrasonographic findings were positive, previous negative findings were considered false-negatives. The sensitivity and the specificity of each diagnostic method were compared.

TABLE 3.—Comparison of Different Diagnostic Methods for Detection of 204 Liver Metastases in 64 Patients

	Sensitivity (%)	Specificity (%)
Preoperative ultrasonography	130/204 (63.7)	214/231 (92.0)
Surgical exploration	146/204 (71.6)	223/231 (96.5)
Intraoperative ultrasonography	192/204 (94.1)	226/231 (97.8)

Sensitivity of intraoperative ultrasonography vs. all other tests: $P < 0.0001$.
(Courtesy of Rafaelsen SR, Kronborg O, Larsen C, et al: Intraoperative ultrasonography in detection of hepatic metastases from colorectal cancer. *Dis Colon Rectum* 38(4):355–360, 1995.)

No. of metastases

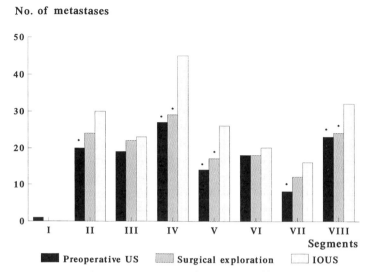

FIGURE 3.—Detection of hepatic metastases according to segmental location. *P < 0.05. (Courtesy of Rafaelsen SR, Kronborg O, Larsen C, et al: Intraoperative ultrasonography in detection of hepatic metastases from colorectal cancer. *Dis Colon Rectum* 38(4):355–360, 1995.)

Results.—There were no complications of IOUS; the usual duration of the study was 8–10 minutes. Curative operations were performed in 216 patients and palliative procedures in 79. Sixty-four of the 295 patients (21.7%) had a total of 204 liver metastases. The sensitivity of IOUS in detecting metastases (62/64) was significantly superior to the findings at surgery (54/64) and to the findings on PUS (45/64). Table 3 compares the sensitivity and specificity of the different diagnostic methods in the 64 patients with 204 metastases. The sensitivity of IOUS was significantly superior to the other diagnostic methods (P < 0.0001) The differences in specificity were not significantly different. Intraoperative ultrasonography was significantly superior to both PUS and surgical exploration in the detection of small and deeply seated metastases and was also significantly superior to PUS in identifying metastatic lesions in the posterior segments of the liver (II, VII, and VIII) and in segments IV and V. In addition, IOUS was superior to surgical exploration in detecting metastases in segments IV, V, and VIII (Fig 3). Intraoperative ultrasonography was superior to liver function abnormalities in 29 patients who had fewer than 4 metastatic lesions.

Conclusions.—Intraoperative ultrasonography is a safe and quickly performed procedure that is superior to PUS and surgical exploration in the detection of liver metastases from colorectal carcinoma. Its use may result in the identification and treatment of patients potentially curable by surgery and in the prevention of unnecessary liver surgery.

▶ This is a large consecutive series that shows intraoperative ultrasonography being superior to either preoperative sonography or intraoperative surgical examination in the detection of liver metastases. In our institution, intraoperative ultrasound has become the standard prior to a patient under-going liver resection for metastatic colorectal tumors. Although new preoperative techniques such as CT portography and newly developed contrast agents are being tested, this simple and safe technique will still be the standard of practice in the prevention of unnecessary liver surgery.

T.J. Eberlein, M.D.

Endoscopic Assessment of Invasion of Colorectal Tumors With a New High-Frequency Ultrasound Probe
Yoshida M, Tsukamoto Y, Niwa Y, Goto H, Hase S, Hayakawa T, Okamura S
(Nagoya Univ, Japan; Toyohashi Municipal Hosp, Japan)
Gastrointest Endosc 41:587–592, 1995   11–16

Objective.—Endoscopic ultrasonography (EUS) has become a useful procedure for preoperative staging of colorectal carcinomas and diagnosis of submucosal tumors. A high-frequency ultrasound probe has been developed to overcome some of the disadvantages of EUS. This probe, used through the biopsy channel of a conventional colonoscope, permits conventional colonoscopy, EUS, and endoscopic resection without the need to change colonoscopes. The value of the new probe for the evaluation of invasive colorectal malignancies was assessed.

Methods.—In an in vitro study, the new probe was used to examine 23 specimens of normal colorectal wall resected from patients with colorectal cancer. A clinical study of 51 patients with colorectal carcinoma and 16 patients with rectal carcinoid tumor was performed as well. In this study, conventional preoperative colonoscopy was followed by examination using the new probe via the biopsy. The probe, which had a small 15-MHz transducer fixed in its tip, was used with a scanner and a specially designed ultrasound generator/display unit. The probe measured 2.4 mm in diameter and 1,980 mm in length. Endoscopic resection was performed in 27 patients and surgical resection in 40, and the histologic and ultrasonographic findings were compared.

Results.—In the in vitro study, both techniques showed the colorectal wall as a 7-layered structure; the imaging achieved with the new ultrasound probe compared favorably with that of conventional EUS. Both carcinomas and carcinoid tumors appeared as an echo-poor region with the probe. Accuracy for depth of invasion of colorectal cancer was 76% overall, 83% for tumors limited to the mucosa, and 90% for those invading the submucosa. Accuracy was lower for tumors invading the muscularis propria and beyond: 50% and 73%, respectively. Accuracy decreased with increasing tumor size. In 4 patients, the new probe could pass through narrow stenoses of the colorectal tract that prevented the passage of conventional colonoscopes. None of the patients with carcinoid tumor had invasion beyond the submucosa, and this was accurately demonstrated by the new probe.

Conclusions.—The new, high-frequency ultrasound probe evaluated in this study is useful in assessing the invasiveness of colorectal cancers. It is particularly helpful in depicting small and flat lesions in which invasion does not extend beyond the submucosa. The new probe can be positioned under exact visual control, can be passed through strictures, and can make the EUS examination easier and more comfortable for the patient.

▶ This study utilizes a new high-frequency ultrasound probe that makes it possible to perform conventional colonoscopy, EUS, and resection without changing the colonoscope. While this technique was useful and accurate for mucosal and submucosal tumors, accuracy diminished with the depth of invasion, thereby limiting its utility. As improved instruments become available in the future, better resolution and improved accuracy with depth of invasion can be anticipated.

T.J. Eberlein, M.D.

Rectal Cancer

The following 6 articles discuss some form of preoperative treatment for rectal cancer.

T.J. Eberlein, M.D.

Conservative Surgery for Low Rectal Carcinoma After High-Dose Radiation: Functional and Oncologic Results
Rouanet P, Fabre JM, Dubois JB, Dravet F, Saint Aubert B, Pradel J, Ychou M, Solassol C, Pujol H (Montpellier Cancer Inst, France)
Ann Surg 221:67–73, 1995   11–17

Background.—Abdominoperineal resection is standard surgical treatment for lower-third rectal carcinoma. As surgical technique has improved, sphincter conservation is now possible for low rectal carcinoma. Concerns of local recurrence and reduced survival have limited the use of conservative surgery. A preoperative radiation dose of 40 Gy has been used for more than 20 years for patients with invasive rectal cancer. Because of evidence of a relationship between radiation dose and locoregional control, an additional dose of 20 Gy for patients with lower-third rectal tumors is proposed. The functional and oncologic results of this treatment are examined.

Methods.—A total of 27 patients with distal rectal adenocarcinoma and a mean age of 65 years were treated with radiotherapy (40 + 20 Gy delivered with 3 fields) and surgery. The distance from the anal verge was between 27 and 57 mm. There were no T1 tumors; 15 patients had T2 tumors and 12 patients had T3 tumors.

Results.—High-dose radiation administered preoperatively did not increase morbidity or mortality. Conservative surgery was performed in 21 patients. After coloanal anastomosis, good results were seen in all patients

TABLE 2.—Functional Results After Coloanal Anastomosis

Kirwan's continence classification	
1) Perfect	10
2) Incontinent to gas	2
3) Occasional minor leak	2
4) Frequent major soiling	0
5) Colostomy	0
Bowel movements	
Constipation	3
1 or 2 per day	9
3 to 5 per day	1
>5 per day	1
Urgency	2
Urinary dysfunction	
Postoperative	12
After 1 month	2
After 3 months	0
Sexual dysfunction (13 men evaluated)	
An erection	4 (30%)
Sexual weakness	3 (23%)
Retrograde ejaculation	13 (100%)

Note: Fourteen patients studied with a mean follow-up of 14 months (range, 3–28 months).
(Courtesy of Rouanet P, Fabre JM, Dubois JB, et al: Conservative surgery for low rectal carcinoma after high-dose radiation: Functional and oncologic results. *Ann Surg* 221:67–73, 1995.)

with a colonic pouch. After straight coloanal anastomosis, 2 patients had moderate results and 1 patient had poor results (Table 2). At a mean follow-up of 24 months, 80% of the patients were disease-free; there were 2 patients with pulmonary metastases, 1 patient with controlled regional recurrence, 2 deaths related to disease, and 1 postoperative death.

Discussion.—High-dose radiation and conservative surgery are possible for low rectal carcinoma. Less morbidity and better local control can result from preoperative radiation than from postoperative radiation. The safety margin for inferior rectal sectioning needs to be readdressed and is discussed.

▶ This is a relatively small, prospective nonrandomized study. It utilizes a boost-dose radiation preoperatively followed by curative surgery. The majority of these patients had coloanal anastomosis. While the follow-up was relatively short, the overwhelming majority of patients were disease free and had excellent functional results. Preoperative radiotherapy is associated with downstaging and most likely decreases local recurrence; however, it is uncertain whether it has a major impact on survival.

T.J. Eberlein, M.D.

Long-Term Results of a Randomised Trial of Short-Course Low-Dose Adjuvant Pre-Operative Radiotherapy for Rectal Cancer: Reduction in Local Treatment Failure

Goldberg PA, Nicholls RJ, Porter NH, Love S, (St Marks Hosp, London)
Eur J Cancer 30:1602–1606, 1994

11–18

Background.—Radiotherapy is a common adjunct to curative surgery in treating rectal cancer. The major cause of cancer-related death after curative resection is metastatic disease. Local treatment failure usually occurs with metastases and is rarely curable. In a large autopsy study, local recurrence without dissemination occurred in only 8% of the deaths from large-bowel cancer. This might explain the failure of adjuvant radiotherapy to lower mortality. It is often reported that surgery can reduce local recurrence to as little as 2%, but experience shows that the rate with surgery alone is actually much higher. The effects of a preoperative, short course of radiotherapy on local treatment failure and survival were investigated in a randomized trial.

Methods.—There were 468 patients between 31 and 94 years old with a potentially resectable adenocarcinoma 12 cm or less from the anal verge. Of these, 228 received radiotherapy in 3 fractions of 5 Gy for 5 days and then underwent surgery, 239 underwent surgery alone, and the treatment group of 1 patient was unknown.

Results.—Follow-up to 5 years or death was completed for 454 patients; a total of 307 patients died. Of the 468 original patients, 21 who had radiotherapy and surgery and 10 who had surgery alone died within 1 month of surgery; the incidence of cardiovascular and thromboembolic complications was higher for patients who received combined treatment than for those who had surgery alone, and the rate of anastomotic leakage after anterior resection or perineal breakdown after total rectal excision was the same for both groups (Table 3). The 5-year survival rate of 280 patients who had curative surgery was 52% for those who had radiotherapy and surgery and 56% for those who had surgery alone. Outpatient clinics were attended by 395 patients at least once. Local treatment failure

TABLE 3.—Mortality and Morbidity

	Radiotherapy and Surgery n (%)	Surgery Alone n (%)	P
n	228	239	
In-hospital mortality	27 (12)	16 (7)	0.056
30-day mortality	21 (9)	10 (4)	< 0.05
Cardiovascular and thromboembolic complications	30 (13)	8 (3)	< 0.001
Anastomotic leak (anterior resection)	18/122 (15)	15/117 (13)	ns
Perineal breakdown (total rectal excision)	21/82 (26)	20/93 (22)	ns

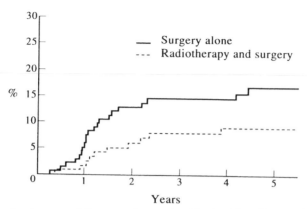

FIGURE 4.—Local treatment failure—curative resection. (Reprinted from *European Journal of Cancer*, vol 30A, Goldberg PA, Nicholls RJ, Porter NG, et al: Long-term results of a randomised trial of short-course low-dose adjuvant pre-operative radiotherapy for rectal cancer: Reduction in local treatment failure, pp 1602–1606, copyright 1994, with kind permission from Elsevier Science Ltd, The Boulevard, Langford Lane, Kidlington OX5 1GB, UK.)

occurred in 17% of the patients who had combined treatment and in 24% of the patients who had only surgery. Of those who had curative resection, local treatment failure occurred in 9% of the patients who had radiotherapy and surgery and in 16% of those who had surgery alone (Fig 4).

Discussion.—In these patients, preoperative, short-course, low-dose radiotherapy resulted in reduced long-term local recurrence and increased perioperative mortality. However, long-term survival was unchanged. Deep vein thrombosis and pulmonary embolism were major causes of morbidity and mortality. During the study period, only 10% of the patients received thromboembolic prophylaxis. More widespread use of prophylaxis today may reduce these complications.

▶ This study used a short course of low-dose preoperative radiation therapy; survival was unaffected. However, local recurrence was reduced, but cardiovascular and thromboembolic complications were more common in the patients treated with radiotherapy and surgery. Thromboembolic prophylaxis was not utilized in this trial; therefore, consideration should be given to using prophylactic therapy in patients with preoperative radiation.

T.J. Eberlein, M.D.

Preoperative Infusional Chemoradiation and Surgery With or Without an Electron Beam Intraoperative Boost for Advanced Primary Rectal Cancer
Weinstein GD, Rich TA, Shumate CR, Skibber JM, Cleary KR, Ajani JA, Ota DM (Univ of Texas MD Anderson Cancer Ctr, Houston)
Int J Radiat Oncol Biol Phys 32:197–204, 1995   11–19

Objective.—In patients with advanced rectal cancers that are tethered or fixed to the pelvic viscera or bones, pelvic tumor recurrence after surgery is correlated with the amount of residual disease. High-dose preoperative radiotherapy (preopXRT) has yielded resectability rates of up to 100% and local control rates of up to 84%. A new preoperative approach— protracted continuous-infusion chemotherapy given during the entire course of irradiation (preop-chemoXRT)—is evaluated in a pilot study.

Methods.—The study included 38 patients with tethered T3 or T4 primary rectal cancer. All received 45 Gy of radiation given in 25 fractions over a 4-week period plus infusional chemotherapy with cisplatin, 5-fluorouracil, or both. Surgical resection was performed in 37 patients; 13 had restorative surgery, whereas the rest had abdominoperineal resection or pelvic exenteration. In 11 patients with adherent pelvic tumors, electron beam intraoperative radiotherapy (EB-IORT), 10 to 20 Gy, was given as well. The results were compared with those of 36 historic control patients who had received preopXRT. The radiation dose in this group was 45 Gy, and 93% had abdominoperineal resection or pelvic exenteration.

Results.—Patients treated with preop-chemoXRT had a local recurrence rate of only 3% as compared with 33% for those treated with preopXRT. The 3-year survival rate was 82% with preop-chemoXRT plus resection vs. 62% for the historic controls. Sixty-four percent of the patients receiving EB-IORT had distant metastases as compared with 19% of those who did not receive an intraoperative boost. The overall 3-year survival rate was 67% with vs. 96% without EB-IORT. The preop-chemoXRT approach had acceptable acute and late toxicity.

Conclusions.—For patients with advanced primary rectal cancer, preop-chemoXRT offers important advantages over preopXRT alone. Control of pelvic disease and overall survival are better with preop-chemoXRT. Acute chemoradiation toxicity is increased, but late morbidity is unchanged. For patients with residual or clinically adherent disease, EB-IORT improves local control. However, survival is worse in these patients than in those who do not receive EB-IORT.

▶ This study from the M.D. Anderson Cancer Center is a relatively small series of patients with tethered T3 or T4 rectal cancer. As might be expected, chemoradiation was better than preoperative radiation alone. While the toxicity was greater, late morbidity was unchanged. Toxicity may be ameliorated by continuous infusion chemotherapy and a bowel exclusion radiotherapy technique. Patients who required electron beam intraoperative radiotherapy because of residual tumor, positive margins, or adherence of tumor seem to have biologically more aggressive disease, poor survival, but improved local control rates when these techniques are used.

T.J. Eberlein, M.D.

The Stockholm I Trial of Preoperative Short Term Radiotherapy in Operable Rectal Carcinoma: A Prospective Randomized Trial

Cedermark B, for the Stockholm Colorectal Cancer Study Group (Stockholm Oncologic Ctr, Sweden; Karolinska Hosp, Stockholm)
Cancer 75:2269–2275, 1995   11–20

Introduction.—Even with "curative" resection, the 5-year survival rate for patients with rectal carcinoma is only about 50%. Many patients die solely as a result of uncontrolled locoregional disease. Randomized trials of adjuvant radiotherapy for patients with rectal cancer have yielded conflicting results. The final results of a randomized multicenter trial of short-term preoperative radiotherapy for rectal cancer are reported.

Methods.—Eight hundred forty-nine patients with clinically resectable rectal adenocarcinoma were enrolled in the trial from 1980 to 1987. The patients were randomized to receive preoperative radiotherapy—25 Gy during the 5 to 7 days before surgery—or surgery alone. The study assessed the effects of preoperative radiotherapy on pelvic recurrence and whether improved local control increased survival.

Results.—The disease-free interval was longer in the preoperative irradiation group, largely because of a lower incidence of local recurrence (Table 4). Six hundred eighty-four patients underwent "curative" surgery. At a median follow-up of 107 months, the incidence of pelvic recurrence was significantly lower in curatively operated patients who also received preoperative radiotherapy. This was so for patients in all Dukes' stages (Table 6). The treatment groups were similar in terms of frequency of distant metastases and overall survival, but time to local recurrence or distant metastasis was significantly longer in the patients who received irradiation (Table 7). Postoperative mortality was significantly higher in patients who received radiotherapy vs. those who had surgery only, 8% vs. 2%.

TABLE 4.—Analysis of Events Among All 849 Randomized Patients

Type of Event	Radiation Therapy*	Surgery*	Relative Hazard (95%) CI	P Value
Pelvic recurrence	61 (14)	120 (28)	0.51 (0.37–0.69)	< 0.01
Distant metastases	128 (30)	159 (37)	0.86 (0.68–1.09)	NS
First recurrence I (pelvic or distant)	158 (37)	210 (49)	0.76 (0.62–0.93)	0.01
First recurrence II (pelvic, distant or death)	297 (70)	304 (72)	0.98 (0.83–1.16)	NS
Death	295 (70)	293 (69)	1.08 (0.98–1.27)	NS
Total no. of patients	424	425		

Note: Relative hazards are estimated with the Cox proportional hazards model. All effects are stratified for clinic. All *P* values are based on the log-rank test, and values less than 0.10 are considered nonsignificant.
Abbreviation: CI, confidence interval.
(Courtesy of *Cancer,* from Cedermark B, for the Stockholm Colorectal Cancer Study Group, copyright © 1995. Reprinted by permission of Wiley-Liss, Inc., a division of John Wiley & Sons, Inc.)

TABLE 6.—Analysis of the Cumulative Incidence of Pelvic Recurrence by Dukes' Classification

Dukes' Level	Treatment	No. of Events	No. of Patients	Relative Hazard (95% CI)	Log-rank P Value
Dukes' A	Surgery	11	111		
				0.61 (0.23–1.61)	NS
	Radiation therapy	7	115		
Dukes' B	Surgery	49	132		
				0.40 (0.22–0.68)	< 0.001
	Radiation therapy	19	122		
Dukes' C	Surgery	45	104		
				0.65 (0.40–1.04)	0.068
	Radiation therapy	29	100		
Total		160	684		

Note: Relative hazards are estimated with the Cox proportional hazards model, with surgery as the reference group. All effects are stratified for clinic. All P values are based on the log-rank test, and values less than 0.10 are considered nonsignificant.

Abbreviation: CI, confidence interval.

(Courtesy of *Cancer*, from Cedermark B, for the Stockholm Colorectal Cancer Study Group, copyright © 1995. Reprinted by permission of Wiley-Liss, Inc., a division of John Wiley & Sons, Inc.)

Conclusions.—For patients with rectal cancer, preoperative short-term radiotherapy decreases the incidence of pelvic recurrence as compared with surgery alone. Disease-free survival and overall survival are improved with preoperative irradiation among patients who undergo curative surgery. However, preoperative irradiation is associated with higher postoperative morbidity (Table 2).

TABLE 7.—Analysis of the Cumulative Incidence of Distant Metastasis by Dukes' Classification

Dukes' Level	Treatment	No. of Events	No. of Patients	Relative Hazard (95% CI)*	Log rank P Value
Dukes's A	Surgery	9	111		
				1.60 (0.64–3.96)	NS
	Radiation therapy	13	115		
Dukes' B	Surgery	52	132		
				0.56 (0.34–0.92)	0.018
	Radiation therapy	27	122		
Dukes' C	Surgery	58	104		
				0.90 (0.60–1.35)	NS
	Radiation therapy	43	100		
Total		202	684		

* Relative hazards are estimated with the Cox proportional hazards model, with surgery as the reference group. All effects are stratified for clinic. All P values are based on the log-rank test, and values less than 0.10 are considered nonsignificant.

Abbreviation: CI, confidence interval.

(Courtesy of *Cancer*, from Cedermark B, for the Stockholm Colorectal Cancer Study Group, copyright © 1995. Reprinted by permission of Wiley-Liss, Inc., a division of John Wiley & Sons, Inc.)

TABLE 2.—Postoperative Complications

Complication	Preoperative Radiation Therapy (n = 424)	Surgery Alone (n = 425)
Wound infection	61 (14)	37 (9)
Wound dehiscence	15 (4)	6 (1)
Anastomotic leak	10 (2)	15 (3)
Bowel obstruction	8 (2)	13 (3)
Hemorrhage	5 (1)	4 (1)
Thrombosis	4 (1)	4 (1)
Other	9 (2)	2 (1)
≥2 complications	23 (5)	16 (4)
Total	112 (26)	81 (19)

▶ This is a very large randomized prospective trial from Sweden, and as was seen with the St. Marks trial (Abstract 140-96-11–18), pelvic recurrence was reduced and there was prolonged survival as compared with surgery alone. While perioperative morbidity was higher in the radiation group, these were primarily due to relatively minor wound problems. The postoperative mortality that was increased in the radiation group may well have been primarily due to age-related cardiovascular disease and did not appear to be due to surgical complications.

T.J. Eberlein, M.D.

Radical and Local Excisional Methods of Sphincter-Sparing Surgery After High-Dose Radiation for Cancer of the Distal 3 cm of the Rectum
Bannon JP, Marks GJ, Mohiuddin M, Rakinic J, Non-Zhou J, Nagle D (Thomas Jefferson Univ, Philadelphia; Univ of Kentucky, Lexington; Jiangsu Inst of Cancer Research, China)
Ann Surg Oncol 2:221–227, 1995   11–21

Background.—Sphincter preservation surgery (SPS) for cancers stemming from the terminal 3 cm of the rectum has traditionally been avoided. However, the authors have selectively used high-dose preoperative external radiation (HDPER) and either radical or local excisional SPS methods for rectal cancer originating between the 0.5- and 3-cm levels above the anorectal ring. Preliminary experience with HDPER and full-thickness local excision (FTLE) and with 3 different methods of radical SPS has been reported. The present report, relates the authors' experience with a single technique of radical excision, transanal abdominal transanal proctosigmoidectomy with coloanal anastomosis (TATA) or FTLE, together with HDPER, for cancers of the distal 3 cm of rectum.

Patients and Methods.—One hundred nine patients enrolled in a prospective rectal cancer management program since 1984 were included in

TABLE 2.—Pattern of Local Recurrence (6/65, 9%) After Transanal Abdominal Transanal Radical Proctosigmoidectomy With Coloanal Anastomosis (Group A)

P/R Favorable	P/R Unfavorable
T0 N0 N = 0/10	T0 N1 N = 0/1
T1 N0 N = 0/2	T2 N1 N = 0/8
T2 N0 N = 0/23	T3 N0 N = 2/11
	T3 N1 N = 2/6
	T3 N2 N = 2/4
Total 0/35 (0%)	6/30 (20%)

Abbreviation: P/R, postirradiated.
(Courtesy of Bannon JP, Marks GJ, Mohiuddin M, et al: Radical and local excisional methods of sphincter-sparing surgery after high-dose radiation for cancer of the distal 3 cm of the rectum. *Ann Surg Oncol* 2:221–227, 1995.)

the analysis. All patients had cancers at or below the 3-cm level. Treatment consisted of HDPER given in doses of 4,500 to 7,000 cGy and a sphincter-preserving radical or local excision method. Sixty-five patients underwent TATA (group A) and 44 patients underwent FTLE. Patients were followed for a mean of 40 months.

Results.—Significant perioperative morbidity occurred in 6 of the group A and 5 of the group B patients. Among group A patients, these included 2 pulmonary embolisms, 1 anastomotic disruption and 1 anastomotic stricture, 1 presacral abscess, 1 case of perianal cellulitis, and 1 pelvic hematoma necessitating a reoperation. In group B patients, wound separation (which healed with nonoperative management) was noted in 2 patients, a rectovaginal fistula in 1, and prolapsing rectal mucosa in 2 patients. There was 1 perioperative death in a group A patient from

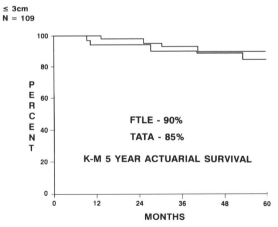

FIGURE 2.—Survival by procedure. *Abbreviations: FTLE,* full-thickness local excision; *TATA,* transanal abdominal transanal with radical proctosigmoidectomy with coloanal anastomosis. (Courtesy of Bannon JP, Marks GJ, Mohiuddin M, et al: Radical and local excisional methods of sphincter-sparing surgery after high-dose radiation for cancer of the distal 3 cm of the rectum. *Ann Surg Oncol* 2:221–227, 1995.)

pulmonary embolism. The local recurrence rate for group A patients was 9%. No local recurrence was observed among the postirradiated favorable-stage cancers (Table 2). Among group B patients, the local recurrence rate was 14%. The Kaplan-Meier 5-year actuarial survival (K-M 5-YAS) rate was 85% for group A and 90% for group B patients. The collective K-M 5-YAS rate was 87% (Fig 2).

Conclusions.—Sphincter preservation surgery using radical or local excision techniques is possible in patients with cancers of the distal 3 cm of rectum. Satisfactory local control and survival can be achieved with HD-PER and adherence to strict selection guidelines.

▶ This is a relatively large series of patients with very distal rectal cancer. Following high-dose preoperative external radiation, the patients undergo either radical resection or FTLE. Survival and functional results are excellent. Local/regional recurrence rates were 9% and were associated with very large tumors with nodal disease. The results are far better than for surgery alone in this patient population. Selection of patients is important and is clearly dependent on experience. Patients treated by FTLE were those with cancers less than 2 cm in diameter and limited to the rectal wall. Unfortunately, even these experienced colorectal surgeons had difficulty with sophisticated imaging techniques for evaluation of rectal nodal disease. This is extremely important in the selection of patients, especially for FTLE, since FTLE would be relatively contraindicated with known perirectal tumor spread.

T.J. Eberlein, M.D.

Preoperative Radiation and Chemotherapy in the Treatment of Adenocarcinoma of the Rectum

Chari RS, Tyler DS, Anscher MS, Russell L, Clary BM, Hathorn J, Seigler HF (Duke Univ, Durham, NC)
Ann Surg 221:778–787, 1995   11–22

Objective.—Rectal carcinoma led to approximately 7,000 deaths in 1994. Although surgical resection can be curative, treatment failure rates

TABLE 2.—Postoperative Complications

Complication	Preoperative Chemoradiation (n = 41)	Control Group (n = 56)
Perineal drainage	20 (49)	5 (9)
Perineal dehiscence	4 (10)	0 (0)
Small bowel obstruction	3 (7)	2 (4)
Operative management	2 (5)	0 (0)
Abdominal wound infection	6 (15)	5 (9)
Abscess—operative drainage	2 (5)	0 (0)

(Courtesy of Chari RS, Tyler DS, Anscher MS, et al: Preoperative radiation and chemotherapy in the treatment of adenocarcinoma of the rectum. *Ann Surg* 221:778–787, 1995.)

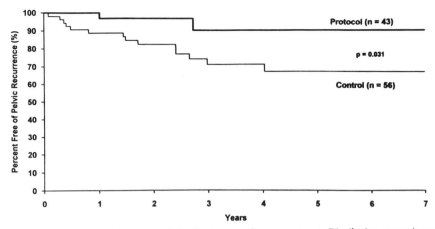

FIGURE 1.—Kaplan-Meier survival distribution according to treatment. Distribution comparisons were made with the Cox-Mantel test. A *P* value of less than 0.05 was considered significant. (Courtesy of Chari RS, Tyler DS, Anscher MS, et al: Preoperative radiation and chemotherapy in the treatment of adenocarcinoma of the rectum. *Ann Surg* 221:778–787, 1995.)

vary from 15% to 70% depending on the stage of the disease. Recent studies have demonstrated that preoperative radiation therapy leads to better locoregional control than does postoperative radiation therapy. This study was conducted to examine the effect of preoperative combined radiation and chemotherapy on local relapse, disease-free survival, and overall survival of patients with rectal carcinoma.

Methods.—A total of 43 patients (12 women) aged 31 to 81 received 5 radiation treatments a week for 5 weeks delivered with a total pelvic dose of 45 Gy by photon irradiation generated by a 6-mV or greater linear accelerator. Chemotherapy consisted of 500 mg/m² of 5-fluorouracil per day for 5 days followed by a half-hour infusion of 20 mg/m² of cisplatin per day. Chemotherapy was repeated during the last week of radiation therapy. All patients had tumors larger than 3 cm involving the entire rectal wall. The control group consisted of 56 patients (21 women) aged 29 to 89 with surgically treated rectal cancer.

Results.—Chemoradiation therapy was well tolerated, and diarrhea was the most common side effect. No lesions progressed during therapy. All patients had reductions in tumor size, and 22 patients had complete clinical responses. Two patients refused surgery. At surgery, 11 of 41 patients were disease free and had negative lymph nodes, 9 had microscopic disease, 21 had residual gross disease, and 35 of 39 had negative nodes. The chemoradiation group had more postoperative complications that did the control group (Table 2). Four patients had positive nodes. At follow-up, 39 of 43 patients are alive, and 1 patient with a complete response had local recurrence and lung metastases. In 6 of 32 patients with residual disease, metastases developed and 3 died. Two of 43 patients had local recurrence.

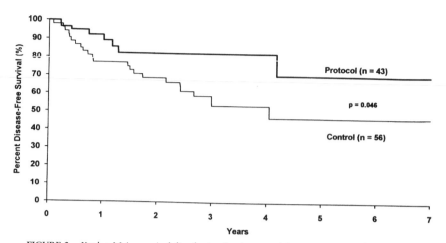

FIGURE 2.—Kaplan-Meier survival distribution for time to pelvic recurrence according to treatment. Distribution comparisons were made with the Cox-Mantel test. A *P* value of less than 0.05 was considered significant. (Courtesy of Chari RS, Tyler DS, Anscher MS, et al: Preoperative radiation and chemotherapy in the treatment of adenocarcinoma of the rectum. *Ann Surg* 221:778–787, 1995.)

Conclusion.—Preoperative chemoradiation therapy provides increased survival (Fig 1), increased disease-free survival, and decreased pelvic recurrence (Fig 2) when compared with the control group. In addition, there was a marked decrease in tumor size and a low incidence of positive lymph nodes, which implies that less radical surgery and preservation of the sphincter may be used in more patients.

▶ This study from Duke University showed significant tumor downstaging with their regimen of 5-fluorouracil, cisplatin, and 4,500-cGy preoperative radiation. As with the other preoperative radiation regimens discussed, this group also found enhanced local control as well as a decreased rate of metastases and increased survival when compared with historical controls.

In summary, I have attempted to select a wide range of various preoperative regimens of radiation therapy in high or low dose, with or without chemotherapy. One can expect, depending on the specific regimen, downstaging, a decrease in tumor size, and an increased ability to preserve the sphincter. Caution is raised with the selection of patients so as to avoid increasing morbidity and/or mortality with these various regimens. Thromboembolic prophylaxis is suggested to prevent mortality, and age-related cardiovascular complications can also be expected.

T.J. Eberlein, M.D.

Adjuvant Radiation Therapy for Rectal Carcinoma: Predictors of Outcome

Myerson RJ, Michalski JM, King ML, Birnbaum E, Fleshman J, Fry R, Kodner I, Lacey D, Lockett MA (Washington Univ, St Louis, Mo)
Int J Radiat Oncol Biol Phys 32:41–50, 1995   11–23

Background.—The benefits of adjuvant radiotherapy (RT) and chemotherapy in rectal adenocarcinoma have been well established. The authors reviewed their experience with adjuvant RT to determine what factors, including pretreatment findings and modalities of therapy, could best be used as predictors of outcome.

Methods.—The records of 307 patients with adenocarcinoma of the rectum who had received RT from 1975 through 1990 were reviewed and analyzed. Of the 307 patients, 251 and 56 had received RT preoperatively and postoperatively, respectively. Forty-one patients with freely movable or slightly tethered lesions received a 5-day course of RT to the pelvis totaling 20 Gy and were operated on immediately. The remaining 210 lesions, which required tumor regression to improve resectability, received a total of 40–50 Gy (mean and median, 45 Gy), followed by surgery in 6 to 7 weeks. Slightly higher doses (40–60 Gy) were administered to those receiving RT postoperatively. Chemotherapy (5-fluorouracil) was administered to 29 of the 56 patients (52%) receiving postoperative RT and to

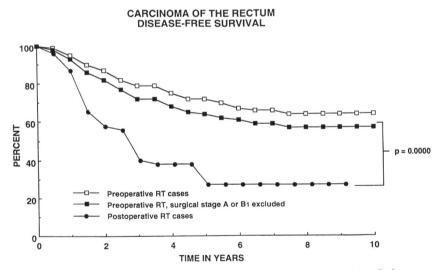

FIGURE 1.—Actuarial disease-free survival (Kaplan-Meier method): preoperative radiotherapy vs. postoperative radiotherapy. Results for all cases as well as the subset of preoperatively treated cases that were surgical stage B2, B3, or C are shown. Even when the (possibly downstaged) A and B1 lesions are excluded, the difference between the preoperatively treated group and the group given postoperative radiation is highly significant (P < 0.0001, Tarone Ware). (Reprinted from *International Journal of Radiation Oncology, Biology, Physics*, vol 32, Myerson RJ, Michalski JM, King ML, et al: Adjuvant radiation therapy for rectal carcinoma: Predictors of outcome, pp 41–50, Copyright 1995, with kind permission from Elsevier Science Ltd, The Boulevard, Langford Lane, Kidlington 0X5 1GB, UK.)

TABLE 5.—Multivariate Analysis (Cox Model), Pretreatment Factors
Only, Preoperative Radiotherapy Cases Only

Factors Considered	Overall Freedom From Disease	Local Control
Colorectal vs. nonspecialist surgeon	0.017	0.026
Grade of Pre-TX biopsy	NS	NS
Tumor circumferential	0.026	0.006
Organ invasion	NS	NS
Tumor near obstructing (lumen ≤ 1 cm)?	NS	NS
Degree of tumor fixation on palpation	NS	NS
Distance from anal verge	0.030	0.026
Preoperative radiation dose	NS	NS
Age	NS	NS
Gender	NS	NS
Race	NS	NS

Abbreviations: RT, radiotherapy; *TX*, treatment.
(Reprinted from *International Journal of Radiation Oncology, Biology, Physics*, vol 32, Myerson RJ, Michalski JM, King ML, et al: Adjuvant radiation therapy for rectal carcinoma: Predictors of outcome, pp 41–50, Copyright 1995, with kind permission from Elsevier Science Ltd, The Boulevard, Langford Lane, Kidlington 0X5 1GB, UK.)

14 of the 251 (6%) receiving preoperative RT. Abdominoperineal resection was performed in 157 patients and a low anterior resection in 128. Other procedures were performed in the remaining 22 patients. Severity of disease was graded according to the degree of tumor fixation, tumor grade, and tumor stage (Astler Coller). Age, radiation dose, and distance from the anal verge were considered to be continuous variables for purposes of multivariate analysis

Results.—Overall, 168 patients were alive and apparently free of disease at the time of their last follow-up. An additional 32 patients had died of unrelated causes and were free of cancer at the time of death. Thus the crude rate of freedom from disease was 200/307 (65%), including 3 patients who had had isolated liver or lung metastases successfully removed. Failures included 69 (22%) with distant metastases, 22 (7%) with both local and distant metastases, and 16 (5%) with disease localized to the pelvis. Multivariate analysis revealed that significant predictor factors for overall freedom from disease included preoperative vs. postoperative RT ($P < 0.001$), colorectal vs. nonspecialized surgeon ($P < 0.007$), grade of tumor in a pretreatment biopsy specimen, ($P = 0.026$), distance from the anal verge ($P = 0.033$), and pathologic stage ($P < 0.001$). Significant predictors for local control included preoperative vs. postoperative RT ($P < 0.001$), grade of tumor in a surgical specimen ($P < 0.001$), and pathologic stage ($P = 0.015$). Factors determined to not be significant for either freedom from disease or local control included the use of adjuvant chemotherapy, the surgical procedure, or the patient's age, gender, or race. Rates of 5-year local control and freedom from disease for the preoperative RT patients were 90% ± 2% and 73% ± 3, respectively. Figure 1 compares disease-free survival in the preoperative and postoperative RT groups and shows the significant superiority of pretreatment RT ($P <$ 0.0001) There was local control in 39 of the 41 patients (95%) who had received the short course of RT. The results of a second multivariate analysis of pretreatment factors performed on pretreatment RT cases is presented in Table 5. The significant pretreatment predictors of outcome were circumferential vs. noncircumferential tumor, experience of the surgeon, and distance from the anal verge.

Conclusions.—This study demonstrates the significant superiority of preoperative adjunctive radiotherapy over postoperative adjunctive radiotherapy in patients with adenocarcinoma of the rectum. Significant predictive factors for outcome included the experience of the surgeon, distance of the tumor from the anal verge, and certain tumor characteristics such as grade, stage, and circumferential vs. noncircumferential.

▶ This large series from St. Louis raises several important issues with respect to selection of patients. Following preoperative radiation therapy, surgery is performed. Those patients having B2, B3, or C surgical stage are treated with chemotherapy. Chemotherapy is added to preoperative radiation therapy if patients have T4 tumors and/or the tumors are circumferential or near obstructing lesions. In patients who have disease with a low surgical stage, it may be useful to identify other biological markers that may help identify subgroups of patients who may benefit from adjuvant chemotherapy. This might include expression of *ras* oncogene, vascular invasion, angiogenesis, and a host of other potential genetic markers.

T.J. Eberlein, M.D.

Distal Spread of Rectal Cancer and Optimal Distal Margin of Resection for Sphincter-Preserving Surgery
Shirouzu K, Isomoto H, Kakegawa T (Kurume Univ, Japan)
Cancer 76:388–392, 1995   11–24

Introduction.—In patients with rectal cancer, lymphatic blockage caused by metastases may result in abnormal retrograde distal spread. This spread is an important consideration in decisions about the distal resection margin from the tumor during sphincter-preserving surgery. Patients with rectal cancer were studied to evaluate the extent and significance of distal rectal spread and the optimal distal margin of resection for sphincter-preserving surgery.

Methods.—The retrospective study included 610 consecutive resection specimens from patients with rectal carcinoma. The specimens were analyzed to determine the extent of distal spread and its effects on prognosis. The International Union Against Cancer stage was I in 150 patients, II in 162, and III in 195. Curative surgery was performed in 505 patients.

Results.—Distal spread was detected in 10% of the patients overall but in fewer than 4% of those undergoing curative surgery. None of the patients with stage I disease had distal spread as compared with 1% of those with stage II disease and 10% of those with stage III disease. This spread was confined within a 1-cm length in all patients with stage II disease and half of those with stage III disease. The rate of distal spread in 103 patients with stage IV disease was 39%.

The 5-year survival rate in patients with stage II disease was 87% for those without distal spread and 50% for those with distal spread. Corresponding figures for patients with stage III disease were 66% and 38%. Most of the patients with distal spread died of distant metastases, even if they had undergone curative surgery.

Conclusions.—In patients with rectal cancer, distal spread appears to be a significant risk factor for distant metastasis. The pathologic findings in this study suggest that a 1 cm margin of resection will be appropriate for most patients. For patients with longer distal spread, a greater resection margin will not necessarily improve prognosis.

▶ This is a very large study correlating the pathologic distal spread of tumor. Most patients had a distal spread of 1 cm; however, abnormal retrograde distal spread more easily develops in patients with stage III or IV disease. Additionally, there appears to be a correlation of survival with distal margin spread (survival being decreased if distal spread of the tumor is greater than 1 cm). This obviously has implications when recommending surgical procedures in patients with rectal cancer; for example, patients who have distal spread longer than 1 cm, may not necessarily have improved survival with more radical resection. While most of us strive to obtain at least a 2-cm margin in rectal cancers as we perform more sphincter-sparing operations, it is comforting to know that a 1-cm margin may be sufficient in most patients.

T.J. Eberlein, M.D.

Local Excision of Rectal Tumours

Banerjee AK, Jehle EC, Shorthouse AJ, Buess G (Eberhard-Karls Universitat, Tübingen, Germany; Royal Hallamshire Hosp, Sheffield, England)
Br J Surg 82:1165–1173, 1995   11–25

Introduction.—Local excision offers the optimal surgical management for palliation in patients with rectal tumors. However, in selected patients, local excision may also offer curative treatment. The currently available methods and their efficacy are reviewed.

Palliative Local Excision.—Two techniques, endoscopic transanal resection and laser and photodynamic therapy, may be used for either palliative or curative purposes. Endoscopic transanal resection is the best palliative treatment for obstructing lesions at or below the peritoneal reflection. Laser and photodynamic therapy can provide safe palliative treatment for lesions above the peritoneal reflection and has a low risk of perforation. Electrocoagulation does not allow good control of the depth of tissue damage, has a high complication rate, and cannot be used on lesions above the peritoneal reflection. Other emerging methods of palliative local excision include cryosurgery and endoscopic injection of alcohol directly into tumor tissue.

Curative Local Excision.—Peranal excision and endoscopic transanal resection are safe and effective in patients with tumors smaller than 3 cm. Studies comparing endoscopic transanal resection with radical surgery have found comparable recurrence and mortality rates. The technique appears to be especially appropriate in elderly, fragile patients with small tumors not penetrating the muscularis propria. Laser excision should be used only for patients unfit for surgery inasmuch as it appears to be appropriate only for symptomatic relief. Transanal endoscopic microsurgery is the most recently developed technique for local excision of rectal and lower colon tumors. It has been shown to be a viable option for submucous, partial-wall, or full-thickness excision and is associated with short hospital stays and few complications. Developments in laparoscopic local excision indicate that this technique may allow excision of more proximal low-grade colonic tumors.

Patient Selection.—Indications for curative local excision are mobile tumors, T_1 tumors, a well or moderately differentiated histologic pattern, and tumors smaller than 3 cm. In patients unfit for surgery, curative local excision may be performed when the tumors are T_2 or T_3, have a poorly differentiated histologic pattern, or are larger than 3 cm. Local curative excision is contraindicated when the tumor is fixed, but palliative local excision can be performed.

▶ This is a very nice review of the indications for local excision of colorectal tumors when they are palliative and when they may be expected to be curative. Any surgeon who treats a large number of patients with colorectal tumors would benefit from this very nice review.

T.J. Eberlein, M.D.

Coloanal Anastomosis for Rectal Cancer: Long-Term Results at the Mayo and Cleveland Clinics
Cavaliere F, Pemberton JH, Cosimelli M, Fazio VW, Beart RW Jr (Mayo Clinic and Mayo Found, Rochester, Minn; Regina Elena Cancer Inst, Rome; Univ of Southern California, Los Angeles)
Dis Colon Rectum 38:807–812, 1995   11–26

Background.—In a previous report of 29 patients with rectal cancer, coloanal anastomosis was found to be associated with acceptable mortality, morbidity, and survival and adequate function. In the present study, the short- and long-term complication rates, incidence of relapse, survival, and functional results of coloanal anastomosis were evaluated in a larger patient population.

Patients.—One hundred seventeen patients with rectal cancer who underwent coloanal anastomosis over a 10-year period were included. The

TABLE 2.—Complications

Complication	% of Patients
Early	
Leakage (symptomatic, 57%)	18
Urinary retention (temporary)	15
Urinary tract infection	4
Late	
Stricture (symptomatic, 60%)	21
Sexual dysfunction	14

(Courtesy of Cavaliere F, Pemberton JH, Cosimelli M, et al: Coloanal anastomosis for rectal cancer: Long-term results at the Mayo and Cleveland clinics. *Dis Colon Rectum* 38(8):807–812, 1995.)

median patient age was 59 years. A straight coloanal anastomosis was performed in the majority of patients, whereas 15% had a J pouch. There were no diverting stomas in 38% of the patients. Endoscopic examination showed that the median distance from the anal verge to the lower edge of the tumor was 6.7 cm. Tumors were noted in the lower third of the rectum in 64% of the patients.

Results.—None of the patients died within 30 days after surgery. Early or late major or minor complications were experienced by 62% (Table 2). Eighteen percent of the patients had anastomotic leakage, 21% had strictures, 15% had temporary urinary retention, and 14% experienced sexual dysfunction. A temporary stoma was required in 6 patients as a result of septic complications. Seventy-eight percent of the patients had satisfactory fecal continence. Frequent incontinence was not observed in any of the

TABLE 3.—Functional Parameters

	Pouch (7)	No Pouch (22)
Incontinence day		
None	5	12
Occasional	2	6
Frequent	0	4
Incontinence night		
None	3	11
Occasional	4	6
Frequent	0	5
Pad		
None	6	11
Occasional	1	7
Frequent	0	4
Stools (daytime)		
Range	0.5–4	1–8
Median	2	3
Stools (nighttime)		
Range	0–1	0–4
Median	1	0
Distinguish stool/gas	5	19

(Courtesy of Cavaliere F, Pemberton JH, Cosimelli M, et al: Coloanal anastomosis for rectal cancer: Long-term results at the Mayo and Cleveland clinics. *Dis Colon Rectum* 38(8):807–812, 1995.)

TABLE 4.—Recurrence

Site	Total (%)	Mayo (%)	Cleveland (%)
Locoregional	6	5	7
Distant	13	14	13
Locoregional and distant	1	—	2
Metachronous tumors	5	7	2
Recurrence	25	27	24

(Courtesy of Cavaliere F, Pemberton JH, Cosimelli M, et al: Coloanal anastomosis for rectal cancer: Long-term results at the Mayo and Cleveland clinics. *Dis Colon Rectum* 38(8):807–812, 1995.)

patients with J pouches (Table 3). Recurrent carcinoma occurred in 25% of all patients, whereas metachronous disease developed in 5% (Table 4). Among individuals with a lower third tumor, local recurrence and distant relapse rates were 7% and 16, respectively; median survival after relapse was 11 months. The 5-year disease-free actuarial survival rate was 69% for the entire patient population.

Conclusions.—Although the risk of complications after coloanal anastomosis is high, long-term survival rates and functional outcomes are excellent. Coloanal anastomosis should thus be considered a reasonable alternative to abdominoperineal resection.

▶ Coloanal anastomosis is associated with a relatively high complication rate and is, therefore best done by experienced surgeons. Functional parameters show fewer complications if a pouch is created. Contraindications to this type of anastomosis are relatively few; however, bulky tumors and/or pelvic extension are contraindications. Again, ensuring the adequacy of mesorectal dissection should be emphasized since if done properly, satisfactory survival and recurrence data can be anticipated; this emphasizes the importance of experience as well as patient selection.

T.J. Eberlein, M.D.

Colonic J Pouch/Anal Anastomosis

The first 2 articles in this section are grouped together because they discuss the ramifications of construction of a J colonic pouch in performing an anal anastomosis.

T.J. Eberlein, M.D.

Prospective Randomized Trial Comparing J Colonic Pouch–Anal Anastomosis and Straight Coloanal Reconstruction
Seow-Choen F, Goh HS (Singapore Gen Hosp)
Br J Surg 82:608–610, 1995   11–27

Background.—Previous studies have reported the effectiveness of a J colonic pouch–anal anastomosis as surgical treatment of low-lying rectal carcinomas. In a prospective, randomized study, the authors compared the intraoperative and postoperative results of a J pouch colonic–anal anastomosis with a straight coloanal reconstruction.

Methods.—Forty patients with rectally palpable, low-lying rectal carcinomas were randomized between J pouch colonic–anal anastomosis and straight coloanal reconstruction. Patients with gross peritoneal or liver metastatic disease or advanced pelvic involvement were excluded. Patients with apparent solitary metastatic liver lesions were included. Follow-up took place 1, 6, and 12 months after closure of the temporary ileostomies. A comparison of multiple efficacy end points was done at these follow-up visits.

Results.—The treatment groups, consisting of 20 patients each, were comparable demographically and clinically. The time duration of the 2 procedures was similar. Four patients had postoperative complications after the pouch-anal anastomosis; 3 with infections and 1 with a pulmonary infection. There were 8 complications after coloanal reconstruction. Three patients had wound infections and 2 had pulmonary infections, 1 of whom also had urinary sepsis. One patient each had prolonged ileus, deep calf vein thrombosis, and drip-site inflammation. Recurrent disease developed in 4 patients who had pouch-anal anastomoses, 3 at about 12 months postoperatively and the other 33 months postoperatively. One patient in this group died 2 months postoperatively of an acute myocardial infarction. Two patients who had undergone coloanal reconstruction had recurrent tumor. Table 1 compares the functional results of the 2 procedures. There was a significantly higher incidence of increased bowel movements per 24 hours in the coloanal reconstruction group than in the pouch-anal anastomosis group. This was noted at 1, 6, and 12 months after ileostomy closure. At 1 month, bowel frequency per 24 hours was 2.5 (range, 0.5–10) in the pouch-anal anastomosis group as compared with 4 per 24 hours (range, 2–20) in the coloanal reconstruction group ($P < 0.03$). At 6 months, the corresponding bowel frequencies were 2 (range, 0.5–6) and 4 (range, 2–20) per 24 hours, respectively ($P < 0.007$). No patient in the pouch-anal anastomosis group required antidiarrheal medication, whereas 10 patients in the coloanal reconstruction group required medication at 1 month and 8 patients required it at 6 months. Thirteen (65%) patients in the pouch-anal anastomosis group and 7 (35%) in the coloanal reconstruction group had 3 or fewer bowel movements per 24 hours. Two patients in the pouch-anal anastomosis group (10%) and 3 in the coloanal reconstruction group (15%) were having 10 or more bowel movements per 24 hours 1 month after ileostomy closure. At 12 months, all patients with a pouch reconstruction (19 of 19) had regained normal continence as compared with 14 of 20 of those who had a straight coloanal reconstruction. There were no significant differences between the 2 groups at 1 and 6 months with regard to urgency, continence, nocturnal leaks, use of pads, constipation, or need for enemas to evacuate.

TABLE 1.—Functional Results in Patients With Pouch-Anal Anastomosis or Straight
Coloanal Reconstruction 12 Months After Ileostomy Closure

	Pouch-anal Anastomosis	Straight Coloanal Anastomosis	P
No. of patients	19*	20	
Frequency of motion per 24 hr (range)	2 (0.5–4)	2 (0.5–10)	< 0.05
Use of antidiarrheal medication	0	9	< 0.008
Urgency			
<15 min	2†	4	NS
>15 min	17	16	NS
Continence			
Liquid incontinence	0	6	—
Air incontinence	0	0	—
Normal continence	19	14	0.01
Nocturnal leakage	1†	5	NS
Pads necessary	1†	3	NS
Constipation	1	1	NS
Need for enema	0	0	NS
No. of motions per 24 hr			
≤3	18 (95)	14 (70)	< 0.05
4–9	1 (5)	5 (25)	—
≥10	0 (0)	1 (5)	NS

Note: Values in parentheses are percentages unless otherwise stated.

* One patient died 2 months after ileostomy closure of acute myocardial infarction.

† One patient with a previous fistulectomy for an anal fistula needed division of a tight anal band before the stapling instrument could be introduced anally.

(Courtesy of Seow-Choen F, Goh HS: Prospective randomized trial comparing J colonic pouch–anal anastomosis and straight coloanal reconstruction, *Br J Surg* 82:608–610, 1995, Blackwell Science Ltd.)

Conclusions.—The 2 operations for low-lying rectal carcinomas, J pouch colonic–anal anastomosis and coloanal reconstruction, were similar in duration of the procedure and intraoperative and postoperative events. There was, however, significantly superior anal function in regard to frequency of bowel movements per 24 hours at 1, 6, and 12 months in the pouch-anal anastomosis group of patients.

▶ This first study from Singapore is a randomized prospective trial comparing J colonic pouch–anal anastomosis with straight coloanal reconstruction. In this series it was very clear that J pouch anastomosis was associated with less frequent bowel movements, less use of antidiarrheal medication, and better continence by 12-months after ileostomy closure. Care in constructing the pouch is important, both with respect to the size and the portion of colon used for creation of the pouch.

T.J. Eberlein, M.D.

Colonic J Pouch: Anal Anastomosis After Rectal Excision for Carcinoma: Functional Outcome

Mortensen NJM, Ramirez JM, Takeuchi N, Humphreys MMS (John Radcliffe Hosp, Oxford, England)
Br J Surg 82:611–613, 1995   11–28

Background.—The formation of a colonic J loop and anastomosing it to the anus have been proposed as a remedy for loss of the rectal pouch that occurs with curative operations for low-lying rectal carcinomas. The authors relate their experience with this procedure in a consecutive series of 23 patients with low-lying rectal carcinomas.

Methods.—The patients were observed postoperatively to monitor surgical complications, frequency of defecation, nocturnal bowel movements, stool consistency, continence, urgency, evacuation problems, and sexual and urologic difficulties. Manometric measurements were performed on the pouch, and threshold and maximum tolerated volumes were determined. The rectoanal reflex and anorectal sensation were evaluated.

Results.—Of the 23 patients studied, 17 were men. The average patient age was 64.4 years with a range of 44–76 years. The mean distance from the anastomotic site to the anal verge was 3.5 cm (range, 2–4.5 cm). One patient died of unrelated causes postoperatively, and recurrences developed in 4 patients—2 in the local structure and 2 in the liver. As presented in Table 2, there were 5 postoperative complications, including 2 instances each of acute heart failure and partial anastomotic dehiscence and 1 instance of obstruction. Table 3 presents the functional outcome in 19 evaluable patients at a mean duration of 7 months after closing the temporary ileostomy. The mean bowel frequency was 2.1 per day (range, 1–4). Four patients had mild fecal leakage up to 3 times a week, and 5 patients had bowel urgency. Seven patients had some degree of incomplete evacuation, 3 had sexual dysfunction, and 1 had urinary dysfunction. Stool consistency was normal in 15 of 16 patients and soft in 1. The results of anorectal physiology in 13 patients disclosed no manometric differences before and after surgery with respect to the maximum tolerated volume or maximum resting pressure. However, maximum squeeze pressure was significantly lower after surgery (mean of 189 cm H_2O before surgery and 132 cm H_2O after surgery, $P < 0.05$).

TABLE 2.—Details of Complications in 23 Patients

	No.
Complications	5
Partial anastomotic dehiscence	2*
Obstruction	1*
Acute heart failure	2†

* Managed conservatively.
† Died within 30 days of surgery.
(Courtesy of Mortensen NJM, Ramirez JM, Takeuchi N, et al: Colonic J pouch: Anal anastomosis after rectal excision for carcinoma: Functional outcome. *Br J Surg* 82:611–613, 1995, Blackwell Science Ltd.)

TABLE 3.—Functional Outcome in 19 Patients

No. of patients	19
Mean (range) stool frequency per 24 h	2.1(1–4)
Stool consistency	
Normal	18
Soft	1
Continence	
Normal	15
Solids	19
Minor seepage	4
Flatus	19
Discrimination between flatus and solid	19
Urgency	5
Incomplete evacuation	7
Sexual dysfunction	3
Urinary dysfunction	1

(Courtesy of Mortensen NJM, Ramirez JM, Takeuchi N, et al: Colonic J pouch: Anal anastomosis after rectal excision for carcinoma: Functional outcome. *Br J Surg* 82:611–613, 1995, Blackwell Science Ltd.)

Conclusions.—Colonic J pouch–anal anastomosis is a safe alternative procedure for curative surgery of low-lying rectal carcinomas. It has the additional advantage of maintaining anorectal physiology in a significant number of patients.

▶ This is a consecutive series of patients detailing the functional results as well as manometric differences before and after surgery. Using a J pouch configuration, over half of the patients had near-normal physiologic pressures. Thus it would appear that coloanal anastomosis is an alternative to more radical surgery and permanent colostomy. Therefore it is an important alternative for sphincter-sparing procedures. A correctly performed J pouch seems to offer the most physiologic and best functional results. Once again, the key is to construct the pouch carefully, without compromise of the vascular supply and care taken to not place excessive tension on it. The latter point usually requires full mobilization of the left colon and splenic flexure.

T.J. Eberlein, M.D.

Epidural Analgesia Shortens Postoperative Ileus After Ileal Pouch-Anal Canal Anastomosis

Morimoto H, Cullen JJ, Messick JM Jr, Kelly KA (Mayo Clinic and Mayo Med School, Rochester, Minn)
Am J Surg 169:79–83, 1995   11–29

Objective.—Although postoperative ileus is a well-recognized complication of open abdominal surgery, its exact mechanism is unknown. Some, but not all studies have suggested that giving epidural rather than systemic analgesia can prevent or ameliorate postoperative ileus. The effects of epidural analgesia on recovery from postoperative ileus were studied in patients undergoing ileal pouch–anal canal anastomosis.

Methods.—The retrospective study included 85 patients undergoing proctocolectomy with ileal pouch–anal canal anastomosis. In 44 patients, postoperative pain was treated with a continuous infusion of epidural fentanyl citrate with supplemental IV morphine as needed. The 41 controls received only systemic morphine as needed. The 2 groups were matched for age and sex and were comparable in terms of their preoperative and operative risk factors and postoperative morbidity.

Results.—There were no operative deaths. Patients receiving epidural fentanyl needed less nasogastric suction and IV fluids. They also had more rapid discharge of fecal content, 3.5 vs. 4.3 days; a quicker return to oral intake, 4.5 vs. 6.2 days; and a shorter hospitalization, 9.6 vs. 12.1 days. The epidural fentanyl group also needed less postoperative morphine.

Conclusions.—In patients undergoing proctocolectomy and ileal pouch–anal canal anastomosis, epidural analgesia with fentanyl citrate can shorten postoperative ileus. The mechanism of this effect is unknown. It does not appear to involve a smaller total dose of opioids, although it may be related to the more continuous pain relief offered by epidural analgesia.

▶ While this series is retrospective, it nicely demonstrates the added benefit of epidural analgesia with fentanyl citrate. The more rapid recovery of the gastrointestinal tract may be related to the fact that opioids in the epidural space do not access the bloodstream and are therefore not available to the α-opioid agonists in the gastrointestinal tract. However, opioid concentrations were not measured in this study.

T.J. Eberlein, M.D.

Colon Cancer

Genetic Linkage Analysis in Hereditary Non-Polyposis Colon Cancer Syndrome

Froggatt NJ, Koch J, Davies R, Evans DGR, Clamp A, Quarrell OWJ, Weissenbach J, Hodgson SV, Ponder BAJ, Barton DE, Maher ER (Cambridge Univ, England; Addenbrooke's Hosp, Cambridge, England; St Mary's Hosp, Manchester, England; et al)

J Med Genet 32:352–357, 1995   11–30

Background.—As many as 10% of colorectal cancers may occur in those genetically predisposed to the disease. The most common familial form is hereditary nonpolyposis colon cancer (HNPCC) syndrome. Previous molecular genetic studies have demonstrated heterogeneous loci. Mutations in 4 genes that encode parts of the mismatch enzyme repair system (*hMSH2, hMLH1, hPMS1, hPMS2*) may be responsible for HNPCC syndrome.

Objective.—The extent of locus heterogeneity was determined by performing linkage studies in 14 families with HNPCC syndrome from eastern and northwestern England. Forty-five affected individuals and 123 relatives and spouses at risk were included in the study.

Findings.—Linkage to *hMLH1* was ruled out in 6 families, each of which was probably linked with *hMSH2*. Linkage to *hMSH2* was excluded in 3 families, each of which was likely to be linked to *hMLH1*. Linkage to these genes could not be excluded in the 5 remaining families.

Discussion.—Locus heterogeneity is a feature of HNPCC syndrome. In the population under study, most large families with HNPCC syndrome exhibit mutations in *hMSH2* or *hMLH1*. There was no obvious correlation between clinical phenotype and the linkage findings in this population. The use of molecular genetic techniques to diagnose HNPCC syndrome will probably rest on directly detecting mutations.

▶ This is a very nice study that looks at HNPCC syndrome, which has been mapped to a locus on chromosome 2p16, subsequently identified as *hMSH2*. Further studies have shown mutations in 3 other genes: *hMLH1* in chromosome 3p21, *hPMS1* in chromosome 2q31-32, and *hPMS2* in 7p22. This study looks at 14 HNPCC families; while this study confirms the heterogeneity in HNPCC, it associates most mutations with *hMSH2* or *hMLH1*. I include this paper to make the reader familiar with these genetic mutations since further identification of other genetic mutations in colon cancer will become a more prominent diagnostic tool as well as a potential therapeutic option for this type of disease.

T.J. Eberlein, M.D.

Restoration of CD44H Expression in Colon Carcinomas Reduces Tumorigenicity
Tanabe KK, Stamenkovic I, Cutler M, Takahashi K (Massachusetts Gen Hosp, Boston; Harvard Med School, Boston)
Ann Surg 222:493–503, 1995   11–31

Background.—CD44, a cell surface glycoprotein in a variety of normal and malignant tissues, exists in a number of isoforms that arise from mRNA alternative splicing. Previous in vitro studies of CD44 have demonstrated its role in several properties required by invasive and metastatic tumor cells. In a previous study of CD44 isoforms, downregulation of CD44H relative to other CD44 transcripts was associated with the transformation of normal colonic mucosa to carcinoma. The functional consequences of this downregulation and the effects of introducing CD44H back into colon carcinoma cell lines were examined.

Methods.—CD44 expression was examined with Western blot analysis in paired tumor and normal colon mucosa tissues from 3 patients and in 7 colon carcinoma cell lines. Two of the colon carcinoma cell lines and mice with colon cancer were transfected with CD44H cDNA and a mutant of CD44H cDNA encoding only a 3–amino acid cytoplasmic domain and

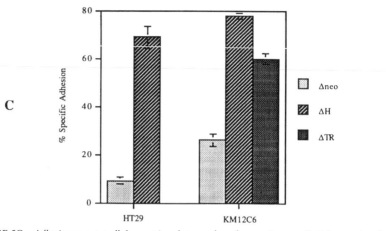

FIGURE 5C.—Adhesion to extracellular matrix substances by colon carcinoma cell. Cells transfected with CD44H cDNA (Δ*H*), CD44TR cDNA (Δ*TR*), and no cDNA (Δ*neo*) were also tested for adhesion to hyaluronate. (Courtesy of Tanabe KK, Stamenkovic I, Cutler M, et al: Restoration of CD44H expression in colon carcinomas reduces tumorigenicity. *Ann Surg* 222:493–503, 1995.)

then studied for adhesion to hyaluronate and in vitro and in vivo tumor growth.

Results.—CD44H was expressed significantly more abundantly in the normal mucosa than in the tumor tissue and was not expressed significantly in the colon carcinoma cell lines. Tumor tissue and cell lines primarily expressed high–molecular weight CD44 isoforms, which were not expressed by normal mucosa. Hyaluronate elicited moderate affinity from the high–molecular weight CD44 isoforms but high affinity from CD44H after transfection with either the normal CD44H or the mutant CD44H lacking the cytoplasmic domain (Fig 5C). Transfection of CD44H reduced tumor growth rates both in vitro and in vivo. Transfection with the mutant of CD44H cDNA reduced tumor growth rates only in vivo (Figs 6 and 7).

Conclusions.—Downregulation of CD44H occurs during the transformation of colon mucosa to carcinoma, and reintroduction of CD44H into tumor cells causes a reduction in tumor growth rate, thus suggesting that CD44H controls tumorigenicity. The differing effects on in vitro and in vivo growth rates of a CD44H protein without the cytoplasmic domain suggest that the inhibition of in vitro cell growth is dependent on cytoplasmic proteins, whereas with the additional environmental elements present in vivo, only the extracellular domain of CD44 is used to reduce cell growth.

▶ This is a very elegant series of experiments by Tanabe and colleagues. These authors previously showed that the isoform CD44H is downregulated during the transformation of normal colon mucosa to carcinoma. In this study, CD44H cDNA was transfected into colon carcinoma cells. This resulted in their in vitro and in vivo growth being significantly reduced. These

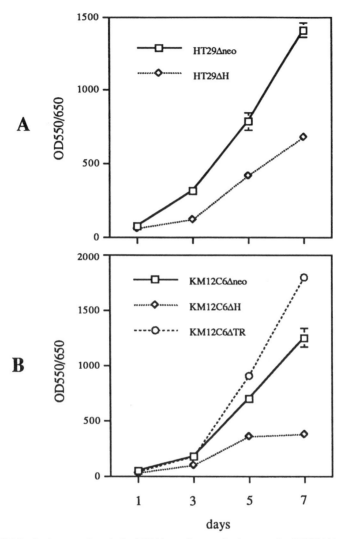

FIGURE 6.—In vitro growth analysis of CD44 transfectants. In vitro growth of HT29 (**A**) or KM12C6 (**B**) cells tranfected with either no cDNA (*Δneo*), CD44H cDNA (*ΔH*), or CD44TR cDNA (*ΔTR*) was measured by the methylthiotetrazole assay. (Courtesy of Tanabe KK, Stamenkovic I, Cutler M, et al: Restoration of CD44H expression in colon carcinomas reduces tumorigenicity. *Ann Surg* 222:493–503, 1995.)

authors have therefore identified a possibly unique role for this cell surface glycoprotein in the regulation and growth of colon cancer and in the transformation of normal colonic mucosa to cancer. It may also provide a new target for novel gene therapeutic interventions.

T.J. Eberlein, M.D.

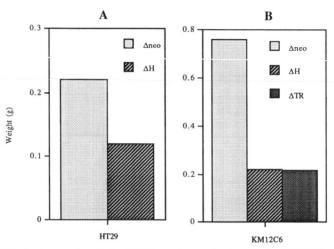

FIGURE 7.—In vivo growth analysis of CD44 transfectants. In vivo growth of HT29 (A) or KM12C6 (B) transfectants was determined through measurement of tumor weights 16 days after subcutaneous implantation of 5×10^6 cells. (Courtesy of Tanabe KK, Stamenkovic I, Cutler M, et al: Restoration of CD44H expression in colon carcinomas reduces tumorigenicity. *Ann Surg* 222:493–503, 1995.)

Gastric Cancer

Expression of Transforming Growth Factor Alpha, Epidermal Growth Factor Receptor and Epidermal Growth Factor in Precursor Lesions to Gastric Carcinoma

Filipe MI, Osborn M, Linehan J, Sanidas E, Brito MJ, Jankowski J (UMDS Guy's Hosp, London; Sta Marta Hosp, Lisbon, Portugal; Herakleion Univ Hosp, Crete, Greece; et al)
Br J Cancer 71:30–36, 1995   11–32

Purpose.—The stepwise process of gastric carcinogenesis begins with molecular changes in normal cells resulting in phenotypic adaptation. The process of gastric carcinogenesis may involve epidermal growth factor (EGF), its related peptide transforming growth factor α (TGF-α), and their common receptor (EGFR), all of which play a role in the control of cell proliferation and differentiation in the gastrointestinal epithelium. Altered expression of EGF, TGF-α, and EGFR was studied in the precursor lesions to gastric carcinoma.

Methods.—Western blot analysis was used to compare the immunohistochemical expression and topographic distribution of EGF, TGF-α, and EGFR in the precursor lesions of gastric carcinoma and in noncancer tissue. One goal of the study was to determine whether immunoreactivity to growth factors and their receptors correspond with normal- or aberrant-sized protein products by Western blotting.

Results.—Areas of normal mucosa and hyperplasia in carcinoma fields showed increased and extended expression of TGF-α as compared with noncancer controls. Specimens of intestinal metaplasia (IM) from carcinoma fields showed increased expression of EGFR. Normal mucosa did not express EGF, and IM expressed it only weakly. When compared with noncancer controls, IM in carcinoma fields showed higher coexpression of TGF-α/EGFR and EGF/EGFR.

Conclusions.—The morphologic changes occurring during gastric carcinogenesis appear to be associated with altered expression of TGF-α/EGFR. Increased TGF-α expression appears to be a very early event that is followed by upregulation of EGFR. Knowledge of the molecular events occurring in precancerous stages may be useful in the early detection of cancer risk and in cancer prevention.

▶ Frequently, gastric carcinoma is seen in advanced stages in patients in this country. I have included this manuscript since study of these growth factors in early tumorigenesis may well lead to earlier diagnosis and, perhaps, prevention. Growth factors have a wide spectrum of biological activity, such as control of cell proliferation, differentiation, apoptosis, transformation, and neovascularization. Epidermal growth factor and TGF-α may regulate the transition rate between the G_2 phase and mitosis of the cell cycle. Increased coexpression of these factors in a precancer stage may play a role in malignant transformation. Additionally, understanding these mechanisms may explain why there appears to be different biological behavior with poorly differentiated tumors and well-differentiated tumors. Further study of these molecular mechanisms may have profound implications in the treatment of gastric cancer in the future.

T.J. Eberlein, M.D.

Pathological Prognostic Factors in the Second British Stomach Cancer Group Trial of Adjuvant Therapy in Resectable Gastric Cancer
Yu CC-W, Levison DA, Dunn JA, Ward LC, Demonakou M, Allum WH, Hallisey MT (Queen Elizabeth Hosp, Birmingham, England; Sismanoglion Gen Hosp, Athens, Greece; St Bartholomew's Hosp, London)
Br J Cancer 71:1106–1110, 1995   11–33

Background.—Gastric carcinoma remains a leading cause of mortality in the United Kingdom despite advances in surgical practice. In an effort to improve disease outcome, the British Stomach Cancer Group has conducted 2 trials of adjuvant therapy. The second trial was a prospective randomized study of adjuvant radiotherapy or cytotoxic chemotherapy after gastrectomy for adenocarcinoma. Ten centers in the United Kingdom participated, with recruitment conducted between 1981 and 1986. A total of 436 patients were randomized to either surgery alone, surgery and chemotherapy, or surgery plus radiotherapy, with follow-up conducted for 5 years or until death. An additional 203 patients referred to the trial who failed to meet trial criteria were also observed in accordance with the trial protocol. The median survival duration was 15 months, with no survival benefits shown for patients receiving either type of adjuvant therapy vs.

TABLE 5.—Summary of the Cox Stepwise Multiple Regression Analysis

Factor	Regression Coefficient (β)	χ² to Remove	P Value	Relative Risk* (95% CI)
Pathological factors assessed by local centers (n = 515)				
Extent	0.49	22.4	< 0.0001	2.66 (1.67–4.17)
Nodal involvement	0.73	37.4	< 0.0001	2.07 (1.61–2.67)
Resection lines	0.62	22.4	< 0.0001	1.86 (1.45–2.40)
Histology	0.12	4.5	0.03	1.62 (1.02–2.52)
Additional pathological factors assessed at review (n = 322)				
Lymphocytic infiltration, MD	0.29	9.26	0.002	1.79 (1.21–2.59)
Histological grade, DL	0.26	5.46	0.01	1.68 (1.07–2.63)
Dysplasia, MD	0.46	11.1	0.0009	1.59 (1.19–2.12)
Combination of factors at local center and review (n = 445)				
Extent	0.49	19.9	< 0.0001	2.66 (1.64–4.41)
Resection lines	0.68	22.6	< 0.0001	1.97 (1.51–2.58)
Nodal involvement	0.67	28.1	< 0.0001	1.94 (1.49–2.54)

* The risk ratios are calculated from the formula $\exp(\beta)^k$, where k is the difference between the high-risk and low-risk groups. In each case, the extreme groups are compared, e.g., for histologic findings: low risk, well; high risk, anaplastic. The groupings used are identical to the groupings shown in the univariate analysis.
Abbreviations: MD, M. Demonakou; *DL,* D. Levison.
(Courtesy of Yu CC-W, Levison DA, Dunn JA, et al: Pathological prognostic factors in the second British Stomach Cancer Group trial of adjuvant therapy in resectable gastric cancer. *Br J Cancer* 71:1106–1110, 1995.)

those undergoing surgery only. As part of the study, various pathologic findings were recorded in detail, and 2 experienced histopathologists independently evaluated the tumors by using the Lauren and Ming classification, as well as a standard grading system based on the extent of differentiation. The extent of infiltration by inflammatory cells was also determined. The prognostic value of these pathologic factors in predicting the outcome after surgery for gastric adenocarcinoma was evaluated by univariate and multivariate analysis.

Findings.—When the pathologic factors collected from the local referring centers were evaluated by univariate analysis, tumor size, macroscopic type, number of involved sites, depth of invasion, involvement of resection lines and lymph nodes, and histologic grade were found to be significant predictors of survival. The Lauren classification and histologic grade, but not the Ming classification, were also identified as significant prognostic factors. Although the degree of lymphocytic and eosinophilic infiltration and the presence of dysplasia evaluated by 1 of the pathologists showed a significant association with survival, interobserver correlation for these parameters and grade was poor. On multivariate analysis, depth of invasion and resection line and nodal involvement were identified as the only significant independent pathologic variables affecting survival (Table 5).

Conclusions.—The prognostic value of conventional pathologic factors in predicting outcome after surgery for gastric adenocarcinoma has been verified in this study, with depth of invasion, lymph node and resection line involvement, and histologic grade identified as the most important independent variables.

▶ This paper was selected simply to emphasize the importance of depth of invasion, resection margins, and nodal involvement as independent variables influencing the survival of patients with gastric cancer. It emphasizes the importance of standardization of pathologic review and the utilization of these parameters in selecting patients for various adjuvant phase I/II protocols.

T.J. Eberlein, M.D.

Intraoperative Radiation Therapy for Gastric Cancer
Abe M, Nishimura Y, Shibamoto Y (Kyoto Univ, Japan; Chest Disease Research Inst, Kyoto, Japan)
World J Surg 19:554–557, 1995   11–34

Purpose.—For patients with gastric cancer, intraoperative radiotherapy (IORT) may lead to more effective control of local disease and thus to better survival. The results of IORT for gastric cancer are compared with those of surgery alone.

Methods.—Histologic classification and survival analysis were performed for 94 of 115 patients with gastric cancer who were treated by IORT. The controls were 127 patients who were treated by surgery alone

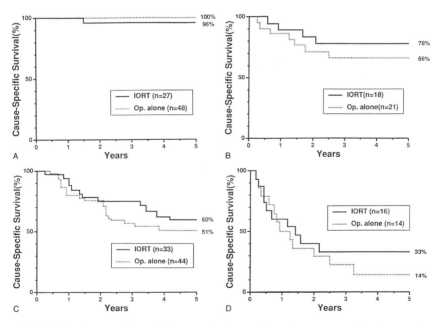

FIGURE 1.—Cause-specific survival curves of patients with gastric cancer treated by intraoperative radiation therapy or by surgery alone. A, survival rates with stage I gastric cancer. B, survival rates with stage II gastric cancer. C, survival rates with stage III gastric cancer. D, survival rates with stage IV gastric cancer. (Courtesy of *World Journal of Surgery*, Intraoperative radiation therapy for gastric cancer, by Abe M, Nishimura Y, Shibamoto Y, vol 19, p 555, Fig 1, 1995, copyright notice of Springer-Verlag.)

during the same period who also underwent histologic classification. Survival was compared in the 2 groups. Survival between groups was also compared according to the presence or absence of serosal invasion and the grade of lymph node metastasis. This analysis included 57 patients in the IORT group and 171 controls.

Results.—There was no difference in survival for patients with stage I disease. For those with more advanced gastric cancer, 5-year survival rates increased by 10% to 20% in the IORT group (Fig 1). For patients with lymph node metastases within N1 or those without serosal invasion, IORT carried no survival advantage. However, IORT was associated with a 10% increase in 5-year survival for patients with serosal invasion and an 18% increase for those with N2 and N3 lymph node metastases.

Conclusions.—Intraoperative radiation therapy improves survival for some patients with gastric cancer, namely, those with stage II to IV disease, those with serosal invasion, and those with N2 or N3 lymph node metastases. There were few significant complications of IORT.

▶ I have included this manuscript because of its provocative nature in showing efficacy for intraoperative radiation therapy (IORT). However, the operative procedure performed, as well as the extent of lymphadenectomy, is not detailed, so it may have had an impact on the results. We have seen promising data, both with pancreas and now with gastric cancer, but what will really be needed is a very well controlled randomized prospective trial to finally answer the question whether IORT is efficacious. This is particularly true in this era of cost-conscious medical care.

T.J. Eberlein, M.D.

Molecular Biology of Gastric Cancer
Tahara E (Hiroshima Univ, Japan)
World J Surg 19:484–490, 1995   11–35

Background.—Gastric cancer has been linked to multiple gene alterations, including oncogenes, growth factor or cytokines, cell cycle regulators, tumor suppressor genes, cell adhesion molecules, and genetic instability. The specific gene changes vary with the histologic type of gastric cancer. Current knowledge of the molecular biology of gastric cancer is reviewed.

Discussion.—Both well-differentiated and poorly differentiated gastric cancers are commonly associated with aberrant expression and amplification of the c-*met* gene, which is rarely noted in colorectal cancers. Inactivation of the p53 gene and CD44 abnormal transcripts are common as well. Gastric cancer of all histologic types may be associated with amplification of the cyclin E gene. There may be decreased expression of the *pic*1 gene independent of p53 mutations. Well-differentiated gastric cancers are more likely to be associated with K-*ras* mutations, c-*erb*B-2 gene amplification, APC gene loss of heterozygosity (LOH) and mutations, LOH of the *bcl*-2 gene, and LOH at the DCC locus. The progression of well-differentiated cancers involves LOH on chromosome 1q.

The genetic changes noted in well-differentiated gastric cancers may be the same as those occurring in precancerous lesions such as hyperplastic polyps, intestinal metaplasia, and adenoma. On the other hand, the carcinogenesis of poorly differentiated gastric cancer may begin with genetic instability. Development and progression of poorly differentiated or scirrhous carcinoma depend on reduction or loss of cadherin and catenins and amplification of the K-*sam* and c-*met* genes. In certain types of stomach cancer, morphogenesis may involve interaction between cell adhesion molecules in the c-*met*–expressing tumor cells and hepatocyte growth factor from stromal cells.

Conclusions.—Well-differentiated and poorly differentiated gastric cancers may involve different genetic pathways, as available research evidence suggests (Fig 2). For well-differentiated cancers, a cumulative series of gene changes similar to those seen in colorectal cancer may be involved. Alterations associated with peritoneal dissemination and metastasis may include LOH on chromosome 7q, reduced nm23 protein, abnormal CD44

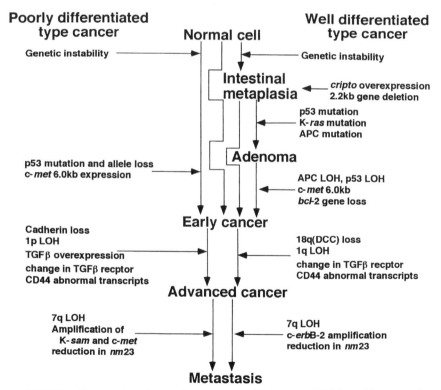

FIGURE 2.—Two genetic pathways of gastric cancer. *Abbreviation: LOH,* loss of heterozygosity. (Courtesy of *World Journal of Surgery,* Molecular biology of gastric cancer, by Tahara E, vol 19, p 487, Fig 2, 1995, copyright notice of Springer-Verlag.)

transcripts, changes in cadherin and catenins, and overexpression of a 31-kd lactoside-binding lectin. Although this knowledge may soon find some clinical application, there is currently no single "molecular" test for clinical use.

▶ This paper by Tahara is a very elegant summary of what is known about the molecular events that occur in the development of well-differentiated, poorly differentiated, and metastatic gastric cancer. Similar to the very elegant work that Vogelstein and others have done with colon cancer, we are beginning to understand on a molecular level the various biological effects of gastric cancer. Obviously, there is a great deal of variability between different tumor populations; therefore, a single molecular model is not yet available. Further definition, however, of these molecular processes will lead to earlier diagnosis, better estimation of prognosis, and therapeutic interventions.

T.J. Eberlein, M.D.

Lymphatic Invasion and Potential for Tumor Growth and Metastasis in Patients With Gastric Cancer

Maehara Y, Oshiro T, Baba H, Ohno S, Kohnoe S, Sugimachi K (Kyushu Univ, Fukuoka, Japan)
Surgery 117:380–385, 1995   11–36

Background.—In previous studies the authors have investigated the influence of serosal involvement, lymph node metastasis, and undifferentiated cell type on the metastatic spread of gastric carcinoma. In the current study the authors report on the relation between lymphatic invasion and the proliferating and metastatic potentials of cancer cells in patients with serosally invasive, advanced gastric carcinoma.

Methods.—Between 1965 and 1987, 324 patients with serosally invasive, advanced gastric carcinoma underwent curative resection. Lymphatic invasion by cancer cells was evident in 214 patients (66%) and absent in 110 (34%). Postoperative follow-up was performed every 3 months for the first year and every 6–12 months thereafter. Cell nuclear DNA content was determined in 53 gastric cancer tissues and graded according to aneuploidy. Tissue sections were stained for proliferating cell nuclear antigen (PCNA) and for the argyrophilic nucleolar organizer region (AgNOR).

Results.—There were no differences in age or in tumor size and location between the groups with and without lymphatic invasion. In those with lymphatic invasion, males were more common, undifferentiated tissue types were less frequent, and vascular involvement was more frequent. Extensive lymph node resections were done in over 90% of the patients in both groups. There was a recurrence of tumor in 49 of the 110 patients without lymphatic invasion (43.6%) and in 138 of 213 (64%) patients with lymphatic invasion (1 patient in this group died postoperatively). In cases of no lymphatic invasion, local and peritoneal metastases were the

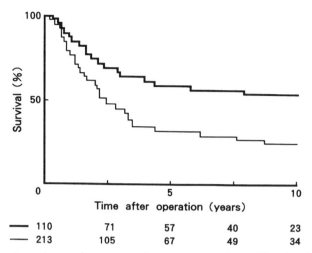

FIGURE 2.—Survival curves for patients with gastric cancer, with or without lymphatic invasion. Numbers of patients eligible for analysis at each point are shown. The survival rate of patients with gastric cancer and lymphatic invasion (*light line*) was significantly shorter than that of patients with gastric cancer and no lymphatic invasion (*dark line*) (P < 0.0001). (Courtesy of Maehara Y, Oshiro T, Baba H, et al: Lymphatic invasion and potential for tumor growth and metastasis in patients with gastric cancer. *Surgery* 117:380–385, 1995.)

predominant areas of recurrence. In patients with lymphatic invasion, recurrences were much more widespread. As shown in Figure 2, the survival rate for patients with lymphatic invasion was poor when compared with that for patients without lymphatic invasion (P < 0.0001). The 5- and 10-year survival rates were 31.0% and 23.8%, respectively, for those with lymphatic invasion vs. 59.3% and 54.1%, respectively, for patients without lymphatic invasion. As shown in Table 6, tumor size, lymph node metastases, and lymphatic invasion were independent important prognostic factors of survival time. Lymphatic invasion was closely

TABLE 6.—Cox Regression Analysis for Patients With Serosally Invasive Gastric Cancer

Prognostic Factor (Observed Value)	P Value	Regression Coefficient	Relative Risk
Tumor size of gastric cancer (per cm)	< 0.05	0.0934	1.10
Lymph node metastasis (none, present)	< 0.05	0.5153	1.67
Lymphatic invasion (none, present)	< 0.05	0.3921	1.48

(Courtesy of Maehara Y, Oshiro T, Baba H, et al: Lymphatic invasion and potential for tumor growth and metastasis in patients with gastric cancer. *Surgery* 117:380–385, 1995.)

related to a higher proliferative activity as indicated by a high ploidy of DNA and higher degrees of PCNA labeling and AgNOR staining.

Conclusions.—Gastric cancers with lymphatic invasion by tumor have higher degrees of proliferating activity and are more prone to distant metastases than are gastric cancers with no lymphatic invasion.

Lymph Node Staging Standards in Gastric Cancer

Bunt AMG, Hogendoorn PCW, van de Velde CJH, Bruijn JA, Hermans J
(Leiden Univ Hosp, The Netherlands)
J Clin Oncol 13:2309–2316, 1995   11–37

Background.—Survival of patients with gastric cancer is better in Japan than in the West. One reason for this may be use of the D2 resection with extended lymph node dissection and thus more diligent pathologic staging by Japanese surgeons. There is no consensus as to the number of lymph nodes that should be examined per N level in the process of tumor-node metastasis staging. Data from the Dutch Gastric Cancer Trial were analyzed to determine the association between the number of nodes examined and the probability of finding metastases.

Methods.—The Dutch Gastric Cancer Trial was a randomized trial comparing Western D1-type gastrectomy and limited N1-level lymphadenectomy with the Japanese D2-type gastrectomy and extended lymph node dissection. The current analysis included 473 patients from that study who underwent curative resection for gastric cancer. The effect of the number of nodes per N level that were histologically examined on the probability of classifying patients as N+ or N− was assessed. Also, the probability of stage migration was evaluated to determine the impact of examining various threshold values for nodal yield per N level on the results of nodal staging.

Results.—Nodal yields ranged from 0 to 67 in the N1 level and from 0 to 43 in the N2 level. There was a significant correlation between nodal yield and N classification: as more nodes were examined, the chances of an N+ classification increased. The probability of detecting positive nodes increased sharply in the lower range of nodal yield but more gradually in the higher range. The results permitted an analysis of the consequences of differing recommendations for the number of lymph nodes per N level that should be histologically examined. Examining 20 nodes in N1 corresponded to a 60% to 65% probability of detecting metastases. In N2, examining 15 nodes corresponded to a probability of 40% to 45%.

Conclusions.—The probability of detecting lymph node metastases per N level should be standardized for individual patients to enhance comparability of treatment results. Such standardization carries some risk of understaging, but this is preferable to the confounding effects of incomparability. The authors recommend histologic examination of 20 nodes in the N1 level and 15 in the N2 level. The precise number can be discussed further, but some consensus should be reached.

▶ Maehara and coauthors show lymphatic invasion being predictive of a higher risk of metastasis to distant organs. This is very similar to the biological results in breast cancer and rectal cancer, where lymphatic vessel invasion is an important, if not bad prognostic sign. Identification of this trait, even in early-stage patients, may provide a selection criteria for adjuvant therapies. Lymphatic vessel invasion appears to have biological behavior similar to that of positive nodes. This has obvious implications in staging gastric cancers. It may also provide selection criteria to treat node-negative patients with adjuvant therapies.

This second paper from The Netherlands, is simply a logical extension emphasizing the importance of standardizing pathologic examination of the lymph node. Obviously, lymph node involvement has great implications in the prognosis and treatment of gastric cancer. We are all aware of the importance of excision of regional lymph nodes along with the primary tumor. This paper simply makes the point that standardization of the pathologic evaluation will make comparison of surgical and adjuvant treatment protocols more accurate.

T.J. Eberlein, M.D.

Pancreatic Cancer

Pancreatic or Liver Resection for Malignancy Is Safe and Effective for the Elderly

Fong Y, Blumgart LH, Fortner JG, Brennan MF (Mem Sloan-Kettering Cancer Ctr, New York)
Ann Surg 222:426–437, 1995   11–38

Background.—Advancements in anesthetic and surgical technique have improved surgical outcomes in elderly patients. However, the current concern with medical expenditure demands that treatment of elderly patients be justified with substantial health benefit. To examine the risk and

TABLE 6.—Multiple Logistic Regression Analysis for the Risk of Complications After Liver Resection in the Aged

Parameter	*P*	Coefficient (SE)	Relative Risk
Liver resection*			
Gender	0.03	1.0	2.6
Extent of resection	0.04	0.9	2.4
Operating room time	0.05	0.9	2.3
ASA = 3	0.06	1.4	4.0
Pancreatic resection†			
Blood loss	0.03	1.2	3.4

* Covariates in this analysis were gender, extent of resection (extended hepatectomy, less than extended hepatectomy), blood loss of 2,000 mL, ASA physical status score, and operative time.
† Covariates in this analysis were gender, extent of resection (pancreaticoduodenectomy/total pancreatectomy vs. distal resection), blood loss greater than 2,000 mL, ASA physical status score, and operative time.
Abbreviation: ASA, American Society of Anesthesiologists.
(Courtesy of Fong Y, Blumgart LH, Fortner JG, et al: Pancreatic or liver resection for malignancy is safe and effective for the elderly. *Ann Surg* 222:426–437, 1995.)

TABLE 7.—Relationship of Age to Outcome After Liver Resection in the Elderly

Age (yr)	Overall	Mortality	Complications
Liver resection			
70–74	74	4 (5%)	35 (47%)
75–79	42	0 (0%)	16 (38%)
≥80	12	1 (8%)	3 (25%)
Pancreatic resection			
70–74	67	5 (7%)	31 (46%)
75–79	47	3 (6%)	21 (45%)
≥80	24	0 (0%)	10 (42%)

(Courtesy of Fong Y, Blumgart LH, Fortner JG, et al: Pancreatic or liver resection for malignancy is safe and effective for the elderly. *Ann Surg* 222:426–437, 1995.)

benefit of liver and pancreatic resection in elderly patients, the perioperative and long-term outcomes of these 2 procedures were studied in relation to age.

Methods.—Data were derived from the surgery department's prospective databases and medical records of 577 patients who underwent liver resection for metastatic colon cancer and 488 patients who underwent pancreatic resection for malignancy. The data included demographic information, pathology of liver lesions, perioperative details, hospital course, and outcome. The outcomes of patients younger and older than age 70 were compared.

Results.—Of the 577 patients who underwent liver resection, 128 were age 70 or older. These elderly patients had a 4% perioperative mortality rate. The median hospital stay was 13 days, with 8% requiring intensive care and 54 patients (42%) experiencing perioperative complications. The independent predictors of complication were gender, extent of the resection, and operative time (Table 6). Among the elderly patients, median survival was 40 months, with a 1-year survival rate of 85% and a 5-year survival rate of 35%. There were no significant differences between the younger and older patients in median hospital stay; rates of complication, mortality, and ICU admission; or long-term survival (Table 7).

Of the 488 patients who underwent pancreatic resection, 138 were age 70 or older. Among the older patients, there was a 6% perioperative mortality rate, a median hospital stay of 20 days, a 19% rate of ICU admission, and a 45% complication rate. Only blood loss greater than 2 L independently predicted complication (see Table 6). The median survival was 18 months, with a 1-year survival rate of 64% and a 5-year survival rate of 21%. There were no significant differences between the younger and older patients in perioperative outcome, but the younger patients had a significantly but not substantially longer long-term survival (see Table 7).

Conclusions.—Both liver and pancreatic resection can be performed in elderly patients with acceptable morbidity and mortality rates, comparable to that of younger patients. Because surgical resection is the only potentially curative therapy for malignancies of the liver and pancreas, resection should be considered the standard treatment for both younger and elderly patients.

▶ This manuscript is included as a reminder that age is relative. This is a very large series with very acceptable results. Two major points, however, need emphasis: to minimize blood loss and to ensure that the patient's temperature stays near normal. Another major caveat with this series of patients is the skills of the authors. However, with appropriate caution and attention to detail, results in elderly patients can duplicate those in younger patients—even for major surgical procedures.

T.J. Eberlein, M.D.

▶ I have grouped the next 3 manuscripts together because they deal with pancreatic resection, prognostic factors, and survival results.

T.J. Eberlein, M.D.

Prognostic Factors for Survival After Pancreaticoduodenectomy for Patients With Carcinoma of the Pancreatic Head Region
Allema JH, Reinders ME, van Gulik TM, Koelemay MJW, Van Leeuwen DJ, de Wit LT, Gouma DJ, Obertop H (Univ of Amsterdam)
Cancer 75:2069–2076, 1995   11–39

Background.—The most common tumors of the pancreatic head region are pancreatic, distal bile duct, and ampullary carcinoma. Pancreaticoduodenectomy is the preferred treatment for these tumors. The resectability rate for pancreatic carcinoma is low. The mortality rate after pancreaticoduodenectomy has decreased dramatically in recent years, but morbidity is still 20% to 70%. Prognostic factors for survival after total or subtotal pancreaticoduodenectomy in patients with carcinoma of the pancreatic head region were determined.

Methods.—There were 176 patients who underwent pancreaticoduodenectomy in a 9-year period. Of these, 67 had ampullary carcinoma, 42 had distal bile duct carcinoma, and 67 had pancreatic carcinoma. Also, 146 patients had subtotal resection and 30 patients had total resection. The median age was 60 years.

Results.—After subtotal pancreaticoduodenectomy, hospital mortality was 4.7%; it was 20% after total pancreaticoduodenectomy. The overall 5-year survival rate was 31%, with a 5-year survival rate of 50% for patients with ampullary carcinoma 24% for patients with distal bile duct carcinoma, and 15% for patients with pancreatic carcinoma. Univariate analysis demonstrated capsular invasion of an involved node to be a negative prognostic factor for the overall group (Table 2). Negative prognostic factors for all subgroups, except those with ampullary carcinoma, were tumor size greater than 2 cm and regional lymph node involvement. A poor tumor differentiation grade was a negative factor for the overall group and for those with bile duct carcinoma but not the other groups. In multivariate analysis, negative prognostic factors for the overall group

TABLE 2.—Prognostic Influence of Preoperative Data and Histologic Findings on Survival After Pancreaticoduodenectomy for Carcinoma of the Pancreatic Head Region

	No.	5-Year Survival (%)	P Value*
Macroscopic vascular invasion			
Yes	37	0	< 0.0001
No	138	38	
Type of resection			
Total PD	30	8	< 0.0001
Subtotal PD	146	36	
Portal vein resection			
Yes	20	<8	0.0001
No	156	34	
Perioperative blood loss			
>2l	59	27	0.04
≤2l	114	34	
Perioperative blood transfusion			
>4 U	52	23	0.008
≤4 U	120	33	
Type/origin of carcinoma			
Ampullary	67	50	< 0.001
Distal bile duct	42	24	
Pancreatic	67	15	
Tumor size			
>2 cm	98	25	0.004
≤2 cm	78	44	
Differentiation grade			
Poor	80	23	0.004
Moderate or good	96	38	
Lymph nodes			
Involved	90	20	0.003
Free	86	42	
Capsular node invasion			
Yes	41	19	0.001
No	135	36	
Resection margins			
Involved	77	4	< 0.0001
Free	99	49	

Note: Results were determined by univariate analysis and log-rank and chi-square tests.
* P value for the chi-square test.
Abbreviation: PD, pancreaticoduodenectomy.
(Courtesy of Cancer, from Allema JH, Reinders ME, van Gulik TM, et al, Copyright © 1995. Reprinted by permission of Wiley-Liss, Inc., a division of John Wiley & Sons, Inc.)

were involved resection margins, macroscopic vascular ingrowth, distal bile duct or pancreatic origin of the carcinoma, and blood transfusion of more than 4 U (Table 4). For the subgroup of patients with ampullary carcinoma, involved resection margins and macroscopic vascular ingrowth were negative prognostic factors.

Discussion.—Independent negative prognostic factors for survival were involvement of resection margins, macroscopic vascular ingrowth, distal bile duct or pancreatic origin of the carcinoma, and perioperative blood transfusion of more than 4 U. Pancreaticoduodenectomy for resectable tumors without major vascular resection offers relatively good prognosis. Perioperative blood transfusions should be limited.

TABLE 4.—Results of Multivariate Survival Analysis With the Cox Regression Model

Multivariate (Cox) Analysis; Negative Prognostic Factors	Overall Group (n = 141)	Ampullary Carcinoma (n = 53)	Distal Bile Duct/ Pancreatic Carcinoma (n = 88)
Involved resection margins	HRR 4.08 (2.44–6.85)	HRR 3.70 (1.38–9.09)	HRR 3.53 (1.92–6.54)
Macroscopic vascular ingrowth	HRR 2.20 (1.32–3.68)	HRR 5.87 (1.45–23.7)	HRR 1.80 (1.03–3.10)
Perioperative blood transfusion >4 units	HRR 1.76 (1.14–2.70)	NS	HRR 2.13 (1.27–3.55)
Distal bile duct/pancreatic origin of carcinoma	HRR 1.93 (1.17–3.20)	—	—

Abbreviation: HRR, hazard rate ratio (95% confidence interval).
(Courtesy of *Cancer*, from Allema JH, Reinders ME, van Gulik TM, et al, Copyright © 1995. Reprinted by permission of Wiley-Liss, Inc., a division of John Wiley & Sons, Inc.)

▶ In the manuscript by Allema and colleagues from the Netherlands, they look at a wide range of prognostic influential factors. Perioperative transfusion was found to be a negative prognostic factor. This obviously deals with the skill and experience of the surgical team in selection of patients for resection, as well as the technical aspects of the procedure. Overall survival in this series was excellent.

T.J. Eberlein, M.D.

Pancreaticoduodenectomy for Cancer of the Head of the Pancreas: 201 Patients
Yeo CJ, Cameron JL, Lillemoe KD, Sitzmann JV, Hruban RH, Goodman SN, Dooley WC, Coleman J, Pitt HA (Johns Hopkins Med Insts, Baltimore, Md)
Ann Surg 221:721–733, 1995   11–40

Background.—Pancreaticoduodenectomy for pancreatic adenocarcinoma has recently been shown to reduce the morbidity and mortality associated with this disease. Some centers have reported 5-year survival rates of approximately 20%, although the factors influencing these improved rates have not been determined. All patients undergoing pancreaticoduodenal resection for adenocarcinoma of the pancreatic head were therefore evaluated in an effort to identify factors affecting long-term survival. The present report represents the largest single-institution experience described in the literature thus far.

Patients and Findings.—Two hundred one patients (mean age, 63 years) with pathologically proven adenocarcinoma of the head of the pancreas were included. Pancreaticoduodenectomy was performed over a 24-year period, with the last 100 resections undertaken between 1991 and 1994. Median follow-up was 12 months. Overall, postoperative in-hospital mortality was 5%. In the most recent 149 patients, however, mortality has been 0.7%. The actuarial 1-, 3-, and 5-year survival rates were 57%, 26%, and 21%, respectively, for all 201 patients. Median survival was 15.5 months (Fig 1). At 5 years, 11 patients were alive. Of the 143 patients with

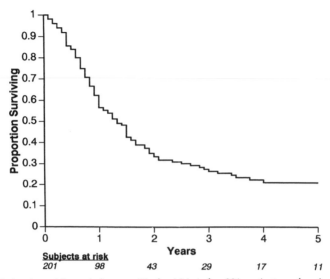

FIGURE 1.—Actuarial survival curve (Kaplan-Meier) for 201 patients undergoing pancreaticoduodenectomy for pancreatic adenocarcinoma. (Courtesy of Yeo CJ, Cameron JL, Lillemoe KD, et al: Pancreaticoduodenectomy for cancer of the head of the pancreas: 201 patients. *Ann Surg* 221:721–733, 1995.)

negative margins (curative resections), the actuarial 5-year survival rate was 26% and median survival was 18 months. Actuarial and median survival was significantly worse among the 58 patients with positive margins (palliative resections): 8% and 10 months, respectively. Improvement in survival has been observed over the study period, with a 14%, 3-year actuarial survival rate noted in the 1970s, 21% in the 1980s, and 36% in the 1990s. Univariate analysis identified tumor diameter less than 3 cm, negative nodal status, diploid tumor DNA content, tumor S phase fraction less than 18%, pylorus-preserving resection (Table 2), less than 800 mL of intraoperative blood loss, less than 2 U of blood transfused, negative resection margins, and use of postoperative adjuvant chemotherapy and radiation therapy as factors significantly favoring long-term survival. Of these, diploid tumor DNA content, tumor diameter less than 3 cm, negative nodal status, negative resection margins, and decade of resection were found to be the strongest predictors of long-term survival on multivariate analysis.

Conclusions.—Survival rates in patients with pancreatic adenocarcinomas undergoing pancreaticoduodenectomy are increasing. Factors most predictive of outcome include DNA content, tumor diameter, and nodal and margin status, although postoperative combined-modality chemoradiation also appears to influence long-term survival rates. The development of improved adjuvant therapy, such as strategies that combine chemoradiation with immunotherapy, may help further increase survival in these patients.

TABLE 2.—Intraoperative Factors Influencing Outcome After Pancreaticoduodenectomy

Parameter (n)	Median Survival (mo)	5-Year Survival (%)	Log-Rank P Value
Type of resection			
Partial pancreatectomy (181)	16.0	20 ⎫	
Total pancreatectomy (20)	10.0	30 ⎭	0.85
Pylorus preserving partial (134)	17.5	24 ⎫	
Classic partial (47)	12.0	9 ⎭	0.02
All pylorus preserving (144)	17.5	25 ⎫	
All classic (57)	10.5	13 ⎭	0.009
Blood loss (median = 800 mL)			
<800 mL (98)	18.0	27 ⎫	
≥800 mL (96)	11.5	17 ⎭	0.03
Packed red cell transfusions			
≤2 units (146)	18.0	26 ⎫	
>2 units (48)	10.5	10 ⎭	0.002
Operative time (median = 7 hr)			
<7 hr (101)	17.5	30 ⎫	
≥7 hr (91)	14.5	10 ⎭	0.07

(Courtesy of Yeo CJ, Cameron JL, Lillemoe KD, et al: Pancreaticoduodenectomy for cancer of the head of the pancreas: 201 patients. *Ann Surg* 221:721–733, 1995.)

▶ Some of the very same issues are raised in the second manuscript by Yeo and colleagues from Johns Hopkins. This institution has, under the direction of Dr. Cameron, developed one of the most comprehensive pancreatic centers in the world. This very large series of patients documents their outstanding results. The factors that these authors found to be important predictors of long-term survival included a diploid tumor DNA content, small tumor size (<3 cm), absence of lymph node metastasis, and negative resection margins. These authors document in their patients an increase in survival by decade, which is not only due to their skills and management, but may also be affected by the number of patients receiving adjuvant chemoradiation.

T.J. Eberlein, M.D.

Long-Term Survival After Resection for Ductal Adenocarcinoma of the Pancreas: Is It Really Improving?
Nitecki SS, Sarr MG, Colby TV, van Heerden JA (Mayo Clinic, Rochester, Minn)
Ann Surg 221:59–66, 1995   11–41

Objective.—Ductile pancreatic adenocarcinoma is almost always fatal. Even after surgical resection the 5-year survival rate is less than 10%. This retrospective study reports increased 5-year survival rates at some centers in patients undergoing curative resection.

Methods.—The medical records of 174 patients with ductile adenocarcinoma aged 34 to 82 who were undergoing curative resection were

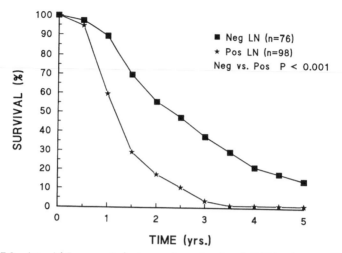

FIGURE 2.—Actuarial 5-year survival rate according to lymph node (*LN*) involvement. (Courtesy of Nitecki SS, Sarr MG, Colby TV, et al: Long-term survival after resection for ductal adenocarcinoma of the pancreas: Is it really improving? *Ann Surg* 211:59–66, 1995.)

reviewed. The average follow-up after surgery was 22 months. Specimens from the 31 patients who survived 3 years were examined histologically.

Results.—Of the total operative procedures, 71% were pancreatoduodenectomies, 20% were total pancreatectomies, and 9% were pancreaticoduodenectomies. Incomplete resections accounted for 16% of the surgeries, 56% of the patients had lymph node involvement, 21% had duodenal invasion, and 12% had perineural invasion. Operative mortality

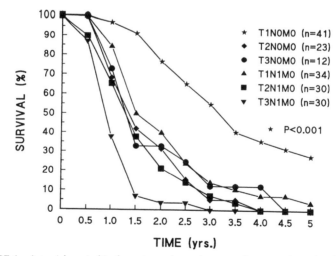

FIGURE 4.—Actuarial survival in the various subsets of tumor-node-metastasis staging. (Courtesy of Nitecki SS, Sarr MG, Colby TV, et al: Long-term survival after resection for ductal adenocarcinoma of the pancreas: Is it really improving? *Ann Surg* 221:59–66, 1995.)

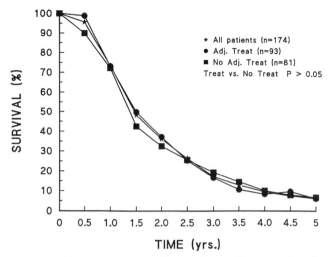

FIGURE 6.—Actuarial 5-year survival according to the use of postoperative adjuvant therapy. (Courtesy of Nitecki SS, Sarr MG, Colby TV, et al: Long-term survival after resection for ductal adeno-carcinoma of the pancreas: Is it really improving? *Ann Surg* 221:59–66, 1995.)

and morbidity rates were 3% and 33%, respectively. The overall 5-year survival rate was 6.8%; medial survival was 17.5 months. Node-negative patients had a significantly greater 5-year survival advantage than did node-positive patients (Fig 2). Patients with smaller tumors had a significantly greater 5-year survival advantage than did patients with large tumors (Fig 4). In the 40% of patients who had complete resections, negative lymph nodes, and no tumor invasion, the 5-year survival rate was 23%. Twelve patients who were originally excluded because they did not have pancreatic cancer had a mean survival of 53 months as compared with the 17.5-month mean survival of patients with pancreatic cancer. The use of adjuvant chemotherapy or radiotherapy had no apparent effect on survival (Fig 6).

Conclusion.—The 5-year survival rate for patients in this study was 7%. In node-negative patients with no invasive tumors, the 5-year survival rate was 23%. Tumor staging is an important prognostic indicator. Pathologic re-review is very important.

▶ The Mayo Clinic series documents a much lower survival in this very carefully performed consecutive series of 186 patients. In addition to re-reviewing all of the histopathology (excluding re-reviewed patients with more favorable histologic findings), these authors included all operations that in the opinion of the operating surgeon were believed to be potentially curative. Obviously, this includes patients who eventually were found to have gross or microscopically involved margins and other more negative prognostic features. Additionally, this large series did not show survival benefit with adjuvant treatment.

In summary, one can conclude that the operative mortality for pancreatic cancer has clearly declined with better perioperative care. Preoperative patient selection may play some role in survival; however, this disease, even in the best of hands, has a relatively poor prognosis and will benefit from a better understanding of the molecular and genetic mechanisms leading to earlier diagnosis and therapeutic intervention (see the next 2 abstracts.)

T.J. Eberlein, M.D.

Consistent Chromosome Abnormalities in Adenocarcinoma of the Pancreas

Griffin CA, Hruban RH, Morsberger LA, Ellingham T, Long PP, Jaffee EM, Hauda KM, Bohlander SK, Yeo CJ (Johns Hopkins School of Medicine, Baltimore, Md)
Cancer Res 55:2394–2399, 1995   11–42

Background.—Pancreatic adenocarcinoma is the fifth leading cause of cancer death in the United States. Like most carcinomas, its etiology has not been identified, nor is much known about the somatic genetic changes that characterize this neoplasm. Identification of acquired genomic alterations would add to the biological understanding of this neoplasm; however, few cytogenetic studies have been conducted thus far. Previously, the authors evaluated 26 primary specimens of pancreatic adenocarcinoma in an effort to identify chromosome abnormalities. Thirty-six additional pancreatic adenocarcinomas have since been studied, and findings from all 62 specimens are reported.

Methods and Findings.—All 62 primary pancreatic adenocarcinomas were obtained from patients undergoing surgical resection over a 3-year period. Specimens were evaluated with standard cytogenetic and fluorescent in situ hybridization techniques. Forty-four neoplasms showed clonally abnormal karyotypes, which were usually complex (more than 3 abnormalities). Both numerical and structural chromosome abnormalities were noted. At least 1 marker chromosome was observed in many of the tumors. Chromosomes 20 and 7 were the most common whole chromosomal gains, observed in 8 and 7 tumors, respectively. Losses occurred with greater frequency, with chromosome 18 lost in 22 tumors, chromosome 13 in 16 tumors, chromosome 12 in 13 tumors, chromosome 17 in 13 tumors, and chromosome 6 in 12 tumors. Structural abnormalities were also common, with 209 chromosome break points observed. With the exception of robertsonian translocations, the most commonly involved chromosomal arms were 1p, 6q, 7q, and 17p, noted in 12, 11, 9, and 9 specimens, respectively, and 1q, 3p, 11p, and 19q, observed in 8 specimens each. In 9 tumors, sections of the long arm of chromosome 6 appeared to be lost. To confirm the evident loss of sections of 6q, 4 tumors with 6q deletions were hybridized with a biotin-labeled microdissection probe from 6q24-ter. In 3 of the 4 tumors, loss of 1 copy of this region was confirmed. Double minute chromosomes were also noted in 8 specimens.

Conclusions.—As far as the authors are aware, these primary pancreatic adenocarcinomas are the first specimens with cytogenetic evidence of gene amplification.

▶ This is a very elegant paper looking at the somatic genetic changes in primary pancreatic adenocarcinomas. Although a specific and consistent chromosome abnormality was not identified, we are beginning to identify and enumerate these very complex changes in chromosomal material. These studies suggest the involvement of several genes in the development of pancreatic cancer. Further research will hopefully identify these genes, similar to the recent identification of *BRCA1* and *BRCA2* in breast cancer.

T.J. Eberlein, M.D.

In Vivo Gene Therapy of a Murine Pancreas Tumor With Recombinant Vaccinia Virus Encoding Human Interleukin-1Beta
Peplinski GR, Tsung K, Meko JB, Norton JA (Washington Univ, St Louis, Mo)
Surgery 118:185–191, 1995   11–43

Introduction.—Recombinant vaccinia virus (VV) encoding human interleukin-1β (vMJ601hIL-1β) has been given by IV as a treatment for cancer. The virus persists in tumor tissues and expresses hIL-1β for at least 9 days, and this significantly slows tumor growth. The antitumor effects of vMJ601hIL-1β, given IV or intratumorally, were compared with those of IV recombinant hIL-1β protein in a mouse model of pancreatic cancer.

Methods.—In the model studied, subcutaneous pancreatic tumors were established in C57BL/6 mice. The animals were randomized in blinded fashion to be treated with IV or intratumoral vmJ601hIL-1β, wild-type VV, saline solution, or IV recombinant hIL-1β protein. The effects were analyzed in terms of toxicity and tumor size.

Results.—Mice treated with intratumoral vMJ601hIL-1β had significant reductions in tumor size when compared with saline-treated control animals (Fig 1). There were no differences in tumor size with IV vs. intratumoral treatment (Fig 2). No antitumor effect was noted with wild-type VV treatment. Animals treated with vMJ601hIL-1β had no significant toxicity and no mortality. Severe toxicity was observed in mice treated with IV recombinant hIL-1β protein, the median lethal dose of which was about 100 µg/kg. At sublethal doses, this agent had no significant antitumor effects.

Conclusions.—In a mouse model of pancreatic cancer, treatment with vMJ601hIL-β results in significant inhibition of tumor growth. This antitumor effect apparently results from local, intratumoral vaccinia infection and production of hIL-1β. vMJ601hIL-β may be given either IV or intratumorally, with no difference in antitumor effect.

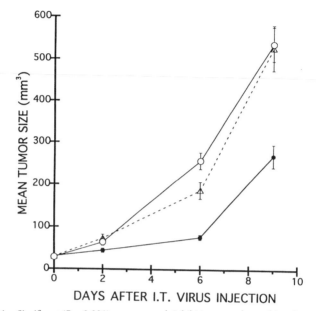

FIGURE 1.—Significant ($P < 0.001$) tumor growth inhibition was observed in mice treated intratumorally with 1×10^5 plaque-forming units of vMJ601hIL-1β (*filled circles*) as compared with wild-type vaccinia virus (*triangles*) and saline-treated controls (*open circles*). *Abbreviation*: I.T., intratumoral. (Courtesy of Peplinski GR, Tsung K, Meko JB, et al: In vivo gene therapy of a murine pancreas tumor with recombinant vaccinia virus encoding human interleukin-1beta. *Surgery* 118:185–191, 1995.)

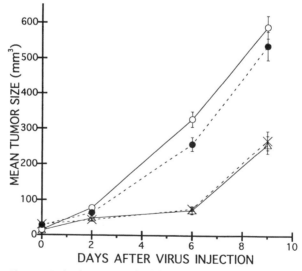

FIGURE 2.—The magnitude of tumor growth inhibition was similar after direct intratumoral administration of 1×10^5 plaque-forming units (PFU) of vMJ601hIL-1β (X's) or after systemic IV injection of 1×10^5 PFU of the same recombinant virus (*triangles*, $P < 0.52$). Tumors grew significantly larger in controls treated by IV (*open circles*) or intratumorally (*filled circles*) with saline solution. (Courtesy of Peplinski GR, Tsung K, Meko JB, et al: In vivo gene therapy of a murine pancreas tumor with recombinant vaccinia virus encoding human interleukin-1beta. *Surgery* 118:185–191, 1995.)

▶ This is a very elegant murine pancreas tumor model that uses vaccinia virus that encodes for the human IL-1β gene. While the effect is only transient, it appears to be secondary to the intratumoral vaccinia infection with resultant production of hIL-1β. Identification of cytokines that may have growth-inhibitory properties as well as the development of vehicles to deliver them to pancreatic cancers may offer hope for a nonsurgical approach to the treatment of this disease.

T.J. Eberlein, M.D.

Hepatocellular Carcinoma

The Role of Intraoperative Ultrasonography in Planning the Resection of Hepatic Neoplasms

Haider MA, Leonhardt C, Hanna SS, Tennenhouse J (Sunnybrook Health Science Centre, North York, Ont, Canada)
Can Assoc Radiol J 46:98–104, 1995   11–44

Background.—The long-term survival of patients with metastatic colorectal cancer and other malignant hepatic lesions can be improved by hepatic resection. However, the quality of life of these patients must not be compromised because their life expectancy may already be limited. Preoperative staging must be accurate to avoid unnecessary surgery. Computed tomography with arterial portography is the preferred imaging modality for patients who may undergo hepatic resection, but flow artifacts can make interpretation difficult. Intraoperative ultrasonography is an alternative, but it prolongs an already lengthy procedure. Also, occult lesions may be detectable by palpating the liver, which is faster than intraoperative ultrasonography. Locating the lesions relative to the major hepatic vessels is vital, and intraoperative ultrasonography may be better at determining the location and maximal extent of these lesions because of

TABLE 2.—Sensitivity, Specificity, Positive and Negative Predictive Values, and Accuracy of Computed Tomography With Arterial Portography and Intraoperative Ultrasonography

Variable	For CTAP	No. of Abnormalities	For US	No. of Abnormalities	Difference (% points)	99% CI for Difference (%)
Sensitivity	87.8%	49*	91.8%	49*	4.0	−11.6,19.8
Specificity	9.1%	11†	100.0%	11†	90.9	68.6, 100
PPV	81.1%	53‡	100.0%	45‡	18.9	5.1,32.7
NPV	14.3%	7§	73.3%	15§	59.0	14.1, 100
Accuracy	73.3%	60‖	93.3%	60‖	20.0	3.2,36.9

* Number of true positives.
† Number of true negatives.
‡ Number of positive results from imaging.
§ Number of negative results from imaging.
‖ Total number of abnormalities analyzed.
Abbreviations: CTAP, CT with arterial portography; *US,* ultrasonography; *CI,* confidence interval; *PPV,* positive predictive value; *NPV,* negative predictive value.
(Reprinted from Haider MkA, Leonhardt C, Hanna SS, et al: The role of intraoperative ultrasonography in planning the resection of hepatic neoplasms, by permission of the publisher, *CARJ,* vol 46, no 2, April 1995.)

its multiplanar capability. The information provided by intraoperative ultrasonography was examined and compared with that from CT with arterial portography.

Methods.—Intraoperative ultrasonography was performed in 22 patients with potentially resectable hepatic lesions as determined by clinical evaluation and CT with arterial portography. The mean age of the patients was 60.1 years. Lesions were examined pathologically or by follow-up imaging and assays for carcinoembryonic antigen.

Results.—In 41% of the patients, the surgical plan based on CT with arterial portography was changed by findings from ultrasonography. Of 60 intrahepatic abnormalities, 49 were malignant lesions and 11 were artifacts. The specificity of intraoperative ultrasonography was 100% and the negative predictive value was 73.3%; the specificity of CT with arterial portography was 9.1% and the negative predictive value was 14.3% (Table 2).

Discussion.—Intraoperative ultrasonography can change the surgical management of the majority of patients undergoing hepatic resection. The specificity of intraoperative ultrasonography is significantly greater than that of CT with arterial portography. Also, ultrasonography can more accurately evaluate the lateral segment of the left lobe. The use of intraoperative ultrasonography is justified in patients undergoing hepatic resection.

▶ This is a very nice paper specifically documenting the change in surgical plan through the use of intraoperative ultrasonography. The authors have utilized CT with arterial portography (CTAP), which has become an excellent preoperative method for documenting the extent of disease in the liver. In spite of this sensitive technique, intraoperative ultrasound alters the approach in a substantial portion of patients. This may be due to the false-positive–related flow artifact of CTAP. As long as surgical intervention remains the primary treatment for most malignancies of the liver, intraoperative ultrasound may well serve as an adjunct to planning or contraindicating surgical intervention.

T.J. Eberlein, M.D.

Criteria for Safe Hepatic Resection
Miyagawa S, Makuuchi M, Kawasaki S, Kakazu T (Shinshu Univ, Matsumoto, Japan)
Am J Surg 169:589–594, 1995   11–45

Objective.—The number of hepatic resections performed has increased in recent years, while the mortality has decreased. Few reports have described the morbidity and mortality associated with hepatic resection. Such an analysis was performed in 172 patients.

Methods.—The patients underwent hepatic resection for primary or secondary liver tumors, biliary cancer, and various benign diseases from

TABLE 5.—Risk Factors in Hepatic Resection (Stepwise Logistic Regression)

Variable	Coeff	SEM	P Value	Stand Coeff
Operation time	0.003	0.001	0.009	0.546
Cardiovascular disease	1.271	0.537	0.019	0.441
Major hepatic resection	1.057	0.517	0.043	0.395

Note: Data are from 172 patients who had surgery performed at the First Department of Surgery, Shinshu University Hospital, Matsumoto, Japan, between January 1990 and December 1992.

Abbreviations: Coef, coefficient; *Stand,* standard.

(Reprinted by permission of the publisher from Miyagawa S, Makuuchi M, Kawasaki S, et al: Criteria for safe hepatic resection. *Am J Surg* 169:589–594, Copyright 1995 by Excerpta Medica Inc.)

1990 through 1992. The criteria for hepatectomy included the presence or absence of ascites, the total serum bilirubin level, and the plasma retention rate of indocyanine green at 15 minutes (ICG 15) in patients with chronic liver disease. Various predictors of morbidity were assessed, including age, sex, preoperative risk factors, total serum bilirubin level, ICG 15, underlying disease, operative blood loss, operative time, blood transfusion requirements, vascular occlusion time, surgical procedure used, and extent of hepatic resection.

Results.—The morbidity rate was 37%, and the hospital and operative mortality rates were 2.3% and 0.6%, respectively. In a multiple logistic model, morbidity risk was increased by 3 factors: longer operation time, major hepatic resection, and preoperative cardiovascular disease (Table 5). There was a 1.2% hospital mortality that was directly related to hepatic resection.

Conclusions.—With the use of simple criteria—including the presence or absence of ascites, total serum bilirubin level, and ICG 15 value—and surgical principles, including a thoracoabdominal approach to ensure a sufficient operative field, minimization of operative blood loss, and decreasing the need for whole blood transfusion, it is possible to reduce the morbidity and mortality of hepatic resection. More work is needed to decrease the operative time in patients undergoing hepatectomy without increasing blood loss and to find new methods of making major hepatectomy safer.

▶ The results of this relatively large study of hepatic resection seem somewhat intuitive. Several additional points from this study need emphasis: the authors stress the importance of adequate exposure and mobilization of the liver as well as control of the vascular structures. This obviously would result in minimizing operative blood loss and the transfusion requirement. An additional point of emphasis is keeping the patient's temperature stable throughout the procedure. Combining all of these aspects will further improve survival of our patients.

T.J. Eberlein, M.D.

Hepatic Resection for Hepatocellular Carcinoma: An Audit of 343 Patients

Lai ECS, Fan S-T, Lo C-M, Chu K-M, Liu C-L, Wong J (Univ of Hong Kong; Queen Mary Hosp, Hong Kong)

Ann Surg 221:291–298, 1995   11–46

Background.—Hepatic resection has generally been viewed as the only treatment option that offers a chance of long-term survival for patients with hepatocellular carcinoma (HCC). Because of early cancer detection and technological advances, strategies for surgical treatment of patients with primary liver cancer have continuously evolved. A 22-year review of the result of hepatectomy for HCC is presented.

Methods.—The analysis included 343 patients with HCC undergoing hepatic resection at a Hong Kong hospital. One hundred forty-nine patients were treated from 1972 to 1987, 128 from 1987 to 1991, and 66 from 1992 to the present; these periods reflect changes in perioperative management. For survival analysis, the patients were stratified into 2 categories: before or after 1987. Seventy-eight percent of the patients had large tumors, 73% had cirrhosis, and 73% had a major hepatectomy. The results were assessed both in the perioperative period and during subsequent follow-up.

Results.—The resectability rate improved from 14% at the beginning of the study period to 23% at the end. The morbidity rate decreased significantly from 73% to 32% and hospital mortality from 22% to 6% (Table 4). Thirty-day mortality decreased nonsignificantly from 14% to 5%. The surgical approach used in the latter part of the series was a significant contributor to the reduced hospital mortality. Survival was significantly better for patients treated after 1987; survival rates at 1, 3, and 5 years

TABLE 4.—Postoperative Morbidity and Mortality of Patients With Hepatocellular Carcinoma Who Had Hepatectomy Between 1972 and 1994

Complication	Before 1987 (n = 149)		1987 to 1991 (n = 128)		1992 to Present (n = 66)		P Value
Chest infection	14		9		1		NS
Pleural effusion	59		23		8		< 0.001
Wound infection	12		4		1		NS
Wound dehiscence	6	(1)	0		0		NS
Intra-abdominal sepsis	28	(7)	11	(2)	2	(2)	< 0.005
Intra-abdominal bleeding	24	(16)	9	(4)	3	(1)	< 0.03
Gastrointestinal bleeding	7	(2)	3		0		NS
Variceal bleeding	3		2		0		NS
Blood loss (L)	3.2 (2.8–3.7)		2.9 (2.4–3.5)		3.3 (2.5–4.0)		NS
Morbidity (%)	73		52		32		< 0.001
30-day mortality (%)	14		9.4		4.5		NS
Hospital mortality (%)	21.5		14.8		6		< 0.02

Note: Numbers of patients with re-exploration for complications are shown in parentheses, except for blood loss, which is expressed as means (95% confidence interval).

(Courtesy of Lai ECS, Fan S-T, Lo C-M, et al: Hepatic resection for hepatocellular carcinoma: An audit of 343 patients. *Ann Surg* 221:291–298, 1995.)

TABLE 5.—Factors Associated With Hospital Mortality of Patients With Hepatocellular Carcinoma Who Had Hepatectomy Between 1972 and 1994 Aside From the Time Period of Hepatectomy

Factors	Survivors (n = 288)	Deaths (n = 55)	P Value
Hemoglobin (g/L)	13.4 (13.1–13.6)	12.6 (11.8–13.4)	< 0.03
Serum albumin (g/L)	40.8 (40.1–41.6)	37.2 (35.7–38.7)	< 0.001
Prothrombin time (sec > control)	1.1 (0.9–1.3)	1.9 (1.5–2.5)	< 0.001
Activated partial thromboplastin time (sec > control)	2.6 (2.1–3.0)	4.3 (3.0–5.6)	< 0.005
Indocyanine green retention rate at 15 min	14 (12.3–15.7)	19.4 (13.9–24.9)	< 0.03
Gamma glutyl transpeptidase (units/L)	130 (111–150)	200 (125–274)	< 0.02
Blood loss (L)	2.8 (2.5–3.1)	4.7 (3.6–5.8)	< 0.001
Percentage with emergency surgery	3.6	12.7	< 0.02
Percentage with large tumor	7.8	18.4	< 0.04
Percentage with morbidity	1.4	26.9	< 0.001

Note: All values are expressed as means (95% confidence interval) unless stated.
(Courtesy of Lai ECS, Fan S-T, Lo C-M, et al: Hepatic resection for hepatocellular carcinoma: An audit of 343 patients. *Ann Surg* 221:291–298, 1995.)

were 68%, 45%, and 35%, respectively, for the more recently treated patients. This improvement in prognosis was attributed to early detection and effective treatment for recurrences. Aside from the time period, 10 factors were found to be significantly associated with hospital mortality (Table 5).

Conclusions.—Technological advances and newer management strategies have improved the results of hepatic resection for patients with HCC. The newer surgical techniques used by the authors include a bilateral subcostal incision, meticulous attention to guard against bleeding and bile leakage, and use of an ultrasonic dissector to transect the hepatic parenchyma. Further improvements in prognosis might be possible through prevention of the frequent recurrences; because of socioeconomic obstacles, liver transplantation is not a viable option for HCC patients in Asia.

▶ This very large series by one of the world's leaders of liver surgery utilizes a bilateral subcostal incision that avoids the necessity of a thoracotomy and therefore eliminates postoperative pleural effusions. An approach I also prefer, although I utilize a "lazy S" type of incision from the xyphoid to near the iliac crest. Meticulous attention to guard against bleeding and bile leak have also diminished abdominal sepsis. Yet there are difficulties, with recurrence frequently seen at long-term follow-up. Surveillance with serial α-fetoprotein and frequent ultrasound is the simplest and cheapest way of following this disease.

T.J. Eberlein, M.D.

Surgical Treatment of Hepatocellular Carcinomas in Noncirrhotic Liver: Experience With 68 Liver Resections
Bismuth H, Chiche L, Castaing D (Paul Brousse Hosp, Villejuif, France; Univ of Paris Sud, Villejuif, France)
World J Surg 19:35–41, 1995   11–47

Objective.—Hepatocellular carcinoma in noncirrhotic liver occurs in fewer than 25% of liver cancer patients. Little is known about the specific clinical findings, prognosis, and surgical management of the disease because it is usually included with other liver cancers in the literature. The surgical treatment and outcome of patients with hepatocellular carcinoma in noncirrhotic liver who had partial hepatectomy are retrospectively analyzed.

Methods.—Between January 1970 and December 1992, 68 patients (25 women) aged 2 to 77 with noncirrhotic liver cancer underwent partial hepatectomy. Four patients had recurrent disease. In 13 patients, liver specimens showed histologic modifications. Five patients had fibrolamellar carcinoma. The mean tumor size was 8.8 cm. Three patients received preoperative embolization, and 13 had chemoembolization. A total of 49

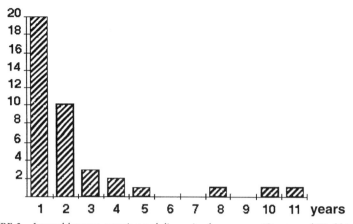

FIGURE 2.—Interval between resection and diagnosis of recurrence. (Courtesy of *World Journal of Surgery*, Surgical treatment of hepatocellular carcinomas in noncirrhotic liver: Experience with 68 liver resections, by Bismuth H, Chiche L, Castaing D, vol 19, p 37, Fig 2, 1995, copyright notice of Springer-Verlag.)

patients had major hepatectomy, and 17 of these required total vascular exclusion.

Results.—Perioperative mortality was 2.9%. Morbidity as a result of bile leakage, subphrenic collections, intraperitoneal bleeding, and pulmonary complications occurred in 19% of the patients. Thirty-nine (59%) of

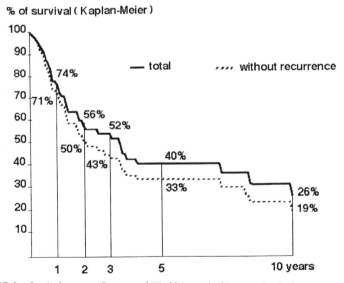

FIGURE 3.—Survival curves. (Courtesy of *World Journal of Surgery*, Surgical treatment of hepatocellular carcinomas in noncirrhotic liver: Experience with 68 liver resections, by Bismuth H, Chiche L, Castaing D, vol 19, p 38, Fig 3, 1995, copyright notice of Springer-Verlag.)

66 survivors had recurrences, 29 of which were intrahepatic (Fig 2). Twelve patients had rehepatectomies. Kaplan-Meier survival rates, with and without recurrence, were determined. (Fig 3).

Conclusion.—Extensive, aggressive surgery is justified in cases of hepatocellular carcinoma in noncirrhotic liver because it prolongs survival. Long-term follow-up to detect late recurrence is necessary.

▶ The excellent results and aggressive recommendations in this manuscript are related to the fact that these patients are noncirrhotic. In the majority of patients, hepatocellular carcinoma is associated with cirrhosis. This is particularly true of patients from the Pacific basin, whether the patient is cirrhotic or not. Ultrasound and α-fetoprotein levels are useful in diagnosing recurrence, which occurs in a high proportion of patients. This recurrence is probably as frequent as in patients with cirrhosis, but frequently occurs later, thereby emphasizing another point in this manuscript that longer-term follow-up is necessary in noncirrhotic patients.

T.J. Eberlein, M.D.

Melanoma

Prognostic Factors in 1521 Melanoma Patients With Distant Metastases
Barth A, Wanek LA, Morton DL (John Wayne Cancer Inst, Santa Monica, Calif; St John's Hosp and Health Ctr, Santa Monica, Calif)
J Am Coll Surg 181:193–201, 1995   11–48

Purpose.—The incidence of malignant melanoma of the skin is increasing rapidly, with 7,200 deaths from metastatic melanoma expected in 1995. However, little prognostic information for patients with metastatic melanoma is available. Variables predicting outcome in melanoma patients with distant metastases were assessed retrospectively.

Methods.—The analysis included 1,521 patients with American Joint Committee on Cancer (AJCC) stage IV melanoma who were treated at 1

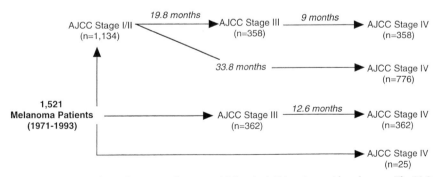

FIGURE 1.—Initial manifestation and pattern of failure in 1,521 patients with melanoma. The 33.8 months represent the median time for progression of stage I/II to stage IV for patients with a known disease-free interval. *Abbreviation*: *AJCC*, American Joint Committee on Cancer. (By permission of the *Journal of the American College of Surgeons.*)

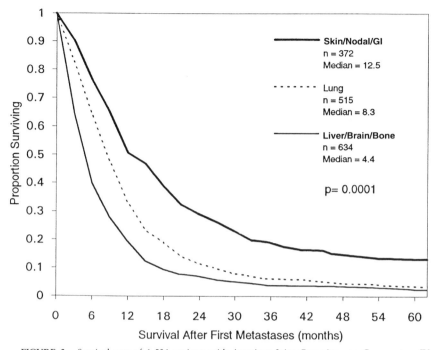

FIGURE 3.—Survival rate of 1,521 patients with American Joint Committee on Cancer stage IV melanoma: 372 patients with skin/lymph node/gastrointestinal (*GI*) metastases, 515 patients with pulmonary metastases, and 634 patients with liver/brain/bone metastases. The 5-year survival rates were 14%, 4%, and 3%, respectively. (By permission of the *Journal of the American College of Surgeons.*)

cancer center from 1971 to 1993. The median age was 51 years, and 61% of the patients were male. The patients received a wide range of different treatments. Ten clinical and pathologic variables were evaluated as potential predictors of outcome by Cox proportional hazard regression analysis. The review also sought to determine whether survival for this patient group had changed over the years.

Results.—Just 2% of the patients had stage IV disease when first seen (Fig 1). The patients had a median survival time of 7½ months and an estimated 5-year survival rate of 6%. Independent predictors of survival were the initial site of metastasis, disease-free interval before distant metastasis occurred, and disease stage before distant metastasis occurred. The site of the initial metastasis could be used to divide the patients into 3 prognostic groups. Those with cutaneous metastases had a median survival time of 12½ months and an estimated 5-year survival rate of 14%; those with nodal metastases had a survival time of 8 months and a 5-year survival rate of 4%; and those with liver, brain, or bone metastases had a survival time of 4 months and a 5-year survival rate of 3% (Fig 3). Survival was significantly longer for patients with a disease-free interval before distant metastasis of 72 months or longer (Fig 4). Across the 22-year experience, the survival rate did not improve significantly.

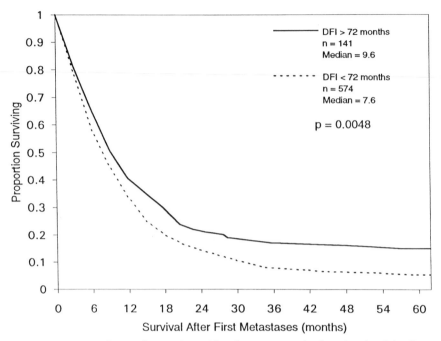

FIGURE 4.—Survival rates of 715 patients with melanoma progressing from American Joint Committee on Cancer stage I/II to stage IV. The 5-year survival rate was 15% for the 141 patients with a disease-free interval (*DFI*) of greater than or equal to 72 months vs. 5% for the 574 patients with a DFI less than 72 months. (By permission of the *Journal of the American College of Surgeons*.)

Conclusions.—The initial site of metastasis, disease-free interval before distant metastasis, and stage of disease before distant metastasis are independent prognostic factors for survival in patients with malignant melanoma. These variables should be taken into account in planning future treatment trials. The last 2 decades have seen no significant improvement in survival for patients with AJCC stage IV melanoma despite advances in diagnostic imaging and the development of new treatment techniques.

▶ This is a very unique series. It is extremely large and it has been managed by a single investigator. The initial site of metastasis, disease-free interval before distant metastasis, and stage of disease before distant metastasis are independent prognostic factors for survival in this patient population. Better survival will result from a more thorough understanding of the basic mechanisms of this disease. Very likely, genetic, molecular biological, and immunologic understanding of this disease will aid in the development of future systemic treatments. In the meantime, consideration of these prognostic features in the design of adjuvant trials will be useful.

T.J. Eberlein, M.D.

Elective Lymph Node Dissection in Patients With Primary Melanoma of the Trunk and Limbs Treated at the Sydney Melanoma Unit From 1960 to 1991

Coates AS, Ingvar CI, Petersen-Schaefer K, Shaw HM, Milton GW, O'Brien C, Thompson JF, McCarthy WH (Royal Prince Alfred Hosp, Camperdown, Australia; Univ of Sydney, Australia)

J Am Coll Surg 180:402–409, 1995

11–49

Background.—The role of elective lymph node dissection in cutaneous malignant melanoma is unclear and controversial. Retrospective studies can be unreliable, and the methods of 2 randomized trials in process have been criticized. One retrospective review of experience of the Sydney Melanoma Unit reported a survival benefit from elective lymph node dissection, particularly in males with tumors 1.6 to 3 mm thick. Since the publication of that report, more than 5,000 patients have been treated at this unit. The experience at this unit was analyzed, and the results of patients who underwent elective lymph node dissection or wide excision were compared.

Methods.—The cases of 1,278 patients treated since 1960 for primary cutaneous melanomas at least 1.5 mm occurring on the trunk or extremities without clinical lymph node involvement were analyzed. Patients were treated with wide excision with or without elective lymph node dissection.

Results.—There were 845 patients treated with elective lymph node dissection and 433 treated with wide excision alone. Median follow-up

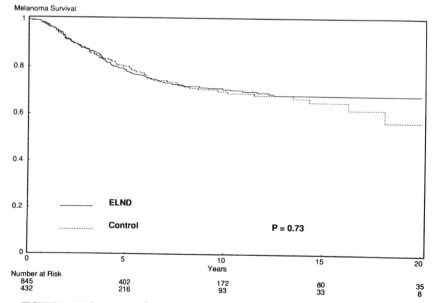

FIGURE 1.—Melanoma-specific survival by treatment for all patients. *Abbreviation:* ELND, elective lymph node dissection. (By permission of the *Journal of the American College of Surgeons.*)

was 58 months. Elective lymph node dissection was performed more often in patients who were younger and who had thicker tumors. In patients with thinner tumors, elective lymph node dissection was performed more often in males than in females. There was no benefit from elective lymph node dissection in any group or subgroup of patients (Fig 1).

Discussion.—A survival benefit from elective lymph node dissection is not supported by this review. To help eliminate selection bias, patients were excluded from analysis if they had undergone wide excision with or without elective lymph node dissection at another facility. Another trial under way involves preoperative lymphoscintigraphy and intraoperative lymphatic mapping with selective lymphadenectomy as an alternative to elective lymph node dissection.

▶ This paper does not show a survival benefit for elective lymph node dissection in patients with intermediate-thickness melanoma. This is not hard to understand since the majority of the patients will have no evidence of metastatic disease or will have disease beyond the lymph node drainage area. It is only the small number of patients who have disease only in the draining lymph nodes and have them excised who will benefit from elective lymph node dissection. This whole area will be dramatically changed by advances, such as that reported in the next abstract.

T.J. Eberlein, M.D.

The Identification and Mapping of Melanoma Regional Nodal Metastases: Minimally Invasive Surgery for the Diagnosis of Nodal Metastases

Godellas CV, Berman CG, Lyman G, Cruse CW, Rapaport D, Heller R, Wang X, Glass F, Fenske N, Messina J, Puleo C, Ross M, Reintgen DS (Univ of South Florida, Tampa; MD Anderson Cancer Ctr, Houston)
Am Surg 61:97–101, 1995   11–50

Introduction.—Elective lymph node dissection (ELND) is the most controversial area of melanoma surgical care. In sentinel node mapping and selective lymphadenectomy, the first node into which the primary melanoma drains is identified and removed; if this node is negative, complete lymphadenectomy is theoretically unnecessary to control occult nodal disease. Optimally, the surgeon would have a map of the position of the sentinel nodes relative to the other nodes in the lymphatic basin. This would permit the procedure to be done with local anesthesia and a small incision; morbidity would be minimal, and the procedure could be performed on an outpatient basis. A protocol for mapping of the sentinel node to allow minimally invasive surgery for the diagnosis of nodal metastases is presented.

Methods.—The study included 29 patients who were candidates for ELND: all had melanomas of more than 0.76 mm in thickness and clinically negative nodes. The sentinel node was marked by preoperative lymphoscintigraphy performed in 2 planes. Intraoperative lymphatic mapping and sentinel node biopsy were then performed in the operating room, followed by complete ELND.

Results.—The sentinel node could not be localized within 5 cm in 33% of the cases. In contrast, lymphoscintigraphy accurately identified the location of the sentinel node in all cases. The patients had no "skip" metastases. Neither mapping technique was associated with any complications.

Conclusions.—Sentinel node histologic studies may be a useful prognostic factor to identify a subgroup of melanoma patients as candidates for ELND. All basins at risk for metastatic disease and the relative locations of sentinel nodes can be identified by means of lymphoscintigraphy. These techniques may allow more widespread use of selective lymphadenectomy in the care of patients with melanoma.

▶ Several important issues in this manuscript need emphasis: lymphoscintigraphy was accurate in identification of the location of the sentinel node 100% of the time. This study also emphasizes the fact that there were no "skip" metastases. This technology therefore provides the operating surgeon with the ability to identify all basins at risk for metastatic disease as well as the ability to mark the location of the sentinel node. Its excision under local anesthesia is therefore appealing. Data from this group and other randomized prospective trials may potentially show that a pathologically negative sentinel lymph node can eliminate the need for elective lymph node dissection. We will anxiously await the results of these randomized trials since this may have a dramatic impact on recommendations for lymph node dissection in this disease.

T.J. Eberlein, M.D.

Soft-tissue Sarcoma

Prognostic Factors Predictive of Survival for Truncal and Retroperitoneal Soft-Tissue Sarcoma

Singer S, Corson JM, Demetri GD, Healey EZ, Marcus K, Eberlein TJ (Brigham and Women's Hosp, Boston; Harvard Med School, Boston; Dana Farber Cancer Inst, Boston)
Ann Surg 221:185–195, 1995   11–51

Background.—For patients with truncal sarcoma and sarcomas of the abdomen/retroperitoneum, the chances of local control and cure depend on complete, wide-margin surgical resection. Debate continues as to the role of adjuvant chemotherapy in truncal and retroperitoneal sarcoma. Toward identifying the patient subgroups most likely to benefit from novel approaches to adjuvant therapy, prognostic factors for survival among patients with truncal and retroperitoneal soft-tissue sarcoma were studied.

Methods.—One hundred eighty-three consecutive patients with truncal and retroperitoneal sarcomas were analyzed. They were drawn from a prospectively compiled database of patients treated from 1970 to 1994.

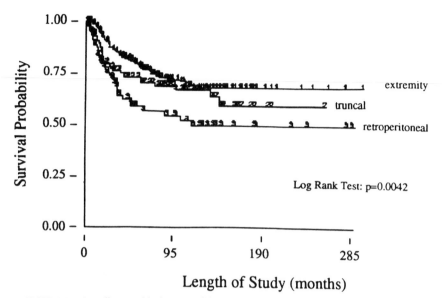

Length of Study (months)

FIGURE 1.—Overall survival by location of the sarcoma. (Courtesy of Singer S, Corson JM, Demetri GD, et al: Prognostic factors predictive of survival for truncal and retroperitoneal soft-tissue sarcoma. *Ann Surg* 221:185–195, 1995.)

Findings.—The 15-year overall survival rate was 68% for patients with extremity soft-tissue sarcomas, 60% for those with truncal sarcomas, and 50% for those with retroperitoneal sarcomas (Fig 1). On multivariate analysis, truncal sarcoma of high-grade histology was associated with an 8-fold increased risk of death as compared with low-grade histology. Other independent prognostic factors included a gross positive margin of resection, a microscopic positive margin, and tumors larger than 5 cm. Patients receiving postoperative radiation therapy for truncal sarcoma

TABLE 1.—Predictors of Survival for Truncal Sarcoma From Multivariate Analysis (n = 100)

Variable	Parameter Estimate	Standard Error	P Value	Risk Ratio
High grade vs. low grade	2.06	0.62	0.001	7.88
Size > 5 cm vs. size < 5 cm	0.92	0.389	0.018	2.51
Gross positive margins vs. clean margins	1.49	0.460	0.001	4.43
Microscopic positive margins vs. clean margins	1.01	0.446	0.023	2.76
Postoperative radiation therapy vs. no adjuvant radiation	−0.86	0.396	0.030	0.42

(Courtesy of Singer S, Corson JM, Demetri GD, et al: Prognostic factors predictive of survival for truncal and retroperitoneal soft-tissue sarcoma. *Ann Surg* 221:185–195, 1995.)

TABLE 2.—Predictors of Survival for Retroperitoneal Sarcoma From
Multivariate Analysis (n = 83)

Variable	Parameter Estimate	Standard Error	*P* Value	Risk Ratio
High grade vs. low grade	1.69	0.64	0.008	5.43
Intermediate grade vs. low grade	1.83	0.70	0.009	6.23
Gross positive margins vs. clean margins	1.63	0.49	0.001	5.09
Microscopic positive vs. clean margins	1.30	0.45	0.004	3.67
Postoperative chemotherapy vs. no adjuvant chemotherapy	1.09	0.43	0.010	2.98
Preoperative chemotherapy vs. no adjuvant chemotherapy	1.52	0.48	0.002	4.56

(Courtesy of Singer S, Corson JM, Demetri GD, et al: Prognostic factors predictive of survival for truncal and retroperitoneal soft-tissue sarcoma. *Ann Surg* 221:185–195, 1995.)

were at a 2.4-fold decreased risk of death when compared with patients receiving no adjuvant therapy after adjustment for other prognostic factors (Table 1).

Retroperitoneal sarcoma with high-grade and intermediate-grade histologic findings increased the risk of death by 5- and 6-fold, respectively. Other independent prognostic factors included gross and microscopic positive margin of resection. When compared with patients receiving no adjuvant chemotherapy, those receiving preoperative chemotherapy were at a 4.6-fold increased risk of death after adjustment for other prognostic factors. Those receiving postoperative chemotherapy were at a 3-fold increased risk of death (Table 2).

Conclusions.—For patients with truncal and retroperitoneal soft tissue sarcoma, histologic grade and the margin of resection are prognostic factors for survival. In truncal but not retroperitoneal sarcoma, tumor size is an independent prognostic factor. Postoperative adjuvant radiation improves overall survival in patients with truncal sarcoma. However, chemotherapy appears to have no such survival benefit.

▶ This is a very large retrospective analysis of truncal and retroperitoneal soft-tissue sarcoma. As with extremity sarcomas, grade and margin of resection are extremely important. Tumor size is important in truncal sarcomas, but not so in retroperitoneal tumors. Although radiation therapy was shown to have a survival benefit in truncal sarcomas, both of these variants of soft-tissue sarcoma are best treated surgically. Often with retroperitoneal tumors, it is very difficult to obtain pathologically negative margins. Hopefully, through the use of genetic markers and other biochemical profiles, we will be able to select the tumors that best benefit from other adjuvant and neoadjuvant therapies.

T.J. Eberlein, M.D.

Molecular Assays for Chromosomal Translocations in the Diagnosis of Pediatric Soft Tissue Sarcomas

Barr FC, Chatten J, D'Cruz CM, Wilson AE, Nauta LE, Nycum LM, Biegel JA, Womer RB (Univ of Pennsylvania, Philadelphia; Children's Hospital, Philadelphia)
JAMA 273:553–557, 1995   11–52

Background.—Soft tissue tumors in children commonly pose diagnostic problems. Several small round cell tumors have been associated with consistent chromosomal translocations, and molecular assays have been developed for the detection of these translocations in clinical specimens. The value of these molecular assays for differential diagnosis was assessed in comparison with standard histopathologic and cytogenetic analysis.

Methods.—The study included frozen tumor tissue and histopathologic slides from 79 patients with soft tissue sarcoma. The reverse transcriptase–polymerase chain reaction (RT-PCR) was used to assay tumor RNA. The chromosomal translocations detected by these assays include PAX3-FKHR and PAX7-FKHR chimeric transcripts in alveolar rhabdomyosarcoma, EWS-FLI1 and EWS-ERG chimeric transcripts in Ewing's sarcoma, and EWS-WT1 chimeric transcripts in desmoplastic small round cell tumor. The PCR results were compared in blinded fashion with the cytogenetic and histopathologic results.

Results.—The RT-PCR assays detected chimeric transcripts in all tumors shown to have translocations by standard cytogenetic study. Chimeric transcripts were also found in additional cases without cytogenetically detectable translocations. Eighteen of 21 alveolar rhabdomyosarcomas showed PAX3-FKHR PAX7-FKHR fusions, as did 2 of 30 embryonal rhabdomyosarcomas and 1 of 7 undifferentiated sarcomas. Six of 8 Ewing's sarcomas and 1 of 7 undifferentiated sarcomas showed EWS-FLI1 or EWS-ERG fusions. All 3 desmoplastic small round cell tumors in the series showed the EWS-WT1 fusion.

Conclusions.—A genetic approach to the differential diagnosis of soft tissue sarcoma in children is possible with molecular assays for specific gene fusions. This study finds close correlation between the genetic findings and the standard histopathologic categories. The PCRs used in these studies are useful tools for routine use in the rapid and objective assessment of pediatric soft tissue sarcomas.

▶ This paper shows the power of PCR assays in providing a specific diagnosis of soft-tissue sarcomas. Two features of this manuscript are particularly attractive: first, these assays can be performed on very small specimens, and second, definitive results can be obtained within 1 day of specimen receipt. This obviously has enormous practical implication in diagnosing and recommending appropriate treatment. As our experience with these techniques improve, they will also be instrumental in providing the ability to follow response to various treatments in the neoadjuvant setting.

T.J. Eberlein, M.D.

Cholangiocarcinoma

Serum Tumor Markers for the Diagnosis of Cholangiocarcinoma in Primary Sclerosing Cholangitis
Ramage JK, Donaghy A, Farrant JM, Iorns R, Williams R (Inst of Liver Studies, London; Royal Naval Hosp, Haslar, Gosport, England)
Gastroenterology 108:865–869, 1995   11–53

Objective.—Cholangiocarcinoma, usually related to primary sclerosing cholangitis (PSC) in patients with colitis, is difficult to diagnose with various imaging modalities or brush cytology. Because approximately half of the patients with symptomatic PSC require liver transplantation, proper diagnosis is very important. Two tumor markers that could possibly be used to detect cholangiocarcinomas are carcinoembryonic antigen (CEA) and carbohydrate antigen 19-9 (CA19-9). The results of a study evaluating the diagnostic accuracy of these 2 markers, singly and in combination, in patients with cholangiocarcinoma and PSC who are candidates for liver transplantation are presented.

Methods.—Three groups of patients with PSC were enrolled. The 15 patients in group A had cholangiocarcinoma, 11 of which were occult. Ten group A patients had liver transplantations. The 22 patients in group B had liver transplantations but no cholangiocarcinomas. The 37 patients in group C had stable PSC.

Results.—There were more men in the cancer group than in the other groups. Mean serum CEA and CA19-9 levels were dramatically higher for group A than for either of the other 2 groups. Using the combined index for the 2 tests (CA19-9 + [CEA × 40]) and a cutoff value of 400 U, 10 of 15 patients in group A, none of the patients in group B, and 1 patient in group C had values above 400. The high value in group C was assumed to be a false-positive result because the patient's condition has not changed in more than 1 year. Six of 11 occult tumors in group A were detected by the markers. The combined index of tumor markers had a sensitivity of 66%, a specificity of 100%, a positive predictive value of 100%, a negative predictive value of 81%, and an accuracy of 86%. Ultrasonography, CT scans, and endoscopic cholangiopancreatography gave poor results.

Conclusion.—The combined tumor marker index has a high sensitivity and accuracy rate for detecting occult cholangiocarcinomas and can be useful in screening patients with PSC who are candidates for liver transplantation.

▶ Making a diagnosis of cholangiocarcinoma, even with the current diagnostic methods of ultrasound, CT scan, or endoscopic retrograde cholangiopancreatography, can be extremely difficult. The use of 2 tumor markers,

CA19-9 and CEA had an accuracy rate of 86%. Patients with nonoccult tumors who undergo liver transplantation have a dismal prognosis. Perhaps, identification of tumor (utilizing these tumor markers) may provide an opportunity to intervene at an earlier stage. Further prospective studies are warranted.

T.J. Eberlein, M.D.

12 Plastic, Reconstructive, and Head and Neck Surgery

Introduction

In contrast to years past, the majority, perhaps the overwhelming majority of papers that this reviewer thought would be of interest to the reader are from the head and neck area, with considerably less representation from the breast and complex wound topics.

The 2 papers selected, however, on breast surgery will be of interest to the reader. The first is on the use of minimally invasive surgery to evaluate breast implants for some of the questions that arise currently. The other breast paper is on transverse rectus abdominis myocutaneous flap reconstruction after irradiation.

The 3 difficult wound papers should be of interest to most general surgeons: the first is on self-inflicted or factitious wounds, the second addresses the issue of sacral and perineal defects after anteroposterior resection and radiation, and the third discusses the use of quantitative culture in complex extremity wounds. The single burn paper discusses a synthetic dermis as researchers and clinicians alike still grapple with the problem of a truly synthetic skin. Included in this group as well is an interesting paper on the use of polytetrafluoroethylene (Gore-Tex) grafts in *micro*vascular surgery.

The head and neck neoplasm papers were very carefully gleaned from a large number of manuscripts submitted and may understandably on occasion reflect the personal biases of the reviewer. To give the reader a complete and multiple-course meal of reading, the topics of prevention, imaging, adjuvant therapy, extirpative surgery, reconstruction, and outcomes were covered. Also included were a half-dozen "basic science" papers. The words "basic science" need to be qualified, however, since 5 of the 6 papers are in actuality molecular biology with very substantial clinical links and interpretations. This group includes a study of preinvasive lesions in nasopharyngeal carcinoma, as well as 2 papers on flow cytometry. If the reader peruses nothing else in this group, my advice would be not to miss the 2 papers by Brennan et al. published in *The New England Journal of Medicine.*

Three papers on imaging have been included: 1 of neck masses by color Doppler and 2 on newer imaging techniques in laryngeal carcinoma, including MRI and positron emission tomography. The adjuvant therapy papers were selected more for new and innovative techniques rather than a rehash of older, established methods and include a paper on linear accelerator radiosurgery for recurrent carcinoma, a paper on the use of intraoperative radiotherapy, and a third paper that reaches a conclusion about adjuvant therapy somewhat in contrast to others in the past.

In the arena of extirpative surgery, an effort has been made to deliver a variety of topics, including the complication rate after organ preservation therapy, some risk factors for complications in head and neck surgery, and the efficacy of central venous pressure monitoring (or absence of the same) in such patients. Included also is a topical antiseptic paper with some very surprising findings. The topic of reconstruction of the head and neck included 2 papers on free flap and mandibular reconstruction, including a discussion of the newly developed Thorp plate, and 2 additional papers that study the use of the free jejunal flap. In this group also is an interesting and informative paper on the general topic of craniofacial reconstruction in cranial base–resected patients.

The last 3 papers on the head and neck are something of a miscellany and include an informative quasi-review of the use of antioxidants as chemopreventive agents, the care of terminal patients in the hospice setting (with some unanticipated conclusions), and an outcome analysis of head and neck cancer surgery in elderly patients.

What we have attempted to accomplish for the reader with this section is not to present esoteric subject material, lengthy review papers, or statistic-laden research that makes for tedious reading, but rather a collection of manuscripts that should attain the goal of the YEAR BOOK, a reading list to bring one the current developments in 1996.

Edward A. Luce, M.D.

TRAM Flap Breast Reconstruction After Radiation Treatment
Williams JK, Bostwick J III, Bried JT, Mackay G, Landry J, Benton J (Emory Univ, Atlanta, Ga)
Ann Surg 221:756–766, 1995   12–1

Background.—The transverse rectus abdominis myocutaneous (TRAM) flap reconstruction technique is widely used after radical mastectomy for breast cancer. Often, patients and surgeons delay TRAM flap surgery until postmastectomy radiaiton therapy is completed. To determine the connection between radiation treatment and flap-related complications, patients who had undergone radiation therapy before reconstruction were compared with those who delayed radiation therapy.

Methods.—Patients undergoing TRAM flap reconstructive surgery (N = 680) between 1981 and 1993 at Emory University Hospital formed the cohort of this study. Several risk factors other than radiation treatment were assessed: obesity, smoking at the time of reconstruction, scarring in the abdominal or flap tissue area, hypertension, age older than 60 years, and type of surgical technique (pedicle type or laterality). Several complications were also assessed: fat necrosis (flap loss), full-thickness skin loss, breast infection, and seromas. Radiation therapy data were characterized and recorded. The development of a complication was defined as the end point of the study. Data were interpreted by using a 2×2 contingency chi-square analysis with Yates' continuity correction.

Results.—Before TRAM flap reconstruction, 108 patients had been treated with radiotherapy. Recurrence that required additional radiotherapy occurred in 88% of these patients. Both obesity and previous radiation treatment were associated with the development of fat necrosis, which was the only statistically significant complication found. Obesity, abdominal scarring, and radiation were associated with infection. In patients with prior radiation treatment, the surgical technique had no effect on the development of fat necrosis. Complete data about radiation treatment were obtained for only 22 patients; 7 of them experienced a major complication. Six of those 7 patients had undergone boost irradiation of the internal mammary chain.

Discussion.—Reconstruction with a TRAM flap is a good first choice for reconstructive surgery. Radiation therapy before TRAM flap reconstruction was associated with increased fat necrosis and infection in the group of patients evaluated in this study. Although fat necrosis was not prevented by use of the bipedicled flap technique, the increased number of complications after boost radiation suggests that this method should be chosen to improve blood supply to the recipient bed in patients who have been treated with radiation.

▶ A solid paper with solid recommendations. One principal value of the paper, however, was almost a sidebar, namely, that 6 out of 8 patients who received a boost dose of radiation to the internal mammary nodes had subsequent complications with flap transfer. Perhaps those patients would be better served by free-tissue transfer.

E.A. Luce, M.D.

Endoscopic Plastic Surgery: The Endoscopic Evaluation of Implants After Breast Augmentation
Beer GM, Kompatscher P (Feldkirch, Austria)
Aesthetic Plast Surg 19:353–359, 1995   12–2

Introduction.—At first the silicone gel bag was accepted as being chemically and biologically inert, but more recently the health risks of silicone breast implants have raised considerable concern. There is a strong trend toward recommending regular checks of these implants, but not all the methods proposed are totally reliable. The only certain method is to directly inspect the implant after reopening the incision, but endoscopic assessment may be a reasonable alternative.

Technique.—Endoscopic studies were first performed when a woman wished to change her implants or when open capsulotomy was planned. An endoscope with 30-degree-angle optics is suitable for inspecting the implant and capsule. An optical system 4 mm in diameter is introduced into a 5.5-mm-diameter, wide-bore sheath bearing stopcocks for the inflow and outflow of fluid. Local anesthesia is added to the system fluid when the capsule is to be inspected. An 8-mm incision is made at the entrance site, which if possible is at an area of previous access. The subcutaneous tissue is cautiously divided with small scissors to approach the capsule.

Advantages.—Endoscopy is a rapid and reliable means of detecting even tiny capsular leaks in women with breast implants. It may be performed under local anesthesia and causes little morbidity.

▶ This paper is something less than a tour de force of scientific investigation and analysis. Yet the authors have imposed an intriguing alternative to our present options in the breast implant controversy. Do implants "wear out" after a set period of time? If so, at that juncture do they pose a health concern? A minimally invasive technique to assess the status of implants would be of considerable value—if in fact the findings are reliable.

E.A. Luce, M.D.

The Factitious Wound: Plastic Surgeon Beware

Méndez-Fernández MA (Mercy Med Center, Redding, Calif)
Ann Plast Surg 34:187–190, 1995   12–3

Introduction.—Chronic factitious wounds are the manifestation of a disorder most likely to be seen by the plastic surgeon. In such cases the wound is produced by the patient because of an underlying psychopathology or a conscious motivation to obtain a secondary gain. Three patients with factitious wounds are presented, together with a discussion of the diagnosis and management of the condition.

> *Case Report 3.*—Woman, 41, employed as a licensed vocational nurse was treated by numerous physicians over a 3-year period. The patient was reported to have been kicked in the anterior tibial surface of the proximal third of the left leg. The resulting chronic wound had been treated medically and by 2 wound revisions, but all methods proved unsuccessful. A review of the patient's history revealed various problems, including multiple surgical procedures, allergies, and depression. The wound was debrided and covered with a fasciocutaneous flap and split-thickness skin graft to the donor site. Healing finally occurred after the patient was placed in

a long cast for 4 weeks. She was later admitted for other unexplained and unrelated medical problems.

Discussion.—Patients with factitious wounds are often young women of higher socioeconomic class. In more than 75% of cases, the patient or a relative works in a health-related field. Psychological traits observed include an introverted and depressed personality, a manipulative and demanding nature, disturbance of body image, itinerant lifestyle, and recent, sudden bereavements. Wounds are generally on accessible areas of the body and tend to be regular in shape. There may be signs that chemicals have been applied to the wound. Patients may be willing to accept invasive procedures and relatively hazardous treatments. A problem should be suspected when the wound heals in a controlled environment and recurs after release. When confronted with the factitious nature of the wound, the patient may abandon treatment or threaten litigation. In some cases, known as Munchausen's syndrome by proxy, a parent inflicts a factitious illness or injury on a child. The diagnosis of a factitious wound is one of exclusion, and management of the problem can be complex.

▶ This is not a common problem, but the diagnosis is rarely made until quite late in the course after repeated operations and failures. Only heightened awareness of the surgeon will lead to a suspicion and pursuit of the correct ideology.

E.A. Luce, M.D.

Management of Sacral and Perineal Defects Following Abdominoperineal Resection and Radiation With Transpelvic Muscle Flaps

Loessin SJ, Meland NB, Devine RM, Wolff BG, Nelson H, Zincke H (Mayo Clinic and Mayo Found, Rochester, Minn)
Dis Colon Rectum 38:940–945, 1995   12–4

Background.—Chronic open wounds commonly occur in patients undergoing abdominoperineal resections because there may not be adequate soft tissue to close the pelvic floor. Such wounds can lead to various complications, including enterocutaneous and vesiculocutaneous fistulas, pelvic abscesses, pelvic osteomyelitis, and the development of persistent sinuses. The rectus abdominis myocutaneous flap has been used in various surgical reconstruction procedures and can also be applied to sacral and perineal defects. Advantages associated with this procedure include a wide arc of rotation based on the deep inferior epigastric vessels, relative ease of performance, and minimal donor site morbidity, among others. Experience with rectus abdominis flaps for the treatment of patients with sacral and perineal defects is described.

Patients and Methods.—Fifteen patients (mean age, 52 years) who had undergone a rectus abdominis flap procedure were evaluated. Reconstruction was indicated for chronic, open pelvic cavities with foul-smelling

wound drainage in patients who had undergone postanteroposterior resection and radiation or for sacral defects in those with locally invasive
chordomas or rectal cancers requiring sacrectomy. Ten patients had undergone previous external-beam radiation therapy, and 4 of the 5 not
undergoing radiation had a fistula or inflammatory bowel disease for
which high doses of immunosuppressants had been prescribed.

Very aggressive debridement of the perineal wound was first performed
so that yield fresh bleeding tissue and healthy bone were exposed. A rectus
abdominis or musculocutaneous flap was then raised as an island flap
connected to the inferior epigastric pedicle. After passing the entire muscle
and skin unit into the pelvis through a 5-cm incision placed in the posterior
sheath/peritoneum, blunt finger dissection was performed to create a 4-fin-
ger-breadth passage in the perineal wound. The pelvic cavity was thoroughly irrigated, bleeding was controlled, and the urinary tract was evaluated for injury. The skin-muscle unit was next pulled and pushed into the
defect and the perineal skin and abdomen were closed (Fig 5). Patients
were permitted to walk on postoperative day 7, and pelvic and abdominal
drains were removed on day 10. Follow-up ranged from 6 to 56 months.

Results.—On average, 5 preoperative debridement or drainage procedures were completed before rectus abdominis reconstruction. One donor
site complication was noted and consisted of a superficial wound seroma/
infection that healed without event. Complications at the recipient site
included necrosis of the small skin island in 2 patients, a ruptured obtu-
rator artery with hematoma in 1, and preoperative membranous urethral

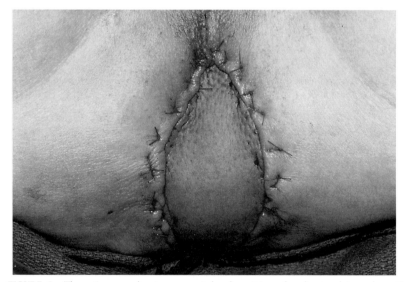

FIGURE 5.—The entire musculocutaneous unit has been trimmed and sutured into place. Note
placement of the suction drainage system well within the pelvic cavity and exit at the posterior portion of
the intragluteal cleft. (Courtesy of Loessin SJ, Meland NB, Devine RM, et al: Management of sacral and
perineal defects following abdominoperineal resection and radiation with transpelvic muscle flaps. *Dis
Colon Rectum* 38(9):940–945, 1995.)

disruption that continued to drain urine out of the deep drains for several days, eventually requiring urinary diversion. The most frequently noted minor complication, occurring in 3 patients, was a persistently draining sinus tract. Local wound care led to successful resolution of these problems. Excellent outcomes were obtained in 14 of the 15 patients. Only 1 patient required continued wound care for more than 12 months postoperatively.

Conclusions.—Sufficient debridement, control of infection, and well-vascularized muscle flaps can lead to successful resolution of postirradiated perineal and sacral wounds. The rectus abdominis flap procedure should thus be considered in these difficult-to-treat patients.

▶ With the institution's large volume of difficult and tertiary patient problems, the Mayo Clinic can often provide us with information for which smaller case numbers would simply be inadequate. Reported here are 15 late reconstructions of chronic postoperative perineal wounds in irradiated patients, an extreme problem for both the surgeon and patient. The presence of an avascular, chronically infected, and irradiated defect is a tremendous challenge to achieve wound healing. The authors were successful in all but 1 case with the use of pedicled muscle flaps composed of the rectus abdominis. Take note, however, that this result was achieved with the price of complications in half of the patients, probably not particularly surprising.

The ideal and *most appropriate* approach is immediate wound closure at the time of the extirpation with a similar technique, the use of a rectus flap to fill the perineal defect. To do so requires preoperative planning and collaboration between the general and plastic surgeon.

E.A. Luce, M.D.

Quantitative Culture Technique and Infection in Complex Wounds of The Extremities Closed With Free Flaps

Breidenbach WC, Trager S (Univ of Louisville, Ky)
Plast Reconstr Surg 95:860–865, 1995   12–5

Background.—A number of studies have found a relationship between a critical quantity of bacteria and infection in simple wounds. The use of quantitative cultures to determine the probability of infection in complex wounds of the extremities is less clear, however. Such wounds involve soft tissue defects that require a flap for wound closure and may be associated with loss of muscle or bone. Fifty consecutive patients with complex extremity wounds covered by a free-tissue transfer were evaluated to determine whether a relationship exists between a critical quantity of bacteria and infection and to compare predictive values of certain laboratory and clinical tests.

Methods.—Parameters compared in all 50 patients were wound position, mechanism of injury, and the presence or absence of a fracture. Twenty-eight patients had quantitative cultures before flap coverage and

16 had swab cultures. Wound management was based on clinical evaluation of the wound and patient and, if culture information was available, on qualitative bacteriology. All patients were evaluated for superficial infection, defined by the presence of cellulitis with minimal drainage, and for deep infection, defined as an infection that produces an abscess, osteitis, or osteomyelitis. Study parameters were evaluated for positive and negative predictive values (PPVs and NPVs), sensitivities, and specificities.

Results.—Eighteen patients (36%) had wound infections. Among patients who had quantitative cultures, the prevalence of infection was significantly greater when bacterial counts were greater than or equal to 10^4 than when less than 10^4. Although lower extremities appeared to have a higher infection rate than upper extremities, the difference was not statistically significant. Infection rates were similar for wounds with positive or negative swab cultures. Quantitative cultures had the best PPV (89%), NPV (95%), sensitivity (89%), and specificity (95%) for predicting wound infection.

Conclusion.—The likelihood of infection in complex wounds of the extremities closed with free flaps can be predicted by quantitative cultures. Infection occurs when a critical level of bacteria equal to or greater than 10^4 is reached. Other parameters thought to be associated with a risk of infection, namely, wound position, mechanism of injury, fracture type, and swab culture, generally had low PPVs, NPVs, sensitivity, and specificity.

▶ This paper is worth reading because of the application of a very useful laboratory technique for wound closure, namely, quantitative culture, that has not been used much in difficult wounds of the extremities. Quantitative cultures seem highly successful in predicting wound infection following closure with a flap. The problem here is the high prevalence of wound infections: over one third of the patients had such complications. Better clinical judgment would have permitted a reduction in this infection rate by one half (not necessarily accusing the authors of poor clinical judgment). The utility value of quantitative cultures would be substantially less.

E.A. Luce, M.D.

Use of an Acellular Allograft Dermal Matrix (AlloDerm) in the Management of Full-Thickness Burns
Wainwright DJ (Univ of Texas Health Sciences Ctr, Houston; Hermann Hosp, Houston)
Burns 21:243–248, 1995 12–6

Background.—The method currently used for replacing burned skin, the meshed split-thickness skin graft (STSG), is associated with scarring and contracture at the wound site. The alternative method of using allograft skin is complicated by a high rate of rejection because of the immune response. To avoid these complications, 2 patients undergoing skin grafting for full-thickness burns were treated with an acellular allograft dermal matrix (AlloDerm). The matrix was derived from fresh human cadaver skin by using a process that results in an acellular dermal matrix with normal collagen bundling and organization plus an intact basement membrane complex. The dermis was processed aseptically and tested for its ability to stimulate lymphoblast proliferation.

> *Case Report.*—Woman, 58, had a full-thickness burn on her forearm. A piece of rehydrated AlloDerm was placed on the wound and covered with a meshed STSG. A control site was treated in the same manner. Sixteen days after surgery, the epithelium from the meshed graft covered the surface of the underlying matrix. A bi-

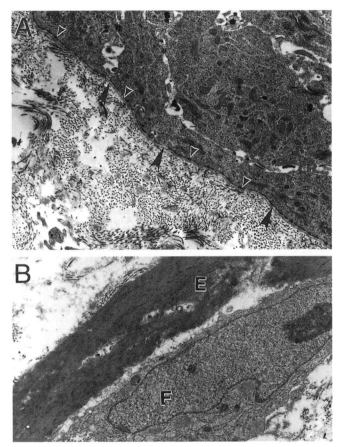

FIGURE 4.—Electron micrograph taken from the test site biopsy at day 16 postsurgery. **A,** intact basement membrane complex (*large arrows*) and normal collagen bundles, keratinocyte attachment, and formation of hemidesmosomes (*small arrows*). **B,** fibroblast infiltrate (*F*) and retained elastin fiber (*E*). The fibroblasts were indicative of a normal synthetic phenotype (*scale bar,* 1 μm). (Reprinted from *Burns,* vol 21, Wainwright DJ: Use of an acellular allograft dermal matrix (AlloDerm) in the management of full-thickness burns, pp 243–248, copyright 1995, with kind permission from Butterworth-Heinemann journals, Elsevier Science Ltd, The Boulevard, Langford Lane, Kidlington 0X5 1GB, UK.)

opsy showed that keratinocytes had spread from the STSG onto the dermal matrix and had migrated beneath the dermal component of the STSG to cover the AlloDerm surface; this finding was corroborated with electron microscopy (Fig 4).

Case Report.—Man, 29, experienced a full-thickness burn to the thigh that was excised and covered with rehydrated AlloDerm and then covered with a meshed 1.5:1 STSG. A control site was treated in the same manner. Epithelialization was complete 15 days after surgery. At day 180, both the patient and surgeon determined that the AlloDerm-treated site had better cosmesis and elasticity than the control site. At days 60 and 90, the control site had blistered, whereas the test site had not. At day 60, the test site had twice the elasticity of the control site; no scarring occurred at the test site by day 90, but there was scarring visible at the control site.

Discussion.—These case reports show that a grafted acellular dermal matrix supports fibroblast infiltration, neovascularization, and epithelialization without an immune response. In this study, AlloDerm demonstrated retention of the basement membrane complex. Cultured epithelial autografts do not show elastin formation 4 months after grafting, whereas normal collagen bundle patterns and elastin formation were seen 16 days after surgery. Superior cosmetic results were obtained with the acellular allograft dermal matrix than with widely meshed, thin autografts. Use of this technique may reduce the amount of donor skin required to treat full-thickness burn injuries.

▶ The "best" skin graft in terms of function is the full-thickness skin graft, the next best is a split-thickness skin graft, the next best a narrow meshed (1.5:1) split-thickness graft, and so on. The common denominator is the amount of dermis transplanted with the epidermis since dermis supplies stability to the ultimate graft. The results presented here are promising, but 2 swallows don't make a summer and 2 patients don't establish a therapeutic modality. Most importantly, the authors failed to inform the readers whether or not they have a financial relationship with the manufacturer of the dermal matrix (AlloDerm) used.

E.A. Luce, M.D.

Clinical Use of Microvascular PTFE Grafts
Lanzetta M (Sydney Hosp, Australia)
Microsurgery 16:412–415, 1995   12–7

Purpose.—The use of autologous vein grafts in microvascular surgery has yielded excellent clinical results so far. However, these grafts can pose problems related to the time needed for preparation, the limited choice of veins, and size matching. Synthetic grafts could be useful in many clinical situations, such as multiple-graft procedures. However, the thrombogenic potential of synthetic materials may pose particular problems with microvascular grafts. Polytetrafluoroethylene (PTFE) is a popular prosthetic graft material with many important advantages. The use of a 1.5-mm-diameter microvascular PTFE graft in a patient with an arterial injury to the hand is reported.

Case.—Man, 41, was brought for microneurovascular repair of a laceration in the palmar area of his dominant hand. A 1.5-cm gap in the superficial palmar arch precluded direct end-to-end repair. A PTFE graft measuring 1.5 mm in diameter and 1.5 cm in length was placed. The graft had a wall thickness of 0.18 mm and a fibril length of 60 μm. The 3M Precise Microvascular Anastomotic System was used for graft implantation on 1 end, and conventional microsurgical technique was used at the other end; these anastomoses took about 3 and 10 minutes, respectively. The patient had no postoperative complications and was discharged from the hospital after 48 hours. He had no foreign body reaction or local inflammation and was able to resume his usual activities 9 weeks after the accident. Twelve-week follow-up angiography confirmed graft patency.

Discussion.—Microvascular PTFE grafts can be used to bridge vascular defects in the arterial system. Initial experience suggests that these grafts provide a durable, safe, and reliable anastomosis and thus serve as a useful alternative to vein grafts for microvascular defects.

▶ The current thought about prosthetic grafts in microvascular surgery is that they don't work, a conclusion that doesn't seem logical. If prosthetic grafts composed of PTFE are applicable to macrovascular surgery, why not microsurgery? The solution might well be, as the author suggests, a matter of selection of the appropriate physical characteristics of fibril length and density to obtain a satisfactory patency rate. The argument and pursuit are something other than academic since the use of vein grafts in microvascular surgery can be difficult from the perspective of donor site availability and size match.

E.A. Luce, M.D.

Association Between Cigarette Smoking and Mutation of the p53 Gene in Squamous-Cell Carcinoma of the Head and Neck
Brennan JA, Boyle JO, Koch WM, Goodman SN, Hruban RH, Eby YJ, Couch MJ, Forastiere AA, Sidransky D (Johns Hopkins Univ, Baltimore, Md)
N Engl J Med 332:712–717, 1995   12–8

Background.—Epidemiologic evidence has linked tobacco and alcohol use with squamous cell carcinoma of the head and neck, but the molecular targets of these carcinogens have not yet been determined. Although some studies have reported an association between p53 mutations and tobacco smoking in squamous cell carcinoma of the head and neck, many of these investigations have involved small numbers of patients and relied on immunohistochemical evaluation—a method that does not always detect p53 mutations because of its high false-positive and false-negative rates. A molecular analysis was thus performed to identify the pattern of p53 mutations in neoplasms from patients with carcinoma of the head and neck and histories of alcohol and tobacco use.

Patients and Methods.—Tumor samples were obtained from 129 patients with primary squamous cell carcinoma of the head and neck. Sequence analysis of the conserved regions of the p53 gene was performed, and correlations between clinical characteristics and gene mutations were determined. Patients who had never used, rarely used, or stopped using tobacco and alcohol more than 20 years before receiving treatment for head and neck cancer were considered nonsmokers and nondrinkers, whereas those who were moderate or heavy users of cigarettes (at least 20 pack-years) and alcohol (1 or more drinks per day) were defined as smokers and drinkers. Perioperative data were also collected and included the tumor-node-metastasis stage of the head and neck cancer, the primary tumor site, and the pathologic grade of the neoplasm on light microscopy.

Results.—There were 102 patients with primary and 27 patients with recurrent squamous cell cancer of the head and neck. Among the newly diagnosed patients, 90 had advanced stage III or IV cancer and 81 either currently smoked cigarettes or had smoked within the past 20 years. Fifty-eight patients also reported moderate to heavy alcohol use within the past 20 years. Among the 27 patients with recurrent cancer, 22 smoked and 8 were moderate to heavy alcohol users. Fifty-four patients were found to have p53 mutations on molecular analysis. No significant associations between the presence or lack of p53 mutations, the tumor-node-metastasis stage, the pathologic tumor grade, or the primary tumor site were noted in patients with newly diagnosed or recurrent cancer on logistic regression analysis. In contrast, 38 of the smokers in the newly diagnosed cancer group had p53 mutations as compared with only 3 of the non-smokers. A significant association between alcohol use and p53 mutations was also noted in patients with primary cancer, with mutations occurring in 32 of the tumors from alcohol users but in only 9 of those from nondrinkers. No significant associations between cigarette and alcohol use and p53 mutations were observed in the patients with recurrent cancer, possibly because of the small number of patients. The proportions and patterns of p53 mutations were nearly identical in patients with primary (42%) and recurrent (50%) cancer. A more detailed analysis of smoking and drinking habits was thus performed after combining the 2 groups. A 58% incidence of p53 mutations was observed in the tumors of patients who smoked cigarettes and drank alcohol as compared with a 33% incidence in patients who smoked but did not drink and a 17% incidence in patients who neither smoked nor drank (Fig 2). Neither of the 2 nonsmoking patients who used alcohol had a p53 mutation.

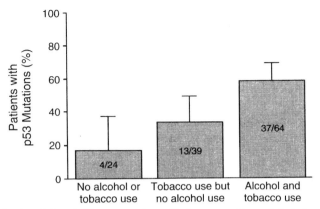

FIGURE 2.—Association of p53 gene mutations with cigarette smoking and alcohol consumption in 129 patients with squamous cell carcinoma of the head and neck. The frequency of p53 gene mutations in patients with invasive squamous cell carcinoma of the head and neck was related to the patients' exposure to cigarette tobacco and alcohol ($P = 0.001$). Cigarette smokers who drank alcohol were 3.5 times more likely than nonsmokers who abstained from alcohol to have mutations of the p53 gene. The *T bars* represent the upper 95% confidence limit. Two nonsmokers who drank were excluded from the analysis (neither had a p53 mutation). (Reprinted by permission of *The New England Journal of Medicine*, from Brennan JA, Boyle JO, Koch WM, et al: Association between cigarette smoking and mutation of the p53 gene in squamous-cell carcinoma of the head and neck. *N Engl J Med* 332:712–717, Copyright 1995, Massachusetts Medical Society.)

Conclusions.—Tobacco and alcohol use is associated with a high frequency of p53 mutations in patients with squamous cell cancer of the head and neck.

▶ The reader will enjoy this article despite the possible daunting effect of the title. The authors very lucidly explain their thesis in terms that a non–molecular biologist can readily comprehend and move forward with results and conclusions. Of course, this paper is a far cry from a total explanation of the relationship between cigarette smoking and squamous cell carcinoma of the head and neck (to which the authors readily admit) and yet provides a significant link. The lack of a relationship seen in some squamous cell carcinomas of the head and neck, in fact half of this group, *without* a p53 mutation needs further elucidation.

E.A. Luce, M.D.

Molecular Assessment of Histopathological Staging in Squamous-Cell Carcinoma of the Head and Neck
Brennan JA, Mao L, Hruban RH, Boyle JO, Eby YJ, Kock WM, Goodman SN, Sidransky D (Johns Hopkins Univ, Baltimore, Md; Johns Hopkins Hospital, Baltimore, Md)
N Engl J Med 332:429–435, 1995   12–9

Objective.—With squamous cell carcinoma of the head and neck, local recurrence rates increase substantially and survival rates decrease if the neoplasm is not completely removed. Lymph node involvement also de-creases survival by approximately 50%. Because micrometastases are eas-ily missed microscopically, this study examined the use of polymerase chain reaction (PCR) to detect microscopic neoplastic cells in surgical margins or lymph nodes.

Methods.—Tumors from 69 patients with invasive squamous cell car-cinoma of the head and neck were examined for p53 mutations by PCR. The cloned PCR products were analyzed by Southern blot analysis.

Results.—There were 30 patients aged 46 to 85 with mutations of the p53 gene. Most of these patients had advanced or recurrent cancer, 29 were heavy smokers, and 25 were heavy drinkers. A total of 72 surgical margins from 25 patients who had no pathologic evidence of microscopic cancer and 33 cervical lymph nodes from 6 patients were probed with the specific p53 assay. Thirteen margins were positive (Fig 1). Microscopic examination of slides from these 25 patients showed 1 positive surgical margin. Microscopic analysis of the cervical lymph nodes identified 5 positive nodes, whereas molecular analysis yielded positive results in 11

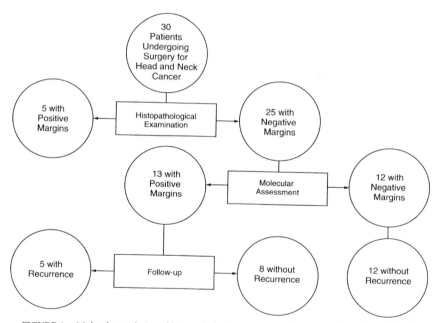

FIGURE 1.—Molecular analysis and histopathologic assessment of the surgical margins of 25 patients with squamous cell carcinoma of the head and neck who underwent resection intended to be curative. Thirteen of the 25 patients (52%) had neoplastic cells in the margins of the resected tissue that were not detected on histopathologic examination. After a median follow-up of 17 months (range, 10–27), 5 of the 13 patients with positive margins by molecular analysis had local recurrences, whereas none of the 12 patients with negative margins by molecular analysis had a local recurrence. All 5 patients with positive surgical margins by histopathologic examination had persistent locoregional cancer. (Reprinted by per-mission of *The New England Journal of Medicine,* from Brennan JA, Mao L, Hruban RH, et al: Molecular assessment of histopathological staging in squamous-cell carcinoma of the head and neck. *N Engl J Med* 332:429–435, Copyright 1995, Massachusetts Medical Society.)

cases, including 6 not identified microscopically. Five patients with positive margins had recurrences at margin sites, but no patients with negative margins had recurrences.

Conclusion.—A large percentage of surgical margins and lymph nodes were found to contain p53 mutations specific for the primary tumor, and these results were correlated with findings of local recurrence. The molecular assay method was more sensitive than light microscopy in detecting micrometastases, but the assay takes 3 days, and p53 mutations were found in only 50% of the head and neck cancers. Other genetic changes in squamous cell carcinomas may provide additional prognostic capability.

▶ This paper is one of several—perhaps the cream of the crop—that have used molecular techniques to assess surgical margins and lymph nodes in patients with head and neck cancer. The ability to better estimate margins, stage the patients, and base treatment rationale, particularly the use of postoperative radiotherapy, is intriguing. There are 2 problems, however: (1) the most well studied oncogene in head and neck cancer, p53, occurs in only about 50% of patients with squamous cell carcinoma of the head and neck; and (2) even in skilled labs the technique requires a minimum of 3 days even after the probe has been synthesized. Even though that permits the implementation of radiation therapy for a positive margin by molecular analysis, a more satisfactory approach would be re-excision of the margin, obviously a much more difficult task if done 3 to 4 days postoperatively rather than at the time of resection. Yet genetic markers are clearly the next era in pathologic assessment of head and neck cancer.

E.A. Luce, M.D.

Overexpression of p53 Predicts Organ Preservation Using Induction Chemotherapy and Radiation in Patients With Advanced Laryngeal Cancer

Bradford CR, Zhu S, Wolf GT, Poore J, Fisher SG, Beals T, McClatchey KD, Carey TE, and the Department of Veterans Affairs Laryngeal Cancer Study Group (Univ of Michigan, Ann Arbor; Hines Dept of Veterans Affairs, Ill)
Otolaryngol Head Neck Surg 113:408–412, 1995   12–10

Background.—Combined radical surgery plus radiation therapy is associated with significant profound functional morbidity in patients with advanced head and neck squamous cell carcinoma. For this reason, clinicians are exploring other avenues of treatment. Induction chemotherapy plus radiation therapy has been identified as an effective alternative to laryngectomy plus radiation therapy in patients with advanced laryngeal cancer, although those individuals likely to respond to chemotherapy cannot yet be predicted. Mutation of the p53 tumor suppressor gene, a frequent genetic alteration found in squamous cell carcinoma of the head

TABLE 1.—Response to Chemotherapy According to p53 Expression

Chemotherapy Response	p53 Expression	
	Positive	Negative
CR, PR	47	26
NR	6	9

Note: No difference was found in chemotherapy response according to p53 (*P* = 0.079).
Abbreviations: CR, complete response; *PR,* partial response; *NR,* no response.
(Courtesy of Bradford CR, Zhu S, Wolf CT, et al: Overexpression of p53 predicts organ preservation using induction chemotherapy and radiation in patients with advanced laryngeal cancer. *Otolaryngol Head Neck Surg* 113:408–412, 1995.)

and neck, may play an important regulatory role in cell proliferation and chemosensitivity. Thus tissue sections obtained from patients with advanced laryngeal cancer were evaluated for immunohistologic expression of p53 in an effort to determine whether p53 overexpression can predict chemotherapy response, organ preservation, and survival.

Patients and Findings.—Tissue sections obtained from 178 patients with advanced laryngeal cancer were evaluated. All patients were enrolled in the Department of Veterans Affairs Laryngeal Cancer Cooperative Study, 94 of whom were receiving induction chemotherapy consisting of cisplatin and 5-fluorouracil plus radiation therapy and 84 of whom were assigned to surgery plus postoperative radiation therapy.

Overexpression of p53 was noted in 61.2% of the larynx carcinoma specimens, the presence of which did not predict survival in either the chemotherapy or surgery patients. Likewise, no differences in disease-free interval were observed in either patient group based on p53 status. Among patients whose tumors overexpressed p53, 88.7% achieved a complete or partial response to chemotherapy as compared with 74.3% of the patients in the p53-negative group. This difference was not statistically significant (Table 1).

A significant association between outcome of larynx preservation and overexpression of p53 was noted, with 74% of the patients overexpressing p53 preserving their larynx vs. 52.2% of those not expressing this gene (Table 2). No difference in survival of patients with larynx preservation could be based on p53 status.

TABLE 2.—Larnyx Preservation According to p53 Expression

Larynx Preservation	p53 Expression	
	Positive	Negative
Yes	40	21
No	14	19

Note: Larnyx preservattion is significantly higher in the p53-positive group (74% vs. 52.5%, *P* = 0.03).
(Courtesy of Bradford CR, Zhu S, Wolf CT, et al: Overexpression of p53 predicts organ preservation using induction chemotherapy and radiation in patients with advanced laryngeal cancer. *Otolaryngol Head Neck Surg* 113:408–412, 1995.)

Conclusions.—Patients likely to achieve successful organ preservation with induction chemotherapy and radiation therapy can be predicted by p53 overexpression. Expression of p53 did not correlate with survival in either of the patient groups and does not predict survival with larynx preservation.

▶ Interesting information continues to come from the VA cancer study group, and this recent paper is an effort to predict those patients who will respond to inductive chemotherapy and radiation. Oncogene p53 findings remain controversial. Other studies have ascertained that overexpression of p53 indicates a higher responsiveness to radiation therapy but a lower overall survival. We haven't found the key for this lock yet. Also, such a huge overlap exists among the 2 groups in this study and others that clinical usefulness is not exactly on the immediate horizon.

E.A. Luce, M.D.

Significance of DNA Ploidy in the Treatment of T1 Glottic Carcinoma
Stern Y, Aronson M, Shpitzer T, Nativ O, Medalia O, Segal K, Feinmesser R (Tel Aviv Univ, Israel)
Arch Otolaryngol Head Neck Surg 121:1003–1005, 1995   12–11

Purpose.—For patients with T1N0M0 glottic carcinoma, radiotherapy yields a high cure rate. However, about 10% of patients do not respond to radiotherapy. These patients may need total laryngectomy after radiotherapy fails, whereas a more limited approach could be used if surgery were the primary treatment modality. There are no reliable histopathologic markers to predict which tumors will recur after radiotherapy. Tumor cell ploidy can be objectively determined by flow cytometric analysis of DNA content. Known radiosensitive and radioresistant glottic carcinomas were studied to find out whether flow cytometric analysis can predict tumor response to radiotherapy.

Methods.—The case-control study used paraffin-embedded tumor specimens from 15 patients with T1 glottic laryngeal carcinoma who had recurrent tumors after radiotherapy and 15 patients in whom the same radiotherapy regimen was curative. The patients were matched for stage, age, sex, and smoking habits. Flow cytometric analysis was performed in each tumor specimen.

Results.—Tumor DNA content was diploid in 16 tumors and aneuploid in 14. Of the 15 patients with recurrence, 10 had diploid and 5 had aneuploid tumors. In the disease-free group, 6 tumors were diploid and 9 were aneuploid. The difference was not significant, although diploid tumors showed a trend toward postradiation recurrence.

Conclusions.—Among patients with T1 glottic carcinoma, those with aneuploid tumors may tend to respond better to radiotherapy. The difference in radiosensitivity between diploid and aneuploid tumors, although nonsignificant in this study, could be related to a mutant form of the p53 gene in aneuploid tumors. Inactivation of p53 by mutation may leave tumor cells more vulnerable to the effects of DNA-damaging agents. A larger study is needed to determine the true value of assessing DNA ploidy in early laryngeal tumors.

▶ This short, concisely written paper brings the reader "up to speed" on the current status of flow cytometry in attempting to prognosticate head and neck cancer. Ploidy did not predict response to radiotherapy in patients with T1 glottic cancer, the very same clinical situation in which a prognostic indicator would be of tremendous value. In fact, the aneuploid tumors had a somewhat lower risk of local recurrence after radiotherapy. What this paper tells me again is that despite early enthusiasm for flow cytometry, we have a long way to go in refining the technique to be of clinical value.

E.A. Luce, M.D.

Clonal Proliferations of Cells Infected With Epstein-Barr Virus in Preinvasive Lesions Related to Nasopharyngeal Carcinoma
Pathmanathan R, Prasad U, Sadler R, Flynn K, Raab-Traub N (Univ of North Carolina, Chapel Hill; Univ of Malaya, Kuala Lumpur, Malaysia)
N Engl J Med 333:693–698, 1995   12–12

Introduction.—Epstein-Barr virus (EBV) plays a key role in development of the epithelial cancer nasopharyngeal carcinoma, with affected patients showing elevated IgA antibodies to viral capsid antigen and other EBV replicative antigens. Few studies have examined premalignant, preinvasive nasopharyngeal neoplasia among patients who go on to have nasopharyngeal carcinoma. Such a study was performed to assess the role of EBV infection in the development of nasopharyngeal carcinoma.

Methods.—Five thousand three hundred twenty-six nasopharyngeal biopsy samples were screened for early malignant changes such as dysplasia and carcinoma in situ. Eleven such preinvasive lesions were identified and tested for the presence of EBV by various assays.

Results.—All 11 lesions showed evidence of EBV infection. Eight of 8 specimens tested with in situ hybridization showed EBV-encoded RNAs, and 6 of 6 samples tested by immunohistochemical staining showed latent membrane protein type 1 (LMP-1). Clonal EBV DNA was detected in 6 of 7 lesions tested for the EBV termini. Most specimens showed transcription of EBV nuclear antigen type 1, LMP-1 and LMP-2A, and the *Bam*HI-A fragment, which are latent EBV gene products, but the viral proteins typically associated with lytic lesions were not present.

Conclusions.—Epstein-Barr virus infection is documented in preinvasive nasopharyngeal lesions. The finding of clonal EBV DNA suggests that the lesions arise from a single EBV-infected cell and that the infection could be an initiating event in the development of nasopharyngeal carcinoma. Expression of LMP-1 as the EBV-transforming gene appears to play a critical role in preinvasive epithelial proliferations.

▶ For many years, EBV has been implicated in a number of neoplasms, including nasopharyngeal carcinoma. The consummate beauty of this paper was the ability of the authors to step back a couple of paces and take a longitudinal perspective of the relationship. What is new is the establishment of perhaps the first link of a *causative* nature to that relationship rather than simply associative.

E.A. Luce, M.D.

Histocytologic Grading of Mucoepidermoid Carcinoma of Major Salivary Glands in Prognosis and Survival: A Clinicopathologic and Flow Cytometric Investigation
Hicks MJ, El-Naggar AK, Flaitz CM, Luna MA, Batsakis JG (Univ of Texas, Houston; Baylor College of Medicine, Houston; Univ of Texas Dental Branch, Houston)
Head Neck 17:89–95, 1995

12–13

Background.—Mucoepidermoid carcinoma (MEC) is the most common malignant salivary gland tumor. A 3-tiered grading system has been introduced for these tumors but has not gained universal acceptance. The relationship between the MEC 3-tiered grading system of Healey et al., as modified by Batsakis and Luna, to flow cytometric and clinicopathologic prognostic parameters was investigated.

Materials.—Tumors were examined from 48 patients with MEC who received primary treatment from 1956 to 1986 at the University of Texas M.D. Anderson Cancer Center. All tumors underwent both histologic and DNA flow cytometric analysis. Among these 48 tumors, 7 were low-grade (LG), 23 were intermediate-grade (IG), and 18 were high-grade (HG) by the 3-tiered histologic rating system. There were 43 tumors of the parotid and 5 of the submandibular glands.

Results.—The mean age was 42 years for patients with LG tumors, 47 years for patients with IG tumors, and 59 years for patients with HG tumors. There was a female preponderance for LG and IG but a male preponderance for HG tumors. The mean tumor stage was 1.4 for LG, 2.4 for IG, and 3.6 for HG. Tumor size increased from 2.1 cm for LG to 3.8 cm for HG. The margins were never involved in LG tumors but were involved in 44% of the IG tumors and 61% of the HG tumors. The lymph nodes were never involved in LG tumors but were involved in 22% of IG and 72% of HG tumors. DNA aneuploidy was not present in LG but was present in 13% of IG and 28% of HG tumors. There were no LG recurrences, but 39% of LG tumors and 61% of HG tumors recurred. Survival decreased significantly with increasing tumor grade.

Conclusions.—Histologic grading of MEC tumors with the modified Healey 3-tiered system correlates with clinical, pathologic, and flow cytometric factors that influence prognosis and survival.

▶ This paper was selected not from a critical aspect of a comprehensive treatment of salivary tumors but rather a concise demonstration of how the DNA flow cytometry technique can be utilized to facilitate and standardize our systems of grading of tumors of the head and neck in a better fashion than what we accomplish today. In conferences and discussions we tend to use the terms "high-grade and low-grade" rather loosely without a more concise description and perhaps reach some clinical decisions as well. Flow cytometry and other cellular techniques may assist us in refinement.

E.A. Luce, M.D.

Predictive Value of MR Imaging–Dependent and Non–MR Imaging–Dependent Parameters for Recurrence of Laryngeal Cancer After Radiation Therapy
Castelijns JA, van den Brekel MWM, Smit EMT, Tobi H, van Wagtendonk FW, Golding RP, Venema HW, van Schaik C, Snow GB (Free Univ Hosp, Amsterdam)
Radiology 196:735–739, 1995   12–14

Background.—Limited surgery for laryngeal cancer offers the possibility of curing the disease while conserving vocal function. When there is a possibility of achieving primary control with radiotherapy, it is necessary to accurately estimate tumor size and assess deep extension. Tumor volume is a key factor influencing local control when only radiotherapy is used. Magnetic resonance imaging is a very sensitive means of demonstrating cartilage invasion and is more accurate than CT.

Objective.—The predictive value of various MR parameters was investigated in 80 previously untreated patients who were to receive radiotherapy with curative intent.

Methods.—Sixty-nine men and 11 women with adequate T1- and T2-weighted MR images were included in the study. In 27 cases, 1 vocal cord was not fully mobile, and in 9 patients at least 1 cord was fixed. Radiation doses ranged from 60 to 78 Gy. Tumor volume was calculated from T1-weighted images. Cartilage invasion was considered present if there was intermediate signal intensity on T1-weighted spin-echo images and high signal intensity on T2-weighted images. Patients were observed for at least 2 years after treatment.

Findings.—Thirty of the 80 patients had recurrences, nearly all of them within 2 years of treatment. Half the patients with impaired cord mobility and about one fourth of the others had recurrences. Invasion of the pre-epiglottic space was not a significant factor predicting recurrence. Invasion of the vocal muscle was associated with recurrence, although not significantly. Recurrences were significantly more frequent when cartilage invasion was present (52% vs. 21%). The average tumor volume was 3.9 cc in patients with and 2.4 cc in those without recurrent disease. A model including cord mobility, tumor volume, and cartilage invasion best predicted the risk of disease recurring.

Conclusion.—Magnetic resonance imaging improves the ability to select patients with laryngeal cancer for either radiotherapy or surgery.

▶ This group of authors from Amsterdam makes a strong case for routine MRI of laryngeal neoplasms. Our practice has been to assess by CT, but not necessarily MRI because of the cost differential. One of the 3 significant parameters, impaired cord mobility, can be assessed as well, if not better clinically than with imaging techniques. A similar correlation with tumor volume by the use of CT scan could be accomplished with a similarly designed type of study as this one. That leaves us with the single parameter of cartilage invasion. Granted, the variability in ossification of the laryngeal cartilage can determine the quality of the CT image, but the interpretation of MRI is also reader dependent. My final "take" is that if the cost differential becomes less, MRI will probably be the preferable method of imaging larynx (and other head and neck cancers) in the quite immediate future.

E.A. Luce, M.D.

Positron Emission Tomography in the Evaluation of Laryngeal Carcinoma

McGuirt WF, Greven KM, Keyes JW Jr, Williams DW III, Watson NE Jr, Geisinger KR, Cappellari JO (Wake Forest Univ, Winston-Salem, NC)
Ann Otol Rhinol Laryngol 104:274–278, 1995   12–15

Background.—Management decisions for patients with laryngeal carcinoma depend on the identification of occult and manifest nodal disease and on the distinction between tumor recurrence and postirradiation soft tissue sequelae. In positron emission tomography (PET), differences in tissue metabolism can be imaged by the use of a radioisotope affixed to a glucose analogue. Other imaging studies, namely, CT and MRI, may fail to correctly predict recurrence of laryngeal carcinoma after radiotherapy. The pretreatment and posttreatment findings of PET in patients with squamous cell carcinoma of the larynx were compared with the findings of CT and MRI.

Methods.—Thirty-eight patients with laryngeal carcinoma were studied with PET. Twenty-five patients were studied before receiving definitive therapy. The other 13 had previously undergone radiotherapy but now had abnormal soft tissue findings that could represent either recurrent cancer or radionecrosis. At the same time the PET studies were performed, CT scans or MR images were obtained.

Results.—Positron emission tomography correctly identified the primary tumor in 88% of the pretreatment group, with 1 false-negative and 2 equivocal results. Correlative studies in 27 surgical neck specimens showed agreement between PET and pathology findings in 81% of the cases. The CT and MRI findings regarding the presence of metastatic disease also agreed with the pathology findings in 81% of the cases. These imaging studies depicted the primary lesion in 88% of the cases, with 1 equivocal and 2 false-negative results.

In the posttreatment group, PET correctly distinguished between recurrent cancer and postirradiation soft tissue changes in 11 of 13 patients. Pathologic examination showed recurrent or residual cancer in 7 patients and no cancer in 1; 5 patients whose larynxes had been salvaged had no cancer at long-term clinical follow-up. In 7 of 12 patients, CT or MRI yielded equivocal results for recurrent or persistent tumor. These 2 imaging studies were 42% accurate in distinguishing radionecrosis from recurrent or residual carcinoma.

Conclusions.—Positron emission tomography, CT, and MRI are comparable in their ability to positively identify primary laryngeal carcinomas, although none is as sensitive as clinical examination. There are many problems with the use of PET for tumor detection and treatment planning, including its limited resolution, lack of anatomical definition, and high cost. In patients who have undergone radiotherapy and now have worrisome soft tissue changes, PET has clear advantages over clinical examination, CT, or MRI. Its accuracy in differentiating between cancer and postirradiation soft tissue changes is 85%. This distinction is most reliably made at least 4 months after treatment.

▶ Positron emission tomography is still an investigative tool in the pretreatment assessment of patients with head and neck cancer, primarily because of cost and difficulty with resolution and definition. In this study, however, PET was superior in differentiating postradiation recurrence from soft tissue changes alone, a difficult diagnostic dilemma in laryngeal cancer. The imaging technique is relatively new and not widely available.

E.A. Luce, M.D.

Differential Diagnosis of Pulsatile Neck Masses by Doppler Color Flow Imaging

Takeuchi Y, Numata T, Suzuki H, Konno A, Kaneko T (Chiba Univ, Japan)
Ann Otol Rhinol Laryngol 104:633–638, 1995   12–16

Purpose.—Patients with the relatively rare finding of a pulsatile neck mass (PNM) must be evaluated carefully. Early recognition of carotid artery aneurysms is essential, and the morbidity and mortality of arteriography should be avoided. Doppler color flow imaging (DCI) has come to be widely used for assessment of the blood vessels of the head and neck. Its use in the investigation of patients with PNMs was evaluated.

Methods.—The study sample comprised 9 patients with PNMs, all of whom underwent DCI as their initial diagnostic study. Further investigations included x-ray CT in 5 patients, MRI in 4, and intra-arterial angiography (IAA) in 2.

Findings.—On physical examination, a bruit could be auscultated from the 7 vascular masses but not the 2 nonvascular masses. However, none of the vascular masses could be distinguished from a carotid artery aneurysm on the basis of the physical findings. In each patient with a vascular mass, DCI was able to make the clinical diagnosis. In 7 of 9 patients, IAA was not needed to confirm the nature of the PNM.

Conclusions.—Doppler color imaging is very useful in the evaluation of patients with PMNs. It permits real-time, noninvasive, and repeated evaluations and, in many cases, can avoid the use of IV digital subtraction angiography and IAA. The authors suggest using DCI as the initial investigation to see whether the mass is vascular. Vascularity can be clarified with x-ray CT or MRI, with angiographic studies reserved for difficult cases or preoperative planning.

▶ Maybe yes, maybe no. The radiology profession is currently grappling with the development of the most effective, efficient, and cheapest method of imaging the vascular system. Vascular MRI may hold great promise for the extremities as recently published elsewhere. One of the difficulties with this study was that unfortunately, angiography was only done in 2 patients as a gold standard comparison. In addition, diagnoses in 5 of the patients and perhaps 6 were of a nature that made diagnosis by Doppler color flow imaging relatively straightforward, but perhaps in other situations such would not be the case, as the author stated. The only way to properly image a tumor mass for feeding vessels is angiography (at least at the present). Finally, the flow of diagnostic options offered would add up to a hefty bill in this era of managed care.

E.A. Luce, M.D.

Linac Radiosurgery for Locally Recurrent Nasopharyngeal Carcinoma: Rationale and Technique
Buatti JM, Friedman WA, Bova FJ, Mendenhall WM (Univ of Florida, Gainesville)
Head Neck 17:14–19, 1995   12–17

Background.—Stereotactic radiosurgery is a means of delivering a single high-dose fraction of radiotherapy to a precisely delimited target. It has been used chiefly in neurosurgery but may also be used to treat recurrent head/neck lesions at the skull base.

Series.—Three patients with locally recurrent nasopharyngeal carcinoma were treated with linear accelerator (linac)-based stereotactic radiosurgery. The lesions were near the clivus and variably involved the cavernous sinus. In each case a single 12.5-Gy fraction of 6-MV photons was delivered to the 80% isodose shell. One patient remained free of disease a year after radiotherapy. Another had further local recurrence 6 months after radiosurgery. One patient deteriorated neurologically 6 months after treatment, but it was not clear whether a complication or recurrent disease was responsible.

Discussion.—Stereotactic radiosurgery is the most accurate means of delivering localized radiotherapy to intracranial sites. Its chief disadvantage is the inability to deliver fractionated treatment. The results achieved in this small series are inconclusive.

▶ This small series of 3 patients is somewhat less than convincing about the value of the gamma knife in extracranial head and neck cancer. Yet the outlook for recurrent nasopharyngeal carcinoma patients is so bleak and the other options, as the authors carefully outline, so limited and ineffective that experimental methods such as this one warrant a report and review. The combination of small-field external-beam therapy to reduce the recurrence to a manageable size for a subsequent single blast by the gamma knife also has some conceptual appeal. More reported experience is needed.

E.A. Luce, M.D.

Simultaneous Radiochemotherapy in the Treatment of Inoperable, Locally Advanced Head and Neck Cancers: A Single-Institution Study
Franchin G, Gobitti C, Minatel E, Barzan L, De Paoli A, Boz G, Mascarin M, Lamon S, Trovò MG (Centro di Riferimento Oncologico, Aviano, Italy; Gen Hosp, Pordenone, Italy)
Cancer 75:1025–1029, 1995   12–18

Background.—Only about 15% of patients with inoperable malignancies in the head/neck region achieve locoregional control for 5 years with radiotherapy alone, and the median survival time is only 1 year. Simultaneous radiotherapy and chemotherapy have been proposed in the hope of increasing the regional control rate and lowering the risk of distant spread.

Study Plan.—A trial of simultaneous radiotherapy and cisplatin chemotherapy was undertaken in 45 patients with primary inoperable head/neck cancer that had not metastasized. The first 21 patients (group 1) received cisplatin and simultaneous radiotherapy in a total dose of 660–7,020 cGy. Cisplatin was given by IV bolus in a dose of 50 mg/m^2 on days 1, 21, and 42 of radiotherapy. A radiotherapy boost was delivered to the lymph nodes if positive. The next 24 patients (group 2) received 5-fluorouracil (5-FU) in addition in a dose of 300 mg/m^2 daily 5 days a week until radiotherapy was completed.

Results.—More complete clinical and pathologic responses occurred in group 2 patients, who received 5-FU in addition to cisplatin chemotherapy (Table 3). The median time to progression in patients who responded completely was 13 months in group 1 and 10 months in group 2. Mucositis developed in all group 1 patients, who were treated as outpatients,

TABLE 3.—Results

	Group 1 (RT + CDDP)	Group 2 (RT + 5-FU/CDDP)
Total no. of patients	22	24
No. of evaluable patients	21	24
Complete response	10	17
Complete response (pathologic)	(3)	(6)
Partial response	8	7
No change	3	0

Abbreviations: RT, radiation therapy; *CDDP*, cisplatin; *5-FU*, 5-fluorouracil.
(Courtesy of *Cancer*, from Franchin G, Gobitti C, Minatel E, et al, copyright © 1995. Reprinted by permission of Wiley-Liss, Inc., a division of John Wiley & Sons, Inc.)

and 4 required hospitalization for this reason. Group 2 patients were hospitalized for the first week of treatment. In 5 cases treatment had to be interrupted for 7–10 days. The median overall survival time was 17 months for group 1 patients and 16 months for group 2.

Conclusion.—Adding chemotherapy to radiotherapy for patients with locally advanced but inoperable head/neck cancer produces more complete responses, but overall survival is not significantly lengthened. The results do not justify the added effort and cost entailed in this treatment or the psychophysical stress imposed on patients.

▶ This is an honest paper that reaches the conclusion that chemotherapy did not add to the efficacy of treatment of advanced inoperable head and neck cancer. Investigations are currently under way to examine the chemotherapy component of chemoradiotherapy organ preservation in advanced head and neck cancer.

E.A. Luce, M.D.

Management of Advanced Cervical Metastasis Using Intraoperative Radiotherapy

Freeman SB, Hamaker RC, Rate WR, Garrett PG, Pugh N, Huntley TC, Borrowdale R (Head and Neck Surgery Assoc Inc, Indianapolis, Ind; Methodist Hosp of Indiana, Indianapolis)
Laryngoscope 105:575–578, 1995   12–19

Introduction.—In patients with advanced metastatic disease in the neck, massively involved lymph nodes make it difficult to achieve adequate operative margins. Nodes fixed to deep tissues, including the carotid artery, and extranodal spread also complicate the management of these patients. External-beam irradiation often fails to eliminate advanced neck disease, or the maximum dose may already have been administered.

Objective.—A combined approach involving aggressive resection and intraoperative radiotherapy (IORT) was evaluated in 75 patients with advanced cervical metastasis, usually of squamous cell cancer, and possible invasion of the deep muscles or carotid artery. All involved nodes were more than 3 cm in diameter, and a majority of them were clinically fixed. One third of the nodes involved the carotid artery. Previous radiotherapy had been given to 61% of the patients.

Management.—Fifty-two patients were treated for recurrent disease, whereas 22 received IORT as part of initial treatment. Radical neck dissection was performed in 49 patients. The involved carotid artery was resected in 15 patients, and in 11 others the adventitia was removed from the vessel. If the margins were involved or were narrow, the patient was taken under IV anesthesia to the radiation oncology department. Current treatment is 2,000 cGy.

Results.—The operative margins were considered close in 42 patients. Seven received IORT for residual gross disease. One fourth of the patients and one third of those with carotid artery involvement had major complications. The 70 patients treated for squamous cell cancer had 1- and 2-year survival rates of 59% and 45%, respectively. Only 14% of the patients with gross residual disease lived 2 years.

Conclusions.—Intraoperative radiotherapy appears to be especially helpful to patients with disease involving the carotid artery. The presence of microscopic disease at the operative margins has not compromised local control or survival.

▶ This paper was included not because of the highly scientific analysis of the results (even the authors admit it was impossible to determine the effectiveness) but rather to alert the reader to a technique that may address a very difficult group of patients. Advanced neck disease, particularly if adventitial peeling of the carotid or resection is required, is often poorly controlled even with external-beam radiotherapy. Intraoperative radiotherapy may be an alternative to that of brachytherapy administered by the catheter and beads technique.

This reviewer has not had experience with intraoperative radiotherapy, but the description of transport to the radiation oncology department under general anesthesia for radiation and then return to the operating room for closure sounds daunting to say the least.

E.A. Luce, M.D.

Surgery After Organ Preservation Therapy: Analysis of Wound Complications
Sassler AM, Esclamado RM, Wolf GT (Naval Med Ctr, Portsmouth, Va; Univ of Michigan, Ann Arbor)
Arch Otolaryngol Head Neck Surg 121:162–165, 1995   12–20

Introduction.—In patients with advanced head and neck cancer, neoadjuvant or induction chemotherapy with radiation therapy may help preserve the structure and function of vital organs such as the larynx better than conventional surgery does. This retrospective survey assessed the incidence and risk factors for the development of major wound complications in patients with squamous cell cancer of the head and neck who had received neoadjuvant therapy.

Methods.—The medical records of 18 patients who required surgery after completing chemotherapy and radiation were reviewed.

Results.—Major wound complications were found in 11 (61%) of 18 patients. Those who had salvage surgery within a year of initial treatment had a 77% incidence of major wound complications, whereas the complication rate for those having surgery a year or more after initial therapy was 20%. Mucocutaneous fistulas occurred in 50% of the patients requiring surgery of the pharynx and neck skin, and the mean time to resolve these complications was 7.7 months. Two of these patients died during the course of treatment, 1 of a carotid blowout and another from postoperative pneumonia.

Conclusions.—Major wound complications in patients who need surgery after chemotherapy and radiation therapy are highest if the surgery is performed within the first year after initial treatment. When chemotherapy is combined with radiation, more wound complications may develop if surgery is needed later. Because of the high rate of complications, organ preservation treatment strategies require careful assessment.

▶ The contemporary impetus is organ preservation by the use of combined chemotherapy and radiation therapy. Yet surgical salvage is necessary in anywhere from 30% to 50% of these patients with advanced-stage disease. This paper outlines that the majority of such patients will sustain wound complications. The postoperative mortality for this group was 11%, a substantial increase over the anticipated result. Even when the upper area digestive tract was not opened in the small number of patients (4), half had complications. Our experience has been that the use of vascularized tissue, either pedicled or more commonly as a free flap, will bring well-vascularized tissue into the field and hopefully minimize wound healing complications.

Just as an aside, these authors found that 10 of the 15 patients in whom they measured thyrotropin were hypothyroid at the time of surgical salvage. Hypothyroid patients don't tolerate major surgery and probably don't heal particularly well either.

E.A. Luce, M.D.

Risk Factors for Complications in Clean-Contaminated Head and Neck Surgical Procedures

Girod DA, McCulloch TM, Tsue TT, Weymuller EA Jr (Naval Hosp, Oakland, Calif; Univ of Iowa Hosps and Clinics, Iowa City; Univ of Washington, Seattle)
Head Neck 17:7–13, 1995   12–21

Introduction.—In patients undergoing major head and neck surgery, the risk of complications is significantly higher if the surgical wound is contaminated by oral secretions, known as clean-contaminated wounds. Major perioperative complications can considerably increase the length and expense of hospitalization. Toward clarification of the preoperative and operative factors associated with perioperative complications—infectious as well as noninfectious—a series of 159 patients undergoing clean-contaminated head and neck operations were reviewed.

Methods.—The study included only patients who had a surgical neck wound that communicated with the oral cavity or pharynx. The investigators examined the effects of both preoperative variables, such as age, sex, weight, height, tobacco and alcohol history, medical illnesses, previous treatments, TNM stage, previous tracheotomy, and nutrition, and operative factors, including surgical procedure, operative time, blood loss and volume replacement, transfusions, reconstructive technique, antibiotic treatment, and perioperative steroid treatment. Perioperative complications were identified as being either infectious or noninfectious and wound related or non–wound related.

Results.—Sixty-three percent of the patients had at least 1 complication. Wound infections, including orocutaneous/pharyngocutaneous fistulas, occurred in 22% of the patients. The most frequent non–wound-related infections were pneumonia and enterocolitis, with rates of 13% and 11%, respectively. Operative mortality was 1.2%. Previous radiotherapy was linked to an increased rate of complications overall and to an increased wound infection rate. None of the other preoperative risk factors were significant.

The complication rate was significantly higher for patients undergoing reconstructive surgery with either a myocutaneous flap or microvascular free tissue transfer, but there was no related increase in the wound infection rate. The complication rate was nonsignificantly elevated in patients who received perioperative steroids. Patients with longer durations of surgery were significantly more likely to have complications and somewhat more likely to have wound infections. These relationships could have reflected either the length of anesthesia or the complexity of the surgical procedures performed. The average duration of antibiotic prophylaxis was 8 days.

Conclusions.—In patients undergoing clean-contaminated major head and neck surgical procedures, preoperative variables are of little help in identifying patients at high risk of complications. Some operative factors are linked to higher rates of overall complications or wound infection, such as previous radiotherapy, myocutaneous flap or microvascular free flap reconstruction, and possibly corticosteroid use. Extended antibiotic prophylaxis does not seem to reduce the incidence of wound infections.

▶ Three aspects warrant discussion:

1. The authors fail to find a correlation between preoperative risk factors (other than radiotherapy), including nutritional status, and the risk of complications. Note that the authors used very crude indices of nutritional and

immune status, albumin and hematocrit. Somehow one intuitively assumes that a well-nourished patient will have fewer complications than a poorly nourished one.

2. Apparently these authors utilized postoperative steroids in the vast majority of such cases (85%) and noted a tendency toward increased complications. Actually the justification for the use of steroids is at best anecdotal and would probably fail a risk/benefit analysis.

3. The authors report a surprisingly high incidence of enterocolitis (10.3%). This increased incidence might be linked to the prolonged duration of antibiotic use in their cases, nearly 8 days on average. In fact, they did not find their regimen to be more efficacious in regard to wound infection rates than 24-hour antibiotic prophylaxis regimens published in the literature.

E.A. Luce, M.D.

The Efficacy of Routine Central Venous Monitoring in Major Head and Neck Surgery: A Retrospective Review
Jensen NF, Todd MM, Block RI, Hegtvedt RL, McCulloch TM (Univ of Iowa Hosps and Clinics, Iowa City)
J Clin Anesth 7:119–125, 1995   12–22

Objective.—Patients undergoing major surgery that is expected to entail large fluid shifts commonly have a central venous pressure (CVP) catheter placed to help assess cardiac function and intravascular volume status. These catheters are often placed in patients undergoing lengthy, major head and neck operations in the hope of improving fluid management. A retrospective pilot study was performed to clarify the role of routine CVP monitoring during major head and neck surgery.

Methods.—The study included a random sample of 104 patients undergoing elective major head and neck surgery. Each procedure lasted at least 4 hours and had an expected blood loss of 500 mL or more. The attending anesthesiologists placed central venous catheters at their discretion. The patients' charts were reviewed to assess preoperative variables, including age, weight, hemoglobin, blood urea nitrogen, creatinine, and history of cardiovascular or renal disease; intraoperative variables, including duration of surgery, estimated blood loss, lowest hourly urine output, intraoperative administration of blood or colloid, and the presence of systolic blood pressures less than 70 mm Hg; and postoperative variables, including hemoglobin, blood urea nitrogen, and oliguria.

Results.—Forty-nine percent of the patients underwent central venous monitoring. The patients who did and did not have CVP catheters placed did not differ in age, weight, preoperative laboratory values, or history of cardiac or renal disease. Nor were there any significant differences in intraoperative or postoperative variables. The patients with and without CVP catheters were no different in their rate of complications related to fluid administration, including pulmonary edema, oliguria, and wound dehiscence.

Conclusions.—Central venous monitoring during major head and neck surgery appears to have little or no impact on perioperative management. A randomized, prospective study is needed to evaluate the efficacy or necessity of placing CVP catheters in this group of surgical patients. The findings highlight the way in which expensive, invasive medical practices are often used in the absence of evidence proving their efficacy.

▶ Please note the retrospective nature of this paper, a point the authors take considerable pains to emphasize as well. Yet within that framework, CVP catheters made little impact on the care of the head and neck patients.

First, if we really need central pressure monitoring—and this should be a very careful and judicious decision—probably a Swan-Ganz catheter rather than simply a CVP monitor would be preferable. Second, as our patients are hospitalized and moved through the process of preoperative, intraoperative, and postoperative care, they are exposed to and interface with a large number of individuals and medical units. We are the sole source of continuity of care and must at times be a buffer against potential adverse and detrimental diagnostic and/or therapeutic practices.

E.A. Luce, M.D.

Topical Antiseptic Mouthwash in Oncological Surgery of the Oral Cavity and Oropharynx

Redleaf MI, Bauer CA (Univ of Chicago; Univ of Iowa Hosps and Clinics, Iowa City)
J Laryngol Otol 108:973–979, 1994   12–23

Objective.—While the use of perioperative IV antibiotics has decreased the rate of wound complications in upper aerodigestive tract surgery, small studies of the effectiveness of topical antibiotics or antiseptic solutions have led to inconclusive results. The outcome of a wound study in 106 patients who underwent head and neck oral and pharyngeal surgery is presented.

Methods.—The results of oral cavity and oropharyngeal surgery were retrospectively evaluated in 106 patients, 43 of whom received a preoperative antiseptic preparation after induction and tracheal intubation and 3 rinses of 10% povidone-iodine. Demographic data and disease characteristics, medical and treatment histories, and type of wound closure were recorded. All but 5 patients were given IV antibiotic treatment preoperatively and postoperatively.

Results.—There were no differences between groups with respect to demographic, medical or treatment history, or type of wound closure. The mouthwash group was significantly younger than the non-mouthwash group. Seven percent of the mouthwash group had poor teeth whereas 24% of the non-mouthwash group had poor teeth. Previous radiation or surgery, disease stage, and use of preoperative mouthwash were significantly associated with less frequent and less severe wound complications.

Primary wound closure and free flap wound closure led to better wound healing than did pedicled flap closure. Dentition and age had no effect on wound outcome. Patients having neck surgery were 25% as likely to have a good wound outcome. Postoperative use of antistaphylococcal antibiotics improved wound healing results.

Conclusion.—Use of preoperative mouthwash, and probably the method of applying it, decreased the likelihood of wound complication by 23 to 40 times. The effect was independent of other factors. Povidone-iodine solution appears to have potentiated the effect of the mouthwash. Antiseptic mouthwash probably reduces the incidence of wound complications by decreasing the concentrations of bacteria and fungi.

▶ First, the critique of this paper is that although prospective, the study was probably not random and certainly not double blinded (see Methods), yet it is a significant effort. These authors used an iodine solution instead of some of the past antibiotic-based materials, and that choice certainly may have contributed to their good results. Regardless, the results are phenomenal and probably little downside exists. Many surgeons don't bother to prep the oral cavity, including myself (at least in the past), but perhaps we should start.

E.A. Luce, M.D.

Laryngeal Preservation for Advanced Laryngeal and Hypopharyngeal Cancers
Clayman GL, Weber RS, Guillamondegui O, Byers RM, Wolf PF, Frankenthaler RA, Morrison WH, Garden AS, Hong WK, Goepfert H (Univ of Texas, Houston)
Arch Otolaryngol Head Neck Surg 121:219–223, 1995   12–24

Background.—A prospective multicenter trial of induction chemotherapy combined with definitive radiotherapy was begun in 1985 to learn whether this is a viable alternative to surgical treatment for patients with stage III/IV squamous cell cancer of the larynx. The interim results suggest no substantial difference in disease-free survival rates. The larynx was preserved in 64% of all patients, as well as 64% of those who remained alive without disease.

Objective.—The effectiveness of laryngeal preservation therapy was examined in 55 patients seen at a single center with stage III or IV squamous cell cancer of the larynx or hypopharynx. Each patient was matched for age, stage, and site of disease with 2 surgical control patients treated in 1975–1990.

Management.—Study patients received cisplatin-based induction chemotherapy that included fluorouracil, with or without bleomycin. Laryngoscopy and CT scanning were done after 2 cycles of chemotherapy. Patients who had at least a partial response received a third cycle, followed by definitive radiotherapy. Otherwise, resection was immediately carried out and postoperative radiotherapy delivered.

Results.—A complete response was documented in 38% of the study patients after chemotherapy and a partial response in 31%; the remaining 31% of patients had stable disease. After chemotherapy and radiotherapy, 64% of the patients had a complete and 22% had a partial response; 14% had stable disease. The larynx was preserved in two thirds of the patients with laryngeal cancer. These patients had a 2-year survival rate of 56%, not significantly different from the 71% rate in their respective surgical controls. The 18 patients requiring salvage laryngectomy had a 2-year survival rate of 75% vs. 80% for matched control patients. Patients with hypopharyngeal cancer had results comparable to those of their surgical controls.

Summing Up.—Laryngeal preservation is feasible in patients with advanced-stage cancer, but the role and cost-effectiveness of chemotherapy vs. radiotherapy alone—remains uncertain.

▶ This study supports the conclusions of other studies that have documented the efficacy of organ preservation in *advanced* laryngeal cancer. Their ability to preserve the larynx in two thirds of the cases is consistent with other studies and should be the impetus to investigate such an approach in the treatment of intermediate-stage (T2 and T3) disease. Please note that this group from M.D. Anderson is similar in experience to others who have yielded such results by the facile detection of local failure and aggressive pursuit of surgical salvage, certainly one of the keys to outcome. As the authors note, the specific role of inductive chemotherapy vs. radiotherapy alone needs further definition.

E.A. Luce, M.D.

Prognosis of Recurrent Laryngeal Carcinoma After Laryngectomy
Yuen APW, Ho CM, Wei WI, Lam LK (Univ of Hong Kong)
Head Neck 17:526–530, 1995   12–25

Background.—Many patients undergoing total laryngectomy for advanced laryngeal carcinoma experience disease recurrence at the pharynx, tracheostome, neck lymph node, or distant sites postoperatively. The efficacy of surgical salvage for recurrent tumor after total laryngectomy was evaluated in the present study.

Patients and Methods.—One hundred sixty-five patients who experienced tumor recurrences after total laryngectomy for laryngeal squamous cell carcinoma between 1971 and 1990 were evaluated. Patients with tumors that could clearly be resected and that permitted tissue reconstruction underwent surgical salvage, whereas those whose tumors were extensively infiltrative, fixed to the prevertebral muscles or bony structures, or extended to the mediastinum received palliative treatment only. Survival was compared between groups.

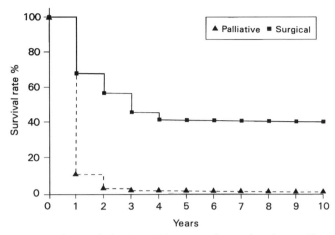

FIGURE 1.—Actuarial survival of patients with recurrent laryngeal carcinoma. (Courtesy of Yuen APW, Ho CM, Wei WI, et al: Prognosis of recurrent laryngeal carcinoma after laryngectomy, *Head Neck*, copyright 1995. Reprinted by permission of John Wiley & Sons, Inc.)

Results.—Thirty-four patients underwent surgical salvage, and 131 were given palliative care. The mean time of detection of recurrence from the date of initial laryngectomy was 12 months in patients undergoing surgical salvage and 11 months in those receiving palliative care. Among the 34 surgical salvage patients, there were 11 pharyngeal, 3 tracheostomal, 15 nodal, and 2 pharyngeal plus nodal recurrences. The remaining 3 patients had pulmonary metastasis from the laryngeal carcinoma. The highest salvage rates were noted for pharyngeal, nodal, and pulmonary recurrences, in that order. Sixteen patients, including all patients with tracheostomal recurrence, had recurrent tumors after surgical salvage, for a rate of 44%. Of all patients undergoing surgical salvage, death occurred as a result of surgical complications in 2, tumor recurrence in 15, and unrelated causes in 4. The remaining 13 patients were alive and tumor free at the last follow-up. Among the 131 patients treated palliatively, only 2 who received chemotherapy for distant metastasis survived for more than 24 months. The 5-year actuarial survival rate was 42% for the surgical salvage patients and 2% for those receiving palliative care, and the median survival duration was 32 months and 7 months, respectively (Fig 1).

Conclusions.—Surgical salvage for recurrent tumor after total laryngectomy is associated with an acceptable prognosis. Careful monitoring of patients after the initial operation is important for early identification of recurrence, a time when surgical salvage is still an option.

▶ Several worthy points arise from this paper, and of these the most important is that locoregional recurrence after total laryngectomy has a dismal outcome. Although the thrust of this article is to advocate radical surgery, actually only 1 out of 5 patients with a recurrence qualified for resection, and fewer than half of those survived 5 years. Another point is to question the benefit of "palliative" chemoradiotherapy for recurrence that is not amenable to resection. The mean survival with chemoradiotherapy was 7 months, and the 5-year survival was essentially zero. The final point has to do with the site of recurrence. Tracheostomal recurrence in these authors' hands, and in this reviewer's experience, is incurable, in contrast to reports by others. Our approach has been to resect the tumor and use postoperative radiotherapy, but recognize the palliative approach in light of mediastinal persistence.

Finally, as this paper advocates, these patients need to be monitored carefully, particularly for the occurrence of dysphagia, which is indicative of a pharyngeal recurrence, because that site is the most likely to be cured by secondary salvage surgery.

E.A. Luce, M.D.

Management of the Recurrent Laryngeal Nerve in Suspected and Proven Thyroid Cancer
Falk SA, McCaffrey TV (Univ of Rochester, NY; Mayo Clinic, Rochester, Minn)
Otolaryngol Head Neck Surg 113:42–48, 1995   12–26

Background.—When a thyroid nodule is associated with paralysis of the ipsilateral vocal cord, invasive cancer is very likely, but occasionally benign disease may be present. The recurrent laryngeal nerve (RLN) should be preserved whenever possible because function may return if benign disease is responsible for the paralysis. Recovery is also possible when lymphoma is treated by irradiation. Conversely, the RLN may be infiltrated even if there is no cord dysfunction.

Objective.—Management and outcome were reviewed for 296 patients given primary treatment for invasive thyroid cancer in 1940–1990. Of the 262 patients with invasive papillary carcinoma, 123 were found to have invasion of the RLN and 24 of these patients lacked invasion of any other structures.

Observations.—Only 5 of the 24 patients with papillary cancer infiltrating the RLN had cord paralysis. These patients and 12 of the 19 with normal vocal cord function had complete tumor excision. Two of 17 patients died after complete excision. One of the 78 patients with incomplete tumor excision died of disease. In a larger series of 480 patients having thyroid surgery for benign or malignant disease (including the 24 study patients), 25 patients had vocal cord paralysis associated with infiltration of the RLN, and 2 (with lymphoma and Reidel's thyroiditis) recovered cord function. Of 6 patients with cord paralysis but an intact RLN, 3 recovered function. Thirty patients with infiltration of the RLN nevertheless retained normal vocal cord function. They included patients with lymphoma, Graves' disease, and thyroiditis.

Recommendations.—Patients with vocal cord paralysis associated with benign or malignant nodules, in whom the RLN is not infiltrated, may recover vocal cord function. When operating on a suspicious nodule in a patient with cord paralysis, the RLN should be identified, but resected only if infiltrated by carcinoma.

▶ A Mayo Clinic–type paper in that the recommendations afforded in the "discussion" portion give the readers some solid and useful clinical information. They also reiterate the point that vocal cord paralysis in benign disease is really quite rare.

E.A. Luce, M.D.

The Free Flap and Plate in Oromandibular Reconstruction: Long-Term Review and Indications
Boyd JB, Mulholland RS, Davidson J, Gullane PJ, Rotstein LE, Brown DH, Freeman JE, Irish JC (Univ of Toronto)
Plast Reconstr Surg 95:1018–1028, 1995   12–27

Objective.—In the present study, the long-term results of oromandibular reconstruction using a radial forearm flap with either the radius or a reconstruction plate for mandibular replacement were compared. Reconstructions using a plate together with a fasciocutaneous flap were also evaluated in an effort to clearly define the role of this plate-flap option. Finally, the durability of the THORP (titanium hollow-screw reconstruction plate) system was compared with the comparable stainless steel product.
Patients and Methods.—Seventy-one consecutive patients with oral cancer necessitating composite resection and reconstruction over a 4-year period were enrolled in 1 of 2 studies. The first study included 31 patients, 15 of whom were assigned to oromandibular reconstruction with a radial forearm osteocutaneous flap and 16 of whom received a radial forearm fasciocutaneous flap along with a mandibular reconstruction plate. Patient demographics were similar between groups. In the second study, 40 patients received a radial forearm fasciocutaneous flap with a reconstruction plate, including a stainless steel plate in 21 and a THORP-type plate in 19. The previously published HCL classification system was used to compare outcomes by mandibular defect in this latter study (Fig 5). All patients were followed prospectively. Successful reconstructions were defined as those not requiring removal. Because these patients also had limited life expectancy, days of life lost, referring to the amount of time a patient spends in the hospital for the initial surgery, as well as for second operative procedures and complications occurring as a result of the original reconstruction, were also evaluated and incorporated into the definition of surgical success.
Results.—The mean follow-up of study 1 patients was 21.4 months. Among patients in the bone group, no perioperative deaths occurred. A

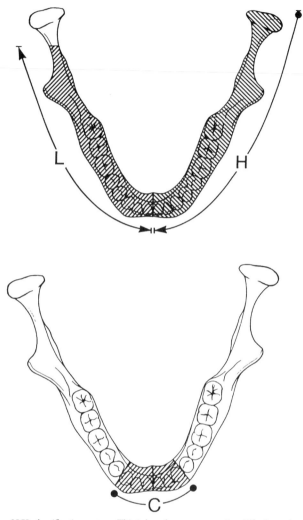

FIGURE 5.—HCL classification system. This is based on reconstructive difficulty rather than on classic anatomical landmarks. C represents the central segment of the mandible containing the canines and the incisor teeth. For C to be included in the designation, the *whole* segment must be present. L represents a lateral segment of *any length* minus the condyle. It may encroach on the C segment but would only be termed *LC* if the entire C segment were part of it. *H* is the same as *L* except that it includes a condyle. Thus there are only 8 possibilities: C, L, H, CL, CH, LCL, HCL, and HCH. To this bony defect the letters *m*, *s*, and *ms* may be added to signify an additional requirement for mucosa, skin, or both, respectively. (Courtesy of Boyd JB, Mulholland RS, Davidson J, et al: The free flap and plate in oromandibular reconstruction: Long-term review and indications. *Plast Reconstr Surg* 95:1018–1028, May 1995.)

general complication rate of 20% was noted, and average days of life lost amounted to 4 days. No reconstructive failures occurred in the bone group patients.

In the plate group, general complications were noted in 42.9%. An overall failure rate of 33.3% was noted for plate and free-flap mandibular

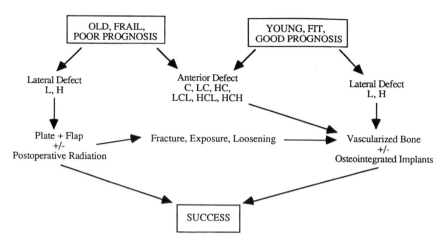

FIGURE 12.—Reconstructive algorithm using the findings from the present study. An additional benefit of using a plate in a patient who is to receive postoperative radiotherapy is that a secondary vascularized bone graft will not be exposed to radiation and will therefore more easily tolerate osteointegrated implants. See Figure 5 for definitions of defects. (Courtesy of Boyd JB, Mulholland RS, Davidson J, et al: The free flap and plate in oromandibular reconstruction: Long-term review and indications. *Plast Reconstr Surg* 95:1018–1028, May 1995.)

reconstructions, occurring on average at 14.3 months postoperatively. In this group, the mean number of days lost because of subsequent surgery was 35.

The average follow-up of study 2 patients was 20 months. Plates were removed in 21% of the patients because of intraoral and extraoral exposure, plate fracture, or loosening at an average of 11.9 months postoperatively. Anterior defects were associated with a failure rate of 35% vs. 5% for pure lateral defects, the difference being significant. The stainless steel and THORP plates failed 23.8% and 15.8% of the time, respectively. Although the difference was not significant, a trend toward better durability was noted with use of the THORP plates.

Conclusions.—The use of vascularized autogenous bone was associated with better reconstructive survival and less days of life lost than was the sole use of metallic plates. An overall success rate of 78.9% was observed for mandibular plate reconstruction, although analysis by anterior and lateral defect types revealed significant differences in failure rates. These findings suggest that plate reconstruction should be performed only for lateral defects among patients with unfavorable prognoses (Fig 12).

▶ This paper is remarkable from a couple of different aspects. First, the authors made the effort to reassess a conclusion reached from a prior paper, namely, that a free flap plus reconstruction plate was adequate for mandibular reconstruction in patients with head and neck cancer. The problem with the prior paper was that the follow-up was only an average of 9 to 12 months. This paper, as you can ascertain, reaches an entirely different conclusion based on a longer follow-up.

The other aspect is the critical sense that this particular group of authors adopt toward their analysis of results. Again, this is another example of a paper that the reader may wish to read in total because of the excellent and concise discussion.

Unfortunately, although the conclusion reached is that the fibula is the optimal donor site for mandibular reconstruction, the skin component is not as reliable, nor does it provide the qualities that radial forearm skin bring to the reconstruction.

E.A. Luce, M.D.

Primary Mandibular Reconstruction With the Titanium Hollow Screw Reconstruction Plate: Evaluation of 51 Cases
Irish JC, Gullane PJ, Gilbert RW, Brown DH, Birt BD, Boyd JB (Sunnybrook Health Science Centre, Toronto; Univ of Toronto)
Plast Reconstr Surg 96:93–99, 1995   12–28

Background.—Methods of surgical reconstruction of the mandible that employ Vitallium or stainless steel autogenous trays packed with cancellous bone have met with failure in hostile irradiated beds. Improved methods of soft tissue coverage have led to the recent success of alloplastic methods in recreating the mandibular arch. A more solid method, the titanium hollow-screw reconstruction plate (THORP), was evaluated for its efficacy in mandibular reconstruction.

Methods.—Ninety percent of the 51 patients undergoing mandibulectomies in this study had surgery for squamous cell carcinoma of the oral cavity. To be included in this study, patients were required to have had a resection of more than 50% of a region (Fig 1). The surgery was a primary method of treatment in 76% of the cases, with 35% undergoing radiation after surgery. The THORP system is composed of hollow titanium screws and a malleable titanium plate. Correctly sized plates were selected for each patient; they were placed after intraoral soft tissue reconstruction. After surgery, plate failure was determined.

Results.—Plate failure was defined as flap necrosis, plate extrusion, plate fracture, or any problem that required subsequent surgical correction. Plate failure occurred in 24% of the patients. The average time before failure was identified was 17 months after surgery. Patients who required more than 6 cm of mucosal resection of tissue had a failure rate of 21%; those requiring resection of 4 to 6 cm of tissue had a failure rate of 22%. Neither the extent nor the location of the bone defect affected plate failure. The incidence of failure increased as the nature of the bone resection became more radical. Four failures were early (<1 month after surgery) and 8 were considered late. The incidence of failure occurring in patients consuming a normal postoperative diet (26%) as compared with those who required a gastrostomy (29%) was not significantly different. Although 61% of the patients undergoing this procedure were alive after 1 year, only 41% survived to 2 years.

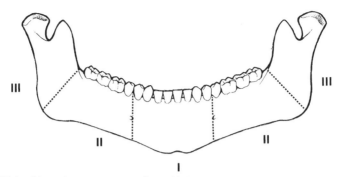

FIGURE 1.—Schematic representation of mandibular regions. (Courtesy of Irish JC, Gullane PJ, Gilbert RW, et al: Primary mandibular reconstruction with the titanium hollow screw reconstruction plate: Evaluation of 51 cases. *Plast Reconstr Surg* 96:93–99, July 1995.)

Discussion.—In an earlier evaluation of the AO system, the investigators found that this plate failed as a consequence of screw loosening or fracture. In this study, they found that the THORP system failed because of fracture at the distal arm. The primary location of the tumor did not affect the failure rate. The investigators conclude that titanium reconstruction in combination with a cutaneous or myocutaneous flap has a high success rate for primary alloplastic mandibular reconstruction. Patients surviving to 18 to 24 months after a first surgery may be candidates for secondary reconstruction.

▶ These authors have had tremendous experience in reconstruction in the head and neck, and the posture taken in this paper, namely, that a reconstruction plate plus flap will suffice for patients with advanced cancer of the head and neck, is a distinct change from past publications from the same group. In essence, they now advocate delay before definitive reconstruction because so many patients will succumb and the reconstruction plate is satisfactory three fourths of the time.

In a somewhat cavalier fashion, however, they suggest reconstruction secondarily at 24 months. That task is easier said than done because most will receive radiation and late reconstruction with free tissue transfer in a heavily irradiated head and neck patient is considerably more difficult than primary reconstruction.

E.A. Luce, M.D.

Morbidity and Functional Outcome of Free Jejunal Transfer Reconstruction for Circumferential Defects of the Pharynx and Cervical Esophagus

Reece GP, Schusterman MA, Miller MJ, Kroll SS, Robb GL, Baldwin BJ, Luethcke DR (Univ of Texas, Houston)

Plast Reconstr Surg 96:1307–1316, 1995   12–29

Background.—Although free jejunal transfer is considered the procedure of choice for pharyngoesophageal reconstruction at many medical facilities, various technique-related concerns have been raised. These include the reliability of the microvascular anastomoses required for free jejunal transfer, a high rate of complications, poor tolerance of postoperative radiation therapy, dysphagia from hyperperistalsis of the transferred jejunum, and unfavorable speech patterns after surgery. Experience with free jejunal transfer reconstruction was therefore retrospectively evaluated in an effort to determine the validity of these concerns.

Patients and Methods.—Ninety-three patients (mean age, 60 years) undergoing 96 free jejunal transfers for repair of circumferential pharyngoesophageal defects over a 5-year period were reviewed. Approximately 50% of the patients had undergone previous surgery and/or preoperative radiation treatment. Although the study was retrospective, data pertaining to patient and tumor traits, adjuvant therapy, defects, reconstruction times, and outcomes were prospectively collected for all patients. Patients receiving a Blom-Singer prosthesis after surgery were evaluated by a speech pathologist at an average of 27 postoperative months. Diet histories were also obtained and cinefluorographic barium examinations performed in all patients 7 to 14 days postoperatively to evaluate swallowing.

Results.—The most common indication for free jejunal transfer reconstruction was immediate repair of pharyngoesophageal defects after laryngopharyngectomy and bilateral lymph node dissection (Table 2). The procedure was completed in 3–12 hours (mean, 6.6 hours). The overall success rate was 97%. Three flaps failed despite salvage attempts, but all 3 were successfully repaired with repeated free jejunal transfer. Major surgical complications were noted in 33 patients, and second surgical

TABLE 2.—Indications for Free Jejunal Transfer Reconstruction

Indication	No. of Cases
Immediate reconstruction	
Laryngopharyngectomy + BLND	89
Pharyngectomy (larynx spared)	1
Delayed reconstruction	
Pharyngocutaneous fistula	2
Failed colon interposition	1
Failed free jejunal transfer	3
Total free jejunal transfers performed	96

Abbreviation: BLND, bilateral lymph node dissection.
(Courtesy of Reece GP, Schusterman MA, Miller MJ, et al: Morbidity and functional outcome of free jejunal transfer reconstruction for circumferential defects of the pharynx and cervical esophagus. *Plast Reconstr Surg* 96:1307–1316, November 1995.)

TABLE 8.—Postoperative Radiation Therapy and Selected Complications

Number of Patients (%)*

Complication	No Postoperative Radiation Therapy† (n = 43)	Postoperative Radiation Therapy‡ (n = 48)	P
Wound-healing problem	12 (28)	8 (17)	0.149
Fistula	9 (21)	8 (17)	0.399
Stricture	8 (19)	6 (13)	0.303
Tube feeding dependence	13 (30)	5 (10)	0.017

* Excludes the 2 patients who died in the perioperative period.
† Mean follow-up of 14 months.
‡ Mean follow-up of 17 months.
(Courtesy of Reece GP, Schusterman MA, Miller MJ, et al: Morbidity and functional outcome of free jejunal transfer reconstruction for circumferential defects of the pharynx and cervical esophagus. *Plast Reconstr Surg* 96:1307–1316, November 1995.)

procedures were needed in 18. The most frequent reconstructive site complication was fistula formation (19%). This occurred with equal frequency at the proximal and distal anastomoses. Fistulas closed spontaneously in 11 patients, whereas 4 patients required surgical closure. In 3 patients with recurrent tumor, the fistula was not repaired. Strictures were also noted in 15% of the patients. The most frequent donor site complication was small-bowel obstruction, with partial obstruction occurring in 3 patients and complete obstruction occurring in 1. All partial obstructions resolved with conservative management.

In patients undergoing tracheoesophageal puncture, voice quality was excellent in 3, good in 7, and poor in 2. Three patients required removal of the Blom-Singer prosthesis because they were unable to manage this device. Seventy-three patients tolerated a regular or liquid diet after reconstruction. Forty-eight patients received postoperative radiation therapy, which did not appear to adversely affect wound healing, fistula or structure formation, or swallowing (Table 8). Fewer patients undergoing postoperative radiation required supplemental tube feedings than did those not undergoing such therapy. A total of 2 perioperative deaths occurred.

Conclusions.—Pharyngoesophageal reconstruction can effectively be accomplished with free jejunal transfer. This technique is associated with acceptable morbidity and low mortality, and postoperative radiation therapy is well tolerated.

▶ This is an exhaustive study by a group of authors who are comfortable with the ultimate techniques in microvascular reconstruction of the head and neck, including the radial forearm, yet have continued to select the free jejunum for reconstruction of the pharynx and cervical esophagus. This paper is not the final answer. Their technical results were superb, with only 3% flap loss, and about 55% to 60% of their patients were able to take a regular diet, about as good as can be expected in this difficult problem. Their complication rate was not exactly trivial; fistulas developed in one fifth of their patients, almost half of whom required surgery whereas the fistulas in the others could not be closed. Yet all series of pharyngeal-esophageal reconstruction report significant complication rates.

The real argument here is between free radial forearm vs. jejunum for reconstruction. The former has undeniably better voice results with tracheoesophageal puncture; the latter has *perhaps* a lower morbidity rate and certainly fulfills the reconstructive credo: "Reconstruct like with like."

E.A. Luce, M.D.

Postoperative Radiation of Free Jejunal Autografts in Patients With Advanced Cancer of the Head and Neck
Cole CJ, Garden AS, Frankenthaler RA, Reece GP, Morrison WH, Ang KK, Peters LJ (Univ of Texas, Houston)
Cancer 75:2356–2360, 1995   12–30

Introduction.—At many centers, free jejunal transfer is the preferred means of reconstructing defects of the hypopharynx and cervical esophagus. The procedure is a relatively rapid one, provides early return of function, and lessens the risk of hospital mortality. Speech rehabilitation is a possibility, and the interval to adjuvant radiotherapy is shortened. Typically the radiation dose limit is 45–50 Gy, but patients with head/neck cancer frequently require higher doses to adequately control local disease.

Patients.—Complications of radiotherapy were examined in 29 patients with free jejunal autografts who received postoperative radiotherapy. Twenty patients had squamous cell cancer of the hypopharynx, 5 of the oropharynx, and 2 of the larynx. Two patients had papillary carcinoma of the thyroid gland. Seventy percent of the patients had pathologic stage T4 disease.

Treatment.—The median interval from surgery to radiotherapy was 34 days. The median dose to the tumor bed and autograft was 63 Gy. Cobalt-60 γ-rays or 6-MV photons were used in all cases.

Complications.—Two of the 29 patients had confluent mucositis involving more than half the graft, and 18 patients had less extensive mucositis. Weight loss was limited by placement of a gastrostomy tube in all but 4 patients. No patient had problems related to viability of the jejunal autograft. All patients but 1 were able to continue taking at least a soft diet. Disease was controlled above the clavicles in 71% of the patients 2 years after treatment.

Discussion.—Patients requiring postoperative radiation for advanced head/neck cancer may safely be treated even if a free jejunal autograft is present. Apparently the displaced small bowel tolerates higher radiation doses than does the in situ organ. The question of late complications remains open.

▶ The paper presents fairly conclusive evidence that postoperative radiation can be given in full therapeutic doses without fear of an enhanced rate of complications. Some authors recently have favored a radial forearm flap rather than free jejunum in these reconstructive situations because of concerns about radiation effects to the jejunum. Actually, the free radial forearm flap wouldn't be particularly happy with these doses either. The next question to be answered, as the authors intimate at the end of the article, is whether more aggressive radiotherapeutic regimens (hyperfractionation) can be tolerated by the free jejunal segment.

E.A. Luce, M.D.

Microvascular Craniofacial Reconstruction in Cancer Patients
Miller MJ, Schusterman MA, Reece GP, Kroll SS (Univ of Texas, Houston)
Ann Surg Oncol 2:145–150, 1995   12–31

Purpose.—In patients with large malignancies of the cranium, scalp, or middle or upper third of the face, resection may necessitate combined bone and soft tissue defects. Some of these defects will involve exposed dura and carry a risk of contamination from the contiguous paranasal sinuses. Conventional reconstruction is often inadequate for some of the more aggressive combined resections performed today. The results of microvascular reconstruction for patients with such craniofacial defects are reported.

Experience.—A total of 54 craniofacial reconstructions were performed in 50 consecutive patients, with a free-flap success rate of 96%. Seven patients had significant wound complications for a rate of 13.5%. The donor site morbidity rate was 11%. Forty of the 50 patients underwent immediate reconstruction. Eight patients had a history of previous treatment with surgery, 4 with radiotherapy, and 34 with both surgery and radiotherapy. Complications and free-flap survival were not significantly affected by the timing or dose of preoperative irradiation or by previous neck dissection.

Discussion.—Good results are reported with free tissue transfer for the reconstruction of large craniofacial defects resulting from cancer resection (Fig 3). These patients require a multidisciplinary approach to management, with close cooperation between the neurosurgery, ablative head and neck surgery, and reconstructive surgery personnel. With a cooperative approach, reconstructive microsurgical procedures can be performed more safely and successfully than ever.

▶ A topical, descriptive paper, worthwhile for the oncologic surgeon who has not been exposed to the versatility of microvascular reconstruction and cranial base resections.

E.A. Luce, M.D.

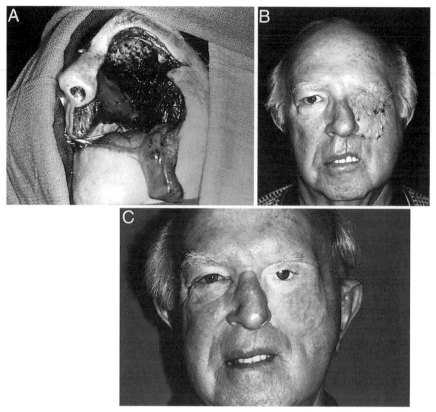

FIGURE 3.—**A,** orbitomaxillary defect including resection of the base of the skull. **B,** result 3 months after reconstruction with a rectus abdominis muscle free flap and split-thickness skin graft. **C,** view with an external prosthesis in place. (Courtesy of Miller MJ, Schusterman MA, Reece GP, et al: Microvascular craniofacial reconstruction in cancer patients. *Ann Surg Oncol* 2:145–150, 1995.)

Modified Neoglottis Reconstruction Following Total Laryngectomy: Long-Term Follow-Up and Results

Brandenburg JH, Patil N, Swift EW (Univ of Wisconsin, Madison)
Laryngoscope 105:714–716, 1995   12–32

Introduction.—Restoration of optimal speech is a major goal in patients requiring total laryngectomy. Previous efforts have been limited to esophageal speech, use of an artificial larynx, and a valved vocal prosthesis used with tracheoesophageal puncture (TEP). An alternative approach, the "Brandenburg neoglottis" procedure, involves constructing a myomucosal shunt to reintroduce air from the trachea into the hypopharynx.

> *Technique.*—An anterior segment of the first 4 tracheal rings measuring about 1 cm in width is removed with heavy scissors and the endotracheal tube moved inferiorly. The walls of the upper

rings are then reapproximated anteriorly with interrupted 3-0 polyglactin sutures, starting with the mucosa. The resultant triangular-shaped tube becomes the neoglottis. A vertical 1-cm incision is made in the midline through the anterior wall of the upper part of the esophagus about 1 cm below the inferior margin of the pharyngostome. The upper end of the neoglottis is placed through this opening, and the esophageal mucosa is joined to the rim of the neoglottis. A second-layer closure includes the muscularis and submucosa. The lower margin of the pharyngostome is reflected on itself and sutured to the anterior and anterolateral part of the upper margin of the neoglottis. Finally A "T" closure of the pharyngostome is done in 3 layers.

Patients.—Forty-five patients have had this operation after total laryngectomy for resection of T3 or T4 squamous cell carcinoma of the larynx. Ten patients were treated for persistent cancer after having first received radiotherapy. Ten other patients received planned postoperative radiotherapy.

Results.—All but 3 of the 45 patients were able to vocalize after surgery, and 35 (78%) were still speaking with a functional neoglottis after an average follow-up of 6 years. Twenty-four of these patients required 1 or more revision procedures because of liquid aspiration persisting for 3 months or longer. In 2 of the earlier patients, hypopharyngeal/cutaneous fistulas developed but healed spontaneously, and 3 had wound infections. Sixteen of the 18 patients interviewed were using their neoglottal voice.

Conclusions.—This neoglottis is a very effective alternative TEP and a prosthetic valve for patients requiring total laryngectomy. The new neoglottis should be shielded from radiotherapy to avoid a dysfunctional shunt.

▶ This is one of very few papers with long-term follow-up on some of the neoglottic techniques for the totally laryngectomized patient. This particular author has performed this technique for almost 20 years, and his paper is worthy of review. Yet the same criticisms that applied when these techniques were first described are still valid today. One significant contraindication in terms of anatomical location of the primary exists, namely, subglottic, some transglottic, most postcricoid, and certainly large piriform sinus lesions would be compromised oncologically by the technique. Second, aspiration remains a problem in this series and in others. In this particular group of patients, over half of the total required secondary procedures for aspiration. Third, the area of neoglottic reconstruction must be shielded postoperatively for the development of satisfactory voice quality. The area to be shielded is actually a significantly high priority for the ports in postoperative radiotherapy, the tracheoesophageal groove. We still don't have a good technique for neoglottic reconstruction, at least in this reviewer's opinion.

E.A. Luce, M.D.

Emerging Role of β-Carotene and Antioxidant Nutrients in Prevention of Oral Cancer

Garewal HS, Schantz S (Univ of Arizona, Tucson; Veterans Affairs Med Ctr, Tucson, Ariz; Mem Sloan-Kettering Cancer Ctr, New York)
Arch Otolaryngol Head Neck Surg 121:141–144, 1995   12–33

Introduction.—Oral cancer is responsible for 42,000 new cases and 12,000 deaths each year in the United States. More than 75% of these cancers are attributed to alcohol and tobacco, so abstinence from these agents is of major preventive importance. There is also considerable evidence suggesting that antioxidants, β-carotene, and vitamin E may play major roles in preventing these cancers. This study reviews the benefits of β-carotene and vitamin E in the prevention of oral cancer.

Discussion.—Low carotenoid intake has been linked to increased cancer risk in several epidemiologic studies. All these studies cite β-carotene as protection for laryngeal and pharyngeal cancers. Other epidemiologic studies of vitamin E also suggest increased protection against oral cancer. Laboratory evidence has shown that retinoids (isotretinoin, retinyl acetate), β-carotene, and vitamin E inhibit cancerous growth in animal models. Although most premalignant lesions of the oral cavity are leukoplakia, their malignant potential is low. However, several interventional trials have attempted to reverse leukoplakia with antioxidants such as β-carotene and vitamin E, but the results of these studies have not definitively proved whether these agents prevent cancer. Leukoplakia studies continue throughout the world, and in all these trials retinoid toxicity remains a serious problem.

Conclusions.—Although the cumulative evidence from epidemiologic, laboratory, and interventional studies suggest that β-carotene and other antioxidants may play key roles in preventing malignancy of the oral cavity, much research is still needed to determine how these agents affect cancer prevention. The results of recent studies are encouraging, and prospective, controlled clinical trials should be given high priority on the national research agenda.

▶ This paper is worth reading because it is an excellent review of the use of antioxidant substances as chemopreventive agents in head and neck cancer. A couple of problems exist. Although β-carotene and vitamin E are relatively innocuous substances, the more powerful retinoid agents (isotretinoin) have significant toxic side effects, including hepatic toxicity, that at present prevent long-term therapy trials. As the authors describe, we need some large-scale prospective clinical trials to examine β-carotene, vitamin E, and other more nontoxic substances as dietary chemopreventive agents.

E.A. Luce, M.D.

Care of the Terminal Head and Neck Cancer Patient in the Hospice Setting

Talmi YP, Roth Y, Waller A, Chesnin V, Adunski A, Lander MI, Kronenberg J (Tel Aviv Univ, Israel)
Laryngoscope 105:315–318, 1995   12–34

Background.—Deciding on where a terminally ill patient wishes to die is a significant concern for physicians, patients, and families. Hospice facilities offer an alternative to the hospital or household setting, and a growing number of patients with terminal head and neck cancer are choosing to end their lives in such facilities. The characteristics of 67 patients with terminal head and neck cancer admitted to a hospice facility were retrospectively analyzed in an effort to better define the problems and needs of these individuals.

Patients and Findings.—Thirty-four men and 3 women were included in the study. The mean age was 65 years for males and 70 years for females. The mean time from detection of disease to hospice admission was 4 years. The mean time from admission to death was 13 days vs. 18 days for the entire hospice population. Tumor sites in patients with head and neck cancer included the oral cavity, thyroid gland, skin, larynx, nasopharynx, maxilla, hypopharynx, major salivary gland, and esophagus (Table 1). Tumor histology was unknown or unrecorded in 5 patients and included squamous cell, anaplastic, undifferentiated, adenoid cystic, melanoma, basosquamous, follicular, medullary, and papillary types in the remainder of the patients. Of the 62 patients treated with curative intent, most had undergone surgery or radiation therapy. Chemotherapy had also been used, but primarily as tertiary treatment. Two patients were not treated, and 3 received palliative treatment only. Weight loss was documented in 63 patients, most of whom experienced moderate to severe losses. Twenty-two patients had feeding problems, and 11 required a feeding tube, gastrotomy, or jejunostomy. Airway problems were noted in 15 patients, and 17 patients had a temporary or permanent tracheotomy. Severe bleeding from the primary or regional tumor site was recorded in 4 patients and massive bleeding in another 2 patients. Despite the high proportion of

TABLE 1.—Tumor Site in Patients With Head and Neck Cancer (N = 67)

Tumor Site	Number of Cases
Oral cavity	16
Thyroid gland	12
Skin	11
Larynx	11
Nasopharynx	7
Maxilla	6
Hypopharynx	3
Major salivary gland	1
Esophagus (second primary in 1 patient)	1

(Courtesy of Talmi YP, Roth Y, Waller A, et al: Care of the terminal head and neck cancer patient in the hospice setting. *Laryngoscope* 105:315–318, 1995.)

physical dysfunction, only 5 patients reported concerns about body image. Pain was the most significant symptom in the majority of patients, and 88% had been receiving chronic pain medication before hospice admission. Sixty percent had problems with severe pain, 22% had light to moderate pain, and 17% had incapacitating pain. A combination of oral and parenteral analgesics was used to alleviate pain in all patients, based on the analgesic ladder recommended by the World Health Organization. Oral or intramuscular morphine and IV dexacort and amitriptyline represented the most commonly used agents. Dosing was liberal, although no patient-controlled anesthesia was available.

Conclusions.—Nearly 50% of patients with head and neck cancer die of their disease. Such patients may receive better palliative treatment and emotional support in the hospice setting, given that patients are managed by physicians and nurses trained in care of the dying. Further studies of hospice care for patients with terminal neck and head cancer are recommended.

▶ This paper focuses on a little-discussed topic in the care of the head and neck cancer patient, namely, the terminal aspect. I relearned a couple things from the authors' experience, namely, the short stay for such patients in a hospice setting (half died within 10 days of admission) and the efficacy of the use of clinical steroids on a short-term basis. The euphoric effect of steroids in my experience is short-lived (10–14 days), but that "window" would benefit the majority of patients in this series.

E.A. Luce, M.D.

Demographic Portrayal and Outcome Analysis of Head and Neck Cancer Surgery in the Elderly

McGuirt WF, Davis SP III (Wake Forest Univ, Winston-Salem, NC)
Arch Otolaryngol Head Neck Surg 121:150–154, 1995   12–35

Objective.—The outcome of surgery for head/neck cancer was reviewed in 217 patients aged 65 years and older. The primary site was the oral cavity in 45% of the patients, the larynx in 25%, and the pharynx in 15%.

Management.—Half the patients had their lesions locally resected, as by parotidectomy or partial glossectomy. Another 41% required extended resectional procedures such as laryngectomy and mandibulectomy, and 9% of the patients had radical neck dissection. Eleven percent of the patients had flap reconstruction. More than one fourth of the patients received radiotherapy.

Observations.—Nearly one third of the patients had postoperative complications, but only 13% died or incurred major complications. The perioperative mortality rate was 4%. Patients more than 75 years of age tended to have more severe complications and were likelier to die perioperatively. Eighty percent of the surviving patients were discharged within 3 weeks of surgery and only 5% were hospitalized longer than 1 month. More than half the patients hospitalized for longer than 2 weeks were 82 years of age or older.

Discussion.—Chronologic age does not in itself predict the mortality risk of surgery in elderly patients with head/neck cancer. Major complications have been infrequent. Early ambulation, adequate nutritional support, and self-care measures should all be emphasized.

▶ Several series of elderly head and neck cancer patients have been published in the past, but this study is noteworthy because of the size, over 200 patients. The authors make a point that deserves re-emphasis, namely, a decision made solely on the basis of age to withhold or compromise therapy or to utilize inappropriate therapies such as radiation when surgery is indicated are terribly inappropriate. A 90-year-old has better than 4 years of life expectancy according to life tables, and if one decides on some type of palliation with the expectation that natural causes will intervene, one will probably then have a 91-year-old with the same or worse cancer problem.

E.A. Luce, M.D.

13 Vascular Surgery

Introduction

A further step was taken this year in resolving the controversy surrounding the value of carotid endarterectomy in the treatment of carotid atherosclerosis. With publication of the Asymptomatic Carotid Artery Stenosis study (Abstract 13–1), carotid endarterectomy was shown to significantly benefit asymptomatic patients with carotid stenoses of 60% or greater when the stroke risk associated with the procedure is less than 3% and the patient survives for 5 years after the procedure. However, using only the degree of stenosis to identify patients who will benefit from treatment of asymptomatic carotid atherosclerosis was inexact as stroke reduction was only 1% per year. Further work will be required to better identify asymptomatic patients at risk for stroke, and transcranial detection of asymptomatic cerebral emboli (Abstract 13–6) may help locate the unstable carotid plaque that puts the patient at risk for ipsilateral ischemic neurologic events. Increasing use of carotid endarterectomy also means increased cost for the health care system, and ways of decreasing the cost associated with the procedure while maintaining good results are being explored (Abstracts 13–2 and 13–3).

Screening of selected populations for abdominal aortic aneurysm and elective surgical repair of these aneurysms has also been shown to decrease mortality in patients who are offered screening (Abstract 13–10). Once this finding is confirmed, elective aneurysm repair will likely be more widely used, even in selected patients over 80 years of age (Abstract 13–9). The potential of endoluminal repair of arterial lesions, particularly abdominal aortic aneurysms, has also stimulated a great deal of interest because of the reduced morbidity associated with this procedure. Parodi, who developed the concept of the stent graft, reported encouraging results this year from his first 50 patients treated with endoluminal stent grafting (Abstract 13–8). However, long-term follow-up of sufficient patients to determine whether stent grafting of abdominal aortic aneurysms will prevent future aneurysm rupture (as does surgical repair) remains to be done, and recent anecdotal reports have demonstrated subsequent rupture of aneurysms treated with endoluminal stent grafts. Thus surgical repair remains the standard treatment of abdominal aortic aneurysms, and identifying methods of decreasing the risk associated with surgical repair, such as avoiding intraoperative hypothermia (Abstract 13–7), remains important.

The success of infrainguinal bypass for the treatment of arterial occlusive disease has traditionally been judged on parameters of hemodynamic improvement and long-term graft patency. However, from the patient's point of view, improvement in lower extremity function is most important, and as the patient's perception of our treatment of peripheral vascular disease begins to be evaluated, some interesting observations are being made. From the patient's perspective, lower extremity function is better after surgical bypass than after balloon angioplasty or noninvasive therapy despite complete recuperation after surgery requiring up to 6 months. In addition, the most important determinant of functional outcome is the level of function prior to treatment (Abstracts 13–17 and 13–16). This suggests that patients should be treated earlier in the course of their disease, such as the use of femorotibial bypass in selected patients who only have intermittent claudication (Abstract 13–13). However, such treatment must still be associated with excellent hemodynamic results and excellent long-term graft patency as the adage remains that "there is no patient who cannot be made worse by arterial surgery."

Use of duplex venous imaging has made detection of venous thrombosis easy and allowed insight into the relatively high incidence of this problem in patients with peripheral vascular disease (Abstract 13–22). However, duplex venous imaging is not cheap, and use of this technique to screen for deep venous thrombosis in all trauma patients is not cost-effective (Abstract 13–21). Rather, screening of high-risk patients and symptomatic patients has been suggested, although this approach is untested. The time required for duplex venous scanning and thus the cost of the procedure can be reduced by not scanning the contralateral leg when deep venous thrombosis is found in the symptomatic leg, and this has been shown to be safe (Abstract 13–23). Finally, demonstration of the efficacy of transesophageal echocardiography in patients suspected of having acute, traumatic aortic disruption (Abstract 13–26) should decrease both the cost and risk associated with treatment of this serious problem as arteriography can be avoided in most patients.

James M. Seeger, M.D.

Cerebrovascular

Endarterectomy for Asymptomatic Carotid Artery Stenosis
Executive Committee for the Asymptomatic Carotid Atherosclerosis Study
(Asymptomatic Carotid Atherosclerosis Study)
JAMA 273:1421–1428, 1995   13–1

Background.—In 1987, the Asymptomatic Carotid Atherosclerosis Study (ACAS) was initiated to determine whether the addition of carotid endarterectomy (CEA) to aggressive reduction of modifiable risk factors and treatment with aspirin would decrease the incidence of cerebral infarction in patients with asymptomatic carotid artery stenosis.

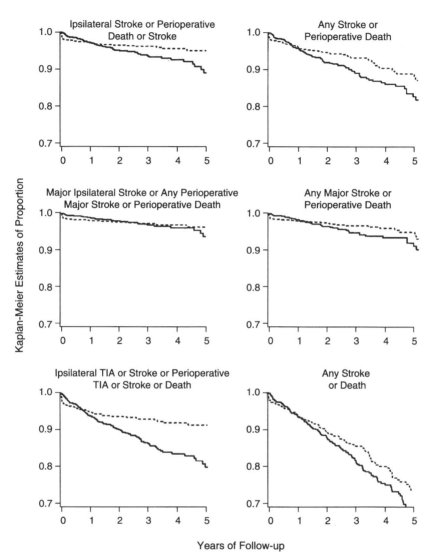

FIGURE.—Proportion of patients without an end point at a given time during follow-up by treatment group using the Kaplan-Meier estimation method. The *solid line* indicates medical patients; the *broken line,* surgical patients. *Abbreviation: TIA,* transient ischemic attack. (Courtesy of *JAMA,* May 10, 1995, 273:1421–1428, Copyright 1995, American Medical Association.)

Patients and Methods.—A total of 1,662 patients (mean age, 67 years) with asymptomatic carotid artery stenosis of 60% or greater were enrolled in the ACAS study, and 1,659 were available for follow-up. All patients received treatment with daily aspirin and medical risk factor management, and 825 were also randomly assigned to CEA. Transient ischemic attack or cerebral infarction in the distribution of the study artery and any transient ischemic attack, stroke, or mortality observed perioperatively were the main outcome measures. During the last 9 months of the study, these were changed to cerebral infarction in the distribution of the study artery or any stroke or mortality occurring perioperatively. Median follow-up was 2.7 years.

Results.—Baseline risk factors for stroke were comparable between the medical and surgical treatment groups. During the perioperative period, 2.3% of the CEA patients had a stroke or died. At the median follow-up, the aggregate risk over 5 years for ipsilateral stroke and any stroke or mortality occurring perioperatively was approximately 5.1% for patients assigned to CEA and 11.0% for those receiving medical treatment only (risk reduction, 53%; $P = 0.004$) (Fig). In men, CEA reduced the stroke rate by 55%, whereas the reduction in women was only 17% ($P =$ NS). This lack of efficacy of CEA in women was largely due to a higher (3.6%) perioperative stroke risk. The degree of stenosis did not influence the likelihood of risk reduction by CEA, although only 29% of the patients in this study had stenoses greater than 80%.

Conclusions.—Carotid endarterectomy performed with less than 3% perioperative morbidity and mortality and combined with aggressive management of modifiable risk factors can help reduce the 5-year risk of ipsilateral stroke in patients with asymptomatic carotid artery stenosis of 60% or greater.

▶ Management of patients with asymptomatic carotid stenosis remains controversial. Although this large, multicenter trial demonstrated the benefit of carotid endarterectomy in patients with asymptomatic stenosis of less than 60%, a significant benefit was not seen in women (largely due to an increased perioperative stroke risk) and the overall stroke risk reduction was modest (11.0% to 5.1%). In addition, the risk of stroke did not increase as the degree of carotid stenosis increased to between 60% and 99%. Thus other markers, such as those described in Abstract 140-96-13–6, will need to be found to allow better identification of patients with asymptomatic carotid stenosis who are most likely to have an ipsilateral stroke without carotid endarterectomy so that endarterectomy will not need to be done in 20 patients to prevent 1 stroke.

J.M. Seeger, M.D.

Early Discharge After Carotid Endarterectomy
Harbaugh KS, Harbaugh RE (Dartmouth-Hitchcock Med Ctr, Lebanon, NH)
Neurosurgery 37:219–225, 1995   13–2

Rationale.—It is expected that carotid endarterectomy will be done increasingly often, which raises concern over the financial consequences of this trend and less intensive postoperative monitoring. Early discharge after carotid endarterectomy can reduce costs but must be safe and effec-

tive. Complications were reviewed in a series of 233 consecutive procedures done in 195 patients under the direction of a single neurosurgeon to
learn whether early discharge and less intensive postoperative monitoring
will compromise the outcome.

Patients.—Men constituted nearly two thirds of the series, the average
age was 69 years, and risk factors for atherosclerotic carotid stenosis were
present in more than 90% of the patients. All but 15 patients were
symptomatic and had a transient or fixed hemispheric or retinal ischemic
deficit. Four patients had previously had carotid endarterectomy. All operations were done under general anesthesia.

Outcome.—No patient died perioperatively, stroke occurred in 5 patients (2.6%) but was ipsilateral in only 3 (1.3%), and myocardial infarction occurred in 3 patients (1.3%). Complications occurred either within
36 hours of surgery or not until 1–2 weeks after surgery. Patients were
discharged after 2.5 days on average, and in the final year of the study the
postoperative hospital time averaged 1.6 days.

Conclusions.—Patients who are neurologically and hemodynamically
stable immediately after carotid endarterectomy may safely be discharged
early.

Short-Stay Carotid Endarterectomy Is Safe and Cost-Effective
Kraiss LW, Kilberg L, Critch S, Johansen KH (Univ of Washington, Seattle;
Providence Med Ctr, Seattle)
Am J Surg 169:512–515, 1995   13–3

Introduction.—The common protocol for performing carotid endarterectomy (CEA) includes a preceding contrast arteriogram, the use of general
anesthesia with cerebral perfusion monitoring, and postoperative admission to the ICU. It would be expected that performing CEA with alternative protocols could be less expensive, provided that safety and effectiveness are maintained. A more streamlined protocol that eliminates routine
preoperative arteriography and postoperative ICU admission and that uses
regional anesthesia was studied.

Methods.—Over a 2-year period, 2 groups of patients underwent CEA
performed with either the alternative protocol (group I, 18 patients) or the
conventional protocol (group II, 178 patients). Group I patients underwent preoperative duplex scans routinely and carotid angiography only
when occlusion or an atypical disease pattern was present. Regional anesthesia was used without cerebral perfusion monitoring. Patients were
admitted to the ICU only when ICU services were clearly needed. Data on
operative risk, perioperative complications, use of vasoactive medication,
ICU admission, hosital length of stay, and charges were compared for the
2 groups.

Results.—The groups had comparable operative risks. There were no
perioperative complications in group I, whereas 1 death (1%) and 6

postoperative strokes (3%) occurred in group II. Twenty-two percent of the patients in group I were admitted to the ICU as compared with 98% of group II, even though only 20% of the patients in group II received vasoactive medication. The average length of stay was 1.3 days for group I and 3.1 days for group II, and average hospital charges were $5,861 for group I and $11,140 for group II.

Conclusions.—These results suggest a favorable complication rate and reduced cost for CEA performed without routine carotid arteriography and ICU admission, but these findings require confirmation with a larger group.

▶ These 2 articles demonstrate that complications after carotid endarterectomy generally occur within 36 hours of the procedure and that CEA done in conjunction with duplex ultrasound for carotid imaging, regional anesthesia, selective ICU admission, and early discharge is both safe and cost-effective. Changes in practice stimulated by cost containment can lead to benefits for the patient.

J.M. Seeger, M.D.

Clinical Outcome in Patients With Mild and Moderate Carotid Artery Stenosis

Johnson BF, Verlato F, Bergelin RO, Primozich JF, Strandness DE Jr (Univ of Washington, Seattle)
J Vasc Surg 21:120–126, 1995   13–4

Objective.—Duplex ultrasonography was used to investigate the rate of progression of mild carotid artery stenosis, defined as narrowing of less than 50%, and moderate stenosis, defined as 50%–79% narrowing.

Methods.—A total of 232 patients who had a carotid bruit and less than 80% luminal narrowing at the outset and no associated symptoms had bilateral carotid duplex studies annually for up to 10 years. Sufficient data for a 7-year life-table analysis were collected.

Results.—The degree of stenosis increased in 23% of the patients during follow-up, and severe (80% or greater) stenosis or occlusion developed in nearly half of these patients. The risk of progression to 50%–79% stenosis or 80%–99% stenosis was 3%/yr and 0.6%/yr for patients with initial stenoses less than 50%, whereas the risk of progression to 80%–99% stenosis or occlusion for patients with initial stenoses of 50%–79% was 3.7%/yr and 2.9%/yr, respectively. The cumulative risk of stroke after 7 years was 6% in patients with mild initial stenosis and 11% for those with moderate initial stenosis. This led to a recommendation of yearly examination for asymptomatic patients with carotid stenoses of 50%–79% and examination every 2 years for those with stenoses less than 50%.

Conclusion.—Monitoring the course of initially asymptomatic carotid stenosis by duplex ultrasonography permits a realistic assessment of the risk that an ischemic cerebrovascular event will take place.

▶ Appropriate follow-up of patients with asymptomatic carotid stenosis has been difficult to determine because the rate of progression of various degrees of carotid stenosis has been unclear. This study demonstrates that patients with stenosis less than 50% can probably be examined only every 2–3 years, while those with stenosis greater than 50% need yearly exams.

J.M. Seeger, M.D.

Perioperative Imaging Strategies for Carotid Endarterectomy: An Analysis of Morbidity and Cost-Effectiveness in Symptomatic Patients
Kent KC, Kuntz KM, Patel MR, Kim D, Klufas RA, Whittemore AD, Polak JF, Skillman JJ, Edelman RR (Beth Israel Hosp, Boston; Brigham and Women's Hosp, Boston; Harvard Med School, Boston)
JAMA 274:888–893, 1995   13–5

Introduction.—The traditional method of evaluating the carotid bifurcation before endarterectomy is contrast angiography. However, some centers now use noninvasive tests instead, such as duplex sonography and MR angiography (MRA). Sufficiently high accuracies must be demonstrated for the noninvasive imaging studies, which are appealing as a replacement for carotid angiography because of their lower cost, because any potential cost advantage or reduction may be offset by false-negative or false-positive results. If a patient with 70% to 99% stenosis does not have carotid endarterectomy because the patient has been identified as having a low-grade stenosis by duplex sonography, the patient has a 15% greater risk of having a stroke. A decision analysis model was used to identify the least morbid approach to preoperative evaluation of symptomatic candidates for carotid endarterectomy and assess the cost-effectiveness of competing diagnostic strategies.

Methods.—Four diagnostic strategies for evaluating 81 potential candidates for carotid endarterectomy were examined for their cost-effectiveness: duplex sonography, MRA, contrast angiography, and the combination of duplex sonography and MRA supplemented by contrast angiography for disparate results. The outcome measure was determined as incremental cost per quality-adjusted year of life gained.

Results.—Of the 4 options considered, the combination of duplex ultrasound and MRA resulted in the greatest quality-adjusted life expectancy. In contrast, duplex sonography alone resulted in the lowest quality-adjusted life expectancy and MRA or contrast angiography alone were not cost-effective. Although the combination of tests was more effective, the combination was more expensive than duplex sonography and incurred an additional cost of $22,400 per quality-adjusted year of life gained.

Conclusion.—Quality-adjusted life expectancy is maximized through the combination of MRA and duplex sonography, with carotid angiography reserved for disparate results. The next least expensive option is duplex sonography.

▶ Avoiding cerebral arteriography with its associated risk of stroke further decreases the morbidity and expense associated with the treatment of carotid disease. However, at present, none of the noninvasive techniques for imaging the carotid bifurcation are as accurate as angiography. This study suggests that combining duplex ultrasound and MRA is the safest and most cost-effective imaging strategy for carotid endarterectomy. This still seems cumbersome and, hopefully, as MRA and duplex ultrasound evolve, one of these techniques alone will be of sufficient accuracy to use for imaging prior to carotid endarterectomy.

J.M. Seeger, M.D.

Cerebral Microembolism and the Risk of Ischemia in Asymptomatic High-Grade Internal Carotid Artery Stenosis

Siebler M, Nachtmann A, Sitzer M, Rose G, Kleinschmidt A, Rademacher J, Steinmetz H (Heinrich-Heine-Universität Düsseldorf, Germany)
Stroke 26:2184–2186, 1995   13–6

Background.—Management of asymptomatic internal carotid artery disease, which has a 1% to 2% annual risk of ischemic stroke, has benefited from the recognition of several risk factors. Recently, the presence of clinically silent cerebral microemboli in the ipsilateral middle cerebral artery has been suggested as an additional risk factor. The clinical importance of cerebral microembolism in asymptomatic patients with high-grade internal carotid artery stenosis was studied.

Methods.—Sixty-four asymptomatic patients with unilateral 70% to 90% internal carotid artery stenosis underwent transcranial Doppler sonography at the start of the study period and at follow-up visits. The end point of the study for a patient occurred when an ischemic symptom or sign developed that could be attributed to the diseased internal carotid artery.

Results.—The mean follow-up period was 72 weeks. Of 154 transcranial Doppler recordings from the 64 patients, 8 recordings from 8 patients revealed 2 or more microemboli per hour in the ipsilateral middle cerebral artery. Ischemic symptoms developed on the appropriate side in 5 patients, 3 of whom had 2 or more microemboli per hour. Thus there was a highly significant association of 2 or more microemboli per hour and a subsequent ipsilateral cerebral or retinal ischemic event, with an odds ratio of 31 (excluding 16 patients who dropped out for reasons unrelated to ischemic symptoms).

Conclusion.—By using a threshold criterion of 2 or more microemboli per hour, transcranial Doppler sonography predicted 3 of 5 cerebral or retinal ischemic events ipsilateral to the stenotic internal carotid artery.

▶ This brief article is intriguing. If emboli detected by transcranial Doppler could be used to identify patients with asymptomatic carotid stenosis at high risk for stroke, carotid endarterectomy potentially could be done only in patients who clearly would benefit.

J.M. Seeger, M.D.

Aid

Hypothermia During Elective Abdominal Aortic Aneurysm Repair: The High Price of Avoidable Morbidity

Bush HL Jr, Hydo LJ, Fischer E, Fantini GA, Silane MF, Barie PS (Cornell Univ, New York)
J Vasc Surg 21:392–402, 1995   13–7

Background.—Hypothermia is a common occurrence during abdominal aortic aneurysm (AAA) repair. Although hypothermia could help protect tissue during the ischemic period caused by aortic cross-clamping, it may also be associated with adverse effects involving decreased oxygen delivery at the microcirculatory level. A retrospective study was performed to evaluate the effects of intraoperative hypothermia on morbidity and mortality after elective abdominal aortic reconstruction.

Methods.—The review included 262 patients undergoing elective AAA repair. Data on core temperature, age, Acute Physiology and Chronic Health Evaluation (APACHE) II and III scores, fluid resuscitation, and perioperative organ dysfunction were collected prospectively. Hypothermia was defined as a temperature of less than 34.5°C.

Results.—The hypothermic and nonhypothermic patients were comparable in their preoperative risk factors, except that women had a higher risk of hypothermia. In the postoperative period, APACHE scores were significantly higher in the hypothermia group (Table 5). Hypothermic patients who died had significantly longer rewarming times, which suggested that marked hypoperfusion was present. Requirements for fluids,

TABLE 5.—Physiologic Status at the End of Surgery

	Normothermic	Hypothermic	Hypothermic Survivor	Hypothermic Nonsurvivor
Temperature (° C)	36.1 ± 0.1	34.0 ± 0.1*	34.0 ± 0.1	33.9 ± 0.2
Rewarming time (hr.)	1.0 ± 0.1	5.8 ± 0.4†	5.4 ± 0.4	9.0 ± 4.3‡
APACHE II	12.8 ± 0.4	17.0 ± 0.9*	15.4 ± 0.6	28.9 ± 4.9§
APACHE III	38.1 ± 1.1	57.1 ± 3.5*	51.1 ± 2.0	100.5 ± 17.1§
APACHE III-T	37.0 ± 1.3	46.5 ± 3.5†	40.5 ± 2.4	90.3 ± 17.3§

Note: The normothermic nonsurvivor group (n = 3) is not described separately because of insufficient numbers for statistical analysis.
 * *P* < 0.0002 vs. the normothermic group.
 † *P* < 0.05 vs. the normothermic group.
 ‡ *P* < 0.05 vs. the hypothermic survivor group.
 § *P* < 0.0001 vs. the hypothermic survivor group.
 Abbreviation: APACHE III-T, APACHE III score adjusted for temperature.
 (Courtesy of Bush HL Jr, Hydo LJ, Fischer E, et al: Hypothermia during elective abdominal aortic aneurysm repair: The high price of avoidable morbidity. *J Vasc Surg* 21:392–402, 1995.)

TABLE 7.—Univariate Analysis of Outcome Variables

	Normothermic	Hypothermic	Hypothermic Survivors	Hypothermic Nonsurvivors
SICU LOS (days)	5.3 ± 0.6	9.5 ± 1.9*	7.2 ± 1.2	25.9 ± 11.8†
Hospital LOS (days)	14.6 ± 0.8	23.1 ± 2.8‡	21.5 ± 2.2	34.6 ± 17.5
Mortality (%)	1.5	12.1‡		

Note: The normothermic nonsurvivor group (n = 3) is not described separately because of insufficient numbers for statistical analysis.
* *P* < 0.05 vs. the normothermic group.
† *P* < 0.01 vs. the hypothermic survivor group.
‡ *P* < 0.01 vs. the normothermic group.
Abbreviations: LOS, length of stay; *SICU*, surgical ICU.
(Courtesy of Bush HL Jr, Hydo LJ, Fischer E, et al: Hypothermia during elective abdominal aortic aneurysm repair: The high price of avoidable morbidity. *J Vasc Surg* 21:392–402, 1995.)

transfusion, vasopressors, and inotropic drugs were all greater in the hypothermic patients. Organ dysfunction occurred in 53% of the hypothermic patients vs. 29% of the nonhypothermic patients. Mortality was 12% vs. 2%. Mean length of stay in the ICU was 9 days for the hypothermic patients vs. 5 days for the nonhypothermic patients, and mean hospital stay was 24 vs. 15 days, respectively (Table 7). The only significant predictor of intraoperative hypothermia on multivariate analysis was female sex.

Conclusions.—The occurrence of hypothermia after AAA repair is associated with various physiologic abnormalities and with increased morbidity and mortality. Although there are many possible interacting etiologic factors in patients undergoing aortic surgery, maintenance of body temperature is one that can and should be controlled.

▶ This observation speaks for itself and shows that some very simple techniques such as keeping the patient warm can make a significant difference in morbidity and mortality after aortic surgery.

J.M. Seeger, M.D.

Endovascular Repair of Abdominal Aortic Aneurysms and Other Arterial Lesions
Parodi JC (Instituto Cardiovascular de Buenos Aires, Buenos Aires)
J Vasc Surg 21:549–557, 1995   13–8

Background.—Elective replacement with a synthetic graft has long been the accepted method to prevent rupture of an abdominal aortic aneurysm (AAA). The increasing number of older patients with severe comorbid medical conditions has led to a search for a simpler and less invasive treatment of this lesion. After a series of experiments in dogs, endovascular graft treatment of AAAs was introduced in the clinical setting. This procedure, which has now been performed on 50 patients with AAAs or aortoiliac aneurysms, is described here and its application also reported for 7 patients with other arterial lesions.

Methods.—Forty-five men and 5 women with an average age of 73 years were treated between September 1990 and April 1994. In all but 3 cases the diameter of the aneurysm was greater than 5 cm; none had ruptured. Other arterial lesions treated included 5 posttraumatic arteriovenous fistulas, 1 infected femoral false aneurysm, and 1 false aneurysm of the right common carotid artery. Associated pathologic conditions were common in the patient group, with severe, chronic heart disease in 25 and severe pulmonary insufficiency in 20. Devices used in endovascular graft treatment consisted of either a Dacron or an autogenous vein graft sutured to a balloon-expandable stent. The stented grafts were placed through remote arteriotomies, advanced under fluoroscopic guidance to predetermined sites, and then secured into position.

Results.—Forty (80%) procedures for AAA or aortoiliac exclusion were judged successful based on complete exclusion of the aneurysm and restoration of normal blood flow. Although 4 patients required a second covered stent to repair an initial leak, recovery after successful graft repair was rapid. Ten AAA procedures were failures, with procedural death in 5 cases and leaks in 5. All 7 patients with arteriovenous fistulas or false aneurysms had a successful outcome. With a mean follow-up of 17 months, the ultimate outcome has been satisfactory in those surviving the procedure.

Conclusion.—Based on these preliminary data and short-term follow-up, endovascular stented graft procedures appear to be feasible for treating AAAs and other arterial lesions. A number of technical problems related to the procedure and the serious complication of microembolization that led to death in 3 of 4 cases are yet to be resolved.

▶ Parodi pioneered this exciting new technique for the less invasive repair of abdominal aortic aneurysms and other vascular lesions. His large experience points out the initial benefits and risks of endovascular repair of abdominal aortic aneurysms. However, sufficient long-term follow-up is not available at present to determine whether these endoluminal grafts will as reliably exclude aneurysms and prevent rupture as standard surgical repair does. Until these data are available, endoluminal repair of arterial lesions with stent grafts must remain experimental so that problems similar to those associated with early widespread use of laser angioplasty will not occur.

J.M. Seeger, M.D.

Ten-Year Experience With Abdominal Aortic Aneurysm Repair in Octogenarians: Early Results and Late Outcome

O'Hara PJ, Hertzer NR, Krajewski LP, Tan M, Xiong X, Beven EG (Cleveland Clinic Found, Ohio)

J Vasc Surg 21:830–838, 1995   13–9

Introduction.—The long-term benefits of any major surgical procedure in the very elderly, abdominal aortic aneurysm (AAA) repair included, raises concerns about quality of life, morbidity, mortality, and financial expenditures. The mortality, morbidity, and late survival rates associated with AAA resection in octogenarians was evaluated to help identify clinical factors that may influence outcome.

Methods.—Retrospective data from 114 consecutive patients aged 80 or older were collected. Eight patients underwent juxtarenal AAA repair and 106 had infrarenal repair. Of these, there were 89 men and 25 women with a mean age of 83 years at the time of surgery. Of 20 patients with symptoms, 11 were admitted with intact AAAs and 9 had ruptured. The mean size of the AAA was 6.7 cm. The AAA repairs consisted of aortic bifurcation grafts in 77, tube grafts in 35, and extra-abdominal procedures in 2. Eighty-one patients were evaluated by coronary angiography sometime before AAA repair. Twenty-four patients underwent coronary artery bypass and 5 had transluminal coronary angioplasty at a mean of 36 months before AAA repair.

Results.—The 30-day mortality rate for these patients was 14% (Table 2). It declined from 23% within the first 5 years to 8% during the second 5 years. Nine of the 94 patients with asymptomatic AAAs had fatal complications, as did 7 of the 20 patients with preoperative symptoms. The early mortality rate was 4% for patients who received myocardial revascularization before AAA repair vs. 12% for those who did not. The cumulative 5-year survival rate for these patients was 48%. The cumulative 5-year survival rate for patients with previous myocardial revascularization was 75%, as compared with 30% for patients who did not have

TABLE 2.—Early (30 Day) Operative Mortality Data

	Entire Series (1984–1993)			First 5 Years (1984–1988)			Second 5 Years (1989–1993)			
	No.	Operative Deaths	%	No.	Operative Deaths	%	No.	Operative Deaths	%	P^*
Asymptomatic	94	9	9.6	41	7	17	53	2	3.8	0.038
Symptomatic	20	7	35	7	4	57	13	3	23	NS
Intact	11	4	36	5	3	60	6	1	17	NS
Ruptured	9	3	33	2	1	50	7	2	29	NS
Total	114	16	14	48	11	23	66	5	7.5	0.028

(Courtesy of O'Hara PJ, Hertzer NR, Krajewski LP, et al: Ten-year experience with abdominal aortic aneurysm repair in octogenarians: Early results and late outcome. *J Vasc Surg* 21:830–838, 1995.)

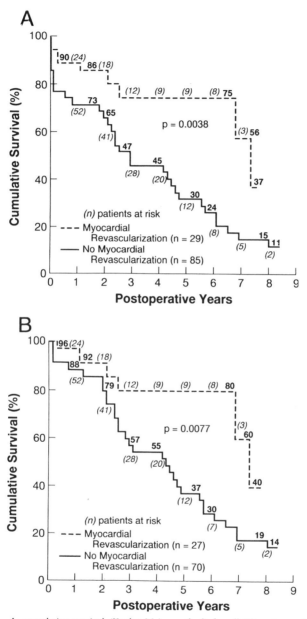

FIGURE 2.—**A,** cumulative survival (Kaplan-Meier method) for all 29 patients who underwent previous coronary artery bypass or transluminal coronary angioplasty before abdominal aortic aneurysm repair (AAA) and for 85 others who did not. Survival distributions are significantly different ($P = 0.0038$, log-rank test). **B,** cumulative survival (Kaplan-Meier method) for 27 operative survivors who underwent previous coronary artery bypass or transluminal coronary angioplasty before AAA repair and for 70 operative survivors who did not. Survival distributions are significantly different ($P = 0.0077$, log-rank test). (Courtesy of O'Hara PJ, Hertzer NR, Krajewski LP, et al: Ten-year experience with abdominal aortic aneurysm repair in octogenarians: Early results and late outcome. *J Vasc Surg* 21:830–838, 1995.)

revascularization (Fig 2, A). A high perioperative homologous blood transfusion requirement was also associated with a deleterious effect on both early and late survival.

Conclusion.—In very elderly patients, AAA repair is relatively safe and this surgery should not be withheld on the basis of advanced age alone. Late survival was favorably influenced by a low perioperative homologous transfusion requirement and a history of previous myocardial revascularization. However, patients in this cohort who undergo AAA must be carefully selected.

▶ Age is no longer an exclusion criterion for AAA repair. However, the mortality associated with AAA repair in patients in their 80s is higher than in younger patients, so careful patient selection is necessary. The improved survival in patients who had undergone myocardial revascularization in this study is in contrast to results in younger patients, where initial cardiac mortality is unaffected by cardiac revascularization. In addition, a previous report from the Mayo Clinic also demonstrated no long-term survival advantages in patients undergoing AAA repair who had also undergone coronary artery bypass.

J.M. Seeger, M.D.

Influence of Screening on the Incidence of Ruptured Abdominal Aortic Aneurysm: 5-Year Results of a Randomized Controlled Study
Scott RAP, Wilson NM, Ashton HA, Kay DN (St Richard's Hosp, Chichester, England)
Br J Surg 82:1066–1070, 1995   13–10

Introduction.—The overall mortality of ruptured aneurysms is 80% to 94%, and in the United Kingdom, ruptured abdominal aortic aneurysm (AAA) is responsible for 1.2% of all deaths in men aged 65 years and older. In contrast, a mortality rate of less than 5% is associated with elective surgery for AAA. Screening for AAA was conducted and compared with a control group to determine the effect of detection and repair of AAA on overall mortality.

Methods.—The study included 15,775 patients aged 65–80 years. The group was divided into 7,888 controls and 7,887 who were invited to be screened with an ultrasound for AAA, 5,394 of whom accepted. An aortic diameter greater than 3 cm was considered aneurysmal, 3.0- to 4.4-cm aneurysms were rescanned at 12-month intervals, 4.5- to 5.9-cm aneurysms were rescanned at 3-month intervals, and 6.0-cm or greater aneurysms were repaired.

Results.—In the screened group, AAAs were found in 218 patients (4% of all patients, 7.6% of the men, and 1.3% of the women). In the screened group 90 had satisfied the criteria for surgery, 35 of whom (31 men) had surgery. Of those who had surgery, 31 had elective surgery with no deaths at 1 year, and 4 had an emergency operation, 3 of whom died. In the group of 2,493 patients who declined screening, 5 died of aneurysm rupture, 4 of whom died without surgery. In the control group, 20 had a rupture and 17 died within 1 year. Therefore, in men invited for screening, the incidence of aortic aneurysm rupture was reduced by 55% in comparison to controls, whereas in women the incidence of rupture was low for both groups. In addition, the mortality rate in the group that refused screening was nearly twice that of the group that accepted screening, 19% vs. 10.4%.

Conclusions.—Ultrasound screen of men aged 65 and older can lower the overall mortality associated with AAA rupture. An ultrasound examination should be conducted in men once at the age of 65 and again at age 70.

▶ The mortality associated with aortic aneurysm rupture has remained constant for the last 20 years. This study demonstrates that screening of selected populations reduces the incidence of abdominal aortic aneurysm rupture and mortality associated with this problem. Because of the high cost associated with treatment of a ruptured AAA, screening and elective repair of AAAs will likely be a cost-effective approach to this difficult problem.

J.M. Seeger, M.D.

Outcome and Expansion Rate of 57 Thoracoabdominal Aortic Aneurysms Managed Nonoperatively
Cambria RA, Glovicki P, Stanson AW, Cherry KJ Jr, Bower TC, Hallett JW Jr, Pairolero PC (Mayo Clinic and Found, Rochester, Minn)
Am J Surg 170:213–217, 1995   13–11

Introduction.—Surgical repair of thoracoabdominal aortic aneurysms (TAAAs) presents a considerable challenge. Mortality rates for elective repair are reported to be as high as 19%, and disabling complications occur in up to 30% of patients in certain subgroups. However, the natural history of patients with TAAAs who do not undergo surgical repair remains unclear. A series of 57 nonoperatively managed patients with TAAAs was reviewed to determine survival and the risk of aneurysm rupture.

Methods.—Patients with TAAAs were identified by reviewing all CT scans performed at the Mayo Clinic from 1987 through 1993 that indicated a diagnosis of aortic disease. Excluded were patients with aortic dissections or ruptured aneurysms or those who proceeded directly to aneurysm repair. The clinical course and CT data of eligible patients were reviewed and the aneurysms carefully measured and classified by Crawford's system. The reason for deferral of surgical repair was also noted. Mean follow-up was 37 months.

Results.—The mean age of the study group was 72 years; 33 patients were men and 24 were women. Nonoperative management of TAAAs was chosen because of aneurysm size being 5 cm or smaller (49%), surgical risk (32%), concomitant illness requiring treatment before TAAA repair

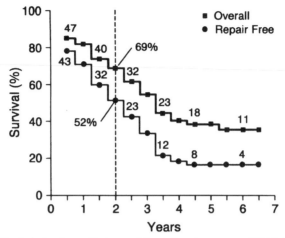

FIGURE 1.—Survival of patients with thoracoabdominal aortic aneurysms (TAAAs) initially managed nonoperatively. Numbers of patients are depicted above each line, and SEM is less than 10% for both lines. Cumulative survival rates in all patients (*squares*) at 2 and 5 years were 69% and 39%, respectively. Survival rates free of TAAA repair (*circles*) were 52% at 2 years (*dashed line*) and 17% at 5 years. (Reprinted by permission of the publisher from Cambria RA, Glovicki P, Stanson AW, et al: Outcome and expansion rate of 57 thoracoabdominal aortic aneurysms managed nonoperatively, *Am J Surg,* 170:312–217, Copyright 1995 by Excerpta Medica Inc.)

(14%), or patient preference (5%). The median diameter of TAAAs at diagnosis was 5.0 cm. Using the Crawford classification, 35% were type I; 14%, type II; 39%, type II; and 12%, type IV. Aneurysms of aortic segments distinct from the TAAA were present in 61% of the patients. Thirty-four (60%) patients died during follow-up. The median survival time for all patients was 3.3 years, and the overall survival rate at 5 years was 39%. Excluding the 15 patients who eventually underwent aneurysm repair, the 5-year survival rate was 23% (Fig 1). The overall risk of aneurysm rupture for patients managed nonoperatively was 12% at 2 years; for those with aneurysms larger than 5 cm, the risk was significantly higher (18%) (Fig 2). No rupture occurred in aneurysms 5 cm or smaller in size, but 5 of 8 ruptures occurred in aneurysms 6 cm or smaller in size. In addition, no ruptures occurred during treatment of a coexisting medical problem before TAAA repair. Twenty-nine of the 57 patients had follow-up CT scans at a mean of 2.4 years after the initial scan, and the mean rate of expansion was 0.2 cm/yr. The rate of expansion was related to the presence of chronic obstructive pulmonary disease, but not to aneurysm size at diagnosis (Fig 3).

Conclusion.—Patients selected for nonoperative management of TAAAs had a high mortality rate, but rupture is uncommon for aneurysms 5 cm or smaller in diameter. Surgical repair should be considered for otherwise healthy patients with TAAAs larger than 5 cm in diameter.

▶ The natural history of TAAAs is not as well defined as that of infrarenal abdominal aortic aneurysms. This, in combination with the significant risk

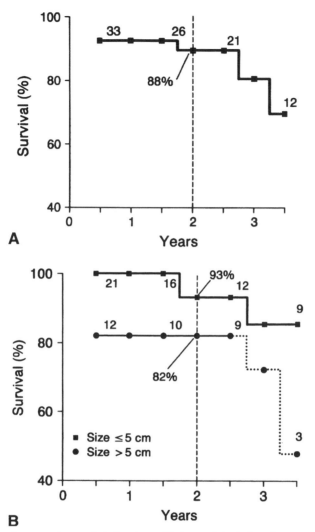

FIGURE 2.—A, rupture-free survival of patients with thoracoabdominal aortic aneurysm, excluding those who eventually had repair. Numbers of patients are depicted above each line, and SEM is less than 10% throughout. The cumulative 2-year risk of rupture was 12%. **B,** rupture-free survival of patients without eventual repair stratified by aneurysm size. Patients with aneurysms 5 cm or smaller in diameter (*squares*) had a significantly higher rupture-free survival (*P* < 0.05, log-rank statistic) than those with aneurysms larger than 5 cm (*circles*). Two-year rupture-free survival risks in both groups are noted at the *dashed line*. The *dotted line* indicates SEM greater than 10%. (Reprinted by permission of the publisher from Cambria RA, Glovicki P, Stanson AW, et al: Outcome and expansion rate of 57 thoracoabdominal aortic aneurysms managed nonoperatively, *Am J Surg*, 170:312–217, Copyright 1995 by Excerpta Medica Inc.)

associated with surgical repair, makes selection of patients for treatment of TAAAs difficult. This paper demonstrates that rupture is uncommon for TAAAs 5 cm or smaller in diameter and that delaying repair while another medical problem is corrected is not associated with undue risk. However,

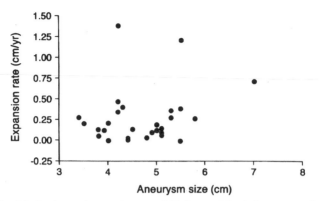

FIGURE 3.—Calculated annual expansion rate of 29 thoracoabdominal aneurysms determined by serial CT examination as related to aneurysm size at initial diagnosis. Note the lack of correlation between aneurysm size and the expansion rate and the propensity of aneurysms to expand at a rate of less than 0.4 cm/yr regardless of their size. (Reprinted by permission of the publisher from Cambria RA, Glovicki P, Stanson AW, et al: Outcome and expansion rate of 57 thoracoabdominal aortic aneurysms managed nonoperatively, *Am J Surg*, 170:312–217, Copyright 1995 by Excerpta Medica Inc.)

mortality for patients treated nonoperatively is high, and repair should be considered for TAAAs larger than 5 cm in diameter.

J.M. Seeger, M.D.

Limb Salvage and Patency After Aortic Reconstruction in Younger Patients

Allen BT, Rubin BG, Reilly JM, Thompson RW, Anderson CB, Flye MW, Sicard GA (Washington Univ, St Louis, Mo)
Am J Surg 170:188–192, 1995   13–12

Introduction.—Recent encounters with young patients with aortoiliac occlusive disease secondary to premature atherosclerosis prompted investigators to review their experience with a group of 56 patients who were 50 years old or younger. These patients were compared retrospectively with a similar group of 128 patients with atherosclerotic vascular disease who were older to determine the influence of age on patient characteristics, treatment, and prognosis after aortic reconstruction.

Methods.—Information on patient characteristics, perioperative course, postoperative graft function, and patient survival was gathered from data from the vascular registry, hospital charts, and vascular surgery office records. At follow-up, data were available on 51 of 56 patients in the younger group and 121 of 128 patients in the older group. About half the patients in the younger group were women.

Results.—There was a significantly larger number of active smokers in the younger group. However, there was a significantly greater number of pack-years in the older group. In contrast, the incidence of hypertension was significantly higher in the older group. No patients in the younger group and 4 patients in the older group died during their postoperative

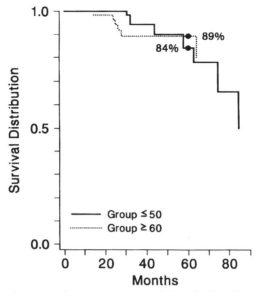

FIGURE 2.—Cumulative secondary patency rates as calculated by life-table analysis. The secondary patency at 60 months was 84% for the younger group and 89% for the older group. These differences were not significant ($P = 0.33$). (Reprinted by permission of the publisher from Allen BT, Rubin BG, Reilly JM, et al: Limb salvage and patency after aortic reconstruction in younger patients, *Am J Surg*, 170:188–192, Copyright 1995 by Excerpta Medica Inc.)

hospital stay or within 30 days of surgery. Cumulative primary and secondary patency rates were equivalent at 5 years in both the younger and older groups (primary patency, 64% and 67%; secondary patency, 84% and 89%, respectively; Fig 2). However, patients in the younger group had a significantly higher rate of revision (29%) than did the older group (8%) (Table). Although not significantly different, the number of revisions needed in the younger group was less after aortoiliac endarterectomy (2/13, 13%) than after aortofemoral bypass (11/29, 38%). Four and 6 patients in the younger and older groups, respectively, required major limb amputation.

TABLE.—Number of Patients With Revision and Mean Time to Revision by Patient Age Group

Age Group (yr)	Patients With Revision	Months to First Revision (Mean ± SEM)†
Group ≤50	15 (29%)	26.4 ± 5.0
Group ≥60	10 (8%)	21.7 ± 6.3

* $P = 0.0003$, chi-square analysis.
† $P = 0.72$, analysis of variance.
(Reprinted by permission of the publisher from Allen BT, Rubin BG, Reilly JM, et al: Limb salvage and patency after aortic reconstruction in younger patients, *Am J Surg*, 170:188–192, Copyright 1995 by Excerpta Medica Inc.)

Conclusion.—Younger patients with severely limiting or limb-threatening ischemia can be recommended to undergo aortoiliac revascularization. If they are willing to participate in a regular program of postoperative surveillance and undergo graft revisions when indicated, they can expect similar patency and risk of amputation as that of older patients.

▶ Young patients with aortoiliac occlusive disease represent a challenging problem. As shown here, they commonly abuse tobacco and have a higher incidence of graft failure. Limb salvage equivalent to that of older patients can be achieved, but only with multiple graft revisions, and both the patient and surgeon must be committed to frequent postoperative surveillance when aortic reconstruction is undertaken in these patients.

J.M. Seeger, M.D.

Infrainguinal

Femorotibial Bypass for Claudication: Do Results Justify an Aggressive Approach?
Conte MS, Belkin M, Donaldson MC, Baum P, Mannick JA, Whittemore AD
(Brigham & Women's Hosp, Boston; Harvard Med School, Boston)
J Vasc Surg 21:873–881, 1995   13–13

Introduction.—The role of infrageniculate arterial reconstructive surgery for claudication remains controversial. During the last 16 years, Brigham and Women's Hospital has liberally used femorotibial bypass procedures in a select group of patients with disabling claudication as part of an aggressive approach to limb salvage. A retrospective review of these procedures was conducted to define a role for tibial bypass in the management of severe claudication.

Patients.—From 1977 to 1993, 53 patients underwent 57 femorotibial reconstructions for claudication, representing 5% of all infrainguinal vein reconstructions. All reconstructions were performed with an autogenous vein conduit, 70% of which involved the greater saphenous vein in situ. Distal anastomoses were constructed to the tibioperoneal trunk in 12%, anterior tibial in 18%, posterior tibial in 47%, and peroneal artery in 23%. The mean follow-up for 45 grafts was 30 months.

Outcome.—There were no perioperative deaths, and major complications occurred in 9%. The overall 5-year survival rate was 54% and no limbs were lost. Cumulative primary and secondary graft patency at 5 years was 81% and 86%, respectively, and these rates were significantly better than those achieved in a concurrent series of tibial bypasses for limb salvage and equivalent to those achieved with femoropopliteal bypass for claudication (Table 4). Furthermore, cumulative successful palliation at 3 years did not differ significantly from that observed for femoropopliteal bypass for claudication. Follow-up interviews indicated that patients reported improved walking distance and a high degree of overall satisfaction with their operation.

TABLE 4.—Comparative 5-Year Results of Infrainguinal Vein Bypass: 1976–1993

	This Series (n = 57 Grafts)	FT/LS (n = 369 Grafts)	FP/CLAUD (n = 261 Grafts)
Survival (%)	54 ± 15	61 ± 4	78 ± 3*
Limb loss (%)	0	25 ± 2†	3 ± 1†
Primary patency (%)	81 ± 6	51 ± 4†	74 ± 3
Secondary patency (%)	86 ± 5	61 ± 4†	81 ± 3
Cumulative palliation (3 yr) (%)	71 ± 9	—	78 ± 3

* $P < 0.055$ vs. this series.
† $P < 0.01$ vs. this series.
(Courtesy of Conte MS, Belkin M, Donaldson MC, et al: Femorotibial bypass for claudication: Do results justify an aggressive approach? *J Vasc Surg* 21:873–881, 1995.)

Conclusions.—Patients at low risk who are severely limited by claudication and have available autogenous vein and suitable tibial outflow to the ischemic muscular bed should be considered for revascularization.

▶ Traditional teaching suggests that femorotibial arterial bypass should be reserved for treatment of patients with ischemic pain or tissue loss. As results improved, this procedure has also been used successfully for treatment of selected patients with severe claudication. However, autogenous conduit, good infrapopliteal vessels, and technical expertise, such as demonstrated by the Brigham group, are necessary before femorotibial bypass should be considered in patients who do not have limb-threatening ischemia.

J.M. Seeger, M.D.

Is Infrapopliteal Bypass Compromised by Distal Origin of the Proximal Anastomosis?
Brothers TE, Robison JG, Elliott BM, Arens C (Med Univ of South Carolina, Charleston)
Ann Vasc Surg 9:172–178, 1995   13–14

Background.—Some patients with severe infrapopliteal arterial occlusive disease will have relative sparing of the superficial femoral and popliteal arteries. For these patients, distal origin of the proximal anastomosis (DOPA) beyond the adductor hiatus can be used to minimize the graft length required and maximize the use of available autogenous conduit. The results of DOPA bypass were reviewed and compared with those of grafts originating more proximally (POPA).

Methods.—From 1986 to 1993, the investigators performed 62 DOPA infrapopliteal revascularizations using autogenous vein for limb salvage and 203 POPA infrapopliteal bypasses. The 2 groups were compared for limb salvage and patency results by life-table analysis.

Results.—At 54 months, primary patency rates were 57% with DOPA and 50% with POPA bypass, secondary patency rates were 78% and 65%, and limb salvage rates were 53% and 66%. None of these differences were significant. In both groups, patients with tissue necrosis had worse limb salvage results than those without this characteristic, 52% vs. 70%. Tissue necrosis was present in 71% of the DOPA group vs. 49% of the POPA group.

Conclusions.—The DOPA approach to infrapopliteal bypass appears to affect long-term patency to a limited degree. However, patients with atherosclerotic disease that involves the popliteal and tibial vessels while sparing the superficial femoral artery are more likely to have tissue necrosis, which is associated with a worse prognosis for limb salvage.

▶ Use of minimally diseased superficial femoral and popliteal arteries as inflow sites for infrapopliteal bypass maximizes use of autogenous conduit. In addition, this approach potentially improves results, as patency of shorter grafts has been suggested to be superior to longer grafts originating from the common femoral artery. This paper reports equivalent results in infrapopliteal bypass regardless of the origin and again demonstrates the adverse effect of tissue necrosis on long-term limb salvage. Obviously, prompt treatment of limb-threatening ischemia prior to development of tissue loss leads to better results—something we need to convey to our primary care colleagues.

J.M. Seeger, M.D.

Preferential Use of Vein for Above-Knee Femoropopliteal Grafts

Wilson YG, Wyatt MG, Currie IC, Baird RN, Lamont PM (Bristol Royal Infirmary, England)
Eur J Vasc Endovasc Surg 10:220–225, 1995   13–15

Background.—Polytetrafluoroethylene (PTFE) grafts are favored for above-knee bypass by many centers. Cited advantages of PTFE include preservation of the vein for subsequent revisions, decreased wound morbidity, and simplification of the surgical procedure. However, the effect of PTFE bypass on the ultimate fate of the limb is unknown because the long-term patency of prosthetic grafts is inferior to that of vein grafts and the utility of preserving vein for subsequent revisions has not been proved. Results are reported for 109 patients who underwent above-knee femoropopliteal bypass between 1983 and 1992 in an attempt to answer these 2 questions.

Patients and Methods.—A total of 112 reconstructions were performed on 109 patients. Vein grafts were used in 87 patients with a mean age of 66 years, and 6-mm unsupported PTFE grafts were used in 23 patients with a mean age of 71 years when vein was absent or inadequate. The rates of diabetes, claudication, and critical ischemia were similar in the 2 groups. The vein graft and PTFE graft groups were compared for primary 3-year graft patency, limb salvage, and survival.

Results.—The initial failure rate was high in both the vein and PTFE groups, and after 3 years of follow-up, the difference in patency rates between the 2 groups was not significant. With a median follow-up of 64 months, occlusion had occurred in 31% of the vein grafts and 48% of the PTFE grafts. Amputation was eventually performed in 9 (32%) of the patients with occluded vein grafts and 6 (55%) of the patients with occluded PTFE grafts. Above-knee amputation was more common in the PTFE group (80%) than in the vein group (20%). Vein was required for only 4 of 17 secondary procedures, and local ipsilateral saphenous vein was used in 2 of these cases.

Conclusion.—Despite equivalent patency for PTFE and vein above-knee femoropopliteal bypass, the consequences of graft failure were more disastrous in the PTFE group than in the vein group. Furthermore, preservation of the vein proved not to be an important consideration, so preferential use of PTFE for above-knee femoropopliteal bypass appears unjustified.

▶ The controversy over the best conduit for above-knee femoropopliteal bypass continues. This paper demonstrates that although graft patency may be equivalent between PTFE graft and vein grafts, the consequences of graft failure are worse with PTFE grafts. This conclusion must be taken in the light of this study being retrospective, but graft patency alone is not an adequate measure of the impact of selection of a prosthetic graft for an infrainguinal bypass.

J.M. Seeger, M.D.

Functional Outcomes for Patients With Intermittent Claudication: Bypass Surgery Versus Angioplasty Versus Noninvasive Management
Reifler DR, Feinglass J, Slavensky R, Martin GJ, Manheim L, McCarthy WJ
(Northwestern Univ, Chicago)
J Vasc Med Biol 5:203–211, 1995   13–16

Introduction.—Traditionally, studies of therapy for intermittent claudication have focused on objective outcome measures such as the limb salvage rate, ankle-brachial index, and vascular patency rate. Recent studies have emphasized patient-reported outcome measures of function and quality of life, which may, after all, be more relevant. Self-reported functional health in patients with intermittent claudication was compared for those treated by bypass surgery, angioplasty, and noninvasive methods.

Methods.—A questionnaire was mailed to 368 consecutive patients with intermittent claudication who were treated at 4 vascular surgery centers from 1988 to 1992. The 4-part survey consisted of the SF-36 Health Survey, the Peripheral Artery Disease (PAD) Walking Impairment Questionnaire, a 16-item comorbidity questionnaire, and a section of original questions addressing such issues as demographics and satisfaction with treatment. Physical functioning of patients who underwent noninvasive management was compared with that of patients who went on to have peripheral bypass and angioplasty procedures. The analysis included an evaluation of whether the results could plausibly be ascribed to the treatment received.

Results.—Excluding patients identified as having died, 187 patients returned their surveys for a response rate of 54%. The response rate was higher for invasively treated patients, but this did not seem to bias the results. Invasive procedures were performed after the initial office visit in 43% of the patients: 39 patients had angioplasty, 28 had bypass, and 13 had both. Patients managed by noninvasive means were older, more likely to be female, and less likely to have aortoiliac disease; however, there was no difference in the mean ankle-brachial index. Seventy-eight percent of the bypass patients and 74% of the angioplasty patients reported improvement in their leg symptoms vs. 25% of the noninvasively treated patients.

Multiple regression analysis demonstrated bypass surgery to be a significant predictor of physical functioning and reported walking distance, whereas angioplasty was not. Physical functioning after treatment was significantly related to pretreatment ankle-brachial index for patients who were managed noninvasively, but not for those undergoing bypass surgery.

Conclusions.—Patients with intermittent claudication who are treated with bypass surgery report better functional status than those treated with angioplasty or noninvasively. The better functional results for bypass patients may reflect improved lower extremity blood flow, but prospective observational studies are needed to confirm this conclusion.

Return to Well-Being and Function After Infrainguinal Revascularization
Gibbons GW, Burgess AM, Guadagnoli E, Pomposelli FB Jr, Freeman DV, Campbell DR, Miller A, Marcaccio EJ Jr, Nordberg P, LoGerfo FW (Harvard Med School, Boston; Harvard School of Public Health, Boston; Surgical Specialists Inc, Pawtucket, RI)
J Vasc Surg 21:35–45, 1995   13–17

Introduction.—Outcome assessment after infrainguinal revascularization has focused primarily on perioperative morbidity/mortality, primary and secondary patency rates, and limb salvage rates, but little from the perspective of patient well-being. To address the latter, functional outcome, symptom relief, well-being, and overall general health perceptions of patients undergoing infrainguinal revascularization were evaluated.

Methods.—Between 1991 and 1992, 318 patients underwent infrainguinal revascularization for severe peripheral arterial occlusive disease. Of these, 156 of 276 (63%) patients completed questionnaires on symptoms, functional status, and well-being before and 6 months after surgery. The mean age of the patients was 66 years; 67% were men. The majority (84%) had diabetes mellitus, and 83% had various heart-related conditions. Distal graft sites were popliteal in 29%, tibial/peroneal in 40%, and pedal/plantar in 31%. The operative morbidity rate was 21%.

TABLE 3.—Patient Health Status Reports at Baseline and Follow-up

	No.	Baseline Mean	Follow-up Mean	Change (P Value)
General health rating*	134	45.0	43.8	NS
Vitality*	124	53.0	61.1	<0.001
Instrumental activities of daily living*	106	53.6	65.6	<0.001
Mental well-being*	126	73.1	76.3	<0.05
Calf cramping†	124	68.9	84.0	<0.001
Leg swelling†	123	70.1	63.4	<0.001
Sores or ulcers†	122	49.5	83.8	<0.001
Toe or foot pain, resting†	119	66.7	80.3	<0.001
Toe or foot pain, walking†	119	62.7	76.8	<0.001

* Scores can range from 0 (least functional) to 100 (most functional).
† Scores can range from 0 (experienced symptom all of the time) to 100 (experienced symptom none of the time).
(Courtesy of Gibbons GW, Burgess AM, Guadagnoli E, et al: Return to well-being and function after infrainguinal revascularization. *J Vasc Surg* 21:35–45, 1995.)

Results.—At 6 months, the cumulative primary graft patency rate was 93%, the cumulative secondary graft patency rate was 95%, and the limb salvage rate was 97%. General health ratings at baseline showed that patients had very low perception of their overall health, and this measure did not improve at the 6-month follow-up (Table 3). All other measures of health status, including instrumental activities of daily living, vitality, and mental well-being, improved after surgery. Symptoms of calf cramping and toe or foot pain when walking and at rest improved, and sores or ulcers healed, but leg swelling became worse. Patients with better functioning or symptom status at baseline reported improved function and well-being at 6 months. However, only 47.4% of the patients reported feeling "back to normal" at 6 months, and many (74%) still required walking devices.

Conclusion.—Health status at baseline is an important predictor of improved function, mental well-being, and resolution of symptoms after infrainguinal revascularization. It appears that earlier intervention toward improving patient function and well-being before surgery may additionally maximize patient benefit from infrainguinal revascularization procedures.

▶ Functional outcome after treatment of lower extremity arterial occlusive disease has only recently been investigated. These 2 studies demonstrate that surgical revascularization improves function better than angioplasty or noninvasive treatment does and that postoperative functional improvement is dependent on the level of impairment prior to treatment. As the goal of lower extremity revascularization is to preserve limbs and restore function, such results are important in selection of appropriate therapy for patients with peripheral vascular disease.

J.M. Seeger, M.D.

Exercise Rehabilitation Programs for the Treatment of Claudication Pain: A Meta-Analysis

Gardner AW, Poehlman ET (Univ of Maryland, Baltimore; Baltimore Veterans Affairs Med Ctr, Md)

JAMA 274:975–980, 1995   13–18

Objective.—Exercise rehabilitation is a noninvasive, inexpensive, and effective treatment alternative for patients with intermittent claudication. Although exercise improves the pain associated with claudication, responses varies widely. A meta-analysis was conducted to identify the most effective components of exercise rehabilitation programs for claudication pain.

Methods.—A careful search of the English-language literature from 1966 through 1994 was performed to identify published studies of exercise rehabilitation programs for patients with intermittent claudication. To be included in the meta-analysis, the studies had to provide pre-exercise and postexercise mean or individual walking distances or times to the onset of claudication pain and to maximal pain on treadmill testing. Two investigators independently abstracted data on walking distances and times and on the components of each exercise program. Treatment effects were estimated for 6 exercise components: frequency, session duration, mode, program length, claudication pain end point used during exercise sessions, and level of supervision. Of 33 studies identified, 21 met the study inclusion criteria. Eighteen studies were unrandomized and uncontrolled and included 548 patients; 3 studies were randomized and included 23 patients.

Results.—Overall, exercise rehabilitation increased the distance to onset of claudication pain by 179%, from 126 to 351 m, and the distance to maximal claudication pain by 122%, from 326 to 723 m. Programs with session durations of more than 30 minutes with exercise frequencies of at least 3 sessions per week, with walking as the main mode of exercise, with near-maximal pain as the claudication end point, and with program lengths of more than 6 months yielded the greatest improvement. The only independent predictors of improved distance were the end point of claudication pain, program length, and type of exercise and together, these 3 variables explained about 85% of the variance in the change in distance. Age was the only baseline characteristic significantly associated with outcome, with older patients showing greater improvement in claudication distances than younger patients.

Conclusions.—Exercise rehabilitation programs appear to improve treadmill distances to onset and maximal claudication pain by 120% to 180%. The optimal exercise program should last at least 6 months and include intermittent walking to near-maximal pain.

▶ Exercise therapy has long been known to improve walking distance in patients with intermittent claudication. This study confirms this observation and demonstrates that the type of exercise and duration of the program influence outcome. A better understanding of other factors that affect the success of exercise therapy and the mechanisms of improvement after exercise training should allow more widespread and appropriate use of this noninvasive treatment of peripheral vascular disease.

J.M. Seeger, M.D.

Venous

Proximal Venous Outflow Obstruction in Patients With Upper Extremity Arteriovenous Dialysis Access

Criado E, Marston WA, Jaques PF, Mauro MA, Keagy BA (Univ of North Carolina, Chapel Hill)
Ann Vasc Surg 8:530–535, 1994   13–19

Objective.—The effects of central venous obstruction on failure of hemodialysis access in the upper extremity were examined in 122 patients who underwent a total of 158 access procedures in a 1-year period.

Findings.—Fourteen patients (11.5%) had marked arm swelling, graft thrombosis, or graft malfunction as the result of central vein obstruction. Lesions included 8 subclavian vein occlusions, 6 subclavian stenoses, 2 internal jugular vein stenoses, and 1 superior vena cava stenosis. All these patients had received temporary bilateral subclavian vein dialysis catheters and all had failed arteriovenous access in the upper extremity.

Management and Outcome.—Twenty-one procedures were done to treat these lesions, including 17 percutaneous transluminal balloon angioplasties (PTAs), 13 of which were accompanied by stent placement, 2 with axillary-to-innominate vein bypasses and 2 with axillary-to–internal jugular vein bypasses. Symptoms resolved in all patients. In 13 (76%) cases PTA was initially successful, and in 4 instances it was not possible to recanalize the vein. One venous angioplasty failed immediately, whereas 8 provided functional hemodialysis access for 2–9 months, restenosis occurred in 2 at 3 and 10 months and redilation was successful, and 2 veins occluded at 2 and 4 months but could not be recanalized. Four patients in whom angioplasty failed underwent venous bypass, and the bypasses remained patent and provided functional access 7–13 months afterward (Fig 1). Six of 9 stenotic vein lesions were successfully dilated with PTA and remained open, but only 2 of 8 occluded veins were successfully opened without recurrent stenosis.

Conclusion.—In patients with arteriovenous access in the upper limb, temporary central hemodialysis catheters produce a significant number of symptomatic central vein stenoses and occlusions. However, access function often can be prolonged by percutaneous dilatation of venous lesions, with or without stent placement and/or surgical bypass.

▶ As use of temporary central hemodialysis becomes more common, the incidence of symptomatic central vein stenoses/occlusions, which can adversely affect upper extremity dialysis access sites, will likely increase. Fortunately, as this study shows, recognition and treatment of this problem

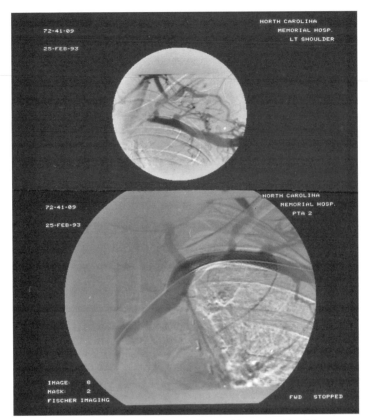

FIGURE 1.—**A,** left subclavian venogram from a 40-year-old woman with a left upper arm arteriovenous fistula and complete subclavian vein occlusion who had massive left arm swelling. **B,** after percutaneous transluminal angioplasty and placement of a 10-mm Wallstent, the swelling improved and the access remains functional 6 months after dilation. (Courtesy of *Annals of Vascular Surgery,* 8(6):530–535, 1994.)

with angioplasty and possibly stenting for stenoses and surgical bypass for occlusion can prolong the function of upper extremity arteriovenous vascular access.

J.M. Seeger, M.D.

Subfascial Endoscopic Ligation in the Treatment of Incompetent Perforating Veins

Pierik EGJM, Wittens CHA, van Urk H (Univ Hosp, Rotterdam-Dijkzigt, The Netherlands)
Eur J Vasc Endovasc Surg 9:38–41, 1995   13–20

Objective.—The efficacy of subfascial endoscopic ligation of incompetent perforating veins was examined in a prospective series of 38 consecutive patients with prolonged or recurrent venous ulcers in 40 lower extremities.

Methods.—Incompetent perforating veins were clinically evident in all extremities and were confirmed by continuous-wave ultrasonography. Incompetent deep veins were also present in 31 legs, and sixteen patients had active ulcers at the time of surgery. Under spinal anesthesia, a short incision is made at the anteromedial border of the proximal third of the lower part of the leg, and after incising the fascia horizontally, a mediastinoscope 18 cm long and 12 mm in diameter is inserted to examine the subfascial region. All communicating veins are ligated with hemoclips and dissected under direct vision. In the early cases, a 10-cm fasciotomy was performed after removing the scope.

Results.—Subfascial infection requiring surgical drainage developed in 2 patients, and 1 had inflammation at the wound site. All active ulcers healed within 2 months, and only 1 of the 38 patients had recurrent ulceration during an average follow-up of nearly 4 years.

Conclusion.—Subfascial endoscopic ligation using a mediastinoscope is a relatively simple and effective means of treating incompetent perforating veins. The cosmetic results are satisfactory, and recurrent ulceration is very infrequent.

▶ This is an ingenious approach to a difficult problem. The successful subfascial ligation of incompetent perforating veins has always been limited by problems with wound healing in an extremity with severe venous stasis disease. This approach should allow more widespread use of a procedure that can help decrease the risk of recurrent ulceration in patients with a difficult problem.

J.M. Seeger, M.D.

Surveillance Venous Scans for Deep Venous Thrombosis in Multiple Trauma Patients
Meyer CS, Blebea J, Davis K Jr, Fowl RJ, Kempczinski RF (Univ of Cincinnati, Ohio)
Ann Vasc Surg 9:109–114, 1995   13–21

Background.—Deep venous thrombosis (DVT) in the lower extremity reportedly develops in about 40% of patients with multisystematic trauma, and the estimated risk of associated pulmonary embolism is approximately 10%. Because of this, prophylactic therapy to prevent DVT and/or surveillance venous duplex examination have been recommended. However, the efficacy and cost-effectiveness of surveillance scans remains unclear.

Methods.—The findings on surveillance venous duplex scanning of the lower extremities were reviewed in 183 multiply injured patients, 122 men and 61 women with an average age of 38 years, who were admitted to intensive care and had a total of 261 scans. All patients received prophylaxis against DVT by either pneumatic compression of the lower extremities or subcutaneous heparin. A large majority of the patients had blunt injuries, and all patients received DVT prophylaxis.

Results.—Six percent of the 261 venous scans were positive for DVT in the proximal region of the lower extremity, and 2% demonstrated thrombus in the calf veins. In one third of the cases, thrombus extended to more than 1 anatomical site. Symptomatic patients were more likely than those without symptoms to have proximal thrombosis, as were patients with spinal injury. However, half of the patients found to have DVT had no symptoms or signs of DVT, and 83% of the patients with DVT limited to the calf veins were asymptomatic but calf vein DVTs showed progression. None of the patients suffered a symptomatic pulmonary embolism. The per-case cost of identifying proximal DVT was $6,688.

Conclusion.—Because of the low incidence of significant proximal DVT and the high cost of routine surveillance scanning of all trauma patients admitted to the surgical ICU ($300 million annually on a national basis), surveillance venous scanning is recommended only for high-risk or symptomatic patients. However, a prospective trial is needed to document the safety and cost-effectiveness of this strategy.

▶ Surveillance venous scanning for deep venous thrombosis in all multiple-trauma patients is simply too costly. More studies like this need to be done to identify risk factors for DVT in these patients so that venous scanning can be used selectively without increasing the risk of pulmonary embolism from an undetected venous thrombosis.

J.M. Seeger, M.D.

Deep Vein Thrombosis Associated With Lower Extremity Amputation
Yeager RA, Moneta GL, Edwards JM, Taylor LM Jr, McConnell DB, Porter JM
(Oregon Health Sciences Univ, Portland)
J Vasc Surg 22:612–615, 1995   13–22

Background.—Although patients undergoing lower extremity amputation are thought to have an increased risk of deep vein thrombosis (DVT), there is little documentation of this. Therefore, the prevalence of DVT among a large cohort of patients undergoing vascular surgery and lower extremity amputation was studied prospectively.

Methods.—Seventy-one men and 1 woman who had amputations over a recent 28-month period were included in the study. The mean patient age was 68 years. Forty-one below-knee and 31 above-knee amputations were done. Duplex scanning for DVT was done perioperatively.

Results.—Nine patients, or 12.5%, were found to have DVT. Venous thromboses were bilateral in 1 patient, ipsilateral in 4, and contralateral to the amputation in 4. In 8 patients, thrombi were detected at or proximal to the popliteal vein, and in 1, thrombi were isolated to the tibial veins, so lower extremity amputation was associated with DVT at or proximal to the popliteal vein in 11% of the patients. Thromboses were found before surgery in 6 patients and afterward in 3. The risk of DVT developing was significantly greater in patients with a history of venous disease and also increased in those with a previous amputation. Heparin anticoagulation was used to treat DVT, and none of the patients had clinical symptoms suggesting pulmonary embolism.

Conclusions.—Deep vein thrombosis is relatively common in patients requiring lower extremity amputation, and in addition, patients with a history of venous disease and pre-existing amputation seemed to be at greatest risk for DVT associated with amputation.

▶ Not surprisingly, deep venous thrombosis is relatively common in patients undergoing lower extremity amputation and is frequently present prior to surgery. Detection and treatment of this problem will hopefully improve outcome in these patients, who have the highest mortality of all patients treated for peripheral vascular disease.

J.M. Seeger, M.D.

Contralateral Duplex Scanning for Deep Venous Thrombosis Is Unnecessary in Patients With Symptoms

Strothman G, Blebea J, Fowl RJ, Rosenthal G (Univ of Cincinnati, Ohio)
J Vasc Surg 22:543–547, 1995   13–23

Background.—Deep vein thrombosis (DVT) involves both legs in 17% to 32% of acute cases, even when the contralateral leg is asymptomatic. As a result, bilateral duplex venous scanning is the recommended evaluation. Because treatment for the symptomatic leg treats the other leg as well, the need for routine bilateral examination has been questioned. This question was evaluated by review of a series of such procedures.

Methods.—All venous duplex scans performed at the institution over a 2-year period were reviewed retrospectively. Demographic patient data, symptoms, scan results, and the incidence of bilateral DVT were recorded.

Results.—Two hundred forty-eight patients with symptoms and acute DVT detected by venous duplex examination were identified. Unilateral DVT was significantly more common in patients with unilateral symptoms (88% of 176 patients), whereas bilateral symptoms were accompanied significantly more often by bilateral disease. However, 66% (44 patients) of those with unilateral symptoms had bilateral DVT. Regardless, every patient with contralateral DVT also had DVT in the symptomatic leg. Thus there was no case of DVT in an asymptomatic limb that would have gone untreated.

Conclusion.—In patients symptomatic for DVT, duplex venous scanning of the symptomatic limb is sufficient because therapy will treat the contralateral limb as well when bilateral disease is present.

▶ This is a useful observation that should decrease the workload of most vascular laboratories. As reimbursement declines, improvements in efficiency, such as can be provided by decreasing the time necessary for a duplex venous scan for deep venous thrombosis, will be necessary for the vascular laboratory to remain financially viable.

J.M. Seeger, M.D.

Miscellaneous

Reducing Perioperative Myocardial Infarction Following Vascular Surgery: The Potential Role of β-Blockade

Yeager RA, Moneta GL, Edwards JM, Taylor LM Jr, McConnell DB, Porter JM (Oregon Health Sciences Univ, Portland)
Arch Surg 130:869–873, 1995   13–24

Introduction.—The leading cause of perioperative mortality after vascular surgery is myocardial infarction. Although many variables that influence the incidence of myocardial infarction after vascular surgery such as age and history of coronary artery disease cannot be modified, others such as the type of anesthetic and selection of perioperative medication can be altered.

Methods.—To determine perioperative variables that could be modified to influence the occurrence of perioperative myocardial infarction, 53 patients with perioperative myocardial infarction after vascular surgery were compared with 106 control patients without perioperative myocardial infarction. The 2 groups were compared for blood pressure, blood loss, length of surgery, heart rate, use of perioperative β-blockers, type of anesthetic, and use of calcium channel blockers, nitroglycerin, angiotensin-converting enzyme inhibitors, and vasopressors.

Results.—In patients with perioperative myocardial infarction, β-blockers were used less frequently than in control patients (30% vs. 50%), and with preoperative and/or intraoperative β-blockade, there was 50% reduction in perioperative myocardial infarction. A maximum intraoperative heart rate of 100 beats per minute or higher and the requirement for a transfusion were also associated with the occurrence of perioperative myocardial infarction.

Conclusion.—Extensive cardiac evaluation has little impact on reducing perioperative cardiac morbidity and mortality in the elderly population having vascular procedures. In contrast, the use of perioperative β-blockade may reduce perioperative myocardial infarction. The use of β-blockers improves myocardial metabolism independently of effects on blood pressure and heart rate. A prospective randomized trial of β-blockers in elderly patients should be conducted.

▶ Myocardial infarction remains a leading cause of perioperative morbidity after vascular surgery. All patients with peripheral vascular disease have coronary atherosclerosis, but why an individual patient has a postoperative myocardial infarction (MI) remains unclear. Preoperative screening for coronary artery disease is costly and ineffective in identifying patients likely to have postoperative MI. In contrast, the use of techniques that limit cardiac stress and improve myocardial metabolism such as β-blockade could potentially reduce the risk of this complication, as the study demonstrates.

J.M. Seeger, M.D.

Diagnosis and Long-Term Clinical Outcome in Patients Diagnosed With Hand Ischemia
McLafferty RB, Edwards JM, Taylor LM Jr, Porter JM (Oregon Health Sciences Univ, Portland)
J Vasc Surg 22:361–369, 1995   13–25

Introduction.—The long-term clinical outcome of patients with hand ischemia caused by digital artery obstruction remains unknown. Forty-four such patients were reviewed in a study of long-term clinical outcome and the role of arteriography and digital photoplethysmography in the diagnosis and classification of hand ischemia.

Patients and Methods.—All patients had symptomatic hand ischemia, a minimum clinical follow-up of 10 years, and digital artery obstruction confirmed by hand arteriography. The average age of the patient group was 44 years at the time of arteriography. Data collected included symptom severity, presence of ischemic finger ulcers, tobacco use, diagnosis of a connective tissue disorder (CTD), and the need for digital amputation during follow-up.

Results.—At study entry, symptoms were classified as moderate in 21 patients and severe in 23. In 17 patients CTD had been diagnosed at the time of arteriography and, in 9 more, during follow-up. With an average follow-up of 15.2 years, symptoms improved in 28 patients, remained unchanged in 15, and worsened in 1. Fifteen of 18 patients without CTD were improved, but only 13 of the 26 with CTD had symptomatic improvement during follow-up. The patient whose symptoms worsened had CTD. Finger ulceration occurred at a significantly higher rate in patients with (65%) than without (22%) CTD, but in only 2 of 25 patients without ulceration initially did subsequent ulcers develop. One patient without and 6 with CTD underwent digital amputation during follow-up. Finger photoplethysmography proved as accurate as arteriography for objectively measuring hand ischemia.

Conclusions.—The long-term prognosis of patients with hand ischemia from digital artery occlusion is generally good, so premature finger amputation should be avoided. Patients with CTD fare poorer, but even in this group, amputation is seldom required.

▶ Hand ischemia is an unusual but devastating problem. This study from the acknowledged experts in the management of this problem demonstrates that long-term outcome is generally good, even in patients with connective tissue disease. Therefore, treatment should be very conservative.

J.M. Seeger, M.D.

Transesophageal Echocardiography in the Diagnosis of Traumatic Rupture of the Aorta

Smith MD, Cassidy JM, Souther S, Morris EJ, Sapin PM, Johnson SB, Kearney PA (Univ of Kentucky, Lexington)
N Engl J Med 332:356–362, 1995   13–26

Background.—Standard chest radiography is useful in the initial screening of traumatic rupture of the aorta. However, diagnosis requires confirmation by aortography, CT, or MRI before surgical repair. This study was performed to determine the safety and efficacy of transesophageal echocardiography in patients with suspected acute traumatic injury to the thoracic aorta.

Study Methods.—Emergency transesophageal echocardiography of the aorta was attempted in 101 patients with possible traumatic rupture of the aorta. Echocardiography and aortography were performed sequentially in each patient.

Findings.—Transesophageal echocardiography was completed successfully in 93 patients. It could not be completed in 7 because of lack of cooperation and in 1 because of maxillofacial trauma. The test was not associated with any complications despite a high mean injury severity score, and the mean time required for the test was 29 minutes. Eleven of the 93 studies showed aortic rupture near the isthmus, which was confirmed by aortography, surgery, or autopsy. One false-positive result occurred on echocardiography. Thus transesophageal echocardiography had a sensitivity of 100% and a specificity of 98% for the detection of aortic injury.

Conclusions.—Transesophageal echocardiography is a very sensitive and specific method for detecting injury to the thoracic aorta. It can be done safely and rapidly in critically injured patients with possible traumatic rupture of the aorta, and the results compare favorably with aortography.

▶ This study clearly demonstrates the value of transesophageal echocardiography (TEE) in patients suspected of having traumatic rupture of the aorta. No patient with a negative TEE study was found to have traumatic aortic rupture, so use of this portable, quick technique should minimize the need for aortography with its attendant risks in these critically injured patients.

J.M. Seeger, M.D.

Accuracy of Disincorporation for Identification of Vascular Graft Infection

Padberg FT Jr, Smith SM, Eng RHK (Univ of Medicine and Dentistry of New Jersey, Newark)
Arch Surg 130:183–187, 1995   13–27

Purpose.—In vascular prosthetic grafting, disincorporation is associated with graft infection; however, failure of graft incorporation may not always represent graft infection. Enhanced microbiologic culture techniques were used to compare the presence and absence of tissue incorporation in vascular prosthetic grafts with the bacterial culture results to determine the reliability of graft incorporation as a marker of graft infection.

Methods.—Samples of vascular prostheses were removed from 113 aortofemoral, extra-anatomic, infrainguinal, and hemoaccess sites at vascular reoperative surgery in 59 patients. All graft samples then underwent gentle sonication followed by quantitative culture. The culture results were predicted from the incorporation or disincorporation status of the prostheses, as assessed at surgery. Any bacterial growth was considered to represent graft infection.

Results.—There were 31 disincorporated prosthetic graft samples, 23 of which were culture-positive and 8 of which yielded no growth. The other 82 graft samples showed good incorporation: 74 were culture negative, but 8 yielded bacterial growth. The rate of incorrect prediction was 14%. Sensitivity, defined as concurrence of disincorporation and a culture positive for bacteria relative to all culture-positive grafts, was 74%. Specificity, defined as concurrence of incorporation and cultures negative for bacteria relative to all culture-negative grafts, varied with the length of graft implantation, being 90% in prostheses implanted for more than 2 weeks and 97% for those implanted for longer than 23 weeks.

Conclusions.—In vascular graft prostheses, the surgical finding of incorporation or disincorporation accurately predicts the bacterial culture results in almost 90% of cases. Graft disincorporation is associated with the presence of bacteria in 71% of cases, whereas graft incorporation excludes the presence of bacteria in 97% of cases.

▶ Confirmation of prosthetic graft infection remains surprisingly difficult, and routine bacterial cultures from apparently infected grafts are negative in up to a third of patients. Incorporation and disincorporation have been presumed to be accurate indicators of the absence or presence of infection, but there has been little objective evidence to confirm this assumption. Using advanced bacterial culture techniques, this study demonstrates that graft incorporation essentially excludes the presence of bacteria on the graft, whereas disincorporation is associated with a positive bacterial culture in 71% of cases. However, previous work by other authors has shown that incorporated portions of infected aortic grafts can subsequently show signs of infection, which suggests that incorporation either interferes with bacterial culture or does not prevent subsequent infection.

J.M. Seeger, M.D.

14 Noncardiac Thoracic Surgery

Introduction

This year's chapter on general thoracic surgery provides an interesting and exciting look at the progress in clinical investigation of video-assisted thoracic surgery. During the past year, we have seen a maturation of studies that assess video-assisted techniques. There has been a progression from feasibility studies in single institutions to multi-institutional clinical trials in which these new, minimally invasive thoracic surgical techniques are evaluated and then compared with standard open procedures.

There have also been some interesting and informative studies in the field of non–small cell lung cancer. These large, randomized, prospective trials represent significant contributions to the surgical approach to this disease. Further, numerous articles covering a broad spectrum of miscellaneous topics of interest to the general thoracic surgeon have been published. Finally, we selected several papers because they provide potentially important findings that suggest innovative therapies for the treatment of a wide range of thoracic malignancies.

David J. Sugarbaker, M.D.

Minimally Invasive Surgical Techniques

As predicted in our previous editions of the YEAR BOOK, thoracic surgical technique is being heavily influenced by the introduction of minimally invasive procedures. During the past 5 years, we have seen a steady progression of these studies from single institution reports, based on a few procedures, to multi-institutional trials that seek to establish firmly the role of minimally invasive techniques in the clinical field of thoracic surgery. Further, video-assisted thoracic surgical techniques are finding their way into the treatment strategies of a number of malignancies. This development is particularly true in the staging and evaluation of patients who have thoracic malignancies, as well as in the interval diagnosis of disease progression.

A number of techniques have been devised to replace standard thoracic surgical techniques. The premise is that a minimally invasive thoracic surgical approach, which limits the size of the incision and number of muscle groups divided during surgery, will provide a long-term advantage in morbidity sustained by the patient as well as rapid recovery and return to occupational activities. Many of these premises are slowly being established in the literature, and some continue to be evaluated prospectively. In any clinical trial, however, there are many limitations, which often frustrate the thoracic surgeon who seeks to evaluate and establish what are intuitively superior procedures within the field. We review 11 very interesting papers that have significantly contributed to the establishment and further development of minimally invasive thoracic surgical techniques in the treatment of a wide variety of diseases in a variety of specific clinical settings. Clearly, it is the appropriate selection of patients for each individual procedure that optimizes clinical outcome in surgery. The following reports help establish appropriate clinical instances in which minimally invasive techniques would be of maximal benefit.

D.J. Sugarbaker, M.D.

Lobectomy: Video-assisted Thoracic Surgery Versus Muscle-sparing Thoracotomy: A Randomized Trial

Kirby TJ, Mack MJ, Landreneau RJ, Rice TW (Cleveland Clinic Found, Ohio; Humana Hosp, Dallas; Univ of Pittsburgh, Pa)
J Thorac Cardiovasc Surg 109:997–1002, 1995   14–1

Objective.—Video-assisted thoracic surgery (VATS) has made it possible to perform minimally invasive lung biopsies, wedge excision of pulmonary nodules, blebectomy, bullectomy, thymectomy, and resection of mediastinal tumors. No studies, however, have demonstrated significant advantages of this approach compared with conventional procedures. In a randomized trial, VATS lobectomy was compared with muscle-sparing thoracotomy (MST) and lobectomy.

Methods.—Muscle-sparing thoracotomy and lobectomy or VATS lobectomy was performed on 55 patients who had non–small cell lung carcinoma.

Results.—There were no significant differences between the 2 groups with respect to operating time, intraoperative complications, blood loss, duration of chest drainage, or length of hospital stay. Sixteen complications, mainly air leaks, occurred among the 30 patients in the MST group, compared with only 6 complications among the 25 patients in the VATS group. Other complications included 3 prolonged air leaks, 1 pulmonary embolism, and 1 case of *Clostridium difficile* colitis. Three patients had disabling pain.

Conclusion.—Although VATS is a safe procedure for early stage I and II non–small cell lung cancer, there is no short-term advantage compared with the MST lobectomy procedure with respect to operating time, intraoperative complications, blood loss, duration of chest drainage, length of hospital stay, or return to work. Because of the additional risk to patients who undergo pulmonary resection in a closed chest, further studies are needed to evaluate long-term survival in patients who undergo a VATS procedure.

▶ This report describes a pilot study in a randomized setting. The results indicate that a VATS lobectomy can be performed with similar morbidity and mortality as a lobectomy performed via MST. It is encouraging that in patients who have early-stage cancer, a VATS lobectomy can be performed without the adverse clinical consequences predicated by some skeptics of this approach.

One might expect that as VATS lobectomy techniques are further refined in the years to come, substantial improvements in morbidity and mortality may be achieved with the use of these techniques. Such expectations are based on the understanding that the conventional techniques are the product of decades of refinement by surgeons who have attempted to reduce morbidity and mortality rates to a minimum. Further, it is clear that instrumentation for VATS surgery is in its infancy when compared with the current conventional instrumentation, which also is the product of decades of refinement and innovation by the surgical community.

D.J. Sugarbaker, M.D.

The Safety and Versatility of Video-thoracoscopy: A Prospective Analysis of 895 Consecutive Cases
DeCamp MM Jr, Jaklitsch MT, Mentzer SJ, Harpole DH Jr, Sugarbaker DJ
(Brigham and Women's Hosp, Boston; Harvard Med School, Boston)
J Am Coll Surg 181:113–120, 1995   14–2

Background.—With the use of video-assisted thoracoscopy, minimally invasive diagnostic evaluation of disease deep to the pleura and definitive resection with the endoscopic technique have been possible. The initial experience with video-assisted thoracoscopy was reviewed by examining prospectively collected data.

Methods.—Preoperative, intraoperative, and postoperative data were collected on all patients undergoing thoracic surgery. Patients who had symptomatic effusive disease of the pleura or pericardium, an indeterminate pulmonary nodule in the peripheral third of the pulmonary parenchyma, or esophageal or mediastinal lesions not evaluable with cervical or anterior mediastinoscopy were eligible for video-thoracoscopy. Procedures were classified as diagnostic and/or therapeutic. Mortality and morbidity rates were analyzed for the entire study population and for 3 high-risk subgroups: patients aged older than 70 years, patients who had impaired pulmonary function, and patients who had significant functional impairment.

Results.—During a 3-year period, 895 patients underwent video-thoracoscopy: 501 had diagnostic procedures, 244 had therapeutic procedures, and 150 had both. The procedures were performed in the lung (63%), pleura (22%), mediastinum (6%), esophagus (5%), and pericardial windows (4%). Fifty-seven percent of patients had malignant disease, and 43% had benign or infectious disease. Overall, the operative mortality rate was 1%, and the operative morbidity rate was 14%. Thirteen patients required conversion to thoracotomy. The most common complications were prolonged air leak, dysrhythmia, and respiratory failure or pneumonia. The subgroup of elderly patients had an operative mortality rate of 1.5% and a morbidity rate of 18.7%. Among those who had impaired pulmonary function, the mortality rate was 2.1% and the complication rate was 29.8%. Patients who had a Karnofsky performance index of less than 8 had a 9.8% mortality rate and an 18% morbidity rate. The median postoperative length of stay was 3 days; patients who underwent purely diagnostic procedures were discharged earlier than those who underwent therapeutic procedures. The length of stay in the study population was significantly shorter than the median postoperative length of stay for all patients undergoing major chest procedures.

Conclusions.—Video-thoracoscopy is associated with a shortened length of stay, a low mortality rate, and an acceptable morbidity rate. Claims of versatility, efficiency, safety, efficacy, and cost containment are supported by these findings.

▶ This study represents a large, prospective analysis of a single institution's experience with video-assisted thoracoscopic procedures. Of note was the improved survival rate relative to historical controls in 3 specific clinical situations. The first situation involved patients at high risk who had a poor forced expiratory volume in 1 second and other indicators of compromised pulmonary function. The second was in the subgroup of elderly patients, who had an operative mortality rate of only 1.5%, which is acceptable when compared with the use of conventional techniques. The third subgroup had a poor Karnofsky performance index of less than 8. Despite an elevated mortality rate of 9.8%, the outcome was still favorable for this subgroup, considering that many of these patients would have been deemed inoperable with conventional techniques. The breadth of this study in terms of the number and range of procedures makes an important contribution to the literature. The identification of these 3 subgroups of patients as target clinical groups for the application of video-assisted thoracic surgery for diagnostic, staging, and therapeutic maneuvers will be the single most important contribution of this report.

D.J. Sugarbaker, M.D.

Video-assisted Thoracoscopy in the Management of Recurrent Spontaneous Pneumothorax

De Giacomo T, Rendina EA, Venuta F, Ciriaco P, Lena A, Ricci C (Univ of Rome "La Sapienza," Italy)
Eur J Surg 161:227–230, 1995   14–3

Objective.—Chest drainage is rapidly effective in most cases of spontaneous pneumothorax. Thoracotomy may be required in patients who have persisting air leaks, incomplete lung expansion, or recurrences. Video-assisted thoracoscopy was recently introduced as an alternative to thoracotomy. Results of the 2 approaches were compared.

Patients.—Between April 1992 and October 1993, 16 men and 4 women (mean age, 30 years) underwent video-assisted thoracoscopy for spontaneous pneumothorax. The results were compared with those of 17 men and 4 women (mean age, 32 years) who had undergone muscle-sparing lateral thoracotomy for spontaneous pneumothorax in 1991.

Results.—The mean duration of chest drainage was 5 days in the thoracoscopy group and 7 days in the control group. The mean hospital stay for the thoracoscopy group was 6 days, compared with 10 days in the control group. Both differences were significant. Only 3 patients (15%) in the thoracoscopy group required postoperative parenteral analgesia, compared with 14 (66%) in the control group. Chest wall paresthesia was the only postoperative complication in 2 patients in the thoracoscopy group; 5 patients (24%) in the control group had minor postoperative complications. After a mean follow-up of 9 months after thoracoscopy and 26 months after thoracotomy, none of the patients had a recurrence.

Conclusions.—Video-assisted thoracoscopy appears to be a superior alternative to thoracotomy in the treatment of spontaneous pneumothorax.

▶ This report seeks to assess the contribution of video-assisted thoracoscopy in the management of recurrent spontaneous pneumothorax. It appears that the management of spontaneous pneumothorax is one of the initial possible applications for video-assisted thoracic surgery and that this approach is preferred when surgical intervention is required. Given similar recurrence rates and reduced length of chest tube drainage and hospital stay with the use of video-assisted techniques, thoracic surgeons should consider this approach as standard therapy in this particular clinical situation.

D.J. Sugarbaker, M.D.

Pathologic Comparison of Video-assisted Thoracic Surgical Lung Biopsy With Traditional Open Lung Biopsy

Kadokura M, Colby TV, Myers JL, Allen MS, Deschamps C, Trastek VF, Pairolero PC (Mayo Clinic and Found, Rochester, Minn)
J Thorac Cardiovasc Surg 109:494–498, 1995   14–4

Background.—Video-assisted thoracic surgical lung biopsy (VATS-LB) is replacing open lung biopsy (OLB) as the procedure of choice for the diagnosis of lung disease. The diagnostic efficacy of VATS-LB was compared with that of OLB in a large series of patients.

Patients.—Between January 7, 1991, and August 3, 1993, 116 consecutive patients were referrred to the Mayo Clinic for lung biopsy. Seventy-one patients underwent VATS-LB, and 42 underwent traditional OLB. The OLB patients had had previous intubation, severe pulmonary dysfunction, or pleural adhesion that precluded VATS-LB.

Results.—The VATS-LB group had more traumatic hemorrhage and neutrophil margination than did the OLB group, but this situation did not affect diagnostic accuracy. Complications developed in 15% of patients in the VATS-LB group and in 17% of those in the OLB group. The operative mortality rates were 8% in the VATS-LB group and 17% in the OLB group. All had preoperative respiratory failure.

Conclusions.—Video-assisted thoracic surgical lung biopsy is a safe and effective alternative to traditional open lung biopsy for the diagnosis of lung disease. Although there was increased hemorrhage and neutrophil margination in patients who received VATS-LB, this tissue damage did not decrease diagnostic accuracy.

▶ These authors compared the pathologic specimens obtained via a VATS-LB with those obtained via the traditional OLB. This carefully performed study notes increased hemorrhage and neutrophil margination in the specimens of patients who underwent a VATS-LB. Careful assessment of the diagnostic accuracy, however, revealed no difference. Given the fact that one can perform a biopsy from 2 or 3 lobes with the use of a video-assisted technique, as opposed to a single lobe for most patients who undergo a standard mini-thoracotomy, one might surmise that the overall diagnostic accuracy from the VATS approach may, in fact, be superior in some cases.

For those unstable patients who make up a large proportion of patients requiring lung biopsy, single-lung anesthesia is not always possible. We have noted in our institution the efficacy of mild CO_2 insufflation in the ipsilateral chest for biopsy. This approach allows for partial atelectasis such that a VATS-LB may be performed without complete unilateral ventilation.

D.J. Sugarbaker, M.D.

▶ The old equation in surgery that seeks to evaluate the morbidity and mortality of a diagnostic technique in light of its presumed efficacy can alter the approach used in patients who have a variety of malignancies. Specifically, the conundrum of the indeterminate or solitary pulmonary nodule has sparked a significant amount of controversy in the surgical community. Past strategies that were based on observation over a period of time have traded off the potential for allowing the development of metastatic disease against the morbidity and mortality of a definitive excisional biopsy. Other means, such as fine-needle aspiration, have been used to minimize the morbidity associated with obtaining a diagnosis but have sacrificed diagnostic accuracy and have still resulted in significant morbidity for a high percentage of patients in whom pneumothorax develops because of the procedure.

These 3 articles evaluate the feasibility and accuracy of thoracoscopic resection of a solitary pulmonary nodule. This procedure permits diagnostic accuracy similar to that of an excisional biopsy but with much reduced morbidity, as compared with standard thoracotomy.

Videothoracoscopy Versus Thoracotomy for the Diagnosis of the Indeterminate Solitary Pulmonary Nodule
Santambrogio L, Nosotti M, Bellaviti N, Mezzetti M (Univ of Milan, Italy)
Ann Thorac Surg 59:868–871, 1995   14–5

Background.—The nature of the solitary pulmonary nodule (SPN) is often difficult to diagnose. In a randomized, prospective trial, video-assisted thoracic surgery (VATS) was compared with lateral thoracotomy (LT) in the diagnosis of indeterminate SPN.

Methods.—Forty-four patients who had SPN were included. Criteria for admission were maximum nodule size of 2.5 cm, location in peripheral third of lung, nodule indeterminate after diagnostic process, low risk of primary lung cancer, and absence of intrabronchial vegetation. The patients were randomly selected to undergo either VATS or LT, from January 1991 to May 1994.

Results.—Thirteen wedge resections, 8 segmentectomies, and 1 lobectomy were performed in the LT group. Nineteen wedge resections, 1 segmentectomy, and 2 lobectomies were performed in the VATS group. Five patients in the VATS group required an access thoracotomy. A final diagnosis was made in all patients in both groups. Neither group had complications. The postoperative stay and the pain reported by patients were both significantly lower in the VATS group than in the LT group.

Conclusions.—The sensitivity and specificity of both VATS and LT were 100% in the diagnosis of SPNs. The use of VATS was associated with less patient discomfort and shorter hospital stay than was the use of LT. Video-assisted thoracic surgery is recommended for analysis of indeterminate SPNs that have a diameter of less than 2.5 cm and are located in the peripheral third of the lung parenchyma.

▶ These authors have nicely described the population of patients in which thoracoscopic resection of a solitary nodule would be feasible. The procedure is particularly suitable for those patients who have a nodule in the outer third of the lung field, i.e., amenable to digital palpation at the time of thoracoscopy. This population, however, does represent a large number of patients. An early thoracoscopic resection would appear to be most appealing for patients in whom a smoking history has been documented and a new nodule has been confirmed by a review of old radiographs.

D.J. Sugarbaker, M.D.

The Solitary Pulmonary Nodule: Update 1995
Libby DM, Henschke CI, Yankelevitz DF (New York Hosp–Cornell Med Ctr)
Am J Med 99:491–496, 1995   14–6

Background.—Although many solitary pulmonary nodules are benign, a significant number represent lung cancer. In the United States, these malignant nodules are the leading cause of cancer death. Prognosis depends on the stage of disease at diagnosis. The results of diagnostic evaluation and the incidence of malignancy in solitary pulmonary nodules in view of the development of improved diagnostic techniques were examined.

Methods.—Complete medical records of 40 patients (mean age, 65 years) who were referred to a pulmonologist between 1990 and 1993 were examined. Solitary pulmonary nodules were defined as a round or ovoid opacity within the lung parenchyma with a diameter of 3 cm or less. Clinical and radiographic characteristics of patients who had lung cancer were compared with those of patients who did not.

Results.—The prevalence of cardiovascular disease and chronic obstructive pulmonary disease was high, but that of tuberculosis was low. The mean diameter of solitary pulmonary nodules was 1.8 cm, and the prevalence of malignancy was 53%. The prevalence of malignancy was 43% in solitary pulmonary nodules 2 cm or less in diameter. In 78% of patients, diagnosis was made by nonsurgical biopsy techniques. Tumor was resectable in 94% of patients who had stage I, II, or IIIa lung cancer in solitary pulmonary nodules; this finding demonstrates the need for early detection. Although the solitary pulmonary nodules were small, the prevalence of malignancy was high.

Conclusions.—No deaths or significant morbidity occurred in these patients, despite their advanced age and the high prevalence of cardiovascular disease and chronic obstructive pulmonary disease. The results demonstrate that better detection of early-stage lung cancer and early therapy can result in favorable prognosis, even in a high-risk population.

▶ This report from a large institution nicely documents the application of video-assisted thoracic resection with very acceptable mortality rates and no significant morbidity, despite the advanced age and high prevalence of cardiovascular disease and chronic obstructive pulmonary disease in this population. This paper further defines that high-risk group of patients in which the definitive diagnosis of a solitary pulmonary nodule would appear to be most appealing with the use of video-assisted techniques. Of note is the fact that a careful preoperative evaluation by the thoracic surgeon and pulmonologist will be required so that the ease of thoracoscopic resection does not become the justification for thoracoscopic resection as definitive therapy. A surgeon must always be aware that most patients who have restricted pulmonary function can undergo anatomical resection, which remains the fundamental procedure for primary carcinoma of the lung.

D.J. Sugarbaker, M.D.

Needle-localized Thoracoscopic Resection of Indeterminate Pulmonary Nodules: Impact on Management of Patients With Malignant Disease
Schwarz RE, Posner MC, Plunkett MB, Ferson PF, Keenan RJ, Landreneau RJ (Univ of Pittsburgh, Pa)
Ann Surg Oncol 2:49–55, 1995   14–7

Background.—Patients who have indeterminate pulmonary nodules (IPNs) present a diagnostic challenge for clinicians. In patients who have had previous diagnoses of cancer, any pulmonary lesion, no matter how small, may represent tumor dissemination. Obtaining tissue is therefore mandatory in these patients, as the identification of either a benign or malignant lesion has a significant effect on their subsequent treatment. The efficacy and therapeutic effect of needle-localized thoracoscopic resection (NLTR) in the treatment of patients who had a history of cancer were assessed.

Method.—From December 1991 to August 1992, 30 patients underwent NLTR of newly discovered IPNs under the guidance of CT. This procedure was followed by thoracoscopic resection. All other attempts to identify these small pulmonary nodules (mean size, 7.9 mm) had failed. In 20 patients, cancer had been diagnosed 1 month to 20 years before NLTR; 10 patients had no history of cancer.

Results.—In all patients, NLTR proved to be a feasible technique and led to a conclusive tissue diagnosis. There were minimal complications directly related to the procedure. Small, asymptomatic, procedure-related pneumothoraces occurred in 50% of patients. There were no associated anesthetic or operative complications. Among the 20 patients who had a previous diagnosis of cancer, 13 had malignant lesions and 7 had benign lesions. In all 20 patients who had a history of cancer, subsequent therapeutic decisions were influenced by the results of NLTR. The procedure also proved to be of value in providing additional histologic information, unobtainable by needle aspiration cytology, that aided in the treatment of select patients. Needle-localized thorascopic resection also allowed for a shorter overall mean hospital stay than did standard thoracotomy (6.7 days vs. 10.5 days).

Conclusion.—Needle-localized thoracoscopic resection is a safe, well tolerated, and highly efficient means of evaluating patients who have IPNs that are not amenable to less invasive diagnostic procedures. The results provided by NLTR can significantly influence the treatment of patients who have a history of cancer. For those patients in whom thoracotomy would be the only available option to perform tissue diagnosis, NLTR has potential advantages compared with the open technique and should be considered an alternative.

▶ This interesting paper outlines a procedure for the preoperative localization of nodules within the lung to aid and facilitate thoracoscopic resection. In these patients, needle localization with the placement of a small wire under the guidance of CT preceded thoracoscopic resection. In our institution, we have found this approach to be somewhat cumbersome and not required for most patients who have outer third solitary pulmonary nodules. Nevertheless, there are clinical situations in which this technique may be of value, and it may be appropriate for surgeons to work with their individual radiologists to perfect this technique so that it may be placed in the armamentarium of surgeons who need to make difficult diagnoses. Again, the appeal of this approach overall is the 100% diagnostic accuracy.

The early detection of primary lung cancer remains the fundamental element to improving survival in 1996. Therefore, the early resection of IPNs particularly in patients who have a history of cigarette smoking, would appear to be the most expeditious way to improve survival and reduce the incidence of metastatic disease associated with this deadly malignancy. As has been noted in breast cancer, where mammographic screening has reduced the size of primary lesions to less than 2 cm in most institutions, the use of aggressive chest radiography and CT in the screening of patients may provide a real possibility of reducing the size of primary lesions at the time of diagnosis and, therefore, significantly affecting overall survival in patients who have bronchogenic carcinoma. The use of video-assisted resection, with its attendant limited morbidity and mortality, would therefore appear to be the most obvious way at present to reduce mortality associated with bronchogenic carcinoma. This approach may therefore become standard for patients who have outer third nodules less than 2 cm in size, particularly in high-risk populations where the complications of needle biopsy would present a formidable morbidity.

D.J. Sugarbaker, M.D.

▶ The next 2 papers seek to find an expanded role for video-assisted thoracoscopy in the pre-resectional staging of patients who have non–small cell lung cancer. This is another example of how video-assisted techniques are beginning to be integrated into the overall management of specific disease processes. These procedures have developed from the feasibility stage to their use in disease management. Particularly during these times of cost containment, with emphasis on lowering the cost of medical care, video-assisted techniques hold the promise of improving quality of care for patients while reducing overall hospitalization and procedural cost.

D.J. Sugarbaker, M.D.

Exploratory Thoracotomy for Nonresectable Lung Cancer

Steinbaum SS, Uretzky ID, McAdams HP, Torrington KG, Cohen AJ (Walter Reed Army Med Ctr, Washington, DC)
Chest 107:1058–1061, 1995   14–8

Objective.—Many patients who undergo thoracotomy for lung cancer are found to have unresectable cancers. The incidence of exploratory surgery in patients who had unresectable disease was investigated retrospectively.

Methods.—Of 335 patients who underwent thoracotomy between July 1983 and February 1992, 35 had unresectable disease. Charts were complete for 28 men and 5 women, aged 45–72 years.

Results.—Five patients were asymptomatic, and 14 had multiple symptoms, including cough, hemoptysis, and pain. Mean forced expiratory volume in 1 second was 2.31. Bronchoscopic findings did not indicate unresectable cancers in any of the 33 patients, but 17 had a preoperative diagnosis of cancer. Eleven patients had N2 disease, 8 had local tumor invasion, 4 had poor pulmonary function, 4 had intrathoracic metastases, and 2 had technically unresectable disease. Two patients underwent thoracotomy to confirm preoperative evaluations, and 1 patient who had suspected non–small cell carcinoma actually had small cell carcinoma.

Conclusion.—Better imaging techniques, such as CT and MRI, and use of video-assisted thoracoscopy could have resulted in 19 fewer thoracotomies. More aggressive surgical approaches to N2 cancers could have resulted in resection of some cancers.

▶ This paper reviewed the records of a group of patients who were found to have unresectable disease at the time of thoracotomy. It is clear from this report that a thoracoscopic evaluation of the chest before thoracotomy would have saved these patients unnecessary attempts at resection. Further, as the multimodality treatment of non–small cell lung cancer becomes more efficacious, particularly in the induction or neoadjuvant setting, the pre-resectional diagnosis of N2 disease with the use of thoracoscopy may provide significant therapeutic benefit to a subset of patients. I would encourage the use of a thoracoscopic examination before any complex intrathoracic resection. Thoracoscopy can be particularly useful in the detection of pleural studding and implants, which would preclude resection for most patients.

D.J. Sugarbaker, M.D.

Videothoracoscopic Staging and Treatment of Lung Cancer

Roviaro GC, Varoli F, Rebuffat C, Vergani C, Maciocco M, Scalambra SM, Sonnino D, Gozi G (Univ of Milan, Italy)

Ann Thorac Surg 59:971–974, 1995   14–9

Purpose.—Videothoracoscopy presents interesting opportunities for the staging and treatment of lung cancer, although its role in the management of this disease is still controversial. By permitting thorough exploration of the chest cavity, video surgery can avoid unnecessary exploratory thoracotomy. The resectability of the lesion can be confirmed by an open approach or, sometimes, by a direct video-assisted approach. The use of videothoracoscopic operative staging was assessed.

Methods.—One hundred fifty-five patients, seen between 1991 and 1994, underwent videothoracoscopic operative staging as the first step of their operation. This evaluation demonstrated the unresectability of the tumor in 8% of patients, mainly because of unexpected conditions noted before surgery. The remaining 142 patients were classified according to the staging of their lesion and their general condition.

Results.—Group A included 13 elderly patients who had small peripheral tumors and could not tolerate lobectomy. These patients underwent thoracoscopic wedge resection instead. The 63 patients in group B had peripheral clinical T1 N0 or T2 N0 tumors. This group underwent 52 videothoracoscopic lobectomies and 4 videothoracoscopic pneumonectomies. In 7 patients, technical problems mandated conversion to thoracotomy. Fifty-one patients had an uneventful postoperative course. Prolonged air leakage developed in 5 patients, and bronchial fistula developed in 1 patient as a result of positive-pressure postoperative ventilation. The 66 patients in group C had stage II or IIIa tumors. The tumor proved unresectable by post-thoracoscopy thoracotomy in 4 patients; the rest underwent radical pulmonary resection. After videothoracoscopic operative staging was adopted, the exploratory thoracotomy rate declined to 2.6%.

Conclusions.—Videothoracoscopic operative staging can reduce the need for exploratory thoracotomy and should therefore be the first step of surgery for lung cancer. It is minimally invasive and provides information equal to that offered by open thoracotomy. The video technique can confirm tumor resectability and, sometimes, permit direct video excision.

▶ This report nicely documents the potential benefit of thoracoscopy in the evaluation of patients for whom the surgeon contemplates extended resection. The use of routine video-thoracoscopic examination of all patients who have lung cancer, however, would appear to be overly enthusiastic in most cases. We would recommend restricting the use of routine thoracoscopic examination to patients in whom pneumonectomy is contemplated, nodal disease is suspected, pleural thickening is detected on preoperative CT scan, or fluid is noted by preoperative radiograph. In these circumstances, thoracoscopic evaluation will yield clinically important information in a large percentage of cases and should minimize operative time while maximizing diagnostic accuracy.

D.J. Sugarbaker, M.D.

Guidelines for Granting Hospital Privileges in Video-assisted Thoracic Surgery
McKneally MF, Lewis RJ, Anderson RP, Fosburg RG, Gay WA Jr, Jones RH, Orringer MB (Toronto Hosp)
Ann Thorac Surg 60:1456, 1995   14–10

Introduction.—The Joint Committee on Video-Assisted Thoracic Surgery has published guidelines for granting hospital privileges in video-assisted thoracic surgery. The committee is sponsored by The American Association for Thoracic Surgery and The Society of Thoracic Surgeons.

Requirements.—Surgeons must be fully able to perform procedures by the open method and to handle complications. Surgeons must produce documentation that they have received education in video-assisted thoracic surgery. This documentation should remain on file at the institution granting privileges. The applicant must successfully perform at least 5 video-assisted thoracic surgery procedures during residency or under observation by a qualified surgeon who certifies the competence of the applicant. Regular documentation of subsequent procedures must be provided. Procedures must be performed in a manner consistent with policies for other operations at the institution granting privileges. The outcome of these procedures must be periodically reviewed by a quality assurance committee, as required by the institution.

Comment.—These criteria are the minimal requirements for granting privileges for performing video-assisted thoracic surgery.

▶ This simple report is included because the issue of appropriate certification for physicians who perform thoracoscopic techniques is often discussed. The performance of a requisite number of video-assisted procedures under observation by a previously certified and qualified surgeon is clearly a *sine qua non*. Documentation and prospective evaluation of a surgeon's performance also represent fundamental elements of quality assurance.

The certification of residents from a variety of different institutions for the performance of thoracoscopic procedures presents a particular challenge in developing a certification strategy. Specific documentation of a resident's thoracoscopic experience is becoming a significant component of the overall training program for thoracic surgeons. Similarly, for general surgeons who perform thoracoscopic procedures, documentation of the quality of these procedures would appear to be essential.

D.J. Sugarbaker, M.D.

Advances in the Understanding of Lung Cancer Therapy

Recent advances in lung cancer therapy have resulted in the use of multiple treatment modalities as primary therapy in a large number of patients. The following papers have explored the appropriate surgical approach to primary lung cancer and evaluated the efficacy of specific thoracic surgical procedures in a variety of settings.

D.J. Sugarbaker, M.D.

Randomized Trial of Lobectomy Versus Limited Resection for T1 N0 Non–Small Cell Lung Cancer
Ginsberg RJ, Rubinstein LV, for the Lung Cancer Study Group (Mem Sloan-Kettering Cancer Ctr, New York)
Ann Thorac Surg 60:615–623, 1995   14–11

Background.—Lobectomy is the standard treatment for early-stage lung cancer. Lesser resections have recently been advocated, however, as treatment for patients who have T1 N0 non–small cell lung cancer (NSCLC). This strategy has the theoretical advantages of preserving pulmonary function, decreasing perioperative mortality and morbidity, and allowing further resections if a second primary lung cancer develops. The efficacy of lobectomy was compared with that of limited resection for the treatment of T1 N0 NSCLC in a prospective, randomized trial.

Methods.—Two hundred seventy-six patients who had a clinical T1 N0 peripheral NSCLC tumor were stratified according to age and pulmonary function and were randomly assigned to surgical treatment with either lobectomy or limited resection (segmentectomy or adequate wedge resection). Two hundred forty-seven of these patients were evaluable. The patients were assessed at 3-month intervals for 2 years, at 6-month intervals for the next 3 years, and annually thereafter.

Results.—There were no significant differences between the 2 treatment groups for the stratification variables and selected prognostic variables. The 2 groups had similar types and numbers of postoperative complications, except that respiratory failure requiring ventilatory assistance developed in 6 patients in the lobectomy group but in no patients in the limited resection group. Compared with the lobectomy group, the limited resection group had a 30% increase in the mortality rate from all causes and a 50% increase in the mortality rate from cancer. In addition, the limited resection group demonstrated a 75% increase in recurrence rate, which was attributable to a tripled locoregional recurrence rate.

Conclusions.—Patients treated with limited resection have a significantly increased risk of local recurrence and a decreased incidence of overall and disease-free survival than do patients treated with lobectomy. Lobectomy with systematic hilar and mediastinal lymph node sampling or dissection is therefore recommended as the continued standard surgical treatment for patients who have T1 N0 NSCLC tumors.

▶ This important study represents a paradigm for thoracic surgical research. The use of a prospective randomized trial yields results of maximal validity. This superior experimental design is noteworthy, because this is the only reported study to document significant advantages of a regional lobectomy compared with limited resection in terms of recurrence rate and long-term survival for most patients who have T1 N0 NSCLC. Interestingly, however, this study did not differentiate between cell types. Previous reports of these data have suggested that the differences noted for T1 adenocarcinomas were not necessarily observed in patients who had T1 squamous cell cancers. Further follow-up of this study will be important in evaluating these differences in prognosis based on cell type. Nevertheless, this study provides further support for the concept that in patients who are medically able to undergo the procedure, lobectomy remains the gold standard for therapy.

D.J. Sugarbaker, M.D.

Concurrent Cisplatin/Etoposide Plus Chest Radiotherapy Followed by Surgery for Stages IIIA (N2) and IIIB Non–Small-Cell Lung Cancer: Mature Results of Southwest Oncology Group Phase II Study 8805
Albain KS, Rusch VW, Crowley JJ, Rice TW, Turrisi AT III, Weick JK, Lonchyna VA, Presant CA, McKenna RJ, Gandara DR, Fosmire H, Taylor SA, Stelzer KJ, Beasley KR, Livingston RB (Loyola Univ, Maywood, Ill; Mem Sloan-Kettering Cancer Ctr, NY; Southwest Oncology Group Statistical Ctr, San Antonio, Tex; et al)
J Clin Oncol 13:1880–1892, 1995   14–12

Background.—When the Southwest Oncology Group phase II study 8805 was designed in 1988, the long-term outcome for unresectable non–small cell lung cancer stage III subsets was poor. Numerous small phase II pilot studies in the 1980s tested various combinations of irradiation, chemotherapy, and surgery. In 1 study, surgery was added to a regimen of chemotherapy plus irradiation for non–small cell lung cancer. The feasibility of this treatment was evaluated.

Methods.—One hundred twenty-six patients who had either positive N2 nodes (IIIa), N3 nodes, or T4 primary lesions (IIIb) were included. Induction consisted of 2 cycles of cisplatin and etoposide with concurrent chest irradiation. If response or stable disease was observed, resection was attempted. If unresectable disease or positive margins or nodes were found, the patient was given a chemotherapy-irradiation boost. Response, resection rates, relapse patterns, and survival for stage subsets IIIa (N2) vs. IIIb were estimated.

Results.—Median follow-up was 2.4 years. The objective response rate to induction was 59%; 29% were stable. For patients who had stage IIIa (N2) disease, resectability was 85%. For patients who had stage IIIb disease, resectability was 80%. In 13% of patients, reversible grade 4 toxicity occurred. There were 13 deaths related to treatment; 19 other patients died of causes unrelated to tumor or toxicity. There were 65 relapses; 11% were locoregional only, and 61% were distant only. There were 26 brain relapses, 19 of which were the sole cause of death. Survival was similar for both groups. Absence of tumor in the mediastinal nodes at surgery was the strongest predictor of long-term survival after thoracotomy.

Conclusions.—The 2-year and 3-year survival rates of 24% and 27% are encouraging. Whether surgery adds more risk than benefit compared with induction with chemotherapy plus irradiation is a question now being addressed by the High Priority Intergroup trial #0139 in a phase III comparison of a revised Southwest Oncology Group–8805 program and a regimen of chemotherapy plus irradiation in patients who have stage IIIa (N2) disease.

▶ This study provides very important insight regarding the appropriate treatment of patients who have IIIa and IIIb non–small cell carcinoma of the lung. Of note was the finding that patients who had T4 lesions when first examined but had resectable lesions after induction chemotherapy and radiation treatment benefited significantly in terms of survival when no nodal disease was present. The second important point is that patients who had N2 disease and were treated with induction chemotherapy and radiation and had an absence of disease in the N2 nodes at the time of resection were the ones who benefited most from an aggressive surgical resection after induction chemotherapy and radiation. This subgroup of patients who are downstaged could expect the most survival benefit from such an approach. Conversely, it may be difficult to justify an extensive surgical procedure in patients who have persistent N2 disease after induction therapy. For these reasons, video-assisted thoracic evaluation of the chest should be considered after induction chemotherapy and radiation. Further, a direct examination of T4 lesions before induction therapy represents another potential application of thoracoscopic techniques in the management of thoracic malignancies.

D.J. Sugarbaker, M.D.

Are Bilobectomies Acceptable Procedures?
Massard G, Dabbagh A, Dumont P, Kessler R, Roeslin N, Wihlm J-M, Morand G (Univ Hosp of Strasbourg, France)
Ann Thorac Surg 60:640–645, 1995   14–13

Introduction.—Lobectomy has long been the standard means of resecting bronchogenic carcinoma. Pneumonectomy generally is done when lobectomy is not practicable, but intermediate procedures, such as sleeve lobectomy, are being increasingly used as compromise procedures. For specific conditions on the right side of the chest, bilobectomy may be a feasible intermediate procedure. The results of bilobectomy were reviewed.

Patients.—One hundred twelve patients who underwent surgery between 1980 and 1992 were included. Most had non–small cell bronchogenic cancer. Ninety-four patients underwent a right lower and middle bilobectomy, and 18 underwent a right upper and middle bilobectomy.

Results.—The operative mortality rate was 3.5%. Forty-nine percent of patients had medical or surgical complications; the most common was pleural-space disease, which occurred in 34%. Three patients required reoperation for this reason. The 92 survivors had 3- and 5-year survival rates of 49% and 40%, respectively. Local recurrences were significantly more frequent in the 44 patients who had stage I tumors and underwent bilobectomy than in 33 similar patients who underwent pneumonectomy. No such difference was apparent in patients who had stage II tumors. In both instances, survival curves were similar after lobectomy and pneumonectomy.

Conclusions.—Bilobectomy is an acceptably safe procedure, but the frequency of local recurrence in patients who have stage I disease brings its efficacy into question. Bilobectomy may be curative in patients who have compromised lung function and are not be able to undergo pneumonectomy.

▶ This paper provides an important answer to a long-asked question regarding the efficacy of bilobectomy. The removal of the upper and middle or middle and lower lobes in the right chest often results in a clinical situation where the lung is not large enough to fill the chest, and one is therefore forced to consider a pneumonectomy. The efficacy of bilobectomy in this clinical setting validates the use of a variety of techniques that seek to reduce the problem of a space in the chest proactively. The basic principle of extending primary resection beyond the scope of the primary tumor with negative microscopic margins, yet retaining as much lung parenchyma as possible after anatomical resection, would provide a rationale for bilobectomy in an appropriate clinical setting. This report establishes the therapeutic efficacy of this approach in a large retrospective series. In our institution, a bilobectomy is performed in preference to a pneumonectomy, particularly when the middle and lower lobes are being resected for a lower lobe tumor. Difficulties with space in the chest are decreased when the upper lobe is retained in a bilobectomy procedure. One should consider the space issues very carefully before attempting to perform a middle and upper bilobectomy with reimplantation of the lower lobe. There are only rare clinical situations in which a very large middle lobe could be preserved by using a sleeve technique with adequate lung parenchyma to fill the ipsilateral chest. In most patients, therefore, a bilobectomy should be performed for lower or middle lobe tumors that require resection of both lobes.

D.J. Sugarbaker, M.D.

Second Primary Lung Cancer

Antakli T, Schaefer RF, Rutherford JE, Read RC (John L McClellan Mem Veterans Hosp, Little Rock, Ark; Univ of Arkansas, Little Rock)
Ann Thorac Surg 59:863–867, 1995   14–14

Purpose.—With a reported incidence of 0.5% to 10%, second primary lung cancer (SPLC) is still less common than second primary tumors of other paired organs, such as the breast or ovary. An experience with SPLC at a Veterans Affairs medical center was reported.

Patients.—Sixty-five SPLCs were detected in 54 patients from 1966 to 1993. The second lesions either had different histology than the first or had the same histology but met other criteria as well, i.e., they were anatomically distinct, had an associated premalignant lesion, occurred without systemic metastases or mediastinal spread, or had different DNA ploidy. The SPLCs represented 4% of a series of 1,572 "curative" resections for lung cancer. Three or more primary tumors were found in 11 patients. Sixty percent of SPLCs were metachronous, and 40% were synchronous. The first and second tumors were found a mean of 55 months apart, and the second and third tumors a mean of 26 months apart. Fifty-eight percent of lesions were squamous cell carcinomas, 31% were adenocarcinomas, and 11% were small cell carcinomas.

In 51% of cases, the SPLC had the same histologic findings as the initial tumor. Seventy-six percent of index tumors were stage I primary tumors, as were 61% of the SPLCs and 72% of the third primary tumors. Forty-four percent of the SPLCs occurred after minimal resection; 37%, after lobectomy; and 13%, after pneumonectomy. Minimal resection did not appear to predispose to SPLC. In the later part of the experience, CT was the main method for diagnosis of SPLCs. Postresection survival rates were 26% at 3 years and 18% at 5 years: 39% and 23%, respectively, for metachronous tumors and 12% and 12% for synchronous tumors.

Conclusions.—In many patients who have survived long-term after curative resection of lung cancers, SPLC will develop. These tumors can be detected early with a high level of awareness and CT scanning; long-term survivors of lung resection need lifetime follow-up. Mini-resections may be the best choice for patients who have limited lung tissue reserve; these procedures do not increase the risk of SPLC.

▶ This paper is important because it establishes the absolute importance of lifelong follow-up of patients who undergo curative resection for lung cancer. It is the subset of patients who have survived a primary lung cancer in which the risk of the development of an SPLC is the highest. Particularly in this era of managed care and restricted access to the thoracic surgeon, the importance of continued thoracic surgical follow-up for patients who undergo primary lung resection for bronchogenic carcinoma must be restated and emphasized. The paper aptly points out that early detection of SPLCs can lead to cure in a large proportion of patients in whom early diagnosis is made. We routinely follow the status of patients every 4 months for 2 years after their primary resection and every 6 months thereafter. The exact nature of the follow-up varies from institution to institution. In our institution, a single chest radiograph and clinical examination provide cost-effective follow-up and long-term evaluation for these patients with the hope of detecting an SPLC early in its clinical course. Indeed, long-term follow-up with bronchogenic carcinoma is primarily directed at the detection of SPLC and not the early detection of recurrent disease, which often adversely affects palliation and quality of life, particularly when no effective therapy is available at this time.

D.J. Sugarbaker, M.D.

Impact of Radical Systematic Mediastinal Lymphadenectomy on Tumor Staging in Lung Cancer
Izbicki JR, Passlick B, Karg O, Bloechle C, Pantel K, Knoefel WT, Thetter O
(Univ of Munich; Central Hosp Gauting, Germany)
Ann Thorac Surg 59:209–214, 1995   14–15

Background.—The extent of lymphadenectomy in the treatment of non–small cell lung cancer (NSCLC) remains controversial. Some authors recommend mediastinal lymph node sampling with resection of only suspicious lymph nodes, whereas others recommend radical, systematic mediastinal lymphadenectomy (LA) to improve survival and achieve a better staging. The effect of LA on nodal staging of NSCLC was investigated prospectively in a randomized, controlled, clinical trial.

Study Design.—A total of 182 patients underwent either conventional lymphadenectomy (LS) or LA. With LS, hilar, interlobal, tracheobronchial, and subcarinal lymph nodes were routinely resected in addition to lymph nodes suspicious of cancer. With LA, resection was combined with a radical systematic en bloc mediastinal lymphadenectomy. Median follow-up period was 26.8 months.

Outcome.—In the LS group, 393 lymph node levels were removed, with metastasis in 55 (13.9%). In the LA group, 590 lymph node levels were removed, with metastasis in 78 (13.2%). Regardless of the type of lymphadenectomy, the percentage of patients who had pathologic N1 or N2 was very similar in the LS (23%) and LA (26.8%) groups. In contrast, the number of patients who had lymph node involvement at multiple levels was significantly increased by LA: only 17.4% of LS patients with N2 disease had more than 1 lymph node level involved, compared with 57.2% of LA patients. Lymph node involvement of more than 1 level was associated with more distant metastases and cancer-related deaths.

Conclusions.—Radical systematic mediastinal lymphadenectomy is not essential to determine the N stage of a patient who has NSCLC. However, LA allows a more detailed staging of the N2 region by significantly increasing the percentage of patients in whom N2 involvement at multiple levels can be detected. Because the latter is associated with worse prognosis, LA is essential as these patients at risk can be identified only by the resection of sufficient number of lymph nodes.

▶ This paper is important because it establishes the effect of systematic lymph node evaluation on the staging of patients who have bronchogenic carcinoma. The detection of disease at multiple levels, and therefore the detection of N2 disease, is important in establishing the definitive stage after resection. Any ongoing evaluation of a treatment strategy should therefore include a systematic lymph node sampling or lymphadenectomy, as outlined in this paper, because it will significantly affect the understanding of the efficacy of induction therapy in a protocol setting. The real impact of systematic lymph node assessment has been debated, but this manuscript establishes the "stage creep" that will occur in a subset of patients in whom systematic evaluation is carried out. The effect of this intraoperative staging should therefore be considered in the construction of clinical trials and in the evaluation of results.

D.J. Sugarbaker, M.D.

Clinical Topics of Interest

This year, we have included a number of interesting clinical topics for the practicing thoracic surgeon. The papers that follow represent topics selected for their individual interest to surgeons. They include particular clinical challenges of performing thoracic surgery in the 1990s and treacherous situations that one needs to avoid. Innovative techniques for solutions to difficult problems are also reviewed.

D.J. Sugarbaker, M.D.

Paraplegia After Thoracotomy: Report of Five Cases and Review of the Literature
Attar S, Hankins JR, Turney SZ, Krasna MJ, McLaughlin JS (Univ of Maryland, Baltimore)
Ann Thorac Surg 59:1410–1416, 1995   14–16

Objective.—Paraplegia after thoracotomy, although rare, can occur after thoracotomy for pleural or pulmonary disease or malignant hypertension. Five such cases were described, and the literature was reviewed.

Methods.—Paraplegia after thoracotomy occurred in 1 patient who had a stab wound of the left chest, in 1 after decortication for tuberculous empyema, in 2 after lobectomy for bronchogenic carcinoma, and in 1 after segmental resection for tuberculosis. A literature search yielded 35 additional examples, including 10 patients who had bronchogenic carcinoma, 3 who had pulmonary tuberculosis, 1 who had bronchiectasis, 1 who had a benign pulmonary lesion, and 10 who had malignant hypertension. Patients with thoracic pathology had 8 lobectomies, 1 bilobectomy, 7 pneumonectomies, 1 decortication, 1 thoracoplasty, 2 neurogenic tumor excisions, 1 drainage of the tuberculous cavity, and 1 Nissen procedure.

Chapter 14–Noncardiac Thoracic Surgery / **587**

Factors thought to contribute to neurologic damage were persistent bleeding of the intercostal vessels at the costovertebral angle in 9 patients, migration of oxidized cellulose into the spinal canal in 9, ligation of intercostal vessels in 6, electrocautery in 6, thrombosis of the anterior spinal artery in 4, epidural hematoma in 2, administration of epidural narcotic in 2, metastatic carcinoma to the spinal canal in 1, and hypotension in 1. The condition of 6 patients improved: Two became fully ambulatory, 2 had slight improvement, 1 had little improvement, and 1 had slight improvement in 1 leg. Ten patients had no improvement, and 5 died.

Conclusion.—Although the precise incidence of paraplegia after thoracotomy is unknown, paraplegia as a complication was associated with posterolateral thoracotomy incision. Excess cellulose pledgets should be removed, and routine ligation of intercostal vessels should be avoided.

▶ Every surgeon who performs open and posterior lateral thoracotomies is concerned about the effects of the thoracic incision on the spinal cord and paravertebral tissues. The group from Maryland has pointed out the treacherous nature of multiple intercostal artery and nerve ligations, which can lead to paraplegia. The uncertainty of the distribution to the spinal cord makes multiple intercostal artery ligation difficult. The indiscriminate use of electrocautery is also to be avoided in the paravertebral region. Thoracic surgery performed when tumor is present in the spinal canal is also a treacherous clinical situation. Finally, the use of cellulose or other packing materials in the thoracic perimeter is to be soundly discouraged. This report, as well as others, discourages the use of gel foam and other materials in the thoracic perimeter. As an alternative, we have found blood patches to be of significant use in this clinical situation.

D.J. Sugarbaker, M.D.

Endobronchial Management of Benign, Malignant, and Lung Transplantation Airway Stenoses
Sonett JR, Keenan RJ, Ferson PF, Griffith BP, Landreneau RJ (Univ of Pittsburgh, Pa)
Ann Thorac Surg 59:1417–1422, 1995   14–17

Objective.—Aggressive endoscopic management can provide symptomatic relief to patients who have anastomotic complications after lung transplantation. Endobronchial stent selection and insertion techniques used to provide symptomatic relief to patients who have benign, malignant, and lung transplantation airway complications were investigated.

Methods.—T tubes, Y stents, bronchial stents, or straight tracheal stents were placed in 23 patients who had endobronchial complications of malignant disease, 10 patients who had benign lesions, and 24 patients who underwent lung transplantation. Patients were aged 41–85 years. Anatomical considerations determined the choice of stent.

Techniques.—Bronchial stents are inserted by using an adult rigid bronchoscope over which a 36F chest tube is inserted to unload and stabilize the stent in the trachea. Tracheobronchial Y stent insertion is accomplished by using a Fogarty catheter placed through the short limb of the Y stent and placed in the airway and into the right segmental bronchus under laryngoscopic guidance. Montgomery T tube stents are inserted through a tracheostomy incision or existing stoma.

Results.—Patients with malignant disease had 26 stents inserted including 13 Y stents, 12 bronchial stents, and 1 T tube. Débridement and stenting were required in 16 patients. In 20 of these patients, symptomatic improvement was achieved, and patients were discharged. The other 3 patients died. Six are still alive at 2–10 months. The 14 patients who died received palliative relief for an average of 10.5 months. Patients with benign disease received 4 T tubes, 3 Y stents, 3 bronchial stents, and 1 straight tracheal stent. Débridement and stenting were required in 4 patients, and dilation and stenting were required in 1. Eight patients had immediate symptomatic relief. The 24 patients who underwent lung transplantation had significant complications that were significantly more common on the left side than on the right. There were 31 stents inserted into 19 patients, 3 of whom needed only temporary placement, 11 of whom needed long-term placement (40–507 days), and 5 of whom died with functioning stents.

Conclusion.—Early endoscopic debridement and stent placement provide safe, palliative treatment of airway obstruction in patients who have benign, malignant, or lung transplantation airway stenosis. All patients had symptomatic relief. Repositioning may be necessary, particularly in patients who undergo lung transplantation.

▶ The use of endobronchial stents in the treatment of benign and malignant bronchial stenoses is a significant advance. Chronic stenosis, particularly after lung transplantation, can result in significant morbidity because of the impaired clearing of secretions leading to chronic pneumonia. The group at Pittsburgh has made a significant contribution by demonstrating the efficacy of conventional T tubes and Y stenting in a variety of clinical situations. At the Brigham and Women's Hospital, we have recently begun to use the Whol stents, which become a permanent part of the endobronchial tissue. More recently, a steel stent with a plastic impervious coating has proved particularly useful in stenting malignant strictures. The impervious coating prevents tumor growth through interstices that cause subsequent obstruction. One must note, however, that all wire stents once deployed are not easily removed, and most become a permanent component of the bronchial tissues.

D.J. Sugarbaker, M.D.

▶ Surgery for Mycobacterium tuberculosis and more commonly resistant strains of tuberculosis is now becoming ubiquitous worldwide. Such surgery is also becoming a more frequent challenge to the thoracic surgeon. Indeed, as more and more strains become resistant to conventional drug therapy, the "old-fashioned" surgical approach remains the only option for these patients. Particularly in the setting of active HIV infection, tuberculosis can present a challenge to the thoracic surgeon.

D.J. Sugarbaker, M.D.

Current Role of Surgery in *Mycobacterium* Tuberculosis
Treasure RL, Seaworth BJ (San Antonio State Chest Hosp, Tex)
Ann Thorac Surg 59:1405–1409, 1995   14–18

Background.—The role of surgery in the modern treatment of *Mycobacterium tuberculosis* (MTB) is unclear. When pulmonary complications of MTB occur, such as empyema, bronchopleural fistula, and large persistent cavities, the long-neglected option of surgery may be needed. A surgical experience in 59 patients who had documented MTB was reported.

Methods.—Forty-four men and 15 women (mean age, 39 years) underwent a total of 65 operations during an 8-year period. The operative indications were multidrug-resistant tuberculosis (MDRTB) in 19 patients, bronchopleural fistula in 12, destroyed lung in 7, solitary nodule in 7, massive hemoptysis in 5, complicated cavity in 4, trapped lung in 3, and empyema in 2. Pneumonectomy with latissimus muscle flap was performed in 15 cases, pneumonectomy in 3, lobectomy in 16, segmental or wedge resection in 11, decortication in 5, window thoracostomy in 3, thoracoplasty with myoplasty in 4, tube thoracostomy in 4, return to the operating room for bleeding in 2, Clagett procedure in 1, and drainage of a cold abscess in 1.

Results.—There was no operative mortality. Five patients had major postoperative complications; 2 had bronchopleural fistula, 2 had postoperative bleeding, and 1 had hypoxic encephalopathy in 1. There were 2 late deaths, both in patients who had MDRTB; 1 patient died with progressive disease and massive hemoptysis and the other with relapsed MDRTB. The remaining 17 patients who underwent surgery for MDRTB have remained culture negative.

Conclusions.—Surgery is an important therapeutic option in the current management of MTB. It can be undertaken with acceptable morbidity and mortality. Depending on the indications, a variety of different procedures may be needed to achieve a cure.

▶ This study shows in detail the reasons why surgery for MTB or MDRTB is to be undertaken only by those experienced in its application to this disease. Five of 65 patients had major postoperative complications. If possible, one should always operate on patients who have been converted to sputum negativity if, indeed, drug sensitivity is noted. The familiarity with such procedures as extrapleural pneumonectomy will be of assistance to surgeons who are contemplating a major resection in multidrug-resistant disease. Early drainage of potential or demonstrated intrathoracic infection remains an important principle in tuberculosis surgery. The use of myoplasty is also an important adjunct in the treatment of these patients.

D.J. Sugarbaker, M.D.

Results of Surgical Management of Tuberculosis: Experience in 206 Patients Undergoing Operation
Rizzi A, Rocco G, Robustellini M, Rossi G, Della Pona C, Massera F ("E Morelli" Regional Hosp, Sondalo, Italy)
Ann Thorac Surg 59:896–900, 1995   14–19

Introduction.—There is no gold standard for the surgical management of pulmonary tuberculosis. Operative decisions are based on the surgeon's expertise. Technical and pleural space problems can lead to serious mortality and morbidity. The 12-year experience at a former sanitarium in Italy was reported.

Methods.—Four hundred patients who had tuberculosis underwent surgical evaluation. After excluding patients who had surgery because of suspicion of cancer and tubercular pleural disease, 206 were finally included. The patients were aged 9–79 years, and the male:female ratio was 5.4:1. More than half the patients had a history of drug resistance or noncompliance. Multiple drug chemotherapy preceded surgery. Preoperative tests included radiographs, respiratory function, ventilation/perfusion scans, CT, bronchoscopy, and, occasionally, bronchography. Operative indications were considered either elective or urgent. Lobectomy was the most common procedure.

Results.—The minimum follow-up was 3 years. Healed patients (90%) had no radiologic signs of the disease after 3 years. Five percent of patients were clinically worse, and 5% died either during the surgery or of tuberculosis-related causes. The overall morbidity rate was 29%. Patients who were sputum positive had the highest morbidity rate and lowest healing rate. Major complications included recurrent tuberculosis, bronchopleural fistula, and aspecific empyema. Minor complications were residual air space, wound breakdown, fever, and hemoptysis.

Conclusion.—Aggressive treatment of drug-resistant tuberculosis is warranted despite the high complication rate. Long-term troublesome complications can be avoided if the disease is eradicated.

▶ This study of a large number of patients who underwent surgical treatment for *Mycobacterium* tuberculosis is very enlightening. Ten percent of patients were either significantly clinically worse off or died during surgery.

The morbidity rate of 29% is not unexpected in the surgical treatment of this disease. Again, this paper points out the important fact that most morbidity and mortality occurred in patients who were persistently sputum positive. Bronchopleural fistula and problems associated with wound healing remain the major sources of morbidity and mortality after surgery for this disease.

D.J. Sugarbaker, M.D.

Hospital-based Group: Ideal Practice for the Future?
Matloff JM, Denton TA (Cedars-Sinai Med Ctr, Los Angeles)
Ann Thorac Surg 60:1476–1480, 1995   14–20

Introduction.—During the past 25 years, the Department of Cardiothoracic Surgery at Cedars-Sinai Medical Center in Los Angeles, has functioned first as a salaried, hospital-based team, then as a contract group. The department has recently returned to being a hospital-based cardiac surgical group. The experience of this group and arguments for and concerns about hospital-based group practice for cardiothoracic surgeons were discussed.

Issues.—Issues that will affect the future of cardiothoracic surgical practice include the quality of work, the ability to predict income, the maintenance of clinical volumes through new strategies for contracting or participating in demonstration projects, the ability to contend with managed care and clinical and financial case-mix changes, and the ability to continue research. Other important issues include malpractice, fraud, and antitrust considerations; networking; telemedicine; changing hospital governance; and practice guidelines, clinical pathways, and patient care protocols.

Future Configurations.—It is believed that technology will be diffused through interdependent regional centers that support new technology and promote specialty practices. Local groups that share responsibilities of clinical care and financing will be related through information and data management technology. These groups, in turn, will relate to a core facility and to each other. Regional groupings will evolve with statewide affiliated hospitals. These statewide networks could relate to other institutions nationwide and around the world.

Concerns.—Good strategies and more patients are not necessarily the only results of being hospital-based. The nature of a hospital-based practice will be determined by the mix of patients that use the hospital. In addition, hospital administrative costs have increased rapidly. Although direct costs can be controlled, indirect costs can get out of hand.

Future Success.—Principles that are critical to successful clinical practice in the future, regardless of how a group is organized, include maintaining superb clinical outcomes; continuing to advocate for patients, regardless of reimbursement; maintaining clinical respect for leaders—business people as middlemen may be problematic; becoming involved in political action committees, if necessary; and, perhaps most importantly, planning for change and becoming part of it.

Discussion.—The hospital-based group practice is viable and supports the preservation of quality work. This relationship helps maintain a steady volume of patients, which enables continuing research. It also provides a means of networking with defined patient referrals, sharing services, and benchmarking with other facilities.

▶ All surgeons are currently under tremendous pressure by the changing health care environment. This study points out some important principles for all of us to consider as we seek to survive, and even thrive, in the new era of health care. Dr. Matloff and his group have been very successful preserving the quality of patient care. Changes and evolution in information systems and practice management are highlighted as the foundation for new relationships in the future that will preserve the quality of care delivered by all health care professionals. A proposed system of advocacy and political activism on the behalf of patients by physicians is an important component of this report.

D.J. Sugarbaker, M.D.

Innovative Therapies and Tumor Biology

The last 6 selections in this year's YEAR BOOK report on interesting new findings regarding the biology of various malignancies. These selections also discuss new treatment interventions that may form the basis of broad new strategies against thoracic malignancies. The thoracic surgeon will find these areas of interest as these new treatment strategies are brought into the clinical arena for study. It behooves all of us in the thoracic surgical community to watch these new developments with care so that we can become enthusiastic supporters of these clinical trials.

D.J. Sugarbaker, M.D.

Lung Tumor Growth Correlates With Glucose Metabolism Measured by Fluoride-18 Fluorodeoxyglucose Positron Emission Tomography
Duhaylongsod FG, Lowe VJ, Patz EF Jr, Vaughn AL, Coleman RE, Wolfe WG (Duke Univ, Durham, NC)
Ann Thorac Surg 60:1348–1352, 1995   14–21

Background.—The growth rate of indeterminate pulmonary lesions is an important determinant of malignancy. Conventional chest imaging techniques delay diagnosis and treatment, and chest radiography and CT have varying sensitivities and cannot provide a definitive diagnosis because they lack sufficient specificity. Positron emission tomography (PET) uses the glucose analogue fluoride-18 fluorodeoxyglucose to detect the enhanced glucose metabolism that is characteristic of neoplastic cells. Whether PET enables lung cancer to be diagnosed promptly, if fluorodeoxyglucose activity correlates with doubling time, was determined.

Methods.—Fluorodeoxyglucose PET imaging was performed in 53 patients who had indeterminate focal pulmonary lesions. Doubling time was calculated. Fluorodeoxyglucose activity in lesions was expressed as a standardized uptake ratio.

Results.—In the 34 patients who had cancer, the mean standardized uptake ratio was 5.9; this ratio was 2.0 in the 19 patients who had benign lesions. The accuracy of PET was 92% when a standardized uptake ratio of 2.5 or greater was the criterion for malignancy. Standardized uptake ratio and doubling time were significantly correlated.

Conclusions.—The growth rate of malignant focal pulmonary lesions correlates with glucose metabolism as measured by fluorodeoxyglucose PET. By quantifying glucose metabolism, this technique can differentiate benign from malignant pulmonary lesions with excellent specificity and sensitivity.

▶ Positron emission tomography works by measuring fluoride-18 fluorodeoxyglucose uptake in tumors. This group at Duke University has led the way in demonstrating the clinical efficacy of this important new radiologic modality. Indeterminate lung masses, as well as enlarged lymph nodes, seen by both CT and MRI have always raised the question regarding malignant vs. benign involvement. By combing radiographic assessment with a metabolic one, this technique holds great promise for diagnosing primary lung cancer at a far earlier stage. Earlier diagnosis remains the only proven method for reducing the mortality rate in patients who have non–small cell lung cancer. We look forward with great enthusiasm to the further evaluation of the PET scanner and its application to clinical practice.

D.J. Sugarbaker, M.D.

Regulation of Lewis Lung Carcinoma Invasion and Metastasis by Protein Kinase A

Young MRI, Montpetit M, Lozano Y, Djordjevic A, Devata S, Matthews JP, Yedavalli S, Chejfec G (Hines VA Hosp, Ill; Loyola Univ, Maywood, Ill)
Int J Cancer 61;104–109, 1995   14–22

Background.—In vitro studies with Lewis lung carcinoma variants have shown that protein kinase A has a positive regulatory effect on the metastatic phenotype of tumor cells. Greater protein kinase A activity and more invasiveness in vitro have been demonstrated in metastatic Lewis lung carcinoma cells than in nonmetastatic cells. The role of protein kinase A in regulating in vitro invasiveness and in vivo metastasis of Lewis lung carcinoma was investigated.

Methods.—Lewis lung carcinoma variants were stably transfected to overexpress the protein kinase A C_α subunit and to have increased protein kinase A activity, or to express a mutant cyclic adenosine monophosphate–resistant protein kinase A $R_{I\alpha}$ subunit leading to blockage of protein kinase A activation.

Results.—Both in vitro and in vivo, wild-type metastatic Lewis lung carcinoma cells were invasive, recurred after excision of the tumor, and metastasized to the lungs. These properties were lost after transfection to express the mutant $R_{I\alpha}$. The Lewis lung carcinoma cells that were noninvasive, nonrecurring, and nonmetastatic could invade, recur after excision of the tumor, and metastasize when transfected to express the C_α subunit.

Conclusions.—These findings show that activation of protein kinase A regulates the capacity in vivo of tumor cells to invade, recur after excision, and metastasize. Protein kinase A did not regulate growth of primary tumors.

▶ Understanding more fully the mechanisms that facilitate tumor growth, as well as those that inhibit tumor growth and metastasis, may provide new targets for therapeutic intervention. This very interesting study demonstrates that when protein kinase A is transfected into Lewis lung carcinoma cells, it imparts to these cells the ability to metastasize and grow. The finding that protein kinase A actively regulates the capacity of in vivo tumor cells to invade, recur after excision, and metastasize may provide a new therapeutic target. This may be particularly applicable after primary excision of the tumor in the adjuvant setting, where the ability to downregulate metastatic potential would be of extreme importance.

D.J. Sugarbaker, M.D.

Cyfra 21-1 as a Biologic Marker of Non–Small Cell Lung Cancer: Evaluation of Sensitivity, Specificity, and Prognostic Role

Wieskopf B, Demangeat C, Purohit A, Stenger R, Gries P, Kreisman H, Quoix E (Hopitaux Universitaires de Strasbourg Cédex France; McGill Univ, Montreal; Institut de Biophysique, Strasbourg Cédex, France; et al)
Chest 108:163–169, 1995   14–23

Background.—Patients with lung cancer generally have a poor prognosis, which worsens considerably in later stages of the disease. Cytokeratin 19, measured in the serum as Cyfra 21-1, is an epithelial marker that has been suggested as a diagnostic and prognostic indicator for squamous cell carcinoma (SCC). Its sensitivity and specificity for various subtypes of non–small cell lung carcinoma (NSCLC), its relationships with other tumor markers, and its independent prognostic value were evaluated.

Methods.—One hundred sixty-one patients who had confirmed lung cancer were studied prospectively during a 4-year period. Seventy-two patients had SCC, 29 had adenocarcinoma, 15 had large cell carcinoma, and 45 had small cell lung carcinoma. Serum levels of Cyfra 21-1, carcinoembryonic antigen (CEA), and neuron-specific enolase (NSE) were assayed in all patients, as was SCC antigen in patients who had SCC. Receiver operating characteristic curves were plotted to determine the ability of the tumor markers to detect specific histologic subtypes.

Results.—By using a Cyfra 21-1 threshold of 3.3 ng/mL, the overall sensitivity was 40.9%, and specificity was 94.4%. Using the same threshold, sensitivity and specificity were 59% and 94%, respectively, for NSCLC and 19% and 94%, respectively, for small cell lung cancer. Its accuracy was significantly greater than that of CEA and NSE and slightly greater than that of SCC antigen. Among patients who had all subtypes of NSCLC, the median values of serum Cyfra 21-1 increased with higher disease stages as follows: 1.05 for stage I–II, 4.15 for IIIa, 5.70 for IIIb, and 12.4 for IV. In multivariate analysis, performance status, stage, and serum concentration of Cyfra 21-1 emerged as the independent prognostic factors.

Conclusions.—Serum concentration of Cyfra 21-1 is a sensitive and specific marker for NSCLC, with particular accuracy for SCC. The level of Cyfra 21-1 correlates with disease stage and functions as an independent prognostic factor.

▶ The use of serum concentrations of Cyfra 21-1 as a marker of disease recurrence and initial prognosis may prove to be a very important finding. The appropriate selection of patients at high risk for recurrence after standard operative therapy could lead to the application of conventional chemotherapeutic regimens in the very near future in patients who have stage I disease. Elevated levels of Cyfra 21-1 may provide an important identifying factor for these patients at high risk. Whether it will become a marker, like CEA, of disease recurrence in patients remains to be determined.

D.J. Sugarbaker, M.D.

Flow Cytometric Analysis of the DNA Content of Adenocarcinoma of the Lung, Especially for Patients With Stage 1 Disease With Long Term Follow-up
Tanaka I, Masuda R, Furuhata Y, Inoue M, Fujiwara M, Takemura T (Japanese Red Cross Med Ctr, Tokyo)
Cancer 75:2461–2465, 1995   14–24

Background.—Tumor, node, metastasis staging is used as a prognostic factor for patients who have malignancies, despite variable outcome within each stage. Flow cytometric analysis has been used to determine prognostic factors in numerous malignancies, and DNA ploidy has been found to be an independent prognostic factor for some malignancies. Results of DNA content analysis in non–small cell lung carcinoma have been conflicting. The prognostic value of DNA ploidy in patients who had adenocarcinoma of the lung was assessed.

Methods.—Paraffin-embedded material from 160 patients who had primary adenocarcinoma of the lung was used to perform DNA flow cytometric analysis. Survival time of patients was determined and analyzed. Follow-up was a median of 7.8 years.

Results.—The results of DNA ploidy revealed that the survival of patients who had stage I disease with diploid tumors was significantly longer than the survival of patients with aneuploid tumors. Differences in outcome of patients with stage II, stage IIIa, or stage IIIb diploid tumors were not significant.

Conclusions.—In patients who have stage I adenocarcinoma of the lung, analysis of aneuploid vs. diploid DNA content is valuable in determining clinical outcome and prognosis.

▶ This study is particularly exciting, because the techniques of flow cytometric analysis are widespread and available in almost every major medical center in the United States. The identification of patients who have aneuploid tumors could also lead to the early treatment of these patients in the adjuvant setting. Ploidy has been shown in other solid tumors to be an accurate predictor of survival. Treatment strategies in early-stage lung cancer may involve flow cytometric analysis to construct an algorithm for adjuvant therapy.

D.J. Sugarbaker, M.D.

E-Cadherin Expression in Primary and Metastatic Thoracic Neoplasms in Barrett's Oesophagus
Bongiorno PF, Al-Kasspooles M, Lee SW, Rachwal WJ, Moore JH, Whyte RI, Orringer MB, Beer DG (Univ of Michigan, Ann Arbor; Harvard Med School, Boston)
Br J Cancer 71:166–172, 1995   14–25

Introduction.—Because esophageal and lung cancers are highly invasive and metastatic, patients with these neoplasms have a poor prognosis. The minimum requirement for cells to metastasize is a change in cell adhesion. These cells must break away from the primary tumor, pass into the circulatory or lymphatic systems, and survive before reattaching to a distant site. The cadherins are cell adhesion molecules that are linked, via α-, β- and γ-catenins, to the actin cytoskeleton, which has a major role in the tight junctions of epithelial tissue. E-cadherin is expressed exclusively on epithelial cells. The relationship between E-cadherin and messenger RNA (mRNA) in the primary tumor and metastases of the lymph system was studied in patients who had esophageal and lung cancer. The expression of E-cadherin before the development of invasive cancer was also examined in patients who had Barrett's esophagus.

Methods.—Tissue was obtained from patients undergoing surgery for either esophageal or lung cancer. Various other samples of normal tissue were also taken. Lymph nodes in which there was a high degree of suspicion regarding metastases were sampled. The tissues were studied histologically and the cancer was staged. Immunohistochemical techniques were used to obtain data on E-cadherin, expression of E-cadherin, mRNA, and transfer RNA.

Findings.—Fifty-nine patients had esophageal cancer, and 52 had lung cancer. Patients who had stage III or IV esophageal cancer showed a reduced and highly disorganized E-cadherin pattern. There were absolute reductions and disorganization of E-cadherin in patients who had stage I, II, and IIIa lung cancer. This pattern was not statistically significant. Patients who had the dysplastic, noninvasive Barrett's esophagus showed an altered expression of E-cadherin. In the 17 patients whose cancer had metastasized to their lymph nodes, a high level of E-cadherin expression was evident. Expression of α-catenin mRNA was found in cells that had an altered expression of E-cadherin.

Conclusion.—Transcriptional and post-translational events were found in cells that had reduced or disorganized expression of E-cadherin. These changes alter cell adhesion. Reductions in E-cadherin can therefore be considered a factor in the invasion and metastases of thoracic neoplasms.

▶ Understanding the mechanism of cell metastases from the primary tumor again may provide new targets for the therapeutic intervention in esophageal cancer. This interesting study has begun to elucidate the role of E-cadherin in the ability of the tumor to break cells free from the primary lesion and deposit them effectively in the remainder of the body. The interruption of this mechanism of metastasis may provide for effective adjuvant therapy in this disease. We look forward to a further translation of these basic findings into the clinical trials enterprise.

D.J. Sugarbaker, M.D.

Expression of Muscle Actins in Diffuse Mesotheliomas
Kung ITM, Thallas V, Spencer EJ, Wilson SM (Heidelberg Repatriation Hosp, Victoria, Australia)
Hum Pathol 26:565–570, 1995   14–26

Objective.—Although fibroblastoid or myofibroblastoid features have been observed in sarcomatoid mesotheliomas, the expression of muscle actins has not been thoroughly studied. The immunoreactivity of epithelial, sarcomatoid, and desmoplastic mesothelioma for muscle-specific actin (MSA) and smooth muscle actin (SMA) was investigated.

Methods.—Specimens from 10 sarcomatoid-desmoplastic mesothelioma (SDM), 12 epithelial, and 5 biphasic mesotheliomas were immunostained and examined to confirm the sensitivity and specificity of each antibody. Results were compared with those obtained with the use of 12 lung cancer specimens and 1 fibrous pleural tumor specimen.

Results.—All SDMs were positive for MSA and SMA. Nine epithelial and 2 biphasic mesotheliomas were positive for MSA. One epithelial mesothelioma was also positive for SMA. Lung tumor epithelial cells were negative for both MSA and SMA, except for 1 tumor that showed a weakly positive reaction for MSA. Stromal cells in both epithelial mesotheliomas and lung cancer tumors were negative for cytokeratin and vimentin and positive for SMA and MSA. Mesothelial and sarcomatoid spindle cells were positive for cytokeratin, SMA, and MSA.

Conclusion.—The presence of SMA and MSA positivity in sarcomatoid mesothelioma and the presence of MSA in some epithelial mesotheliomas differentiate these tumors from lung cancers.

▶ The identification of MSA and SMA proteins in mesothelioma may provide a new immunotherapeutic target for subsequent therapy in this disease. In addition, the presence of SMA and MSA positivity in sarcomatous mesothelioma and the presence of MSA in some epithelial mesotheliomas may help in the diagnosis of these tumors as differentiated from adenocarcinoma.

D.J. Sugarbaker, M.D.

Subject Index*

A

Abdomen, 96: 350
  gunshot wounds, laparoscopy in,
    96: 109
  intra-abdominal
    extravasation complicating parenteral
      nutrition in infant, 96: 246
    infections study, of surgical infection
      society, management techniques
      and outcome, 94: 107
  surgery
    bile duct injury during, medicolegal
      analysis of, 95: 319
    decreasing carbohydrate oxidation
      and increasing fat oxidation in,
      growth hormone for, in total
      parenteral nutrition, 94: 201
  transplant
    multivisceral, 96: 181
    organ cluster, five year experience
      assessment, 96: 183
  trauma
    blunt, causing small intestine rupture,
      CT for early diagnosis, mesentery
      streaky density in, 96: 352
    blunt, emergent abdominal
      ultrasound after, 96: 111
    blunt, ultrasound results in, 95: 102
    massive, delayed gastrointestinal
      reconstruction after, 94: 89
    penetrating, aztreonam clindamycin
      superior to gentamicin clindamycin
      for, 95: 111
    penetrating, celiotomy for, early small
      bowel obstruction after, incidence
      and risk factors, 96: 107
  wall
    defects, acute, planned ventral hernia
      for, 95: 429
    defects, in infant, survival and
      implications for adult life, 96: 359
    repair, reherniation after, with
      polytetrafluoroethylene, 95: 431
Abdominoperineal
  resection
    for early rectal cancer, 95: 375
    and radiotherapy, sacral and perineal
      defects after, transpelvic muscle
      flaps for, 96: 485
Ablation
  of Barrett's esophagus epithelium,
    squamous mucosa restoration after,
    94: 242

Abscess
  liver, pyogenic, current management
    results, 96: 155
  "undrained," of multiple organ failure,
    and gastrointestinal tract, 94: 103
Academic
  health consortium, surgical resource
    consumption in, 95: 9
  medicine, and Health Security Act,
    94: 10
  role models, women surgeons as,
    94: 12
  surgical group practice, and health
    reform, 95: 19
Acetylcholine
  receptor number changes in muscle, in
    critical illness, with muscle
    relaxants, prolonged paralysis after,
    96: 47
Achalasia
  esophagus (see Esophagus, achalasia)
  pneumatic dilatation for, causing
    esophageal perforation, surgical
    repair, 94: 253
Acinar cell
  injury, in hypercalcemia causing
    pancreatitis, acute, 96: 343
Actin
  muscle, expression in mesothelioma,
    96: 597
Acute illness
  of medical patients, mortality and
    hypomagnesemia, 94: 52
Acyclovir
  high dose, vs. ganciclovir for
    cytomegalovirus prophylaxis after
    liver transplant, 96: 160
Adenocarcinoma
  adrenal, case review, 95: 196
  cardia, Barrett's metaplasia as source of,
    95: 282
  lung, flow cytometry of DNA in,
    96: 595
  pancreas (see Pancreas,
    adenocarcinoma)
  rectum, preoperative radiotherapy with
    chemotherapy in, 96: 424
  stomach, erbB-2 expression in,
    predicting shorter survival after
    resection, 95: 399
Adenoma
  parathyroid

All entries refer to the year and page number(s) for data appearing in this and the previous edition of the YEAR BOOK.

Author Index

A

Abbott W, 234
Abe M, 445
Abouljoud MS, 177
Abu-Elmagd K, 175, 181
Achrafi H, 202
Ackermann RJ, 26
Adams M, 243
Adunski A, 527
Adzick NS, 272, 273, 290
Aguilar PS, 372
Aguilar-Nascimento JE, 225
Ahmad S, 375
Ajani JA, 418
Åkerström G, 191
Albain KS, 581
Alessiani M, 183
Alkalay AL, 259
Al-Kasspooles M, 596
Al-Kawas FH, 303
Allaben RD, 120
Allema JH, 453
Allen BT, 548
Allen MS, 572
Allum WH, 443
Almond PS, 172
Ames JE, 171
Ancona E, 319
Anderson CB, 548
Anderson JR, 335
Anderson RP, 579
Andreassen TT, 285
Andrew M, 243
Andrews DF, 353
Andrews HG, 349
Ang KK, 522
Annibali R, 354
Anscher MS, 424
Anselmino M, 319
Antakli T, 584
Anthone GA, 325
Antonacci AC, 82
Apelgren KN, 365
Archibald SD, 208
Arens C, 551
Argenta PA, 290
Armato U, 92
Arnold MW, 408
Aronson M, 497
Arrhenius-Nyberg V, 251
Arrillaga A, 109
Asanuma K, 197
Asch DA, 50
Ashley DW, 26
Ashley SE, 396

Ashton HA, 544
Astiz ME, 68
Atiles L, 88
Attar S, 586
Aubert A, 311
August DA, 400
Aust JB, 242
Avanoglu A, 302
Aversano TR, 186
Awane M, 73
Ayala A, 131

B

Baba H, 448
Bacelar TS, 144
Badihi Y, 51
Baildam AD, 399
Bain A, 217
Baird RN, 552
Bakamjian V, 195
Baldwin BJ, 520
Banerjee AK, 430
Bang C, 285
Bankey PE, 97
Bannon JP, 422
Baracos VE, 239
Barakat RR, 401
Bardram L, 268
Barie PS, 30, 539
Barisoni D, 92
Bark T, 219
Barkun JS, 356
Barnoud D, 263
Barr FC, 478
Barrow RE, 89
Barth A, 470
Bartlett DL, 256
Bartlett RH, 58
Barton DE, 438
Barton JR, 334
Barzan L, 504
Bassin A, 366
Batsakis JG, 499
Batts KP, 379
Bauer CA, 510
Baum P, 550
Baxter C, 88
Baxter JN, 335
Beals T, 495
Beart RW Jr, 431
Beasley KR, 581
Beau P, 263
Becker DA, 316
Beer DG, 596
Beer GM, 483

Bein T, 176
Belcher K, 103
Beliah M, 263
Belkin M, 550
Bell DM, 6
Bellaviti N, 573
Benedetti E, 172
Benjamin SB, 303
Benton J, 482
Beremn CG, 325
Bergelin RO, 536
Berman CG, 474
Bernard GR, 66
Berne TV, 344
Bertagnolli ME, 303
Berthélemy P, 341
Bessey PQ, 85
Beven EG, 542
Biegel JA, 478
Bieski M, 51
Biffl WL, 63
Billi JE, 16
Bills EA, 16
Birnbaum E, 427
Birt BD, 518
Bismuth H, 468
Bixler EO, 316
Black RE, 381
Black TL, 312
Blair JE, 353
Blanton JW, 171
Blebea J, 559, 561
Block RI, 509
Blockx P, 313
Bloechle C, 585
Blohme I, 170
Blumberg D, 287
Blumgart LH, 451
Boccu C, 319
Boden BP, 296
Bodily KC, 29
Bohlander SK, 460
Boltz-Nitulescu G, 228
Bona S, 320
Bonavina L, 319, 320
Bongiorno PF, 596
Bonnet I, 147
Bonneterre J, 403
Borrowdale R, 505
Bossuyt A, 266
Boston VE, 361
Bostwick J III, 482
Botens S, 95
Bouisson M, 341
Boulanger BR, 111, 265
Bouletreau P, 263
Bourge RC, 186

677